Comprehensive
Cancer Nursing Review

Jones and Bartlett Series in Oncology

Comprehensive Cancer Nursing Review

Second Edition

Edited by

Susan L. Groenwald, RN, MS
Assistant Professor of Nursing—Complemental
Department of Medical Nursing
Rush University College of Nursing

Rush-Presbyterian-St. Luke's Medical Center
Chicago, Illinois

Margaret Hansen Frogge, RN, MS
Executive Vice President, Administration
Coordinator, Community Cancer Program

Riverside Medical Center
Kankakee, Illinois

Michelle Goodman, RN, MS
Assistant Professor of Nursing
Rush University College of Nursing
Oncology Clinical Nurse Specialist
Section of Medical Oncology
Rush Cancer Institute

Rush-Presbyterian-St. Luke's Medical Center
Chicago, Illinois

Connie Henke Yarbro, RN, BSN
Editor, *Seminars in Oncology Nursing*
Director, Nursing Resource Development
The Regional Cancer Center

Memorial Medical Center
Springfield, Illinois

JONES AND BARTLETT PUBLISHERS
Boston   **London**

Editorial, Sales, and Customer Service Offices:
Jones and Bartlett Publishers, Inc.
One Exeter Plaza
Boston, MA 02116
617-859-3900
1-800-832-0034

Jones and Bartlett Publishers International
7 Melrose Terrace
London W6 7RL
England

Library of Congress Cataloging-in-Publication Data
Comprehensive cancer nursing review / edited by Susan L. Groenwald...
   [et al.]. -- 2nd ed.
      p.   cm.
   Companion to: Cancer Nursing, 3rd ed. c 1993
   ISBN: 0-86720-720-5
   1. Cancer --Nursing--Outlines. syllabi, etc. 2. Cancer--Nursing-
-Examinations, questions, etc.   I. Groenwald, Susan L.   II Cancer
nursing.
      [DNLM: 1. Neoplasms--nursing--examination questions.   WY 18.2
c737 1995]
RC266.C356   1993 Supp.
610.73'698'076--dc20
DNLM/DLC
for Library of Congress   95-6863
                                                              CIP

Printed in the United States of America
99 98 97 96 95   10 9 8 7 6 5 4 3 2

Contents

Preface

This review guide was written from and for *CANCER NURSING: Principles and Practice,* Third Edition, by Groenwald, Frogge, Goodman, and Yarbro. It can be used effectively by nurses preparing for the Oncology Nursing Certification Examinations, by students who have been assigned the Groenwald et al. text for course reading, by teachers to aid in preparation of course materials, and by others who wish to review or test their knowledge of cancer nursing.

Although this guide can be used independent of the text, users will find its instructional value enhanced if it is studied alongside the text. For example, throughout the guide there are frequent references to figures, tables, and other summary materials appearing in the text. This was done to take advantage of the text's superlative graphics, and in recognition of the pedagogic value that tables and figures can have to students and others attempting to master a subject as comprehensive and difficult as cancer nursing. At the same time, most of the core information contained in the Groenwald et al. text appears in this guide without direct reference to the text.

Each chapter in the guide contains three items: a **Study Outline,** a set of **Practice Questions,** and **Answer Explanations** for the Practice Questions.

The **Study Outline** parallels the topical organization of the corresponding text chapter, but is presented in a highly structured, understandable, and concise format. **Key terms, definitions, distinctions, and ideas are bold-faced for emphasis.** As noted above, references are made to materials in the text whenever such information might be useful to the reader's understanding of a topic. Throughout, the authors have attempted to highlight those facts and concepts that a cancer nurse will be expected to know in practice, in class, and on the Oncology Nursing Certification Examinations.

Practice Questions derive from the outline and test the reader's mastery of information presented in the outline and text. The format of these questions is similar (though not identical) to that of the ONCC exams, and items range from simple and factual to challenging and applied.

Answer Explanations serve three important functions: (1) they provide the letter of the correct answer to each Practice Question; (2) they repeat and reinforce information covered in the Study Outline; and (3) they cite the page or pages in the textbook on which a more detailed discussion of the answer may be found. These explanations should help clarify points the reader may have overlooked or misunderstood in the text, especially many important distinctions between closely related terms or concepts.

Questions and answers may be used without reference to the outlines, of course. This fact may have relevance to users who are pressed for time, or who are using the guide without the text.

Please write to the publisher at the following address if you have any comments about the guide or any suggestions for improving its value to cancer nurses:

Jones and Bartlett Publishers
One Exeter Plaza
Boston, MA 02116

Contributors

Sandra A. Mitchell Beddar, RN, MSN, OCN
Rosewell Park Cancer Institute
Buffalo

Karla Beckman, RN, MSN, OCN
West Roxbury Veterans
Administration Medical Center
Boston

Phyllis Beveridge, RN, EdD, OCN
Boston College School of Nursing
Boston

Douglas Haeuber, RN, MSN, OCN

Karen Ingwersen, RN, MSN, OCN
Beth Israel Hospital
Boston

Susan E. Jaster, RN, MSN, OCN
Massachusetts General Hospital

Contributors to *Cancer Nursing: Principles and Practice, Third Edition*

Barbara Barhamand, RN, MS, OCN
Oncology Clinical Nurse Specialist/Manager
Hematology-Oncology Consultants, Ltd.
Naperville, Illinois

Connie Yuska Bildstein, RN, MS
Director of Medical/Oncology Nursing
Northwestern Memorial Hospital
Chicago, Illinois

Barbara D. Blumberg, ScM.
Director of Education
Baylor-Susan G. Komen Breast Center
Dallas, Texas

Deborah McCaffrey Boyle, RN, MSN, OCN
Oncology Clinical Nurse Specialist
Fairfax Hospital
Fairfax, Virginia

Donald P. Braun, PhD
Associate Director, Section of Medical Oncology
Rush-Presbyterian-St. Luke's Medical Center
Associate Professor of Medicine and Immunology/
    Microbiology
Rush Medical College
Chicago, Illinois

Patricia C. Buchsel, RN, MSN
Senior Research Associate
University of Washington
School of Nursing
Seattle, Washington
Bone Marrow Transplant Consultant
Critical Care of America
Westborough, Massachusetts

Dawn Camp-Sorrell, RN, MSN, FNP, OCN
Oncology Clinical Nurse Specialist
University of Alabama Hospitals and Clinics
Birmingham, Alabama

Brenda Cartmel, PhD
Research Instructor
Department of Family and Community Medicine
University of Arizona and
    The Arizona Cancer Center
Tucson, Arizona

David F. Cella, PhD
Associate Professor of Psychology
Rush Medical College
Director, Division of Psychosocial Oncology
Rush Cancer Institute
Chicago, Illinois

Diane D. Chapman, RN, MS
Coordinator, Comprehensive Breast Center
Rush Cancer Institute
Rush-Presbyterian-St. Luke's Medical Center
Faculty (Complemental)
Rush University
Chicago, Illinois

Jane C. Clark, RN, MN, OCN
Clinical Nurse Specialist, Oncology
Emory University Hospital
Atlanta, Georgia

Rebecca F. Cohen, RN, EdD, MPA, CPHQ
Assistant Professor, Department of Nursing
Rockford College
Rockford, Illinois

Mary Cunningham, RN, MS
Clinical Nurse Specialist
Department of Neuro-Oncology
Pain and Symptom Management Section
M.D. Anderson Cancer Center
Houston, Texas,

Vincent T. DeVita, Jr., MD
Attending Physician and Member
Program of Molecular Pharmacology and
    Therapeutics
Benno C. Schmidt Chair in Clinical Oncology
Memorial Sloan-Kettering Cancer Center
New York, New York

Kathleen A. Dietz, RN, MA, MS
Clinical Nurse Specialist
Memorial Sloan-Kettering Cancer Center
Associate, Columbia University School of Nursing
New York, New York

Michele Girard Donehower, RN, MSN
Adult Nurse Practitioner
University of Maryland Cancer Center
Baltimore, Maryland

Diane Scott Dorsett, RN, PhD, FAAN
Director
Comprehensive Support Services for Persons
    with Cancer
Associate Clinical Professor
University of California
San Francisco, California

Susan Dudas, RN, MSN
Associate Professor
College of Nursing
University of Illinois at Chicago
Chicago, Illinois

Henry J. Durivage, PharmD
Associate Director
Clinical Affairs
Theradex
Princeton, New Jersey

Jan M. Ellerhorst-Ryan, RN, MSN, CS
Nurse Clinician
Critical Care America
Cincinnati, Ohio

Ellen Heid Elpern, RN, MSN
Vice President, Nursing
Illinois Masonic Hospital
Assistant Professor of Nursing
Rush University
Rush-Presbyterian-St. Luke's Medical Center
Chicago, Illinois

Jayne I. Fernsler, RN, DSN
Associate Professor
College of Nursing
University of Delaware
Newark, Delaware

Betty R. Ferrell, RN, PhD, FAAN
Associate Research Scientist, Nursing Research
City of Hope National Medical Center
Duarte, California

Anne Marie Flaherty, RN, MS
Clinical Nurse III
Urgent Care Center
Memorial Sloan-Kettering Cancer Center
New York, New York

Arlene E. Fleck, RN, MNEd
Clinical Specialist Oncology Nursing
Hahnemann University Hospital
Philadelphia, Pennsylvania

Marilyn Frank-Stromborg, RN, EdD, NP,
    FAAN
Professor, Oncology Nursing
School of Nursing
Northern Illinois University
DeKalb, Illinois

Margaret Hansen Frogge, RN, MS
Executive Vice President, Administration
Coordinator, Community Cancer Program
Riverside Medical Center
Kankakee, Illinois

Sue L. Frymark, RN, BS
Manager, Cancer Rehabilitation
Comprehensive Cancer Program
Good Samaritan Hospital and Medical Center
Legacy Health Care System
Portland, Oregon

Barbara Holmes Gobel, RN, MS
Oncology Clinical Specialist
Lake Forest Hospital
Lake Forest, Illinois
Instructor (Complemental)
Rush University College of Nursing
Chicago, Illinois

Michelle Goodman, RN, MS, OCN
Oncology Clinical Nurse Specialist
Section of Medical Oncology
Rush Cancer Institute
Assistant Professor of Nursing
Rush University College of Nursing
Rush-Presbyterian-St. Luke's Medical Center
Chicago, Illinois

Marcia Grant, RN, DNSc, FAAN, OCN
Director of Nursing Research
City of Hope National Medical Center
Duarte, California

Betty Greig, RN, CETN
Enterostomal Therapist
University of Southern California
Kenneth Norris, Jr. Cancer Hospital
    and Research Institute
Los Angeles, California

Susan L. Groenwald, RN, MS
Assistant Professor of Nursing, Complemental
Rush University College of Nursing
Rush-Presbyterian-St. Luke's Medical Center
Chicago, Illinois

Robin R. Gwin, RN, MN, OCN
Coordinator, Bone Marrow Transplant Program
Emory University Clinic
Atlanta, Georgia

Gloria Hagopian, RN, EdD
Associate Professor of Oncological Nursing
University of Pennsylvania School of Nursing
Clinician Educator
Department of Radiation Oncology
Hospital of the University of Pennsylvania
Philadelphia, Pennsylvania

Beverly Hampton, RN, MS, ET
Department of Nursing Staff Development
Division of Nursing
M.D. Anderson Cancer Hospital
Houston, Texas

Laura J. Hilderley, RN, MS
Oncology Clinical Nurse Specialist
Private Practice of Philip G. Maddock, MD
Radiation Oncology
Warwick, Rhode Island

Barbara Hoffman, JD
Private Consultant: Cancer Survivorship and
    Discrimination
Princeton, New Jersey

Patricia F. Jassak, RN, MS, CS, OCN
Oncology Clinical Nurse Specialist
Loyola University Medical Center
Maywood, Illinois

Judith (Judi) L. Bond Johnson, RN, PhD,
    FAAN
Nursing Director, Special Projects
North Memorial Medical Center
Minneapolis, Minnesota

Barbara Kalinowski, RN, MSN, OCN
Oncology Clinical Nurse Specialist
Faulkner Breast Centre
Boston, Massachusetts

Marsha Ketchum, RN, OCN
Clinical Research Nurse, Hematology and
    Oncology
Arizona Cancer Center
University of Arizona
Tucson, Arizona

Paula R. Klemm, RN, DNSc, OCN
Assistant Professor
University of Delaware
College of Nursing
Newark, Delaware

M. Tish Knobf, RN, MSN, FAAN
Assistant Professor
Yale University School of Nursing
Oncology Clinical Nurse Specialist
Yale-New Haven Hospital
New Haven, Connecticut

Kathy Kravitz, RN, MS
Oncology Nurse Specialist
North Colorado Medical Center
Greeley, Colorado

Linda U. Krebs, RN, MS, OCN
Oncology Nursing Program Leader
University of Colorado Cancer Center
Denver, Colorado

Lori A. Ladd, RN, MSN
Oncology Clinical Nurse Specialist
H. Lee Moffet Cancer Center and
    Research Institute
Tampa, Florida

Luana Lamkin, RN, MPH, OCN
Executive Director
The Queen's Medical Center Cancer Institute
Honolulu, Hawaii

Jennifer M. Lang-Kummer, RN, MN
Clinical Assistant Professor
School of Nursing
East Carolina University
Greenville, North Carolina

Susan Leigh, RN, BSN
Cancer Survivorship Consultant
Tucson, Arizona

Julena Lind, RN, MN, PhD cand.
Interim Chair
Department of Nursing
University of Southern California
Los Angeles, California

Ada M. Lindsey, RN, PhD
Dean and Professor
School of Nursing
University of California
Los Angeles, California

Lois J. Loescher, RN, MS
Director, Cancer Control Education Research
Cancer Prevention and Control
Arizona Cancer Center
University of Arizona
Tucson, Arizona

Jeanne Martinez, RN, MPH
Clinical Nurse Manager
Northwestern Memorial Hospice Program Chicago,
Illinois

Mary B. Maxwell, RN, CS, PhD
Oncology Clinical Nurse Specialist
Nurse Practitioner
Veterans' Administration Medical Center
Adjunct Assistant Professor of Nursing
Oregon Health Sciences University
Portland, Oregon

Deborah K. Mayer, RN, MSN, OCN
Oncology Clinical Nurse Specialist
Ontario Cancer Institute
Toronto, Ontario, Canada

Mary Ellen McFadden, RN, MLA, OCN
Clinical Coordinator
The Johns Hopkins Oncology Center
Baltimore, Maryland

Rose F. McGee, RN, PhD
Professor
Nell Hodgson Woodruff School of Nursing Emory
University
Atlanta, Georgia

Deborah B. McGuire, RN, PhD, FAAN
Assistant Professor
Nell Hodgson Woodruff School of Nursing
Emory University
Atlanta, Georgia

Joan C. McNally, RN, MSN, OCN
Director, Health Care Services
Michigan Cancer Foundation
Detroit, Michigan

Mary Ann Miller, RN, PhD
Associate Professor
College of Nursing
University of Delaware
Newark, Delaware

Ida Marie (Ki) Moore, RN, DNSc
Assistant Professor
College of Nursing
University of Arizona
Tucson, Arizona

Theresa A. Moran, RN, MS
AIDS/Oncology Clinical Nursing Specialist
University of California, San Francisco/San
    Francisco General Hospital
Assistant Clinical Professor
Department of Physiological Nursing
University of California
San Francisco, California

Marion E. Morra, MA, ScD
Associate Director, Yale Comprehensive Cancer
    Center
Associate Clinical Professor, Yale University
    School of Nursing
Associate Research Scientist, Yale University
    School of Medicine
New Haven, Connecticut

Lillian M. Nail, RN, PhD
Associate Dean for Research/Associate Professor
University of Utah College of Nursing
Salt Lake City, Utah

Sharon Saldin O'Mary, RN, MN
Cancer Care Coordinator
Stevens Cancer Center
Scripps Memorial Hospital
LaJolla, California

Edith O'Neil-Page, RN, BS
Nursing Supervisor
Hoag Memorial Hospital Presbyterian
Newport, California

Diane M. Otte, RN, MS, ET
Administrative Director
St. Luke's Hospital Cancer Center
Davenport, Iowa

Geraldine V. Padilla, PhD
Associate Professor
Associate Dean for Research
School of Nursing
University of California
Los Angeles, California

Patricia A. Piasecki, RN, MS
Clinical Coordinator
Orthopaedic Oncology and Tissue Bank
Rush-Presbyterian-St. Luke's Medical Center
    and Regional Organ Bank of Illinois
Chicago, Illinois

Sandra Purl, RN, MS, OCN
Oncology Clinical Nurse Specialist
Section of Medical Oncology
Rush Cancer Institute
Complemental Faculty
Rush University College of Nursing
Rush-Presbyterian-St. Luke's Medical Center
Chicago, Illinois

Mary Reid, RN, MPH
Research Specialist
Department of Family and Community Medicine
University of Arizona
Tuscon, Arizona

Patricia E. Reymann, RN, MSN, OCN
Director, Gordon L. Ross Cancer Center
Princeton Baptist Medical Center
Birmingham, Alabama

Kathleen S. Ruccione, RN, MPII
Division of Hematology/Oncology
Children's Hospital of Los Angeles
Los Angeles, California

Vivan R. Sheidler, RN, MS
Clinical Nurse Specialist in Neuro-Oncology
The Johns Hopkins Oncology Center Department
    of Nursing
Baltimore, Maryland

Carol A. Sheridan, RN, MSN, OCN
Albert Einstein Cancer Center
Montefiore Medical Center
Bronx, New York

Annalynn Skipper, RD, MS, CNSD
Coordinator, Nutrition Consultation Service
Instructor, Department of Clinical Nutrition
Rush University College of Health Sciences
Rush-Presbyterian-St. Luke's Medical Center
Chicago, Illinois

Debra J. Szeluga, RD, MD, PhD
The Johns Hopkins Medical Center
Baltimore, Maryland

David C. Thomasma, PhD
The Fr. Michael I. English, S.J. Professor of
    Medical Ethics
Director, Medical Humanities Program
Loyola University of Chicago Medical Center
Maywood, Illinois

Steven Wagner, RN, BSN
Nurse Clinician
Northwestern Memorial Hospice Program
Chicago, Illinois

Janet Ruth Walczak, RN, MSN
Clinical Nurse Specialist
The Johns Hopkins Oncology Center
Clinical Associate
The Johns Hopkins University School of Nursing
Baltimore, Maryland

Jo Ann Wegmann, RN, PhD
Associate Professor
Graduate Coordinator
Statewide Nursing Program
California State University
Dominques Hills
Carsen, California

Maryl L. Winningham, RN, PhD, FACSM
Assistant Professor
University of Utah College of Nursing
Salt Lake City, Utah

Debra Wujcik, RN, MSN, OCN
Clinical Nurse Specialist
Oncology/Bone Marrow Transplant
Vanderbilt University Hospital
Adjunct Instructor of Nursing
Vanderbilt University School of Nursing
Nashville, Tennessee

Connie Henke Yarbro, RN, BSN
Director, Nursing Resource Development
The Regional Cancer Center
Memorial Medical Center
Springfield, Illinois
Editor, *Seminars in Oncology Nursing*

John W. Yarbro, MD, PhD
Director, The Regional Cancer Center
Memorial Medical Center
Springfield, Illinois

1   Cancer Control and Epidemiology

STUDY OUTLINE

I.   **INTRODUCTION**

    1.   **Epidemiology** is **"the study of the distribution and determinants of disease frequency."**

    2.   Cancer epidemiology examines the **frequency** of occurrence of cancer, the role of certain **risk factors,** and **the interrelationships** that exist among the **host, environment,** and any **other contributing conditions.**

    3.   **See Table 1-1, text pages 4–5,** for a glossary of epidemiologic terms.

II.   **BASIC CONSIDERATIONS IN EPIDEMIOLOGIC RESEARCH**

    1.   **Six** components considered in the evaluation of an epidemiologic research project are **study design, population definition, eligibility criteria, definitions of the disease and exposures** related to the research hypothesis, **statistical plan** measuring the association between exposure and disease, and **identification of bias sources.**

    2.   Research designs commonly used in epidemiologic research are **experimental, ecologic, cross-sectional, case-control, cohort, and clinical trials** studies.

    3.   **Factors** considered in study design include the frequency of the disease or condition in the general population and in the defined population to be studied, the length of time it takes for the disease to develop and the anticipated size of the study sample.

    A. **STUDY DESIGNS**

        1. **Experimental studies**

          a. An experimental study design tests a **research hypothesis by attempting to control the variability of all factors except the exposure of interest.**

          b. Experimental studies typically use **animal models in laboratory settings** and are conducted when a research hypothesis is being developed.

        2. **Ecologic studies**

          a. These designs investigate hypotheses further by examining trends in **disease distribution** among humans across ecologic or geographic areas.

        3. **Cross-sectional studies**

          a. The cross-sectional study design assesses **disease rates** and **exposure** in a population.

          b. Cross-sectional studies cannot establish a causal relationship between the exposure and the disease.

        4. **Case-control studies**

          a. The case-control study design should be considered if the disease is **rare** in the population, if the investigation is **preliminary,** and/or if other **study designs** are prohibited by time and funding limitations.

          b. The **association** between disease and exposure is explored in case-control studies.

          c. Cases of the disease being studied are compared to non-cases or **control subjects.**

          d. Control subjects do not have the disease but have the same opportunity to be diagnosed with the disease as the case subjects. Selection of a control group tends to be the **major challenge** in case-control studies.

          e. In an attempt to make the two groups (cases and controls) comparable, **matching** is sometimes done. Demographic characteristics of the cases are matched to those of the controls in order to minimize demographic differences.

    f. An alternative to matching is the recruitment of more than one control subject for each case subject. This technique increases statistical power without limiting the variables that can be investigated.

5. **Cohort studies**

    a. A cohort study may be initiated to test the **research hypothesis** once an association between a disease and an exposure has been established.

    b. Cohort studies can be **retrospective, prospective,** or **ambidirectional.**

    c. Retrospective studies use a **previously defined cohort** and, through review of records, identify individuals that have developed the disease and assess their level of exposure.

    d. **Prospective** studies involve selecting disease-free individuals in a current population and measuring the exposure(s). This population is followed into the future and evaluated for disease development.

    e. An ambidirectional cohort study begins with a previously established cohort and continues subject follow-up into the future.

6. **Clinical trials and intervention studies**

    a. The clinical trial or intervention study tests the effect of an intervention on the rates of disease development.

    b. The study population consists of a treatment group (receiving the treatment) and a control group (receiving the placebo or the current therapy).

    c. A **double-blind** study involves keeping the assignments to the treatment group and to the group receiving the intervention from the subjects and from immediate clinical personnel, to control potential biasing.

    d. A major limitation of the clinical trial design is the **lengthy time frame** often needed for subject follow-up in order to see significant changes.

B. DEFINING THE POPULATION

1. The **source population** for a study is the **larger population** from which a subgroup of study subjects is chosen.

2. **Eligibility criteria**

    a. Study subjects are chosen based on defined **eligibility criteria** intended for creation of a study subject group with sufficient disease prevalence to test the hypothesis and for whom the intervention is safe.

    b. Eligibility criteria include **age, race, gender, disease stage, life expectancy, absence of other cancers or chronic diseases, exposure to certain drugs or treatments,** and **current health status.**

3. **Defining the disease and the exposure**

    a. The disease is **defined** as specifically as possible, including pathologic criteria, specific blood chemistries, histologic characteristics, specific test results, and physical symptoms.

    b. The exposure is clarified. **Exposure** is the contact a subject has with the study variable that may influence the development or improvement in disease status. It includes variables such as **dose** and **duration** of the exposure, as well as the **characteristics** specific to the exposure.

C. STATISTICAL PLAN

1. Epidemiologic research enables the investigator to examine relationships of disease to defined exposures.

2. A main goal is to make inferences to the larger population based on information obtained about the study population.

D. POTENTIAL SOURCES OF BIAS AND CONFOUNDING

1. Sources of bias are examined to determine if differences between study groups can be explained by influences other than the research hypothesis.

E. DATA SOURCES

1. **See Table 1-4, text page 10,** for a list of data sources for epidemiologic research.

III.   **ENVIRONMENTAL FACTORS ASSOCIATED WITH CANCER CAUSATION**

   A.   **HOW DO WE DECIDE WHAT CAUSES CANCER?**

   1.   Causes cannot be determined from one study; many sources of information are required. The criteria to be considered are **magnitude** of association between exposure and disease, **consistency** of findings, **biological credibility,** and **temporal association** between the risk factor and disease.

   2.   **Tobacco**

   a.   Tobacco is the most important **known cause of cancer** in the United States.

   b.   Tobacco causes about **30% of cancer deaths,** and cigarette smoking causes **90% of lung cancers.**

   c.   Tobacco has been associated with many cancer types. There is a clear **linear relationship** between the number of cigarettes smoked and the risk of lung and oropharyngeal cancers.

   d.   The risk of dying from lung cancer decreases in the ex-smoker but is dependent upon **cumulative smoking exposure,** the **age** at which the patient began smoking, and the degree of **inhalation.**

   e.   The overall increase in risk for developing lung cancer is estimated at **30% for nonsmoking women** married to smokers and **70%** for those associated with **heavy passive smoking.**

   f.   The overall prevalence of smoking is **decreasing** in the United States. The decrease is not equal in all sociologic groups. Educational level appears to be the strongest indicator of smoking status.

   3.   **Diet**

   a.   Case-control and cohort studies of diet and cancer present a number of design problems. See **text page 11** for a list of **methodological problems.**

   b.   **Colon cancer and fat intake**

   (1)   Although a strong relationship has been shown to exist between **meat consumption** or **dietary fat** and the incidence of **colorectal cancer** a causal association **cannot** be assumed because it is difficult to differentiate among the effects of fat, protein, and total calories.

   c.   **Colon cancer and fiber intake**

   (1)   The majority of studies support the hypothesis that **high fiber intake is protective for colon cancer.** However, when source of fiber is examined, cereals as a source of fiber are less supportive of a protective effect against colon cancer than are vegetable sources of fiber.

   d.   **Colon cancer and calcium intake**

   (1)   Some studies have shown a **protective role of high calcium intake against colon cancer.** The recommended daily intakes of calcium suggested for reduction of colorectal cancer risk are similar to those for prevention of osteoporosis and hypertension.

   e.   **Breast cancer and fat intake**

   (1)   Ecologic studies using data from many countries show a strong **positive relationship** between per capita fat intake and breast cancer mortality rates.

   f.   **Cancer, micronutrients, and intake of fruits and vegetables**

   (1)   Epidemiologic studies support a protective effect of **fruits and vegetable**s against cancers, but the specific protective nutrient, non-nutrient, or combination is still under study.

   (2)   See **Table 1-5, text page 13,** for a list of chemoprevention trials investigating the role of certain micronutrients in cancer prevention.

   4.   **Alcohol**

   a.   Approximately **3% of cancer deaths** are attributable to alcohol. It has been linked to cancers of the **breast, oral cavity, pharynx, larynx, esophagus, liver, and rectum.**

   5.   **Physical activity**

   a.   Epidemiologic studies of physical activity suggest that **increased activity** is protective against colon cancer and precancerous polyps, breast cancer, and prostate cancer.

   b.   **Accurate measurement** of physical activity and difficulty separating lack of physical activity from obesity and diet, two factors associated with many cancers, make the role of physical activity in relation to cancer risk difficult to assess.

   6.   **Occupational exposures**

   a.   The **lung** is the most common site of cancer leading to death due to its exposure to occupational carcinogens.

    b. Epidemiologic studies of industrial populations are conducted to **identify unusual disease patterns** that might **indicate exposure to previously unidentified carcinogens, monitor safe levels** of identified carcinogens, and **monitor exposure** to mixtures of chemicals that have probably not been tested in animal experiments.

7. **Pollution**
   a. **Air pollution** has been studied mainly in relation to the risk of lung cancer; however, data are insufficient to quantify the risk.
   b. **Water pollution** and site-specific cancer risks are unproven.
   c. **Chlorofluorocarbons (CFCs)** may indirectly increase cancer risk since they are destroying the ozone layer, allowing an increased amount of ultraviolet light to reach the earth, thereby causing more skin cancers.

8. **Reproductive factors and sexual behavior**
   a. Reproductive and sexual factors that may have an impact on development of cancer in women include **age of onset of menarche, age at menopause, age at first pregnancy, obesity, nulliparity,** and **multiplicity of sexual partners (see Table 1-7, text page 15).**

9. **Viruses and other biological agents**
   a. Epidemiologic evidence for viral influences on cancer incidence is relatively strong for **hepatocellular carcinoma, cervical cancer, Burkitt's lymphoma, adult T-cell leukemia-lymphoma, Kaposi's sarcoma, non-Hodgkin's lymphoma,** and **bladder cancer.** See **Table 1-8, text page 15.**

10. **Radiation**
    a. **Ionizing radiation**
       (1) **Eighty percent** of the earth's exposure to ionizing radiation is from natural sources.
       (2) **Breast, thyroid,** and **bone marrow cancers** are particularly sensitive to ionizing radiation. The level at which the exposure occurs is not determined.
       (3) **5000–20,000 lung cancer deaths** annually in the United States may be due to radon exposure in the home.
       (4) Occupational exposure to ionizing radiation is highest among underground uranium miners, commercial nuclear power plant workers, fuel fabricators, physicians, flight crews, industrial radiographers, and well loggers.
    b. **Ultraviolet radiation**
       (1) Ultraviolet radiation (UVR) is the **major cause of nonmelanoma skin cancer,** with cumulative exposure being predictive of risk.
       (2) Individual exposure to UVR is dependent upon **latitude, altitude, humidity,** and **personal behaviors.**
    c. **Nonionizing radiation**
       (1) Nonionizing radiation is generated from **electrical power, radar, and microwave sources.**
       (2) **Residential exposure** is associated with an increased risk of leukemia in children, and occupational exposure is associated with an increased risk of leukemia in adults.
       (3) **Measurement** of exposure to nonionizing radiation is difficult.

11. **Drugs**
    a. Antineoplastic drugs damage normal cells, which can cause the late effect of a second malignancy resulting most commonly in **hematologic or lymphatic malignancies.** See **Table 1-9, text page 16,** for a chart of antineoplastic agents that have been implicated in the development of second malignancies.

12. **Exogenous hormones**
    a. Exogenous hormones are most commonly prescribed for women.
    b. **Vaginal** and **cervical cancers** have been associated with being the daughter of a woman treated with diethylstilbestrol 10–30 years ago, whereas **decreased risk of endometrial and ovarian cancer** is associated with use of oral contraceptives.
    c. **Oral contraceptives** have been associated with an increased risk of liver cancer in young women.

IV. **HOST CHARACTERISTICS INFLUENCING CANCER SUSCEPTIBILITY**

    A. **AGE**

        1. Age is an important **determinant** of cancer risk.

2. The risk of cancer development is **10 times greater in people over 65 years of age** than in those under 65.
3. The increased incidence with advanced age is not uniform for all cancer sites.

B. **SEX**

1. **Lifestyle differences** yield a lower incidence of cancer in women (excluding gender-specific cancers). See **Figure 1-6, text page 20,** for the mortality rates of the five leading cancer sites.

C. **GENETIC PREDISPOSITION**

1. The ability to study **genetic markers** in large populations has increased epidemiologic studies of genetic predisposition to cancer.
2. Individuals with rare autosomal recessive and X-linked recessive syndromes are at higher risk for certain cancers (see **Table 1-12, text page 19**).
3. **Familial polyposis** of the colon is an autosomal dominant syndrome in which individuals develop colon cancer at an early age.
4. Some **gene defects** may increase a person's risk for cancer because they affect the person's carcinogen metabolism.
5. **Familial aggregation** of cancer may be due to common familial exposure or to inherited susceptibility.

D. **ETHNICITY AND RACE**

1. Since ethnicity and race are often assessed in epidemiologic studies, the potential for **misclassification** needs to be considered.
    a. **Race** may be difficult to determine since individuals can often be classified in many ways, depending upon their heritage.
    b. Since **ethnicity and race** are often correlated with socioeconomic status, distinguishing an ethnic or racial effect from a socioeconomic effect can be difficult.
2. Assessment of biological or genetic differences and cultural differences that may decrease or increase the risk of cancer development is important.
3. For most cancer sites, African Americans have higher incidence rates than non-Hispanic Caucasians. Hispanics and Native Americans have lower incidence rates overall.

E. **SOCIOECONOMIC STATUS**

1. Socioeconomic status (SES), is assessed by data on income, education, and percent below the **poverty level.**
2. SES has been found to be associated with some cancers, **independent of race.**

V. **OTHER APPLICATIONS OF EPIDEMIOLOGY IN ONCOLOGY**

A. **SURVIVAL**

1. Survival analysis is the calculation of the **probability that a person with a specific disease will be alive at a specific period of time after diagnosis.** The time frame commonly used is 5 years.
2. Survival rate is **affected by** the stage of disease at diagnosis and by the histology of the disease.
3. **Effectiveness of new treatment modalities** is assessed by comparing patient survival following those treatments to patient survival following standard treatment.

VI. **CANCER CONTROL**

1. Cancer control is the reduction of cancer incidence, morbidity, and mortality through research conducted in an orderly and systematic way.
2. Cancer control encompasses cancer prevention.
3. See **Figure 1-5, text page 23,** for phases of cancer control research. These phases are conducted in order to guide a national strategy for cancer control.

A. **SCREENING**

1. Screening is the process of **disease detection** through the use of tests, examinations, or other procedures before symptoms develop.
2. The assumption regarding screening is that early detection will lead to better prognosis and survival.

B. **BARRIERS TO PARTICIPATION IN SCREENING PROGRAMS**

1. Factors that prevent individuals from benefiting from screening programs include patient characteristics of culture and knowledge, as well as cost, availability, discrimination, and time.
2. **Behavioral change**
    a. Public knowledge about a risk factor for cancer does not automatically result in behavioral change.
    b. Programs that attempt to change the public's behavior must incorporate intervention strategies as well as education.
3. **Government policy**
    a. **Cancer control** is strongly influenced by national, state, and local government. Examples of legislation include restrictions on smoking in public places and rules for labeling food products.

VII. **THE APPLICATION OF EPIDEMIOLOGY TO NURSING PRACTICE**

1. **Nursing roles** in cancer prevention and control are numerous and extend beyond education.
2. Epidemiologic data and research principles are applied in three phases of nurses' work: the **development** phase, the **planning** phases of research and prevention programs, and the **evaluation** phase.

PRACTICE QUESTIONS

1. Why is an understanding of epidemiologic techniques and findings essential to oncology nursing?
    (A) because epidemiologic studies are fundamental to any understanding of the genetic bases of cancer
    (B) because epidemiology involves the analysis of all communicable diseases, including those with no single causative factor
    (C) because recognizing factors that affect health is necessary to plan and evaluate nursing strategies
    (D) because most practical aspects of oncology nursing are based on epidemiologic research

2. An epidemiologic study determines that in a given year approximately 1 of every 12,000 American men suffers from prostate cancer. This figure represents a(n)
    (A) incidence rate.
    (B) mortality rate.
    (C) prevalence rate.
    (D) survival rate.

3. The strength of the association between a factor (such as a suspected carcinogen) and an outcome (such as a type of cancer) is measured by
    (A) prospective risk.
    (B) attributable risk.
    (C) retrospective risk.
    (D) relative risk.

4. The relative risk and the frequency of a suspect etiologic factor in an entire defined population are known, and a case-control study is conducted. What is the study **most** likely to be seeking to establish?
    (A) causation
    (B) attributable risk
    (C) a survival risk
    (D) prevalence

5. The purpose of a cross-sectional study design is to assess
    (A) demographic data.
    (B) the rates of disease and exposure in a population.
    (C) causal relationships between exposures and diseases.
    (D) trends in disease distribution.

6. In cohort studies, the cohort, or group of subjects, consists of
    (A) a cross section of the general population.
    (B) individuals who have the disease of interest.
    (C) individuals who do not have the disease of interest.
    (D) family members of individuals who have the disease of interest.

7. A primary goal of cohort studies is to
    (A) evaluate the effect of time on the emergence of some outcome.
    (B) relate clusters to a common etiologic agent or to genetic or cultural factors.
    (C) reconstruct descriptive data from available historical documents.
    (D) trace changes in cancer incidence that occur through migration.

8. An epidemiologic study is to be conducted on workers in asbestos mines who are free of any cancer. Subjects are to be followed over a 10-year period, and the incidence rates of certain types of cancers are to be determined. This design is an example of a
    (A) prospective study.
    (B) retrospective study.
    (C) historical prospective study.
    (D) historical retrospective study.

9. Compared with a prospective study, a retrospective study has the advantage of being
    (A) less subject to bias from individuals' knowledge of the disease.
    (B) less subject to bias from incomplete or faulty medical records.
    (C) more powerful, less expensive, and quicker.
    (D) more generalizable to the population from which it is drawn.

10. Risk of developing which of the following cancers is directly correlated with the number of cigarettes smoked?
    (A) bladder cancer
    (B) pancreatic cancer
    (C) oropharyngeal cancer
    (D) kidney cancer

11. The rate of decline in former smokers' risk of developing lung cancer is determined by the cumulative smoking exposure prior to cessation, the age when smoking began, and the
    (A) degree of inhalation.
    (B) amount of passive smoke previously exposed to.
    (C) brand of cigarettes smoked.
    (D) amount of time that has passed since quitting.

12. Which of the following sources of fiber has been shown to provide the **most** protection against colon cancer?
    (A) cereals
    (B) vegetables
    (C) fruits
    (D) bread

13. Which of the following cancers is specifically associated with beer intake?
    (A) oropharyngeal cancer
    (B) liver cancer
    (C) esophageal cancer
    (D) rectal cancer

14.   Increased physical activity has been consistently found to be protective against
    (A)   head and neck cancer.
    (B)   esophageal cancer.
    (C)   colon cancer.
    (D)   bone cancer.

15.   Sources of ionizing radiation include
    (A)   air.
    (B)   lightbulbs.
    (C)   plants.
    (D)   microwaves.

16.   Which of the following variables appears to be the **best** descriptive determinant of cancer risk?
    (A)   gender
    (B)   age
    (C)   ethnicity or race
    (D)   genetic predisposition

17.   Which of the following host characteristics does **not** influence susceptibility to cancer?
    (A)   age
    (B)   ethnicity
    (C)   sex
    (D)   hair color

18.   Which of the following is the **best** example of the role of genetic predisposition in the development of cancer?
    (A)   The mortality rates for Japanese Americans with stomach cancer are significantly higher than those for the white American population.
    (B)   As more women smoke, more women are developing lung cancer.
    (C)   A study of Johns Hopkins medical students found that 55 students who later developed cancer perceived themselves as less close to their parents than did their healthy counterparts.
    (D)   Familial aggregates of cancer have been found to occur.

19.   Effective cancer control is influenced **most** by which of the following?
    (A)   government policy
    (B)   routine chest X rays
    (C)   hygiene
    (D)   a low-fat diet

ANSWER EXPLANATIONS

1.   **The answer is (C).**   An understanding of epidemiologic methods can enhance the nurse's assessment skills, and the knowledge gained from findings can give the nurse insight into the magnitude of risk for cancer that is inherent in the individual or community being served. Epidemiologic methods are also valuable in nursing research. (4, 24)

2.   **The answer is (C).**   The prevalence rate is the total number of cases—new and existing—in a given population during a specific time period, in this case 1 year. It is a function of both incidence and duration. In other words, the higher the survival rate (duration) for a type of cancer, the higher its prevalence rate will be. (4)

3.   **The answer is (D).**   Relative risk is expressed as a ratio comparing the rate of the disease among exposed individuals with the rate of the disease among unexposed individuals. A high relative risk suggests a strong correlation between the exposure and the disease. Unlike attributable risk, however, relative risk is not intended to measure the probability that an exposed person will develop the outcome. (5)

4.   **The answer is (B).**   Attributable risk is the difference in the decease rates between the group exposed to some factor and unexposed groups. It is used to evaluate the magnitude of change in an outcome (e.g., respiratory cancer) with the removal of the suspect antecedent fact (e.g., smoking). Provided that the

relative risk and the frequency of the suspect factor in the entire defined population are known, attributable risk can be estimated from a case-control study. Otherwise, it must be calculated directly from a prospective study. (4)

5. **The answer is (B).**   The cross-sectional study is another design that allows an investigator to assess the rates of disease and exposure in a population. A one-time view of a population is taken, and the rates of existing (prevalent) cases of the disease, the degree of exposure, and other demographic characteristics of interest are measured. Although they cannot establish a causal relationship between the exposure and the disease, cross-sectional studies do provide descriptive statistics for the population. (7)

6. **The answer is (C).**   The cohort, or group of subjects, that is included in this type of study design represents individuals who do not have the disease of interest. An initial cross-sectional study or assessment of a population can identify and eliminate all active cases of the disease. Once the cohort is selected, the exposures of interest are assessed, and the subjects are monitored for a designated period of time to record development of the disease. (8)

7. **The answer is (A).**   A cohort is a defined group of persons with similar characteristics or some common exposure in a particular period. In cohort studies, several cohorts are compared at the same time to evaluate the effect of time on the emergence of some outcome, often mortality. This method is used to determine whether common exposure to a suspected etiologic factor resulted in an increased incidence of disease and to measure how prevention or treatment has altered the course of the disease over time. (8)

8. **The answer is (A).**   In this prospective study, subjects (miners) are being selected with varying degrees of exposure to the suspected factor (asbestos). They have not experienced the outcome thought to be associated with the factor (lung cancer or some other cancer). They are then being followed over time to see whether the outcome (e.g., a type of cancer) occurs. (8)

9. **The answer is (C).**   A well-done retrospective study is statistically more powerful, more economical, and quicker than a prospective study, but it is subject to bias from several sources, including the effect of subjects' knowledge of the disease on their recollection of factors associated with the condition, incomplete medical records, and the determination of the risk associated with exposure to some factor. It is also harder to generalize the conclusions of a retrospective study to the population from which it is drawn. (8)

10. **The answer is (C).**   Active tobacco use has been linked to many cancer types (lung, oropharyngeal, bladder, pancreatic, cervical, and kidney), and a clear linear relationship exists between the number of cigarettes smoked and the risk of lung and oropharyngeal cancers. (11)

11. **The answer is (A).**   There is a gradual decrease in the former smoker's risk of dying from lung cancer; eventually the risk is almost equivalent to that of a nonsmoker. The rate of decline of risk after cessation of smoking is determined by the cumulative smoking exposure prior to cessation, the age when smoking began, and the degree of inhalation. (11)

12. **The answer is (B).**   A majority of studies of differing epidemiologic designs support the hypothesis that high fiber intake is protective against colon cancer, although not all studies are supportive. In studies where the source of fiber has been examined, the data for cereal fibers are less supportive of a protective effect. (12)

13. **The answer is (D).**   Alcohol has been causally linked to cancers of the oral cavity, pharynx, larynx, esophagus, and liver, and it may be linked to cancers of the breast and rectum. It is estimated that 3% of cancer deaths are attributable to alcohol. For most cancer sites, alcohol appears to act synergistically with smoking. Although cancers at most sites do not appear to be associated with any particular type of alcohol, rectal cancer appears to be associated specifically with beer consumption. (13)

14. **The answer is (C).**   Increased physical activity consistently has been found to be protective against colon cancer and precancerous colon polyps. Increased physical activity also may be protective against breast cancer. Increased physical activity is known to be protective against heart disease, and a general increase in physical activity throughout the population would be beneficial. (13)

15. **The answer is (A).**   For most of the earth's population, over 80% of exposure to ionizing radiation is from natural sources, such as the food chain, air, water, minerals on or near the earth's crust, and cosmic

rays. Human-made sources include X rays, fallout from nuclear explosions, and emissions and waste from nuclear power stations. (15)

16.   **The answer is (B).**   The vulnerability of the host to different cancers changes throughout each phase of the life cycle, with an overall sharp and steady increase in cancer incidence occurring from childhood to old age as a result of intrinsic psychological states and exposure to different social, cultural, and environmental conditions. (17)

17.   **The answer is (D).**   Cancer is very much a disease of the elderly, with those over age 65 being ten times more likely than those under 65 to develop cancer. The incidence of cancers that are not sex-specific is generally lower in females, in part because of the differences in lifestyle between the sexes. Ethnicity and race can be important issues to assess in epidemiologic research, and they are often highly correlated with socioeconomic status. (17–19)

18.   **The answer is (D).**   Data from a number of sources, including familial patterns, have been studied in an attempt to elicit features of genetic predisposition to cancer. (18–19)

19.   **The answer is (A).**   The degree to which an individual takes advantage of screening opportunities influences effective cancer control. The national, state, and local governments have an impact on cancer control through legislation. Cancer control efforts are affected by the monies specifically appropriated to cancer control in the National Institutes of Health budget. The government can influence advancement in this area by setting national goals for cancer control, such as those in the Healthy People 2000 document. (23)

Milestones in Our Understanding of the Causes of Cancer

STUDY OUTLINE

I. **INTRODUCTION**

    1. **Carcinogenesis** requires **clonal selection.**
       a. A **mutation** in a cell may confer a survival advantage.
       b. If a descendant of that cell is hit by a second **mutation that also confers a survival advantage,** the next clone grows even more vigorously.
       c. A sequence of such events leads to the selection of a clone with the **characteristics of a neoplasm.**
       d. **Subclones** progress to ever greater stages of virulence characterized by invasion, metastatic spread, drug resistance, and other characteristics that ultimately lead to the death of the host.
    2. Animals have evolved an elaborate set of controls **regulating cellular growth** and repair.
       a. Signals turn growth on and off as needed.
       b. Complex **fail-safe mechanisms** prevent the overgrowth of a mutant clone.
    3. **Cancer** overcomes this protection against uncontrolled growth.
       a. Mutations that lead to cancer are mutations of the very **same genes** that regulate normal growth.
    4. Two types of **growth-control genes** that have been identified are oncogenes and anti-oncogenes.
       a. **Oncogenes and proto-oncogenes** code for proteins that stimulate growth.
       b. **Anti-oncogenes,** or cancer suppressor genes, code for proteins that block the action of growth-promoting factors.
    5. There are two types of cancer-causing **mutations.**
       a. **Somatic mutations** are mutations of the ordinary cells of the various organs. They are acquired throughout a lifetime due to various carcinogens.
       b. **Germ cell mutations** are mutations that are transmitted to the next generation at birth and are responsible for hereditary (familial) cancer.
       c. Many human cancers result from a **combination of acquired** and **inherited mutations** with alterations of both oncogenes and anti-oncogenes.
    6. **Carcinogenesis** may result from exposure to chemicals, radiation, asbestos, or viruses.
       a. Oncogenes must be mutated to be **activated,** and cancer-suppressor genes must be mutated to be inactivated.

II. **"THERE IS NO TREATMENT"**

    1. The earliest description of cancer dates back to the seventeenth century B.C.
       a. The oldest written description of a patient with cancer indicated "there is no treatment."
       b. One thousand years later, Hippocrates formulated his rules for medical practice that included his cardinal rule: **"First, do no harm."**
          (1) Hippocrates also applied the first word for cancer, the Greek word for crab, *karkinos.*
    2. In the first century A.D., Celsus compiled in Rome an **encyclopedia of medicine** containing accurate clinical descriptions of cancer.
       a. **Distinctions** were made between benign and malignant disease, and treatments were recommended.

3. Galen, who lived in the second century A.D., was the central medical authority for over a thousand years.
4. **The Middle Ages saw attempts at radical surgery in Byzantine.**

III. **"THERE IS NO IMPROPRIETY IN REMOVING IT"**

1. The advent of the Renaissance signaled the beginning of **medical progress** in Europe.
2. Harvey's *De Mortu Cordis* in 1628 described the **circulation** of the blood and thus heralded the beginning of scientific cardiology.
3. Surgery for cancer was documented in the eighteenth century, despite the fact that anesthesia would not be developed for another century.

IV. **"CAUTIONS AGAINST THE IMMODERATE USE OF SNUFF"**

1. John Hill of London published a description of his observations of the dangers of tobacco in 1761, only a few decades after tobacco had become popular in London.
2. The oft-cited description of scrotal cancer in chimney sweeps by Percival Pott of St. Bartholomew's Hospital in London was the third in a series of reports that launched the field of cancer epidemiology.

V. **"WE MIGHT SUPPRESS IT COMPLETELY IN AN EARLY STAGE"**

1. At the beginning of the nineteenth century, a committee of English physicians and surgeons formed to **investigate** the nature of cancer. Thirteen questions were formulated whose research significance is instantly recognized by any cancer scientist today.
2. A **systematic approach** to cancer biology laid a foundation for scientific progress in the nineteenth century.
3. The nineteenth century saw the birth of scientific oncology as **science** shifted from anatomy to pathology.
   a. Early in the century a **microscope** of sufficient quality for research on tissues became available.
   b. Johannes Muller applied this instrument to cancer research and began to **correlate cellular pathology with clinical symptoms.**
   c. Subsequently Rudolph Virchow, described as the founder of cellular pathology, carried on this work and provided the basis for the modern **pathological study** of cancer.
4. Wilhelm Waldeyer did not agree that cancer metastases resulted from some kind of noncellular infectious substance; he felt **embolic transfer** through the blood or lymph channels was the mechanism.

VI. **"THIS IS NO HUMBUG!"**

1. In 1846 John C. Warren performed the **first reported operation under anesthesia** on a patient anesthetized with ether by a dentist.
   a. Prior to this time anesthesia had bordered on quackery, and it was not immediately accepted.
2. Anesthesia allowed the rapid **progress** in surgery that caused the next 100 years to be called the "century of the surgeon."

VII. **"THERE IS NO SUCH THING AS AN INEVITABLE INFECTION"**

1. Florence Nightingale gave the hospital the **professional** nurse and instituted the tradition of scholarship and dedication that continues today in oncology nursing.
2. Nightingale advocated **preventive medicine** policies far ahead of her time.

VIII. **"AMPUTATION OF THE SHOULDER JOINT MIGHT ERADICATE THE DISEASE"**

1. Halsted was one of the surgical giants whose work led to the **"cancer operation"** designed to remove all of the **tumor en bloc** as well as the lymph nodes that normally drained the region where the tumor was located.
2. Halsted, at Johns Hopkins University, developed the **radical mastectomy** during the last decade of the nineteenth century.
3. Handley believed that **cancer spread centrifugally** through the lymphatics in continuity with the original growth.

IX.   **"THE SEED AND THE SOIL"**

    1.   Stephen Paget drew the conclusion that cells from a primary tumor are able to grow in only certain other organs—not simply in any organ in which they happen to come to rest.

X.   **"ALL VESTIGES OF HER PREVIOUS CANCEROUS DISEASE HAD DISAPPEARED"**

    1.   The potential for **systemic treatment** for cancer can be traced to the end of the nineteenth century when Beatson correlated ovarian function with breast cancer and performed oophorectomies in women with advanced breast cancer, resulting in tumor regression.

XI.   **"A NEW KIND OF RAY"**

    1.   Roentgen published information on the **X ray** as a second modality of cancer therapy. Within three years of presenting his work, radiation therapy was being used in the **treatment of cancer.**

    2.   Within months of the publication of Roentgen's article, systems were being devised to use X rays for diagnosis.

    3.   It was in France that it was discovered that delivering radiation over a **protracted period** of time by use of daily fractions would greatly improve therapeutic response.

XII.   **"FROM A BIT INOCULATED INTO BREAST MUSCLE OF A SUSCEPTIBLE FOWL"**

    1.   **Radiation, viral,** and **chemical carcinogenesis** were demonstrated in the early 1900s.
       a.   **Radiation** was recognized as a carcinogen only seven years after Roentgen's discovery.
       b.   Peyton Rous described a sarcoma in chickens caused by what later became known as the **Rous sarcoma virus.**
       c.   **Cancer was induced in laboratory animals for the first time by coal tar applied to rabbit skin.**

XIII.   **"WE GOT IT ALL"**

    1.   In the first half of the twentieth century, cancer surgical procedures consisted of radical removal of tissue and the graining of lymph nodes; systemic therapy was nonexistent.

    2.   Knowledge of cancer biology was thwarted because of lack of understanding of multistage carcinogenesis and of the relationship of clonal selection during progression to the metastasis of cancer.

XIV.   **"THESE TEND TOWARD MALIGNANCY FROM THE BEGINNING AND ATTAIN IT BY A CONTINUOUS SERIES OF ALTERATIONS"**

    1.   In 1911, Peyton Rous made the key discovery of multistage carcinogenesis by describing a difference between initiation of carcinogenesis and promotion of carcinogenesis in both virus-induced rabbit papilloma transformed to a malignant lesion and coal tar applied to the skin to induce skin cancers.

    2.   These classic experiments were confirmed by Berenblum and Shubik, using croton oil as the promoter.

    3.   Progression to the metastatic phenotype was subsequently well elucidated in modern biological terms by Fidler.

    4.   Evidence obtained 20 years after the work of Rous indicated that
       a.   **Initiation** is irreversible and is characterized by damage to DNA.
       b.   **Promotion** does not involve damage to DNA but rather stimulation of cellular proliferation. Promotion is reversible and exhibits a distinct dose-response and measurable threshold.
       c.   **Progression** leads to morphologic change and to increased grades of malignant behavior such as invasion, metastasis, and drug resistance.

XV.   **"THE CLINICAL RESULTS WERE SOMETIMES DRAMATIC"**

    1.   The term **chemotherapy** took on the present meaning of cytotoxic agents used in the treatment of cancer when nitrogen mustard was developed by the chemical warfare research division of the U.S. Army during World War I.

XVI.   **"CARCINOGENS ARE MUTAGENS"**

    1.   In 1944 **DNA** was demonstrated to be the chemical mediator of heredity.
        a.   It came to be understood that covalent binding within the cell was required for carcinogenic activity.
        b.   The active metabolites of carcinogens were identified as electrophilic reactants bound to DNA.
    2.   An **assay test to measure carcinogens** is known as the **Ames assay system.** The Ames assay identifies only mutagens. And although "carcinogens are mutagens," not all carcinogens are mutagens and not all mutagens are carcinogens.
    3.   **Cancer biology** was beginning to take form.

XVII.   **"I'M NOT SAYING IT. THE DATA ARE SAYING IT"**

    1.   Recognition of the **futility of radical surgery** in the management of cancer began with randomized trials in breast cancer and malignant melanoma.
    2.   Fisher and Veronesi led the way to the overthrow of the classic "cancer operation" by their demonstration that **survival** in breast cancer and melanoma is independent of the extent of radical resection.
    3.   Recognition that treatment methods needed to change led to reevaluation of the notion of the anatomical containment of cancer. This led to the understanding that it is our biology, not our anatomy, that restricts cancer spread.
    4.   What was not understood by those for whom anatomy was central to cancer spread was that the cancer cells had spread throughout the body from the time that the first capillaries had been attracted into the growing tumor by angiogenesis factor secreted by the tumor cells.

XVIII.   **"CARCINOGENS, IRRADIATION, AND THE NORMAL AGING PROCESS ALL FAVOR THE PARTIAL OR COMPLETE ACTIVATION OF THESE GENES"**

    1.   Increasing numbers of oncogenic viruses were discovered in **animal systems.** Originally called type C viruses, they were later called **retroviruses** because they were RNA viruses that were converted to DNA by reverse transcriptase.
    2.   Heubner and Todaro focused attention on the word *oncogene* in 1969 when they proposed that **RNA viruses somehow placed viral genes in the human genome** that were then genetically transmitted.
    3.   See **text page 36,** column 2, for an account of how genes are designated and coded.
    4.   Oncogenes **found in retroviruses** are the same as the growth factor and growth receptor genes found in normal cells.
    5.   The basic experiments in retroviral carcinogenesis used animal systems and cell culture systems to demonstrate that the intact virus and isolated genes were able to induce malignant transformation.
    6.   There was strong support for the hypothesis that the oncogenes found in retroviruses were the same as the **growth factor** and **growth factor receptor genes** found in normal cells.
    7.   Retroviral oncogene research did allow the identification of many human oncogenes that code for normal growth-promoting substances and improved our understanding of the way in which oncogenes promote normal and neoplastic growth.
        a.   Oncogenes have been identified for many **cell signals** in addition to growth factors and growth factor receptors, including signal amplification and transmission within the cell and signal reception within the nucleus.
    8.   It is now known that it is the **human growth-control genes,** first identified as oncogenes in retroviruses, that are the long-sought-after targets of the mutating chemicals and radiation that contribute certain critical lesions leading to human cancer.

XIX.   **"THE FIRST DEMONSTRATION OF A PHYSICAL LINK BETWEEN AN ONCOGENE AND AN ANTI-ONCOGENE"**

    1.   Oncogenes of DNA viruses are not recently captured cellular genes, but their products **react** with the products of human genes.
    2.   Work with the oncogenes of the DNA viruses led to discovery of **several viruses causing human cancer** and to a better understanding of normal cellular control mechanisms.

     a. This is because the products of DNA oncogenes interacted with and blocked the action of normal growth-regulating cellular proteins.

XX.   **"GENES I HAVE CALLED ANTI-ONCOGENES"**

    1. While there are oncogenes that code for proteins that induce malignant growth by "turning on" cell division, there are proteins that "turn off" cell growth.
       a. These suppressor proteins were discovered because the oncogenic DNA viruses had oncogenes whose products bound to and inactivated them.
          (1) Since the genes coding for these proteins had a function opposite to that of oncogenes, they were called **anti-oncogenes;** and because they **suppressed malignant growth,** they were also called **cancer-suppressor genes.**
    2. It is believed that cancer results from a **combination** of genetic changes that must include both the absence of the protein products of cancer-suppressor genes and the presence of abnormal products of oncogenes.

XXI.   **"THERE ARE TOO MANY MUTATIONS IN HUMAN CANCERS"**

    1. The number of mutations involving the oncogenes and cancer-suppressor genes was exceedingly large in all human tumors—too large, in fact, to be explained by the simple action of carcinogens on human cells.
    2. The **p53 gene,** located at chromosome 17p13, is the most commonly altered gene in human cancer, being altered in as many as half of the common neoplasms.

XXII.   **"THE GUARDIAN OF THE GENOME"**

    1. The **p53 cancer-suppressor gene** accumulates when cellular DNA is damaged by radiation or chemotherapy, and the cells are arrested in phase G1 so that they do not enter mitosis until the DNA is repaired.
       a. When normal p53 genes are inserted into cancer cells, they may **induce** programmed cell death.
       b. DNA viruses must knock out p53 in order to move into the cell into S phase, which they need for replication, so DNA viruses produce proteins that inactivate the p53 protein.
          (1) This explains why people with inherited mutant p53 genes are predisposed to an increased risk of cancer.

XXIII. **EXAMPLES OF HUMAN TUMOR CARCINOGENESIS**

    1. Even though carcinogenesis is usually classified as **familial, viral, physical, or chemical,** it probably results from a combination of factors.
    2. **Tobacco, our principal mutagen,** is responsible for over a third of all cancer deaths.
       a. Asbestos exposure **greatly multiplies** the effect of smoking, and radon in the home contributes to a degree yet to be determined because the level of exposure is not yet known.
       b. Many commonly mutated genes have been identified in lung cancer.
          (1) Carcinogenesis in this common cancer results from **mutations of oncogenes and cancer-suppressor genes** by **chemical agents** and from **familial factors.**

A.   **FAMILIAL CANCER**

    1. **Defective genes** can be inherited.
       a. Hereditary retinoblastoma results when a child inherits a defective retinoblastoma gene. Analysis of chromosome 13 has revealed that the chromosome lost during tumorigenesis is the one from the nonaffected parent, whereas the one retained is from the affected parent, proving dominant inheritance.
       b. The proliferative disease predisposing to both breast cancer and early-onset breast cancer is inherited. There is a **13% familial aggregation in breast cancer.**
       c. The Li-Fraumini syndrome results from inheritance of a defective p53 gene.
    2. Most inherited cancer syndromes behave as autosomal dominants but are rare.

B. **VIRAL CARCINOGENESIS**

1. The one clearly established human tumor due to a retrovirus is a **human T lymphoma/leukemia due to the HTLV-1.**
    a. A small proportion of patients with Sezary syndrome and mycosis fungoides also have evidence of HTLV-1.
    b. Hairy cell leukemia is a disease of B-lymphocytes for the most part, but a small portion of the cases involve T-lymphocytes, and HTLV-2 has been isolated.
2. **Human papillomaviruses (HPV)** infect squamous epithelium, and some strains cause genital warts. There are strong data supporting an etiological role for some strains of HPV in cervical cancer.
3. **Hepatitis B (HBV) virus** is etiological in hepatocellular carcinoma.
4. **Epstein-Barr virus (EBV)** is a cause of Burkitt's lymphoma in Africa and infectious mononucleosis in the U.S. and is associated with nasopharyngeal cancer in Chinese people, regardless of where they live.

C. **PHYSICAL CARCINOGENS**

1. Physical carcinogens exert their action on genes by **physical rather than chemical means.**
2. **Ultraviolet radiation (UV) from the sun damages DNA,** causing pyrimidine dimer formation that if not properly repaired leads to mutations.
    a. Basal cell and squamous cell carcinomas of the exposed areas are the result.
    b. The most dramatic example of UV carcinogenesis is seen in patients with **xeroderma pigmentosum,** an autosomal recessive disease in which DNA repair of UV damage is defective, resulting in a high incidence of skin cancer, including melanoma.
3. Estimates are that about 3% of all cancer deaths are due to natural radiation (excluding radon).
4. The risk of **medical radiation exposure** has probably been exaggerated.
5. **Asbestos,** a carcinogenic fiber, is thought to be related to about 2000 cases of mesothelioma annually in the United States.

D. **CHEMICAL CARCINOGENS**

1. Although numerous chemicals can lead to cancer in animals, there are few (other than tobacco and chemotherapeutic agents) that give strong evidence of cancer causation in the human.
2. Occupational causes account for approximately 4% of cancer deaths in the United States.

XXIV. **CONTROVERSIES IN CARCINOGENESIS**

A. **ESTROGENS AND CARCINOGENESIS**

1. There are conflicting data on the role estrogen therapy plays in the development of **breast cancer,** whether for postmenopausal replacement or contraceptive use.
    a. In view of the known benefits of postmenopausal estrogen in the prevention of osteoporosis and the reduction of cardiovascular risk by up to half, any decision that estrogen is contraindicated based on a theoretical or poorly documented breast cancer risk must be carefully evaluated.
    b. The effect of contraceptives on breast cancer risk is not clearly established, with most of the studies showing no relationship. The preponderant opinion is that contraceptives are safe.

B. **INVOLUNTARY (PASSIVE) SMOKING**

1. Although there are insufficient data to confirm passive smoking's role in the cause of cancer, **lung cancer mortality may be about one-third higher in spouses of smokers** than in spouses of nonsmokers.
2. **Sex** of the nonsmoker may also be a factor, men being more sensitive than women.

C. **ENVIRONMENTAL CARCINOGENESIS**

1. The risk of cancer development is better correlated with our **lifestyle** than with any environmental cause. In particular, it is the food and alcohol consumed and the use of tobacco.

D. **DIET AND CARCINOGENESIS**

1. There is a correlation between **fat consumption and/or total calories consumed early in life** and the development of colon and breast cancer.
2. Stomach cancer is believed to be correlated with foods that are pickled, cured, smoked, salted, and preserved.
3. Perhaps one-third of all cancers could be explained by dietary factors.
4. Radical dietary changes would be required early in life to effect substantial reductions in the incidence of cancer.
5. It is difficult to prescribe a reasonable diet that is certain to reduce cancer incidence.
    a. A **diet rich in fruits, fiber,** and **cruciferous vegetables** and low in animal fat is desirable for many health reasons and may perhaps reduce the risk of cancer.

PRACTICE QUESTIONS

1. Cancer-suppressor genes code for proteins that _____ the action of growth-promoting factors.
    (A) enhance
    (B) block
    (C) duplicate
    (D) fuel

2. Carcinogens are generally categorized into three classes. They are
    (A) chemical, radiation, and lifestyle.
    (B) chemical, radiation, and physical.
    (C) chemical, physical, and viral.
    (D) chemical, viral, and radiation.

3. Which of the following statements correctly describes the effect of passive smoke on spouses of active smokers?
    (A) Lung cancer mortality rates are higher in men regardless of exposure to passive smoke.
    (B) The lung cancer mortality rate of nonsmoking spouses is similar to the lung cancer mortality rate of their smoking spouses.
    (C) There is no difference in lung cancer mortality rates among spouses of smokers and spouses of nonsmokers.
    (D) Lung cancer mortality rates may be about one-third higher in spouses of smokers than in spouses of nonsmokers.

4. Hepatitis B virus (HBV) is etiological in
    (A) liver cancer.
    (B) breast cancer.
    (C) colon cancer.
    (D) esophageal cancer.

5. Although research in the correlation of diet and cancer development is still needed, which of the following dietary patterns is recommended for modestly reducing the risk of cancer?
    (A) high fat, high fruit, high fiber
    (B) high fruit, high fiber, high cruciferous vegetables
    (C) moderate fat, low protein, high cruciferous vegetables
    (D) low fat, high fruit, high fiber

6. Which of the following cancer-causing mutations is transmitted to the next generation at birth?
    (A) oncogene mutations
    (B) germ cell mutations
    (C) somatic mutations
    (D) anti-oncogene mutations

ANSWER EXPLANATIONS

1. **The answer is (B).**   Two types of growth-control genes have been identified: oncogenes and anti-oncogenes, or cancer-suppressor genes. The cancer-suppressor genes are recessive genes that code for growth proteins that block the action of growth-promoting factors. (29)

2. **The answer is (D).**   Carcinogenesis may result from exposure to chemicals, such as those in tobacco; radiation, such as cosmic rays or radon from natural sources; asbestos; or various types of viruses. In all cases the final common path of action of such agents is through oncogenes and cancer-suppressing genes. (29)

3. **The answer is (D).**   Although there are insufficient data to allow firm conclusions regarding passive or involuntary smoking as etiological in lung cancer, spousal exposure provides some information. Lung cancer mortality may be about one-third higher in spouses of smokers than in spouses of nonsmokers. This has served as the basis for estimates that exposure of nonsmokers in proximity to smokers may account for 20% of nonsmoker lung cancer deaths (or 2400 deaths) each year. (41)

4. **The answer is (A).**   Hepatitis B virus (HBV) is endemic in Asia and Africa and is etiological in hepatocellular carcinoma. There may be other factors that increase risk, such as aflatoxin, to which there are heavy exposures. (40)

5. **The answer is (D).**   There is a striking correlation between the amount of fat a nation consumes and the incidence of colon cancer and breast cancer and a similar correlation between meat consumption and colon cancer. There is a correlation between fat consumption and/or total calories consumed early in life and the development of colon and breast cancer. Radical dietary changes would be required early in life to effect substantial reductions in cancer incidence. It is difficult to prescribe a reasonable diet that is certain to reduce the incidence of cancer. A diet rich in fruits, fiber, and cruciferous vegetables and low in animal fat is desirable for many health reasons and may perhaps reduce the risk of cancer. (41–42)

6. **The answer is (B).**   Germ cell mutations are mutations that are transmitted to the next generation at birth and are responsible for hereditary (familial) cancer. Most human cancers result from a combination of acquired and inherited mutations with alterations of both oncogenes and anti-oncogenes. (29)

3 Differences between Normal and Cancer Cells

STUDY OUTLINE

I. **INTRODUCTION**

    1. Fundamental goals of cancer research are to identify **what factors or events cause a cell to become aberrant, how cancer cells differ in appearance and behavior** from normal cells, and how that information can be used to prevent and cure cancer.

II. **RESEARCH MODELS**

    A. **LIMITATIONS OF STUDY OF HUMAN TISSUES**

        1. A **technical problem** in studying the differences between normal and cancer cells is that researchers cannot be sure in their identification of the normal cell counterparts of human cancer cells.

    B. **TRANSFORMED CELL MODELS**

        1. For the cancer cell prototype, normal cells derived from normal tissue are established in culture under controlled conditions.
            a. Cells all derive from a **single cell** and are therefore fairly uniform.
            b. Cell lines become permanent or continuous cell lines when they acquire the **ability to be propagated** indefinitely in tissue culture.
            c. These cells can be transformed into cells that **behave like malignant cells when they are exposed to chemical, viral, or radiation carcinogens.** This process is called **transformation,** and the cell lines are called transformed cells.
        2. **Transformed cells** are used to study the differences between normal cell and cancer cell behavior.
        3. The **ultimate criterion** is whether the cells form a tumor when injected into an animal.
        4. Two factors—**uncontrolled growth** and **immortality**—are observed in all cancer cells.
        5. The assumption is made that transformed cells and actual cancer cells share many identical features and that what we have learned about transformed cells can be applied to human cancer.

III. **DIFFERENCES IN GROWTH OF NORMAL AND CANCER CELLS**

    1. The primary feature of a cancer cell is its **uncontrolled growth.**
        a. Cancer cells **continue to divide,** not necessarily at a faster rate, but continuously and without regard to the needs of the host.
        b. Cancer tissues that develop as a result of the continual replication of cancer cells are **without structure** and **organization.**
        c. The fraction of cells dividing provides a net increase in cells, so in contrast to the balance maintained in normal tissues, in cancer tissues the number of new cells is greater than the number of cells lost, resulting in a tumor mass.
    2. The **uncontrolled cancer growth** of tumors occurs as a result of several properties of cancer cells: **cancer cell immortality, loss of cell-to-cell contact inhibition, diminished serum requirements of cancer cells, the ability of a cancer cell to multiply without being in contact with a surface,** and **loss of the restriction point.**

A.   **IMMORTALITY OF CANCER CELLS**

    1.   **Senescence** is the programmed death of all normal cells upon reaching 50–60 divisions, or generations.

    2.   Cancer cells are immortal.

B.   **LOSS OF CONTACT INHIBITION**

    1.   When normal cells are placed in a culture dish containing liquid growth medium, the cells fall to the bottom of the vessel, attach to the surface, and begin to divide, spreading out as they divide, until the cells reach the sides of the dish. At this point the dish has been covered in a monolayer of cells.

        a.   It was thought that cell contact was the signal for the **turning off of cell division,** and the phenomenon was named **contact inhibition of growth.**

    2.   **Density-dependent growth** refers to the same monolayer phenomenon, but it also suggests that when cells crowd each other, their access to nutrients is inhibited and this is why cell division stops.

    3.   In contrast to normal cells, when cancer cells are placed in the same culture medium, they continue to divide, crowding the space they occupy until the cells are piled on each other in an unorganized mass.

        a.   Reasons for lack of contact inhibition:

            (1)   Transformed cells are **held less firmly to adjacent cells** than are normal cells and seem to move about with more frequency than do normal cells.

            (2)   Cancer cells require **lower concentrations of many necessary substances,** so their growth may be less affected than normal cells' growth by contact.

        b.   In addition to contact inhibition of growth, normal cells exhibit contact inhibition of movement, whereas the movement of cancer cells is not inhibited by contact with other cells.

C.   **DIMINISHED GROWTH FACTOR REQUIREMENTS OF CANCER CELLS**

    1.   **Growth factors** facilitate normal cell growth in culture.

    2.   Cancer cells and transformed cells are able to multiply in medium containing about **one-tenth the usual concentration of serum.**

        a.   Some cancer and transformed cell lines will even grow in the absence of serum.

        b.   These transformed cells seem to make their own growth factors.

D.   **ABILITY TO DIVIDE WITHOUT ANCHORAGE**

    1.   **Anchorage-dependent growth** refers to the fact that normal cells need a surface to which they can attach and then spread out and multiply.

    2.   Cancer cells and transformed cells are able to grow in suspension or gel, and this property is most closely associated with the ability to form tumors.

E.   **LOSS OF RESTRICTION POINT IN CELL CYCLE**

    1.   Cellular proliferation occurs as a result of **two coordinated events:** the **duplication of DNA** within the cell and mitosis, the **division of the cell into two** daughter cells with identical complements of DNA.

        a.   The two events combined make up what is known as the **cell cycle.**

            (1)   The G_0 **phase** is the resting state.

            (2) G_1 is the phase during which protein synthesis takes place in preparation for the **S phase** of DNA synthesis.

            (3) G_2 is the phase during which further protein synthesis takes place in preparation for the **M phase,** wherein mitosis takes place.

    2.   Most **differentiated cells** in the adult body are in a resting, or G_0, phase unless called to divide because of cell death or injury.

    3.   The decision by the cell to enter G_0 or to continue in G_1 occurs at a point in G_1 called the **restriction point.**

        a.   Once a cell passes this point, it must continue through all phases of the cell cycle and return to G_1.

4. Neither the biochemical events that regulate the normal cell cycle nor the nature of the transition to G_0 are known.

IV. **DIFFERENCES IN THE APPEARANCE OF NORMAL AND CANCER CELLS**

1. Transformed cells contain the subunits of proteins, but the proteins are not polymerized, causing transformed cells to have **variable sizes** and **shapes (pleomorphism).**
2. There are other important differences in the appearance of cancer cells and normal cells.
    a. The nuclei of cancer cells **stain darker** and are **disproportionately larger.**
    b. Cancer cells exhibit a variety of **abnormal mitotic figures.**
3. See **Figure 3-5, text page 51,** for differences in appearance of normal cells and cancer cells.

V. **DIFFERENCES IN DIFFERENTIATION OF NORMAL AND CANCER CELLS**

1. As the human organism develops from the fertilized egg into an adult person, cells become different and specialized for various structural and functional purposes.
2. The **more differentiated** a cell becomes, the more its potential is restricted.
    a. Fully differentiated cells are often incapable of **replicating** and are committed to performing the functions of the particular tissues that they compose.
3. Cancer cells may arise at any point during differentiation.
4. Cancer cells tend to be **less differentiated** than cells from surrounding normal tissue.
    a. Some cancer cells are so poorly differentiated **(anaplastic)** that the tissue of origin cannot be identified.
5. During the change from normal cells to neoplastic tissue, a sequence of tissue alterations occurs consisting of **metaplasia, dysplasia, carcinoma in situ,** and finally **invasive carcinoma.**

VI. **DIFFERENCES IN THE CELL SURFACES OF NORMAL AND CANCER CELLS**

1. The most elementary cell membrane consists of two layers of lipid molecules called a **lipid bilayer.**
    a. Various proteins and glycoproteins are embedded in the lipid bilayer.
2. The **cell membrane** is a loose structure with many fluid-like properties, and proteins and glycoproteins move both laterally and between the layers, albeit slowly.
3. The fluid nature of the membrane and the existence of mobile proteins within the membrane and on the surface have been described as the **fluid mosaic model.**

A. **GLYCOPROTEIN ALTERATIONS**

1. Cell transformation is almost always associated with profound **changes in cell-surface glycoproteins,** mostly related to lower protein content.
2. **Fibronectin**
    a. Fibronectin is a large glycoprotein found on normal cell surfaces.
        (1) Together with various proteoglycans, collagen, and elastin, fibronectin **forms the matrix** in which cells are embedded and that anchors cells in place within tissues.
        (2) For many cell types to grow in culture, fibronectin must be present in the serum.
    b. Cancer cells and transformed cells have **low levels** of fibronectin, causing them to attach poorly to the surface of the culture vessel; however, they continue to grow.
    c. Since fibronectin plays important roles in cellular organization, cell-to-cell adhesion, and cytoskeletal structure, the lack of fibronectin in cancer cells is an important factor in cancer metastasis.
3. **Proteases**
    a. Transformed cells have been shown to secrete a variety of **protein-degrading enzymes.**
    b. Proteases are involved in **metastasis** through local invasion of the extracellular matrices of surrounding tissue rather than in transformation itself.
    c. The proteolytic enzymes may degrade both the attachment proteins as well as components of the extracellular matrix.
    d. In addition to producing their own proteolytic enzymes, tumor cells may also **induce adjacent host cells to secrete enzymes.**

B. **GLYCOLIPID ALTERATIONS**

1. **Cell-surface changes** in glycolipids are another attribute of transformation.
2. In general, the content and complexity of glycolipids are **reduced** in transformed cell membranes.
3. Transformed cells have less and/or altered glycosphingolipids on their cell surfaces, increasing the responsiveness of the transformed cells to growth factors.
4. Glycosphingolipids have been shown to serve as components of surface markers involved in cell-cell recognition.

C. **CELL-SURFACE ANTIGENS**

1. Many of the proteins and glycoproteins on the surface of the cell can be detected by **immunological assay;** they are referred to as surface antigens.
2. In animals and transformed cells, antigens have been identified that are not found on any normal cell; these antigens are **tumor-specific antigens.**
3. The great majority of antigens identified in human tumors are tumor-associated antigens that have relative rather than absolute specificity for cancer cells.
4. Tumor-associated antigens are of two basic types.
    a. **Tumor-associated transplantation antigens (TATAs)** are antigens that appear on the surfaces of cells transformed by viral, chemical, or radiation carcinogens.
    b. **Oncofetal antigens** (embryonic antigens) are antigens normally found on embryonic cells that are re-expressed on certain tumors.
    c. Examples of oncofetal antigens:
        (1) **Alpha-fetoprotein (AFP)** is found in liver cancers and in some testicular, pancreatic, and gastrointestinal tract tumors.
        (2) **Carcinoembryonic antigen (CEA)** is found in cancers of the gastrointestinal tract, pancreas, liver, and lung.
5. Tumor-associated antigens are used clinically as **tumor markers for detection of tumors, monitoring of patient prognosis,** and **evaluation of treatment measure**s.

D. **ALTERED PERMEABILITY AND MEMBRANE TRANSPORT**

1. Transformed cells transport materials across the cell membrane at **higher rates** than normal cells.

VII. **BIOCHEMICAL DIFFERENCES BETWEEN NORMAL AND CANCER CELLS**

A. **CYCLIC AMP AND CYCLIC GMP**

1. **Cyclic adenosine monophosphate (cAMP)** participates in the regulation of a large number of intracellular biochemical reactions.
    a. cAMP **reduces the rate of division of some normal cells and some transformed cells** in culture.
    b. Because cAMP is critical in cell regulation, it is especially interesting to cancer researchers. It may prove to be a key to autonomous cell growth.
2. **Cyclic guanosine monophosphate (cGMP)** also restricts growth.

B. **NUTRIENTS**

1. In culture, cancer cells take up nutrients such as sugars and amino acids at rates that are greatly increased over those exhibited by untransformed cells of the same type.

C. **CHALONES**

1. Chalones are proteins that inhibit multiplication of normal cells in the skin, lung, liver, bone marrow, lymph nodes, kidney, and uterine lining.
2. Chalones are thought to be responsible for the fact that organs grow to only a certain size.
3. Cancer tissues have a **lower concentration** of chalones than do normal tissues.
    a. Cancer cells have a defect in their ability either to manufacture chalones or to respond to them.
    b. Chalones are found in low levels in cancer cells.

D. **GROWTH FACTORS**

1. In normal cells, growth factors produced by one cell type bind to membrane receptors on another cell type to **initiate a cascade of metabolic events leading to cell division.**
2. Malignant and transformed cells have been shown to have receptors for growth factors on their cell surfaces, as well as the ability to synthesize growth factors.
3. Cancer cells develop an independence from growth factors, probably as a result of release of autocrine growth factors as well as a lack of response to inhibitory controls.
4. **Epidermal growth factor (EGF)**
    a. EGF stimulates a wide variety of cell types and is involved in a variety of physiologic interactions unrelated to cell growth.
    b. It binds to specific receptors on the cell surface of most epithelial cells.
5. **Transforming growth factor-alpha (TGF-alpha)**
    a. TGF-alpha is produced by human tumor cells of diverse origin and binds to the same receptors as EGF.
6. **Transforming growth factor-beta (TGF-beta)**
    a. TGF-beta stimulates the growth of fibroblasts and inhibits the growth of a wide variety of cell types of mesenchymal, myeloid, epithelial, lymphoid, and endothelial origin.
7. **Platelet-derived growth factor (PDGF)**
    a. PDGF is a protein released into serum from blood platelets during the coagulation cascade, promoting growth, though its activity is limited to fibroblasts and smooth muscle cells of arteries.
8. **Basic fibroblast growth factors (bFGF)**
    a. bFGF is produced by both normal and malignant cells of mesodermal and neuroectodermal origin.
9. **Insulinlike growth factors (IGF) I and II**
    a. IGF-I and IGF-II have autocrine functions in human colon carcinoma, lung carcinoma, pancreatic carcinoma, and neuroblastoma cell lines.

VIII. **GENETIC DIFFERENCES BETWEEN NORMAL AND CANCER CELLS**

1. Most neoplasms arise from a single altered cell that acquires a heritable and selective growth advantage over other cells.
2. The initial change in the cell is the alteration of a regulatory gene by a carcinogen that provides the cell with a growth advantage.
    a. As the cell divides and produces offspring, each daughter cell inherits the genetic defect that provides it with the capacity to invade, metastasize, grow without regard to inhibitory growth controls, lose responsiveness to hormones, and so on.
3. Tumor cells are genetically unstable compared to normal cells.
4. Tumor progression results from additional mutations in cells within the clone, involving either growth-regulatory genes or genes responsible for other characteristics of the tumor cells.

PRACTICE QUESTIONS

1. Problems arise when experimental transformed cell models are applied to human cancer because
    (A) transformed cells do not have features identical to those of cancer cells.
    (B) transformed cell lines are characterized by uncontrolled growth and immortality.
    (C) human cancers evolve because of exposure to chemical, viral, or radiation carcinogens.
    (D) there are too many human cancers to develop transformed cell lines.

2. The phenomenon of normal cell division ceasing upon achievement of a monolayer across a petri dish or vessel is called
    (A) density-dependent growth.
    (B) senescence.
    (C) cell-cell growth.
    (D) prototype development.

3. The "decision" of the cell whether to enter G_0 (the resting state) or to continue in G_1 occurs at a point in G_1 called the
    (A)   anchorage-dependent growth phase.
    (B)   restriction point.
    (C)   contact inhibition point.
    (D)   differentiation point.

4. What is the name given to transformed cells that have variable sizes and shapes because of unpolymerized proteins?
    (A)   transforming growth factors
    (B)   hyperchromaticism
    (C)   pleomorphism
    (D)   unequal segregation

5. Which of the following statements about cell differentiation is true?
    (A)   Cancer cells are more differentiated than normal cells.
    (B)   Cancer cells are less differentiated than normal cells.
    (C)   Cancer cells are completely undifferentiated.
    (D)   Cancer cells are at the same level of differentiation as the tissues from which they arise.

6. Fibronectin is a glycoprotein found on the surface of normal cells and in low levels on cancer cells. Which of the following is one of its numerous functions in normal cells?
    (A)   It provides constant sources of nutrients.
    (B)   It inhibits cell responsiveness to growth factors.
    (C)   It promotes cell-to-cell adhesion.
    (D)   It degrades attachment proteins.

7. A tumor-specific antigen that can be assayed for some cancers and is normally found only on embryonic cells is
    (A)   human chorionic gonadotropin.
    (B)   alpha-fetoprotein.
    (C)   testosterone.
    (D)   estrogen.

8. The proteins that inhibit multiplication of normal cells in certain organs of the body, are responsible for the fact that organs grow to only a certain size, and are in lower concentrations in cancer tissues are
    (A)   cyclic guanosine monophosphate.
    (B)   basic fibroblast growth factor.
    (C)   suppressor oncogenes.
    (D)   chalones.

ANSWER EXPLANATIONS

1. **The answer is (A).**   For the cancer cell prototype, normal cells derived from normal tissue are established in culture under controlled conditions. These cells can be transformed into cells that behave like malignant cells when they are exposed to chemical, viral, or radiation carcinogens. Not all transformed cell lines exhibit all the characteristics generally found in transformed cells. Two factors—uncontrolled growth and immortality—are observed in all cancer cells. While transformed cells provide the best model for studying the differences between normal and malignant cells, the model is not a perfect duplication of what actually occurs in a human being. (48–49)

2. **The answer is (A).**   Density-dependent growth refers to a monolayer of cell growth in a vessel or culture that ceases growing upon achievement of the monolayer. Recent experiments have shown that when cells crowd each other, their access to nutrients necessary for cell division is inhibited. This phenomenon may explain why normal cells stop dividing when a contained area is filled with a monolayer of cells. (49)

3. **The answer is (B).**   The cell's decision whether to enter G_0 or to continue in G_1 occurs at a point in G_1 called the restriction point. Once the cell passes this point, it must continue through all phases of the cell cycle and return to G_1. (50–51)

4. **The answer is (C).**   Normal cells have a well-organized and extensive cytoskeleton made up of bundles of microfilaments and microtubules. These bundles consist of polymerized subunits of proteins that provide the structure and shape of the cell. Transformed cells contain the subunits of proteins, but the proteins are not polymerized, which causes transformed cells to have variable sizes and shapes, a condition known as pleomorphism. (51)

5. **The answer is (B).**   As the human organism develops, cells become different and specialized for various structural and functional purposes. This process is called differentiation. Cancer cells may arise at any point during differentiation. Cancer cells tend to be less differentiated than cells from surrounding normal tissue, and some cancer cells are so poorly differentiated (anaplastic) that the tissue of origin cannot be identified. (52)

6. **The answer is (C).**   Fibronectin is a large glycoprotein found on normal cell surfaces. Together with various proteoglycans, collagen, and elastin, fibronectin forms the matrix in which cells are embedded and that anchors cells in place within tissues.

7. **The answer is (B).**   Alpha-fetoprotein (AFP) is an oncofetal antigen normally found on embryonic cells that are re-expressed on certain tumors. AFP can be found in liver cancers and in some testicular, pancreatic, and gastrointestinal tract tumors. (54)

8. **The answer is (D).**   Chalones are proteins that inhibit multiplication of normal cells in the skin, liver, lung, bone marrow, lymph nodes, kidney, and uterine lining. The chalones are synthesized by the cells in the specific tissue, and inhibition of mitosis is tissue-specific. Chalones are thought to be responsible for the fact that organs grow to only a certain size. Cancer tissues have a lower concentration of chalones than do normal tissues. Cancer cells have a defect in their ability either to manufacture chalones or to respond to them. (54)

4 Invasion and Metastasis

STUDY OUTLINE

I. **THE CLINICAL PROBLEM OF METASTASIS**

1. Metastasis is the most frequent cause of cancer treatment failure.
2. Sixty percent of individuals with solid tumors have metastasis (microscopic or gross) at the time of diagnosis.

II. **FACTORS CONTRIBUTING TO METASTATIC POTENTIAL**

1. **Less than 0.01%** of cells in a primary tumor ultimately are able to initiate a successful metastatic deposit.
2. For invasion and metastasis to occur, an **imbalance in the regulation of motility and proteolysis** is required, in addition to **loss of growth control.**
   a. At every stage of the metastatic process, cancer cells must avoid host immune mechanisms.
   b. **Angiogenesis** is required for expansion of the primary tumor, as well as for establishment of a metastatic colony.

A. **TUMOR CELL FACTORS**

1. **Oncogenes**
   a. Progression of tumors from benign to malignant is exemplified by structural alterations in genes and by changes in gene expression that cause proteins to function abnormally, inappropriately, or at improper concentrations, resulting in circumvention of normal controls that regulate cell division and differentiation.
   b. **Suppressor genes** have been identified that normally suppress tumor growth and proliferation.
      (1) These suppressor genes have been shown to be underexpressed in certain types of cancers.
   c. **Transfection** of certain oncogenes into an appropriate recipient cell can induce the complete phenotype of invasion and metastasis, although much research remains to be done to link specific oncogenes and suppressor genes with the metastatic state.
   d. The specific family of genes necessary for metastasis appears to be different for each histologic type of tumor.
   e. Aberrant gene expression and genetic alterations of the *ras* and *myc* gene families have been shown to be important in the progression of human cancers and may be useful as prognostic indicators.
2. **Heterogeneity**
   a. Tumor cells are **heterogeneous** within a tumor, among different cancers of different histologic origin, and among tumors of the same histologic origin but in different individuals.
   b. Not all cells of the primary tumor are metastatic, and varying degrees of metastatic potential exist among the cells of a primary tumor.
   c. Recent research with genetic markers has shown that the **metastatic subpopulation of cells dominates the primary tumor mass** early in its growth.
      (1) A measure of the metastatic propensity of cells extrapolated from a sample of the primary tumor can be **correlated with clinical parameters** of metastasis and recurrence.

    d. Tumor cell heterogeneity explains why one person's tumor may disseminate at a very early stage of growth while another person's tumor of similar size and histologic appearance may continue to grow to a large size without metastasizing.

    e. If there is a 99.9% cell kill achieved with treatment of a 1-cm^3 lesion consisting of 1 billion cells, a significant number of nonresponsive cells will remain to continue growing and developing further diverse populations of cells.

  3. **Production of growth factors**

    a. Peptide growth factors are found in platelets, macrophages, and lymphocytes and are also produced by transformed cells (autocrine growth factors).

    b. Platelet-derived growth factor (PDGF) was the first peptide growth factor to be directly implicated in oncogenesis.

      (1) Peptides resembling PDGF have been found in many different types of cancer cells.

    c. Aberrant synthesis of growth factors by the tumor may be a source of signals that stimulate subpopulations of metastatic cells to proliferate and diversify.

    d. Some growth factors, such as fibroblast growth factors, may promote angiogenesis as well as tumor growth.

    e. Lack of response of tumor cells to inhibitory peptides potentiates these responses.

  4. **Production of angiogenic factors**

    a. Once a tumor has been initiated, any subsequent increase in tumor cell population must be preceded by an increase in new capillaries that converge on the tumor.

    b. The growth and development of new capillaries are initiated and supported by a group of peptide proteins called **angiogenic factors.**

  5. **Motility**

    a. Once tumor cells detach from the primary tumor, they must infiltrate into adjacent tissue and migrate through the vascular wall into the circulation and out again into the tissue at a secondary site.

    b. **Motility factors** produced by tumor cells and normal cells influence the tumor cells to move out into the surrounding host tissue.

  6. **Specific cell surface receptors**

    a. Cells express specific **cell surface receptors** that recognize a vast array of proteins, including extracellular matrix proteins.

    b. One family of cell surface receptors, the **integrins,** are the proteins that serve as receptors for fibronectin and other components of the extracellular matrix.

      (1) This process is altered in malignant cells.

    c. Other receptors for proteins, such as fibronectin, collagen type I, and vitronectin, may also play a role in **tumor cell invasion** and **migration.**

  7. **Invasiveness**

    a. Metastasizing tumor cells meet a variety of host connective tissue barriers as they make their way through various tissue compartments.

    b. Through a series of complex biochemical interactions, tumor cells have the ability to **penetrate epithelial basement membranes** and enter the underlying interstitial stroma, where they gain access to lymphatics and blood vessels for further dissemination.

B. HOST FACTORS

  1. **Deficient immune response**

    a. Throughout the metastatic sequence, tumor cells are subject to attack by the host immune system.

    b. It is thought that some defect in the immune system—in its components or its functioning—may contribute to the development of cancer and metastases.

  2. **Intact hemostatic system**

    a. Normal platelet function is required for tumor cell metastasis, and platelets play a central role in the metastatic process, though their exact role is unknown.

      (1) During metastasis, tumor cells enter the circulation and come in contact with platelets.

      (2) Thus it may be that platelets **secrete proteins** that encourage tumor cell adhesion to vessel walls and subsequent destruction of the basement membrane.

    b. Some studies have shown that tumor cells directly **activate** platelets.

    c. Research has shown that **antiplatelet drugs greatly inhibit experimentally induced cell metastases** in mice.

    d.   Studies have shown that the platelet-secreted protein **thrombospondin** potentiates tumor cell metastasis by encouraging tumor cell adhesion to vessel walls.

    3.   **Favorable target organ environment**

        a.   **Secondary tumor growth** in certain organs is a result of a favorable environment afforded by such tissues.

        b.   Such tissues exert **growth-promoting or growth-inhibiting effects on cancer cells** that make the microenvironment within certain organs more or less conducive to neoplastic growth than the microenvironment in other tissues.

III.   THE METASTATIC SEQUENCE

    1.   Metastasis is a series of **sequential but interwoven steps** involving complex interactions between tumor cell and host and ending in the establishment of one or more secondary tumors at a site apart from the primary tumor.

    2.   **The six steps of metastasis:**

        a.   Tumor growth and neovascularization.

        b.   Tumor cell invasion of the basement membrane and other extracellular matrices.

        c.   Detachment and embolism of tumor cell aggregates.

        d.   Arrest in distant organ capillary beds.

        e.   Extravasation.

        f.   Proliferation within the organ parenchyma.

A.   TUMOR NEOVASCULARIZATION AND GROWTH

    1.   **Neovascularization**

        a.   Cancer originates from the genetic transformation of a single target cell and requires subsequent alterations in the cellular DNA to initiate a series of processes that lead to **autonomy from normal growth regulatory mechanisms, uncontrolled proliferation,** and **growth advantages over adjacent host tissues.**

        b.   Tumor cells are capable of releasing angiogenic factors that stimulate growth of new blood vessels **(angiogenesis),** establishing a capillary network from the surrounding host tissue.

        c.   The onset of angiogenic activity precedes tumor formation and correlates with the transition from hyperplasia to neoplasia.

        d.   Angiogenesis is an invasive process that represents a sequence of events performed by vascular endothelial cells in response to angiogenic stimuli.

            (1)   The same sequence of events takes place whether the angiogenic stimulus is physiological, immunological, or tumor-derived.

        e.   New capillaries arise from **preexisting capillaries** or venules, never from arteries, arterioles, or veins.

        f.   At the onset of tumor angiogenesis, **local shedding of cancer cells into the tumor venous drainage** can begin.

    2.   **Tumor growth**

        a.   As a tumor grows, necrotic areas of the tumor release **chemotactic products** that attract host cells and cellular enzymes that help degrade surrounding structures, alter immune responses, and in general contribute to the emergence of specialized tumor cells capable of surviving in a hostile growth environment.

        b.   The ability of cancer cells to **break away** and **establish secondary sites** perpetuates the neoplastic continuum.

        c.   Tumor invasion and metastasis involve some cellular functions that are quite **distinct** from those involved in tumor growth.

B.   INVASION OF THE BASEMENT MEMBRANE AND OTHER EXTRACELLULAR MATRICES

    1.   Metastasis begins with local invasion of the surrounding host tissue by cells from the primary tumor.

    2.   **Destruction of the basement membrane** is a critical element at this stage in the sequence of metastasis, as well as at later points in the sequence.

    3.   Type IV collagen and laminin are the most important structural components of the basement membrane because they are the main components of the basement membrane and are found only in basement membrane.

4. A number of distinct changes occur in the organization, distribution, and quantity of the epithelial basement membrane during the transition from benign to invasive carcinoma.
   a. The basement membranes of invasive tumors are lost uniformly because they are actively dissolved by the **proteolytic enzymes** secreted by and/or potentiated by the invading tumor cells.
   b. The loss of basement membranes in human cancers significantly correlates with an increased incidence of metastasis and with poor 5-year survival.
   c. Proteolytic enzymes have been implicated in the loss of basement membrane associated with tumor invasion.
      (1) These proteolytic enzymes **overcome natural protease inhibitors,** such as the tissue inhibitors of metalloproteinases, or plasminogen activator inhibitors.
      (2) Synthesis and secretion of proteolytic enzymes and their inhibitors are **regulated by growth factors and cytokines.**
   d. The process of invasion and penetration of basement membranes has been described in terms of three distinct biochemical events: **attachment, degradation of the basement membrane,** and **locomotion.**
5. **Attachment**
   a. Invasive tumor cells possess specific cell surface receptors that facilitate their attachment to vascular basement membrane.
   b. Since invasive tumors have lost their basement membrane, cell surface receptors are exposed, facilitating their attachment to vascular basement membrane.
   c. **Laminin** has been shown to potentiate tumor cell metastasis by increasing cell adhesion to the capillary wall.
6. **Degradation**
   a. Once attached to laminin or type IV collagen, the tumor cell either secretes or causes the secretion by the host of proteases and other hydrolytic enzymes such as type IV collagenase that mediate penetration of the basement membrane by the tumor cells.
   b. The interaction of monocytes and tumor cells produces growth factors, interleukins, interferons, and tumor necrosis factor-alpha for initiation of angiogenesis and invasion.
   c. The host responds to the invasive tumor by forming **a dense and hard fibrous reaction** called **desmoplasia,** which is responsible for the clinically appreciable hard lump that leads to presentation of many cancers.
7. **Locomotion**
   a. The third step in tumor cell invasion is movement by the tumor cell into the area of the matrix altered by proteolysis.
   b. Early movement of the tumor cell is by **pseudopodia protrusion.**
      (1) The stimulation for pseudopodia locomotion and the direction taken by the tumor cells may be **mediated by chemotactic factors released through cell degradation.**
      (2) Pseudopodia act as "sense organs" to determine which direction the cell should take, to physically move the cell, and to induce local matrix proteolysis to help the tumor cell penetrate the matrix.
   c. The direction of the tumor cells is influenced by host chemoattractants produced by the organ to which the tumor cell subsequently travels.

C. **DISSEMINATION**

1. **Direct extension**
   a. Rapid proliferation of cells within a circumscribed space will cause **pressure within the space,** forcing fingerlike projections of cells into nearby body cavities and tissues.
      (1) Local damage from the pressure of an expanding tumor can result in pain, bleeding, bone fractures, or loss of function—depending on the tissues involved and the extent of damage.
   b. Tumor cell invasion of serous cavities is often referred to as **"seeding"** and can result in ascites or pericardial and pleural effusions.
2. **Lymphatic dissemination**
   a. Tumor cells that enter the lymphatic system are transported passively from the site of detachment from the primary tumor to the first draining lymph node.
   b. A mass at the site of the regional lymph nodes draining a tumor may be the first clinical sign of metastasis.

3. **Hematogenous dissemination**
   a. Because of the numerous connections between the lymphatics and the vascular system, most tumor cells that enter the lymphatic system eventually find their way into the vascular system; thus **lymphatic metastasis and hematogenous metastasis are not separate and distinct processes.**
   b. Subsequent to their release into the circulation, tumor cells frequently **adhere** both to other tumor cells and to blood cells, especially platelets, helping to protect the tumor cell from circulating immune cells and to produce enlarged emboli that increase the likelihood that tumor cells will arrest in the target organ.

D. **ARREST**

1. It is estimated that 50%–60% of metastatic distribution can be predicted from the anatomic route followed by the disseminating tumor cell.
2. The site of arrest of metastatic cells in the parenchyma of organs seems to be selective and to depend on a match between the tumor and the organ.
3. Certain tumors have a predilection for metastasis to specific organs, independent of vascular anatomy, rate of bloodflow, or number of tumor cells delivered to each organ.
4. The distribution of metastases is probably determined by a combination of several mechanisms: selective target adhesion, selective and directed chemotaxis mediated by tissue-specific chemotactic factors, and response of metastatic cells to growth factors differentially expressed in different organs and tissues.

E. **EXTRAVASATION**

1. Once the tumor cell arrests in the capillary bed of the target organ, it must find its way to the organ parenchyma by extravasating through the capillary wall.
   a. **Degradative enzymes** produced by tumor cells break down the basement membrane of the capillary, allowing the tumor cell to penetrate through the capillary into the organ tissue.

F. **NEOVASCULARIZATION AND GROWTH OF METASTASIS**

1. As in the growth and development of the primary tumor, any increase in cell population in the metastatic deposit is dependent first on establishment of a blood supply.
2. The metastatic tumor accomplishes this by the process of angiogenesis in the same manner as did the primary tumor.
3. Subsequent proliferation of the tumor within the organ parenchyma completes the metastatic process.
   a. See **Figure 4-1, text page 64,** for visualization of the metastatic sequence.

IV. **ANTIMETASTASIS THERAPY**

1. Failure of any step in the metastatic cascade completely abrogates the metastatic continuum.
   a. It may appear that the **prevention of metastasis** lies in our ability to **interrupt** one or more steps in the metastatic cycle.
   b. "Prevention" presumes that metastasis has not yet occurred, and for most individuals with cancer, metastasis has already occurred by the time the tumor is first diagnosed.
2. The only real prevention of metastasis will be the total destruction of all tumor cells with adjuvant therapy.

A. **PREVENTION OF TUMOR INVASION**

1. **Tumor cell invasion occurs at least twice** during the metastatic cascade.
   a. It occurs first at the site of the **primary tumor,** when tumor cells invade the surrounding tissue, eventually penetrating blood and lymph vessels for their dissemination to distant sites.
   b. Invasion occurs a second time **after tumor cells arrest at distant sites** and extravasate from the blood vessels into the target organ parenchyma.
2. **Proteolytic enzymes** capable of degrading basement membranes or extracellular matrix molecules are key factors in the process of invasion.

B. **ANTIADHESIVE THERAPY**

1. Based on the premise that binding of malignant cells to the glycoproteins fibronectin and laminin in the basement membranes promotes their invasiveness, substances have been studied for their ability to **inhibit the interaction of fibronectin and laminin with specific tumor cell surface receptors.**

C. **MONOCLONAL ANTIBODIES**

1. Studies have shown a **diminished ability** of tumor cells to form metastases after the use of monoclonal antibodies, presumably because the antibodies bind to the tumor cell surface receptors for which they are specific, preventing the tumor cell from binding to and invading the basement membrane.
2. Antibodies to type IV collagenase may also serve as **markers for metastasis** of the tumor cell and may be useful in development of new **diagnostic procedures** for identifying occult metastases.
3. Monoclonal antibodies could **inhibit the uncontrolled proliferation** of malignant cells.
4. Antibodies may be developed to bring cytotoxic agents **directly to tumor cells** that express high levels of the receptor for which the antibody is specific.

D. **MODULATION OF TUMOR VASCULARIZATION**

1. Since growth and development of both the primary tumor and the metastatic deposit depend on the development of an adequate blood supply, it follows that **prevention of angiogenesis** would abrogate this process.

E. **ANTICOAGULATION THERAPY**

1. **Tumor cell aggregation with platelets** assists the tumor cells in their arrest and extravasation into distant organ parenchyma and helps protect them from immune cells as they disseminate throughout the circulatory system.
2. Research findings in this area:
    a. **Agents that inhibit platelet aggregation** decrease cancer metastasis in some experimental tumors.
    b. **Intravenous injection of intact tumor cells induces a decrease** in platelet count.
    c. **Emboli** containing fibrin, platelets, and tumor cells can be detected in the circulation shortly after release of tumor cells into the circulation.
3. Researchers have attempted to inhibit tumor metastasis experimentally by using **heparin** and its related compounds.

F. **GENETIC MANIPULATION**

1. An understanding of what genes regulate tumor cell growth and metastasis may provide important directions for treating cancer and for monitoring prognosis of cancer.

G. **BIOTHERAPEUTICS**

1. **Altering the microenvironment** in which the tumor thrives may deprive the tumor of the factors that stimulate and support its growth.
2. Therapies that **remove growth factors** from the vicinity of the tumor, or somehow block the receptors on tumor cells that stimulate cell division and diversification in response to growth factors, may inhibit tumor growth.
3. **Lymphokine activation of macrophages** leads to macrophage recognition and selective destruction of tumor cells.
    a. In addition, the adoptive transfer of lymphokine-activated immune effector cells (LAK) has shown therapeutic promise.
4. **Interferon** has been shown to enhance the expression of the class I major histocompatibility complex antigens and tumor-associated transplantation antigens, leading to enhanced tumor cell recognition and destruction by T-lymphocytes.

V.   **CLINICAL APPLICATION**

1.   Although research has shown that promise exists for therapies that interrupt the metastatic process, we unfortunately do not yet know enough about the specific biochemical processes in each step of the metastatic cascade to justify widespread use of such therapies.
2.   The fact that **most individuals with cancer have metastases at the time of initial diagnosis** makes prevention of metastasis a moot issue.
3.   Because of the problems of **tumor cell heterogeneity** and the **complexity** of the metastatic process, multiple antimetastatic agents used in combination with conventional cytotoxic therapies will be required for maximum clinical efficacy.
4.   Clinical challenges that the problem of cancer metastasis poses:
     a.   **Accurate identification of the metastatic potential** of a primary tumor.
     b.   **Diagnosis and localization of clinically silent micrometastases** at the time of initial diagnosis of cancer.
     c.   **Complete eradication of all tumor cells** in a heterogeneous tumor with primary tumor treatment.
     d.   **Selective eradication of metastases during treatment** of a primary tumor.
     e.   **Prevention** of invasion and metastasis.

PRACTICE QUESTIONS

1.   What percentage of individuals have metastatic disease at the time of diagnosis?
     (A)   10%
     (B)   30%–40%
     (C)   60%
     (D)   80%

2.   In order for metastasis to occur, a sequence of events takes place. The initial mechanism in the metastatic sequence is
     (A)   loss of control over growth.
     (B)   access to the circulatory system.
     (C)   the completion of differentiation.
     (D)   that motility factors become available.

3.   The role of oncogenes in the progression of tumors from benign to malignant is
     (A)   monitoring cell differentiation.
     (B)   providing nutrients to tumor cells.
     (C)   altering protein function.
     (D)   increasing tumor cell proliferation.

4.   The correct term for tumor cells' creation of capillaries and development of a circulatory system is
     (A)   proliferation.
     (B)   diversification.
     (C)   angiogenesis.
     (D)   intravasation.

5.   In order to enter underlying interstitial stroma and gain access to lymphatics and the bloodstream, tumor cells must first
     (A)   invade epithelial basement membranes.
     (B)   choose an organ to metastasize to.
     (C)   differentiate.
     (D)   enter the progression phase of metastasis.

6.   The three biochemical events describing the process of invasion and penetration by tumor cells during metastasis are
     (A)   attachment, degradation, and locomotion.
     (B)   division, differentiation, and motility.
     (C)   division, attachment, and locomotion.
     (D)   differentiation, attachment, and division.

7. What is the **most** common metastatic cause for clinical symptoms of pain, bleeding, and fractures?
    (A) circulatory support of tumor cells
    (B) tumor cell proliferation within confined spaces
    (C) tumor cell motility within the lymphatic system
    (D) differentiation of tumor cells similar to host tissue

8. Extension of tumor cells into serous cavities can result in clinical problems such as malignant effusions. The term commonly applied to tumor cells that break off and spread over the serous membrane is
    (A) attachment.
    (B) degradation.
    (C) seeding.
    (D) locomotion.

9. Which of the following block(s) basement membrane degradation?
    (A) proteolytic enzymes
    (B) protease inhibitors
    (C) laminin
    (D) glycoproteins

10. Cells of the immune system are capable of responding to tumor cells. Research utilizing immunomodulators is referred to as
    (A) chemotherapy.
    (B) alternative therapies.
    (C) clinical trials.
    (D) biotherapeutics.

ANSWER EXPLANATIONS

1. **The answer is (C).**   Although many tumors are now treated successfully by surgery alone or in combination with chemotherapy, radiotherapy, or immunotherapy, metastasis is the most frequent cause of cancer treatment failure. It is estimated that up to 60% of individuals with solid tumors have metastasis at the time of their initial diagnosis, even though many of the metastases are microscopic lesions that remain undetected until later in the individual's disease course. (59)

2. **The answer is (A).**   In order to understand the complicated process of metastasis, researchers have separated invasion and metastasis into a series of defined, sequential steps and have studied the cellular processes and interactions responsible for each step. In cancer, genetic changes result in an imbalance of growth regulation that leads to uncontrolled proliferation. Unrestrained growth does not by itself result in invasion and metastasis. In fact, tumorigenicity and metastasis have both overlapping and separate features. For invasion and metastasis to occur, an imbalance in the regulation of motility and proteolysis is required, in addition to loss of growth control. Loss of growth control is the initial mechanism in the metastatic sequence. (59)

3. **The answer is (C).**   Progression of tumors from benign to malignant is exemplified by structural alterations in genes and by changes in gene expression that cause proteins to function abnormally, inappropriately, or at improper concentrations, resulting in circumvention of normal controls that regulate cell division and differentiation. (59)

4. **The answer is (C).**   Once a tumor has been initiated, any subsequent increase in tumor cell population must be preceded by an increase in new capillaries that converge on the tumor. Angiogenesis is the production of capillaries and a circulatory system around tumor cells in order to provide necessary nutrients. The growth and development of these new capillaries are initiated and supported by a group of peptide proteins called angiogenic factors. (60–61)

5. **The answer is (A).**   Metastasizing tumor cells meet a variety of host connective tissue barriers as they make their way through various tissue compartments. Through a series of complex biochemical interactions, tumor cells have the ability to penetrate epithelial basement membrane and enter the underlying interstitial stroma, where they gain access to lymphatics and blood vessels for further dissemination. Invasion of epithelial basement membranes is the most critical step in tumor cells' gaining access to

interstitial stroma and host tissue parenchyma. This ability is also central to the basic mechanisms of cancer invasion and metastasis. (60)

6.   **The answer is (A).**   Metastasis begins with the local invasion of the surrounding host tissue by cells from the primary tumor. Destruction of the basement membrane is a critical element at this stage in the sequence of metastasis, as well as at later points in the sequence. The process of invasion and penetration of basement membranes has been described in terms of three distinct biochemical events: attachment, degradation of the basement membrane, and locomotion. (62)

7.   **The answer is (B).**   Rapid proliferation within a circumscribed space will cause pressure within the space, forcing finger-like projections of cells into nearby body cavities and tissues. Local damage from the pressure of the expanding tumor can result in bleeding, pain, bone fractures, and loss of function—depending on the tissues involved and the extent of damage. (63)

8.   **The answer is (B).**   When malignant cells invade a serous cavity such as the peritoneal, pleural, or pericardial spaces, tumor cells can break off and spread over the serous membranes. This tumor "seeding" in body cavities is a major clinical problem that may lead to ascites or to pericardial and pleural effusions. (63)

9.   **The answer is (B).**   Proteolytic enzymes capable of degrading basement membranes or extracellular matrix molecules are key factors in the process of invasion. Several in vivo and in vitro studies have documented that significant reduction in tumor metastasis can be achieved by systemic administration of protease inhibitors. (65)

10.   **The answer is (D).**   Biotherapeutics addresses the complex host-tumor interactions and offers what may be the most promising approach to the treatment of cancer. Altering the microenvironment in which the tumor thrives may deprive the tumor of the factors that stimulate and support its growth. (66)

5 Relation of the Immune System to Cancer

STUDY OUTLINE

I. **INTRODUCTION**

    1.   The immune system is capable of responding to the presence of malignant disease.

        a.   **The earliest evidence for this contention was based on the histopathologic presentation of tumors, many of which were highly infiltrated with round mononuclear cells.**

    2.   **The presence of tumor-associated antigens was demonstrated, and an inverse relationship between immune competence and the development of malignant disease was inferred.**

    3.   **Investigation in the 1970s and 1980s produced a substantial increase in knowledge and understanding both of the immune system and of neoplasia.**

        a.   **These separate bodies of information come together topically in the field of modern tumor immunology.**

II. **TUMOR-ASSOCIATED ANTIGENS**

    1.   Tumor cells are capable of provoking immune reactions in immunocompetent hosts because of the expression of different antigenic determinants on the surface of the malignant cells.

    2.   Researchers demonstrated that animals immunized with a chemically induced tumor could reject a subsequent graft of that tumor and the antigens responsible for the tumor. Rejections observed were referred to as tumor-specific transplantation antigens (TSTAs).

        a.   Tumors induced by oncogenic viruses also express TSTAs.

    3.   The antigens that can be identified on malignant cells in human antigens do not show the same specificity as do most of the TSTAs in animals.

    4.   The great majority of human antigens known today that are capable of provoking immune reactions against tumor tissue are called **tumor-associated differentiation antigens (TADs).**

        a.   These tumor-associated antigens are used clinically as **tumor markers for diagnostic purposes** and, in some cases, for cancer patient management by monitoring prognosis and response to therapy.

A. **NORMAL TISSUE ANTIGENS ASSOCIATED WITH DIFFERENTIATION**

    1.   The expression of normal cellular differentiation antigens by tumors permits a **definitive identification** of their tissue of origin, information that is often fundamental to selection of an appropriate treatment plan.

        a.   These antigens may include the production of a specific hormone, a specific enzyme, or a specific cell-surface protein.

        b.   One of the best examples of the use of a differentiation-associated antigen for cancer patient management is the application of monoclonal antibodies to lymphocyte markers for B- and T-lymphocytes, resulting in extensive reclassification of leukemias and lymphomas.

    2.   Many of the markers identified by monoclonal antibodies are called **cluster designations (CDs).**

        a.   A given CD number (such as CD3) represents a group of peptide markers of differentiation of a common subpopulation of B- or T-lymphocytes.

        b.   Since many B-cell tumors secrete immunoglobulin peptides or fragments into the circulation, levels of these proteins can be used to monitor total tumor burden and responsiveness to therapy.

B.   **VIRAL-ASSOCIATED ANTIGENS**

1. The **expression of antigens specified by either RNA or DNA** virus genetic material is common on many different animal and human tumors.
   a. **Immunization** with killed tumor cells induced by a particular virus can protect susceptible hosts against different tumors induced by the same virus, which suggests the existence of one or more common tumor-associated viral antigens.
2. A role for **viruses in the induction of certain tumors** in humans is suggested by histopathologic and epidemiologic evidence.
3. A **strong association** between the development of tumors and viral infections has been found in the following cases:
   a. Hepatitis B virus and hepatocellular carcinoma.
   b. Epstein-Barr virus and certain B-cell lymphomas.
   c. Human papillomaviruses and cervical carcinoma.
   d. HTLV-1 and acute T-cell leukemias.

C.   **ONCOFETAL ANTIGENS**

1. **Oncofetal antigens** are proteins that are present normally during fetal development but are then suppressed to low but still detectable levels in the adult.
2. These proteins are **expressed on tumor tissues** and reappear in the circulation of patients with malignant disease.
3. The most familiar examples of oncofetal antigens include the **carcinoembryonic antigen (CEA)** and **alpha-fetoprotein (AFP).**
   a. Increased levels of CEA in the circulation are associated with a variety of **epithelial tumors** (breast cancers, lung tumors, colorectal tumors).
   b. Increased levels of AFP in the circulation are associated with **hepatocellular carcinomas** and certain **germ cell tumors.**
4. Oncofetal antigen levels have been most useful in clinical situations as **markers** for following the development of tumors.

III.   **IMMUNOLOGIC REACTIONS AGAINST TUMOR CELLS**

A.   **T-LYMPHOCYTE RESPONSES**

1. Eighty percent of circulating lymphocytes are T-lymphocytes that originate in the bone marrow, migrate to the thymus, and differentiate into cells that express a complex polypeptide surface structure known as the **CD3 complex.**
   a. The antigenic specificity of the T-lymphocyte is also determined in the thymic environment and is reflected by the expression of antigen-specific receptors.
   b. The T-lymphocyte receptor is found in close association with the CD3 complex, which stabilizes the interaction between the receptor and its specific antigen.
2. T-lymphocyte receptors are capable of enormous diversity in antigen recognition.
3. Further **differentiation of T-cells** in the thymus leads to cells that express either the CD4 antigen or the CD8 antigen.
   a. CD4+ T-lymphocytes are the first T-lymphocytes to become activated when antigen (including tumor-associated antigen) is encountered.
   b. Their **principal role** is to function as helper/inducer T-lymphocytes responsible for activating and amplifying the production of other immune cells, including CD8+ T-lymphocytes.
4. The **class II molecules** (which are designated HLA-DR determinants in humans) expressed on antigen-presenting cells are encoded by the genes of the major histocompatibility complex (MHC).
   a. Thus, helper T-lymphocytes are said to be **MHC-restricted** in their ability to become activated by the need to recognize both specific antigen and "self" class II molecules on the surface of the antigen-presenting cell.
5. When a macrophage degrades an antigen such as a tumor cell, peptides from that tumor cell (tumor-associated antigens) become complexed with class II molecules and are then displayed on the macrophage surface.

a. The **helper/inducer T-lymphocytes** become activated when they engage both the tumor-associated antigen and the class II molecules on the surface of the antigen-presenting cells.
    b. If either of these recognition events is disturbed, T-lymphocyte activation is aborted.
6. The **principal outcome** of a successful activation event by the CD4+ T-lymphocytes is the production and secretion of numerous peptides that have potent biological effects and are known collectively as **lymphokines.**
    a. Lymphokines are largely responsible for immune cell **activation, proliferation,** and **regulation.**
7. One of the principal targets of the lymphokines made by activated CD4+ T-lymphocytes is the CD8+ T-lymphocyte.
    a. CD8+ T-lymphocytes can be further subdivided into functionally distinct cytolytic killer T-lymphocytes or immunoregulatory suppressor T-lymphocytes.
8. **Cytolytic or killer T-lymphocytes** can interact with tumor-associated antigens on the surface of antigen-presenting cells or directly with tumor-associated antigens on tumor cell surfaces and can secrete different cytolytic peptides that are capable of mediating tumor cell lysis.
9. Virtually all differentiated tissues in the body express **class I molecules.**
    a. It is the expression of class I molecules that **restricts** the tolerance of the immune system to "self."
    b. Tumor cells, being derived from self tissues, also express class I molecules.
10. In the presence of activated antigen-specific, CD8+ T-lymphocytes, tumor-associated antigens on the surface of tumor cells that express class I molecules are engaged by T-lymphocyte receptors and CD8 complexes, respectively, on the surface of activated cytolytic T-lymphocytes.
    a. The **outcome** of this interaction is the lysis of the tumor cell.
    b. If the expression of either the tumor-associated antigens or the class I molecules on the surface of tumor cells is abnormal, cytolytic T-lymphocyte function is impaired.
11. The other class of T-lymphocytes relevant to tumor immunology is the CD8+ suppressor T-lymphocyte.
    a. This class of T-lymphocyte functions to attenuate or suppress the development of immune cell activation.
12. Like the CD8+ cytolytic T-lymphocytes, the suppressor T-cells are **restricted by the need to recognize tumor-associated antigens together with class I molecules** and thus are **MHC-restricted.**
13. The antigens recognized by suppressor T-lymphocytes are thought to be different from those recognized by either the helper/inducer T-lymphocytes or the cytolytic T-cells.
14. When the suppressor T-lymphocytes recognize a different class of tumor-associated antigens on the surface of a tumor cell, the outcome of that event is **suppression of immune cell activation.**
15. Nonantigen-specific suppressor T-lymphocyte events are responsible for much of the immune deficiency seen in patients with cancer.

B. NATURAL KILLER CELLS

1. **Natural killer (NK)** cells are large granular lymphocytes that account for between 10% and 15% of the total circulating lymphocytes.
    a. NK cells are thought to represent a distinct lineage.
    b. The surface receptor glycoprotein CD16 allows NK cells to interact with IgG antibodies in a mechanism known as antibody-dependent cellular cytotoxicity.
    c. NK cells have azurophilic granules that contain esterase and other enzymes that participate in the cytolysis of target cells.
2. NK cells like cytolytic T-lymphocytes are capable of **lysing a broad range of tumor cells.**
    a. Unlike T-lymphocytes, NK cells do not require sensitization by prior exposure to tumor antigens to exert their cytolytic effects against tumor cells.
3. NK cells are capable of conjugating to tumor cells and lysing susceptible tumors within 4 hours after conjugation.
    a. If conjugation is disrupted after 30 minutes, the lysis of the tumor cells can still proceed normally, indicating that a "lethal hit" can be delivered by the NK cell during the first 30 minutes of target cell binding.
4. NK cells are **not MHC-restricted.**
5. NK cells are also active **secretors of lymphokines** with potent biological effects.
    a. They include **interleukin-1 (IL-1), IL-2, tumor necrosis factor-alpha, interferon-alpha,** and several different **hematopoietic colony stimulating factors.**

b.   These secretory products of NK cells can participate in **inhibiting the growth of some tumor cells directly** and also participate in **promoting and regulating the development of antitumor immunity by other cells.**

C.   LYMPHOKINE-ACTIVATED TUMOR CELL KILLING

1.   Incubation of mononuclear cells from the peripheral blood of healthy individuals with the lymphokine interleukin-2 (IL-2) elicits a **potent tumor-killing response** known as **lymphokine-activated killing (LAK).**
2.   The ability to **mediate** LAK function has been shown for both NK cells and T-cells.
3.   When purified NK cells are incubated with IL-2, the mechanism for their killing effect is identical to what is seen with normal NK-mediated cytolysis; however, the range of tumor target cells that can be killed is **increased** greatly.
4.   NK cells incubated in IL-2 can kill virtually all tumor cell lines.
5.   When purified T-lymphocytes are incubated with IL-2, the LAK exhibited differs from that of classic cytolytic T-lymphocytes in that the tumor-killing effects are **not restricted to MHC-matched tumor cells.**
     a.   This form of T-lymphocyte-mediated tumor killing **does not require prior exposure** to tumor antigens.

D.   MACROPHAGE-MEDIATED TUMOR CELL KILLING

1.   Of all the immune cells capable of participating in tumor immunity, cells of the mononuclear phagocyte series, generally known as macrophages, show the **greatest diversity** in effects.
2.   Of the more complex macrophage functions described, some of the most important for tumor immunology are the processes of **tumor antigen presentation, regulation of other immune cell types,** and the **capacity to destroy tumor cells.**
3.   The process of activating macrophages to the point where they can kill tumor cells depends upon lymphokines.
     a.   When macrophages are incubated with **interferon-gamma,** they undergo a complex series of biochemical changes that culminates in the ability of the macrophages to destroy a wide variety of tumor cells.
4.   Tumoricidal macrophages are extremely **specific for tumor cells,** and normal tissues are not affected.
5.   Macrophage-mediated tumor cell killing is not restricted to MHC-matched tumor cells.
6.   Following tumor cell conjugation, the destruction of the target tumor cells occurs via secretion of various effector molecules from the macrophages into the tumor cells.
7.   A number of discrete effector molecules have been isolated from activated macrophages that mediate the cytotoxic effects on tumor cells.
     a.   **Cytotoxic factor (CF),** a neutral serine protease, is extremely potent against susceptible tumor cells.
     b.   **Tumor necrosis factor-alpha (TNF-alpha)** is isolated from activated macrophages with the capacity to mediate tumor killing.
8.   Activated macrophages have a remarkable capacity to **mediate** tumor cell cytostasis events.
9.   Activated macrophages often induce cytostasis in neoplastic cells prior to tumor cell death.
     a.   This can come about through the macrophages causing tumor cells to undergo a **"reductive division"** wherein the tumor cell continues to divide in the absence of DNA synthesis, ultimately resulting in cell death.
     b.   Lymphokines are needed to activate macrophages to the point where they can kill.
     c.   Tumoricidal macrophages are tumor-cell-specific, and normal tissues are not affected.

E.   ANTIBODY-DEPENDENT TUMOR CELL CYTOTOXICITY

1.   Tumor cells, like most nucleated mammalian cells, are relatively resistant to complement-dependent cellular cytotoxicity.
2.   The exquisite recognition capabilities of antibodies facilitate tumor cell destruction in collaboration with different immune effector cells.
     a.   This sort of mechanism is referred to generally as **antibody-dependent cellular cytotoxicity** and is mediated almost exclusively by antibodies of the IgG class.

3. Both NK cells and macrophages have the capacity to interact with IgG antibody-coated tumor cells, leading to tumor cell lysis.
4. The ability of antibodies coated on tumor cell surfaces to increase tumor cell lysis in collaboration with NK cells or macrophages is based on two factors.
   a. Antibodies on tumor cells increase the possibility of binding between immune cell and tumor cell and the affinity of this interaction.
      (1) The range of tumor cells that can be recognized by NK cells or macrophages is increased when antitumor antibodies are present and the interaction between the cells is stabilized.
   b. The binding of the Fc portion of antibodies to the receptors on NK cells or macrophages provides an activation signal to these immune effector cells.
      (1) This activation signal leads to increased killing function on the part of the immune cells in a manner analogous to the action of lymphokines on NK cells or macrophages.

IV. HOW TUMOR CELLS EVADE THE IMMUNE SYSTEM

1. The outcome of the neoplastic process is determined, at least in part, by the balance between the capacity of the immune system to destroy tumor cells and the capacity of tumor cells to evade immune-mediated destruction.
   a. Support for this idea in humans comes from epidemiological studies that demonstrate a strong correlation between **age, immune competence,** and **cancer incidence.**
   b. Immune deficiency resulting from genetic predisposition or acquired as a result of drug treatment or viral infection is associated with an increased incidence of malignancy.
2. It is also clear that tumors do arise in immunocompetent individuals and that immune stimulation that leads to significantly increased antitumor immunity is not sufficient to destroy the vast majority of spontaneous tumors in humans.
3. Tumor cell escape from immunological destruction is a **fundamental property of most human malignant diseases.**

A. MECHANISMS THAT DISTORT TUMOR CELL RECOGNITION

1. Tumor cells evade recognition in two ways:
   a. Tumor cell antigenic modulation includes both the loss of membrane-associated tumor antigens and the modulation of membrane-associated antigenic structures.
      (1) Tumor-associated antigen loss on tumor cells is thought to come about as a result of increased membrane biosynthesis and turnover by tumor cells, producing a relatively unstable membrane on many tumor cells and often resulting in membrane proteins being shed from tumor cell surfaces into the circulation.
   b. Tumor cell recognition can also be distorted by factors that sterically **block or mask tumor-associated antigens.**
      (1) Such **"blocking factors"** inhibit the ability of sensitized immune effector cells to recognize and conjugate to tumor cell surfaces.
      (2) The most important blocking factors are **antibodies.**

B. MECHANISMS THAT SUPPRESS ANTITUMOR IMMUNITY

1. The other way in which tumors escape immunological destruction is by **suppression of antitumor immunity.**
2. Suppression of antitumor immunity appears to come about through two principal mechanisms.
   a. The **secretion of suppressor factors from tumors.**
   b. The **hyperactivation of suppressor T-cells** and **suppressor macrophages during progressive tumor growth.**
3. The activation of suppressor T-cells by tumors is thought to reflect immunological responses to **"suppressogenic"** epitopes on tumors.
   a. There is no convincing evidence for the existence of suppressogenic epitopes on human tumors as yet.
   b. But there is an extensive literature that demonstrates that suppressor T-cells are activated during the course of tumor growth in humans.

4. **Suppressor macrophages** have also been shown to be hyperactivated during progressive tumor growth in animal systems and in humans.

   a. The principal way in which cancer is thought to affect macrophages suppressor function is by altering macrophages cellular arachidonic acid (AA) metabolism.

V. **THE IMPORTANCE OF THE IMMUNE SYSTEM FOR SPECIFIC ASPECTS OF NEOPLASIA**

   A. **THE ROLE OF THE IMMUNE RESPONSE IN CARCINOGENESIS**

   1. **Initiation**
      a. The **initiation phase of carcinogenesis** requires the production of a mutation in the genetic material of a cell, resulting in a permanent alteration of the cell's growth characteristics.
      b. The mutation(s) in question must be **nonlethal,** must be **heritable from generation to generation of cells,** and must **confer on the cell the characteristics of malignant cell growth.**
   2. **Promotion**
      a. Neoplastic **cell promotion** represents the phase of the carcinogenic process in which initiated clones of cells become adapted to a particular microenvironment, producing a malignantly transformed clone of cells capable of growing in that microenvironment.
      b. The outcome of the promotion event is the production of a malignant tumor.
      c. Most promoting agents are known to affect the immune system and to suppress natural immunity to varying degrees.
      d. The antitumor immune functions of large granular lymphocytes (NK cells and LAK cells) and macrophages during the promotion phase of the carcinogenic event are most responsible for any immune surveillance against developing cancers.
   3. **Progression**
      a. The final phase of the neoplastic process is the progression phase.
      b. In the **progression phase** a tumor that arose during the promotion phase behaves in a malignant, uncontrolled fashion.
      c. The progression phase includes the **expansion of the tumor as well as the spread** of this tumor by different means.
      d. During the progression phase, the potential for further modification of the tumor cell's biologic characteristics as a result of immunostimulation or immunosuppression is great.
      e. By **modifying the existing host environment** with antineoplastic therapies, progression may be modulated.
      f. Thus, the progression phase of malignant disease can be greatly influenced by immune reactions, but this influence can be both positive or negative.

   B. **THE ROLE OF THE IMMUNE SYSTEM IN METASTASIS**

   1. The metastatic process is the most significant biologic behavior of most malignant tumors since it is **metastasis that kills the host** in the overwhelming majority of instances.
   2. **Invasion of vessels**
      a. In metastatic tumors, invasion comes about through a combination of (1) increased tissue pressure exerted by local tumor growth and (2) the production of different degradative enzymes, produced both by tumors and by inflammatory cells of the immune system.
      b. Inflammatory macrophages that are activated in response to local tumor growth produce enzymes such as collagenase, hyaluronidase, and cathepsin B that participate in the destruction of vessel barriers.
   3. **Arrest from circulation**
      a. The question of **tumor cell survival within the circulatory environment** is not insignificant since cells in the circulation are subjected to shear forces that are exerted by the passage of different cells within the rapidly moving bloodstream and are capable of disrupting tumor cell membranes.
      b. To facilitate survival within these fluids and to facilitate trapping in capillary beds at distant sites, tumor cells have the capacity to form emboli in collaboration with platelets, polymorphonuclear leukocytes, and macrophages.

4. **Intravasation to the tissues**
   a. Intravasation through the capillaries needs to occur by **direct intravasation through thin-walled capillaries** or by the **production of enzymes that cleave the proteoglycans of basement membranes.**

VI. IMMUNODEFICIENCY IN CANCER

1. In general, there is a hierarchy of immune deficiency development with advancing stage of disease.
   a. The first sort of immunological function to be eliminated, often very early in the tumor's development, is the **capacity to develop T-cell immunity to a novel antigen.**
   b. The next form of immune function that is eliminated with advancing disease is the **capacity to develop a primary antibody response against novel antigens.**
      (1) This is followed by the **loss of memory antibody synthesis.**
   c. The last immunological function that is eliminated—generally only in patients with widespread disseminated disease—is recall T-cell immunity to ubiquitous environmental fungal or mycobacterial pathogens.
2. The investigation of immune competence in individuals with cancer can also be used to gauge the results of attempted definitive therapy.
3. When groups of patients are analyzed statistically, immune deficiency is found to **correlate with both the clinical stage of disease** and the **histopathological tumor cell grade.**
4. The most **common patterns of immunological deficiency** that have been associated with tumor stage and grade include the following:
   a. Decreased lymphocyte counts in association with relative monocytosis.
   b. Decreased inflammatory cell chemotaxis.
   c. Decreased antigen processing and presentation.
   d. Decreased proliferative responses to antigen and nonspecific stimulants.
   e. Decreased NK function.
   f. Decreased helper and cytotoxic T-cell function.
   g. Increased suppressor T-cell function.
   h. Variable macrophage-mediated cytotoxicity.
   i. Increased macrophage suppressor function.
   j. Variable effects on cytokine synthesis.
5. It has also become apparent that the response of patients to cytotoxic chemotherapy may be influenced by immune deficiency.
6. The capacity of individuals to respond to different immunotherapeutic manipulations such as the interferons, interleukin-2, monoclonal antibodies, and tumor cell vaccines is directly influenced by the level of immune competence in the patient.

VII. PATTERNS OF ANTITUMOR IMMUNITY AND CLINICAL COURSE

1. Apart from the changes in general immunocompetence that have been observed in individuals with cancer, recent studies have also addressed the relationship between the presence or absence of specific antitumor immunity and the clinical course of the disease.

VIII. CRITICAL ISSUES FOR THE FUTURE OF TUMOR IMMUNOLOGY

1. A wide array of immunological functions will continue to be assessed in diverse oncologic settings, and the results of these investigations will be used to guide the development of therapies aimed at stimulating specific kinds of immune function in cancer patients.
2. Recent studies in individuals with cancer have focused on **extending immunologic investigations into microenvironments** that are more intimately associated with tumor tissues than the peripheral blood, and these studies need to be continued.
3. Since numerous studies have demonstrated that different immunologic reactions actually facilitate tumor growth and progression, it is imperative to define **which immunological reactions are most beneficial,** and **which are least beneficial or even undesirable,** for specific clinical cancer settings.

PRACTICE QUESTIONS

1. Tumor cells are capable of provoking immune reactions because of _____ on the surface of the malignant cells. Fill in the blank.
    (A) antibodies
    (B) hormones
    (C) immunomodulators
    (D) antigens

2. A strong association between the development of tumors and viral infections has been established with certain diseases. Which of the following matches is a correct association?
    (A) human papillomaviruses and breast cancer
    (B) Epstein-Barr virus and Burkitt's lymphoma
    (C) hepatitis B virus and renal cell carcinoma
    (D) HTLV-1 and nasopharyngeal cancer

3. Alpha-fetoprotein (AFP) and carcinoembryonic antigen (CEA) are examples of antigens that are normally found on embryonic cells and are re-expressed on certain tumors. What is the term applied to these antigens?
    (A) oncofetal antigens
    (B) tumor-specific transplantation antigens
    (C) surface antigens
    (D) tumor-associated differentiation antigens

4. T-lymphocytes differentiate into cells expressing complex structures that become activated when antigens are encountered. The antigenic specificity of the T-lymphocyte is determined in the
    (A) thymus.
    (B) bone marrow.
    (C) peripheral blood.
    (D) spleen.

5. Lack of immune competence combined with what other variable is associated with the increased incidence of cancer development?
    (A) sex
    (B) age
    (C) race
    (D) health history

6. Which of the following are produced and secreted after successful activation by CD4+ T-lymphocytes and collectively are largely responsible for immune cell activation, proliferation, and regulation?
    (A) lymphokines
    (B) CD3 complexes
    (C) macrophages
    (D) tumor-specific antigens

7. Choose two effector molecules that mediate cytotoxic effects of macrophages on tumor cells.
    (A) lymphokine-activated killer cells and tumor necrosis factor-alpha
    (B) natural killer cells and lymphokine-activated killer cells
    (C) cytotoxic factor and tumor necrosis factor-alpha
    (D) interleukin-2 and lymphokine-activated killer cells

8. "Blocking factors" that restrict the ability of sensitized immune effector cells to identify and conjugate to tumor cell surfaces represent one mechanism that
    (A) suppresses tumor cell proliferation.
    (B) distorts tumor cell recognition.
    (C) enhances CD4+ T-lymphocyte activity.
    (D) destroys tumor cells.

9. Which phase of the carcinogenic process is represented by clones of cells adapting to a particular microenvironment and producing a malignantly transformed clone of cells capable of growing in that microenvironment?
    (A) initiation
    (B) promotion
    (C) progression
    (D) proliferation

10. A fundamental property that distinguishes most malignant cells from most benign cells is the ability of the malignant cells to
    (A) survive without nutrition.
    (B) proliferate into large numbers of cells.
    (C) develop collateral circulation.
    (D) metastasize.

ANSWER EXPLANATIONS

1. **The answer is (D).**   Tumor cells are capable of provoking immune reactions in immunocompetent hosts because of the expression of different antigenic determinants on the surface of the malignant cells. Antigens facilitate identification of tumor types and serve as markers. The great majority of human antigens known today that are capable of provoking immune reactions against tumor tissue are called tumor-associated differentiation antigens. (71)

2. **The answer is (B).**   A role for viruses in the induction of certain tumors in humans is suggested by histopathologic and epidemiologic evidence. The existence of tumor-associated viral antigens in humans does not directly implicate that virus in the development of a particular malignant disease. The genetic mechanism(s) by which viruses can induce tumors in humans are poorly understood, and the effects produced by a virus can be either direct or indirect. (72)

3. **The answer is (A).**   Oncofetal antigens are proteins that are present normally during fetal development but are then suppressed to low but still detectable levels in the adult. These proteins are expressed on tumor tissues and reappear in the circulation of patients with malignant disease. CEA is a glycoprotein expressed in adults at low levels by tissues of the GI tract; AFP is an alpha-globulin that is similar in structure and function to albumin and is expressed at low levels primarily in the liver. Increased levels of CEA in the circulation are associated with a variety of epithelial tumors, and increased levels of AFP in the circulation are associated with hepatocellular carcinomas and certain germ cell tumors. (72)

4. **The answer is (A).**   T-lymphocytes are derived from bone marrow lymphocyte progenitors that migrate to the thymus and differentiate into cells that express a complex polypeptide surface structure known as the CD3 complex. The antigenic specificity of the T-lymphocyte is also determined in the thymic environment and is reflected by the expression of antigen-specific receptors. (73)

5. **The answer is (B).**   Epidemiologic studies have demonstrated a strong correlation between age, immune competence, and cancer incidence. Tumor cell escape from immunological destruction is a fundamental property of most human malignant diseases. (75–76)

6. **The answer is (A).**   The principal outcome of a successful activation event by the CD4+ T-lymphocytes is the production and secretion of numerous peptides that have potent biological effects and are known collectively as lymphokines. One of the principal targets of the lymphokines made by activated CD4+ T-lymphocytes is the CD8+ T-lymphocyte, which can be further subdivided into functionally distinct cytolytic killer T-lymphocytes and immunoregulatory suppressor T-lymphocytes. (73)

7. **The answer is (C).**   A number of discrete effector molecules have been isolated from activated macrophages that mediate the cytotoxic effects on tumor cells. Cytotoxic factor is a neutral serine protease and is extremely potent against susceptible tumor cells. Tumor necrosis factor-alpha is isolated from activated macrophages with the capacity to mediate tumor killing. (75)

8.   **The answer is (B).**   Tumor cell recognition can be distorted by factors that sterically block or mask tumor-associated antigens. Such "blocking factors" hinder the efforts of sensitized immune effector cells to recognize and conjugate to tumor cell surfaces. The most important blocking factors are antibodies. Thus, antibodies can play opposing roles in tumor cell recognition, either facilitating recognition and destruction by immune cells or aborting such recognition. (76)

9.   **The answer is (B).**   The initiation phase of carcinogenesis requires the production of a mutation in the genetic material of a cell, resulting in a permanent alteration of the cell's growth characteristics. Neoplastic cell promotion represents the phase of the carcinogenic process in which initiated clones of cells become adapted to a particular microenvironment, producing a malignantly transformed clone of cells capable of growing in that environment. The final phase of the neoplastic process is the progression phase, in which a tumor that arose during the promotion phase behaves in a malignant, uncontrolled fashion. (77)

10.   **The answer is (D).**   The metastatic process is the most significant biologic behavior of most malignant tumors, because in the overwhelming majority of instances it is metastasis that kills the host. (78)

6   Factors Affecting Health Behavior

STUDY OUTLINE

I.   INTRODUCTION

1.   Promotion of positive health behavior is an important aspect of cancer care since personal choices with regard to diet, tobacco use, alcohol consumption, and sun exposure affect the prevention of cancer.

II. NATIONAL INITIATIVES

1.   Influencing people's health behaviors is a major initiative of the American Cancer Society (ACS), the National Cancer Institute (NCI), and the U.S. Department of Health and Human Services.
     a.   The NCI's goal is to **reduce cancer mortality by 50%** by the year 2000.

III. DEFINITIONS

A.   HEALTH BEHAVIOR

1.   **Health behavior** involves personal habits, beliefs, characteristics, motives, values, and perceptions that influence what people do or don't do to improve, maintain, or restore health.
2.   **Health protective behavior** consists of actions taken by people to protect, promote, or maintain their health.
3.   **Health promotion** is not disease-specific avoidance behavior but rather is active behavior directed toward increasing a person's well-being.

B.   ILLNESS BEHAVIOR

1.   Illness behavior is **"any activity undertaken by a person who feels ill, to define the state of his health and to discover a suitable remedy."**
2.   Illness behaviors are undertaken to understand and explain the meaning of signs and symptoms.

C.   SICK ROLE BEHAVIOR

1.   Sick role behavior consists of actions taken to get well once individuals believe they are ill. It usually involves acceptance of treatment.

D.   See **Figure 6-1, text page 89,** for various types of health behaviors and their determinants.

IV. MODELS AND THEORIES OF HEALTH BEHAVIOR

1.   A number of theories and models to explain health behavior have been developed during the past 20 years.
2.   Because there is no single unifying theory, health practitioners choose the model that best fits a specific health behavior in order to select an intervention to stimulate behavior change.

A.   **SOCIAL LEARNING THEORY**

1.   Bandura's social cognitive theory analyzes health behavior in terms of a **"continuous, mutual interaction among cognitive, behavioral, and environmental determinants."**
2.   A person's environment provides the social and physical situation within which the person must function, and it subsequently provides the incentives and disincentives for his or her actions.
3.   **Sources of influence**
    a.   Three interdependent sources that influence behavior are **antecedent determinants, consequent outcomes, and cognitive determinants.** According to Bandura, individuals need to anticipate potential consequences of different events and then adjust their behavior accordingly.
    b.   Most behavior is maintained by anticipated consequences rather than by immediate consequences.
    c.   The **positive or negative reactions** of others become influential predictors of consequences and evolve into incentives.
4.   **Efficacy and outcome expectations**
    a.   An **outcome expectation** is a personal belief that certain behaviors will lead to certain outcomes.
    b.   An **efficacy expectation** is one's belief that one can successfully perform a specific behavior in order to produce a specific outcome.
    c.   **Efficacy expectations are the most important prerequisite for behavior change.** Stronger efficacy expectations produce more active and sustained efforts, even in the face of adverse conditions.
    d.   The most powerful source of efficacy expectations is **personal experience,** followed by seeing **what others have experienced** and accomplished in similar circumstances.
    e.   **Verbal persuasion,** although of short duration and likely to be weak, is a third source of efficacy expectations.
    f.   A fourth source of efficacy is one's **physiological state or emotional arousal.**
5.   **Application of beliefs about self-efficacy to cancer care**
    a.   Applying social learning theory to understanding an individual's behavior entails understanding that individual's beliefs about targeted health problems or behaviors.
    b.   The decision to engage in healthful behavior is strongly influenced by **one's belief in one's ability** to carry out a required activity.

B.   **HEALTH BELIEF MODEL (HBM)**

1.   The HBM originated in the 1950s and evolved to encompass the value that individuals attach to a given outcome and their expectation that a particular action will result in that outcome. People usually choose behaviors that will produce the maximum number of positive outcomes and the least amount of negative outcomes.
2.   See **Table 6-1, text page 91,** for variables of the HBM.
3.   Perceived barriers, perceived susceptibility, and perceived benefits are strong predictors of behavior, with perceived barriers being the most powerful single predictor.
4.   Perceived severity is the weakest predictor but seems strongly related to behaviors associated with the sick role.
5.   **Application of the Health Belief Model to health behavior**
    a.   The HBM attempts to explain health behavior and is guided by the assumption that people can accept the possibility that they may have an illness.
    b.   The underlying premise of the HBM is that people value health. Variations in behaviors can usually be explained by attitudes and beliefs.
6.   **Application of the Health Belief Model to cancer care**
    a.   The HBM has been used to identify individuals who engage in behaviors to prevent and detect cancer.
    b.   Health motivation and perceived barriers are predictors of people's intentions and behaviors related to cancer prevention and screening activities.

C.   **THEORY OF REASONED ACTION**

1.   The theory of reasoned action is a value-expectancy theory used to predict whether a person will perform behavior in a specific situation.

2. Influence of the social environment and attitude toward the behavior contribute to whether someone intends to perform a behavior. See **Figure 6-2, text page 93.**
3. Factors such as personality traits and demographic characteristics can indirectly influence an individual's intention and behavior.
4. **Application of the Theory of Reasoned Action to cancer care**
   a. The theory of reasoned action has been used in research on BSE; women's beliefs, attitudes, and behaviors regarding Pap tests; and women seeking care for breast cancer symptoms.

D. **SOCIAL SUPPORT**

1. The relationship that individuals have with others constitutes their social or personal network. According to Kahn, the components of supportive transactions are **affirmation, affect, and aid.**
2. Several hypotheses about the mechanism of action whereby social support contributes to health can be reviewed on **text page 93.**
3. **Relevance of social support to health behavior**
   a. There is evidence that family support has a positive influence on compliance with medical advice.
4. **Application of social support to cancer care**
   a. Research has indicated that social support may be more influential with preventive behavior than with detective behavior.

E. **LOCUS OF CONTROL/HEALTH LOCUS OF CONTROL**

1. **Locus of control**
   a. **Internal locus of control** is the perception of individuals that events in their lives are a consequence of their own actions and are controllable.
   b. **External locus of control** is the perception that events in one's life are unrelated to one's behavior and are hence beyond one's control.
2. **Health locus of control**
   a. **Health locus of control** is a generalized expectation about whether health is controllable by one's own behavior or by forces external to oneself.
   b. **External locus of control** is represented by two constructs: chance and powerful others, such as health professionals.
3. **Application of health locus of control to cancer care**
   a. In studies of breast self-examination behavior, BSE was practiced more frequently by women who exhibited an internal locus of control, in combination with belief in high susceptibility and benefits.

F. **ATTRIBUTION THEORY**

1. Attribution theory involves the explanations that individuals use to understand what is happening to them.
2. Attributions can predict behavior, feelings, and expectations. They can maintain self-esteem and reduce anxiety. See **Table 6-2, text page 95,** for dimensions and consequents of attribution theory.
3. **Application of Attribution Theory to cancer care**
   a. Some studies suggest that adjustment may be associated with attribution of the cause of cancer to one's own behavior.
   b. Other studies suggest that not making strong causal attributions may be a positive factor in patient adjustment.

V. **RELATED FACTORS**

A. **SOCIODEMOGRAPHICS**

1. **Knowledge and education level**
   a. Knowledge regarding a specific cancer or screening measure is positively related to health behaviors but is not consistently associated with positive health behaviors.
   b. Although knowledge and education level can influence health behaviors positively and negatively, other factors in a person's life can override those influences.

2. **Socioeconomic status**
    a. Socioeconomic status has a strong association with health behaviors, with people of low socioeconomic status often having more **negative** health behaviors.
3. **Age**
    a. Age is an important influence on health behaviors.
4. **Race**
    a. Examining the influence of race is not easy, although differences in cancer incidence, mortality, and survival rates among different races is being studied.

B. **FAMILY FACTORS**

1. **Family ethnicity, family support, and families in the child-bearing years** have more positive relationships with health behaviors.

C. **SOCIAL FACTORS**

1. Social support has a **positive influence** on preventive health behaviors, whereas social roles may influence health behavior positively or negatively.
2. Social stigmas associated with certain health behaviors or diseases can influence individuals' decisions to participate in prevention, screening, and detection activities.
3. Cultural factors may also play a part.

D. **INSTITUTIONAL FACTORS**

1. **Health care delivery systems, government services, health care providers, and social resources** influence people's health behavior.

VI. **IMPLICATIONS FOR NURSING PRACTICE**

1. Applying principles and concepts of health behavior models can support the nursing process through guidelines for assessment, nursing diagnosis, intervention, and evaluation.

PRACTICE QUESTIONS

1. The **best** reason for the promotion of positive health behaviors is that
    (A) the prevention of cancer is determined by people's health behaviors.
    (B) smoking is the biggest cause of lung cancer.
    (C) health care costs are soaring with the growing number of patients affected by cancer.
    (D) health promotion is not disease specific.

2. What is the term applied to actions taken by people to protect, promote, or maintain their health?
    (A) illness behavior
    (B) sick role behavior
    (C) health protective behavior
    (D) information seeking

3. The action of seeing a physician and pursuing answers, in response to symptoms a person is experiencing, is an example of
    (A) social learning theory.
    (B) illness behavior.
    (C) cancer control.
    (D) environmental influence.

4. The **majority** of health behavior is maintained by
    (A) immediate consequences.
    (B) delayed consequences.
    (C) anticipated consequences.
    (D) outcome consequences.

5. The **most** important prerequisite for behavior change that involves an individual's beliefs is
    (A) reactions of others.
    (B) verbal persuasion.
    (C) outcome expectation.
    (D) efficacy expectation.

6. The **most** powerful source of efficacy expectations is
    (A) personal experience.
    (B) what others have experienced.
    (C) verbal persuasion.
    (D) physiologic state.

7. The Health Belief Model attempts to explain health behavior and is guided by
    (A) the assumption that an individual's subjective perception of the environment determines behavior.
    (B) the assumption that people expect treatment and care.
    (C) the assumption that people change their behaviors in response to familial pressures and familial patterns of disease.
    (D) the assumption that people will perform a specific behavior in response to intense education and peer pressure.

8. Predictors of behaviors are determined by three variables. These variables are
    (A) belief in self, perceived susceptibility, and support systems.
    (B) support systems, perceived barriers, and perceived benefits.
    (C) perceived barriers, perceived benefits, and belief in self.
    (D) perceived barriers, perceived susceptibility, and perceived benefits.

9. Which aspect of social support has a positive influence on compliance with medical advice?
    (A) work relationships
    (B) peer relationships
    (C) family relationships
    (D) the patient-physician relationship

10. In studies of women who practiced breast self-examination behaviors, those who did so more frequently were found to have
    (A) external locus of control, low perceived susceptibility, and high perceived benefits.
    (B) internal locus of control, low perceived susceptibility, and high perceived benefits.
    (C) external locus of control, high perceived susceptibility, and high perceived benefits.
    (D) internal locus of control, high perceived susceptibility, and high perceived benefits.

11. Factors that influence health behaviors include knowledge and education level, socioeconomic status, race, and
    (A) residential location.
    (B) marital status.
    (C) age.
    (D) employment status.

ANSWER EXPLANATIONS

1. **The answer is (A).**   Because personal lifestyle choices affect morbidity and mortality, they must be incorporated into any legislative, motivational, or educational attempts at cancer control.

2. **The answer is (C).**   Health protective behavior consists of actions taken by people in order to protect, promote, or maintain their health.

3. **The answer is (B).**   Illness behavior is any activity that a person who feels ill undertakes to define the state of her or his health and to discover a suitable remedy.

4. **The answer is (C).**   Anticipated consequences, rather than immediate consequences, determine most health behaviors.

5.   **The answer is (D).**   Efficacy expectations are the most important prerequisite for behavior change since stronger efficacy expectations produce more active and sustained efforts in the face of adverse conditions.

6.   **The answer is (A).**   Personal experience is the most powerful and dependable source of efficacy expectations, followed by seeing what others have experienced and accomplished in similar circumstances.

7.   **The answer is (A).**   The Health Belief Model attempts to explain health behavior and is guided by the assumption that people can accept the possibility that they may have an illness.

8.   **The answer is (D).**   Perceived barriers, perceived susceptibility, and perceived benefits are strong predictors of behavior; perceived barriers are the most powerful single predictor. Perceived severity is the weakest predictor but appears to be strongly related to sick role behaviors. (91)

9.   **The answer is (C).**   Family relationships and support have a positive influence on compliance with medical advice.

10.   **The answer is (D).**   In studies of breast self-examination behavior, women who practiced breast self-examination more frequently were those who perceived an internal locus of control in combination with beliefs in high susceptibility and benefits.

11.   **The answer is (C).**   Age has an influence on health behaviors.

7   Cancer Risk and Assessment

STUDY OUTLINE

I.   INTRODUCTION

1. Precise prediction of disease or mortality by any means is currently unattainable because of **incomplete knowledge of the total set of risk factors, their time-dose levels, and the true functional form of their contribution to risk.**
   a. Risk models can differentiate high-, medium-, and low-risk individuals and can estimate relative risk.
   b. But they are much less successful in estimating actual risk in individuals or across populations.
   c. Measurements applied to individuals are also more accurate than those used only in correlational studies, where random errors can offset one another.
2. **Health risk assessment (HRA)** has a number of desirable qualities for clinicians and health educators. A major concern, however, is the value of quantitative estimates of absolute risk.

II.   DEFINITIONS OF RISK

1. **Risk** is the potential realization of unwanted consequences of an event. It is best thought of as the "downside of a gamble," implying that risk and some potential gain are often associated.
2. Risk involves both a **probability of occurrence of an event** and the **magnitude of its consequences.**
3. A person's cancer risk means a factual estimate of the likelihood and severity of adverse effect, or the odds of incurring cancer.
4. After risks are estimated, decisions must be made about whether to **accept the risks** or to **reduce them by reducing their source or taking protective actions.** This process is called **risk evaluation.**

III.   CANCER RISK FACTORS

1. The **two major areas** of cancer prevention strategies are:
   a. **Identification** of the **contributors** to the **cause(s)** of cancer.
   b. The **action taken in response** to this knowledge.
2. **Identification** of the contributors to cause(s) of cancer is the function of the researcher.
3. **Action** in response to the identification is by **behavior modification, legislative control,** or **voluntary actions** taken on the part of concerned individuals.
4. **Cancer risk factors** are specific risk factors or individual characteristics that are associated with an increased cancer risk.
5. They may be **under a person's control** (e.g., cigarette smoking) or **outside a person's control** (e.g., genetic makeup or family traits).
6. They may be **unique to an individual** (e.g., exposure to radiation or drugs) or they may be **shared by a group of persons from the same geographic residence or occupation.**
7. Categorizing risk factors is important for several reasons.
   a. It provides a **data base** from which to develop an individual's cancer-risk profile, make recommendations about risk factors, and plan specific interventions for risk reduction.
   b. It emphasizes the many **causative factors** and the **complex etiology** of cancer.

8. The two biggest challenges for the cancer research establishment are:
   a. Implementation of interventions to prevent cancer from known or proven causes.
   b. Verification of highly suspected causes of major cancers.
9. See **text page 104,** column 1, for a list of all cancer risk factors.

IV. **CANCER RISK FACTORS IN MINORITY POPULATIONS**

A. **MULTIFACTORIAL ASPECTS**

1. **African Americans** have an 11% greater risk of developing cancer and a 25% lower 5-year survival rate than the general population.
2. The cancer death rate among African Americans is 27% higher than for the general population.
3. **Asians and Hispanics** within the United States have a lower cancer incidence rate per 100,000 than either whites or African Americans.
4. Rate differences among ethnic groups may be attributable to **behavioral, social, and environmental factors** rather than to biological or genetic characteristics.
5. **Differences in dietary patterns** have been suggested as the major contributor to rate differences among African Americans and Hispanics.
6. **Delayed diagnosis** is believed to contribute most to mortality differences among ethnic groups.
7. See **Table 7-1, text page 105,** for a list of high-incidence cancers for specific ethnic groups.

B. **SOCIOECONOMIC/EDUCATIONAL FACTORS**

1. Americans living below the poverty level have a 5-year cancer survival rate that is 10%–15% lower than that for other Americans.
2. Four critical issues involving cancer and the poor are:
   a. The poor face substantial obstacles with health insurance and often do not seek care if they cannot pay for it.
   b. The impoverished must make personal sacrifices to obtain and pay for health care.
   c. Outreach and education efforts are irrelevant to many poor people.
   d. The poor often have a fatalistic attitude about cancer.

C. **RACIAL FACTORS**

1. Racial differences are seen when cancer is diagnosed in people at ages 20–54, but few such differences are found in people older than 65 years.
2. Five aspects of poverty affect early detection, treatment, and survival.
   a. **Unemployment.**
   b. **Inadequate education.**
   c. **Substandard housing.**
   d. **Chronic malnutrition.**
   e. **Diminished access to medical care.**
3. See **text pages 105–106** for 11 recommendations made by the American Cancer Society Special Report to reduce the disproportionate effect of cancer in the socioeconomically disadvantaged.

V. **RISK FACTORS FOR SPECIFIC CANCERS**

1. The **actual risk** from a single factor depends on:
   a. The number and intensity of other coexisting factors in an individual.
   b. The intensity of the factor itself.
2. As age advances, more factors accumulate and potentiate each other.
3. See **Table 7-2, text pages 106–108,** for a list of specific cancer risk factors for each type of cancer discussed below.

A. **BLADDER CANCER**

1. In general, the strongest risk factors for bladder cancer involve **occupational exposure** (e.g., exposure to carcinogenic chemicals) and **lifestyle practices** (e.g., cigarette smoking).
2. In the United States, risk factors for bladder cancer involve primarily occupational exposures and tobacco use.

3.   Workers exposed to aromatic amines have a fourfold greater risk of bladder cancer.
     a.   High-risk occupations include apparel, textile, and leather workers, workers in the dye industry, rubber workers, metal workers, and painters.
4.   Smokers develop bladder cancer 2–3 times more often than nonsmokers.
5.   There can be a latency period of as much as 18 years before bladder tumors develop after exposure to carcinogens.

B.   **BREAST CANCER**

1.   The primary risk factors for breast cancer are a **family history of breast cancer, history of benign breast disease, late age at first live birth, nulliparity, early age at menarche, late age at menopause, higher socioeconomic status, being Jewish,** and **being single.**
2.   There are conflicting data on the relationship between breast cancer and alcohol and between breast cancer and birth control pills.
3.   Data on the relationship between breast cancer and **dietary fat** are more conclusive.
4.   See **Table 7-3, text page 109,** for risk factors.

C.   **CERVICAL CANCER**

1.   The major risk factors are **race, personal factors such as multiple sexual partners,** and **venereal disease.**
2.   Black women in the United States have a twofold higher risk than white women, while certain religious groups have lower incidence rates.

D.   **COLORECTAL CANCER**

1.   Important risk factors include a **sedentary lifestyle, a low-fiber/high-fat diet, age, familial and hereditary factors,** and having **ulcerative colitis, Crohn's disease, a past history of colon cancer, or intestinal polyps.**
2.   Many of these factors are associated with highly developed countries.

E.   **LIVER CANCER**

1.   The incidence of **hepatocellular carcinoma (HCC) increases** with age and is greater in men. HCC occurs most often between the ages of 30 and 50.
2.   Although rare in the United States, it is the most common worldwide cancer for men.
3.   Risk factors include: **hepatitis B and C virus, cirrhosis,** and the **chemical vinyl chloride.**
4.   **Chronic hepatitis B virus infection is probably the leading cause of HCC throughout the world, accounting for 75%–90% of the world's cases.**

F.   **LUNG CANCER**

1.   The major risk factors are **geographic location, social class, occupation,** and **tobacco use.**
2.   **Cigarette smoking** may contribute to at least 80% of all lung cancers in American males and 40% in females. Many others die from environmental tobacco smoke.
3.   **Indoor radon exposure** causes about 10,000 deaths a year. Most of the risk from radon occurs in smokers, suggesting a synergistic relationship between the two carcinogens.
4.   Many **industrial substances** have been linked to lung cancer (e.g., asbestos and polycyclic hydrocarbons).

G.   **ORAL CANCER**

1.   **Chewing or smoking tobacco** is a major risk factor, as are **excessive alcohol intake, poor nutrition,** and **long-term exposure of the lip to the sun.**

H.   **OVARIAN CANCER**

1.   The risk factors for ovarian cancer are less well known than those of the other gynecologic cancers.

2.   Risk factors such as delayed age at first pregnancy and a smaller number of pregnancies suggest an abnormality of endocrine secretion.
3.   Oral contraceptives may give protection.

I.   **ENDOMETRIAL (UTERINE CORPUS) CANCER**

1.   The risk factors for cancer of the uterus are well known. (See **Table 7-2, text page 108.**)
2.   The use of oral contraceptives containing both estrogen and progesterone appears to offer protection.

J.   **PROSTATE CANCER**

1.   **Age** and **race** are significant risk factors. Both the **elderly** and **African Americans** are at much higher risk.

K.   **SKIN CANCER**

1.   Basal and squamous cell carcinomas and melanomas are related to **exposure to ultraviolet radiation.** Melanomas involve several other risk factors as well, including **familial predisposition, hormonal factors, and dysplastic nevus syndrome.**
2.   Light-skinned people who spend considerable time in the sun are at greatest risk.

L.   **TESTICULAR CANCER**

1.   As with prostate cancer, **race** and **age** are significant risk factors. White men between the ages of 20 and 40 are at highest risk.
2.   Another risk factor is undescended testicles.

M.   **VAGINAL CANCER**

1.   Both **diethylstilbesterol (DES)** and **radiation of the cervix for cancer** are known risk factors. Refer to **Table 7-3** for additional information.

VI. **CANCER RISK ASSESSMENT**

1.   The purposes of a **cancer risk assessment** include
     a.   Providing individuals with information about their health-related behaviors that may increase cancer risk.
     b.   Educating patients about the relationship between risk factors and the likelihood of cancer.
     c.   Stimulating individuals to participate in activities aimed at changing lifestyle and improving health.
     d.   Helping patients identify their options so they can make realistic decisions about their health care.
     e.   Helping physicians in the development of health regimens that are tailored to each individual's risk and tolerance for living with that risk.
2.   The average risk serves as a baseline against which individuals can measure the magnitude of their increased risk, if any.
3.   One problem in risk assessment is that many people's fears, worries, and other emotions make them unwilling to consider what their risks might be.
     a.   Through **self-understanding** and **education,** people can learn to deal with their emotions and to accept the importance of risk assessment.
     b.   People who receive information about risk are more likely to schedule regular checkups and undergo necessary diagnostic procedures.
4.   Health care consumers should understand what "high" or "low" risk means. They should also understand the concepts of risk assessment in order to understand what it can and cannot do and how to use the data obtained.
5.   A **comprehensive risk analysis** should include
     a.   The **identification of risk** and the **estimation of the likelihood and magnitude of the risk occurring.**
     b.   An **evaluation that measures risk acceptance** (the acceptance level of societal risk) and **risk management** (the control of risks, including methods of reducing and avoiding risk).

A.   **EVALUATION**

1. See **text page 113,** column 1, for a list of factors that should comprise a **health history.** Most of this information can be supplied by the patient on a questionnaire form.
    a. The health history helps detect both early symptoms and symptoms that a patient might deny if asked outright.
    b. It also helps identify factors, such as a family history of genetic susceptibility, that may increase an individual's risk of specific cancers.
2. A complete **physical examination** then provides objective data that can complement and verify the health history's subjective data.
3. Evaluation can lead to several outcomes.
    a. High-risk patients should be **advised about avoiding additional exposure to carcinogens.**
    b. **Rigorous intervention** may be needed (e.g., removing a dysplastic nevus to prevent progression to melanoma).
    c. In high-risk patients, **screening** may be carried out more frequently and in greater detail (e.g., mammograms for women at high risk of breast cancer).
4. See **text page 119** for the American Cancer Society's (ACS) recommended schedule of prevention and detection procedures for the general population.

VII.   **EDUCATION**

1. **Cancer education** attempts to maintain positive health behavior or to interrupt a behavior pattern that is linked to increased risks of cancer (e.g., smoking, high-fat diet, sexual promiscuity).
2. A cancer education program seeks to **prevent disability, illness, or death** or to **enhance quality of life through voluntary change of cancer-related behavior.**
3. Educational programs should encompass all major areas, including tobacco, alcohol, occupations and cancer, environmental pollutants, sexual activity, radiation, infective and genetic factors, and diet.
4. Each area should be discussed from several perspectives, including
    a. The risks they impose for certain types of cancers.
    b. Actions to reduce risks.
    c. Signs and symptoms of specific cancers.
    d. Screening and detection methods.
    e. Personal responsibility in prevention.
5. Reassurance should also be given that some forms of cancers respond well to treatment.

PRACTICE QUESTIONS

1. In general, health risk assessment models are **most** effective in estimating what type of risk?
    (A) relative risk
    (B) quantitative risk
    (C) empirical risk
    (D) absolute risk

2. Risk involves two important components. One of these is the probability of occurrence of an event. The other is the
    (A) consequences if the event does not occur.
    (B) magnitude of the event itself.
    (C) protective reactions to the event.
    (D) magnitude of the consequences of the event.

3. Risk factors may be under a person's control or outside of it, and they may be unique to an individual or shared by a group of persons. An example of a risk factor that is both individual and outside of the individual's control is
    (A) cigarette smoking.
    (B) exposure to asbestos.
    (C) air pollution.
    (D) familial polyposis.

4. Which factor is believed to contribute **most** to mortality differences among ethnic groups?
    (A)   socioeconomic status
    (B)   educational level
    (C)   delay in diagnosis
    (D)   lack of access to medical care

5. A type of cancer that has been associated with occupational exposure to a carcinogen is
    (A)   bladder cancer.
    (B)   colorectal cancer.
    (C)   testicular cancer.
    (D)   cervical cancer.

6. Which of the following individuals is likely to be at **greatest** risk of developing cervical cancer?
    (A)   an African-American woman with multiple sexual partners
    (B)   a white woman who first became pregnant at age 41
    (C)   a white teenaged woman who takes oral contraceptives
    (D)   a woman who used diethylstilbesterol (DES) during pregnancy

7. The leading cause of liver cancer throughout the world is
    (A)   chronic hepatitis B virus.
    (B)   chronic hepatitis C virus.
    (C)   chronic cirrhosis.
    (D)   chronic hepatitis A virus.

8. Long-term exposure to the sun has been associated with skin cancer and also with
    (A)   colorectal cancer.
    (B)   testicular cancer.
    (C)   cancer of the lip.
    (D)   prostate cancer.

9. The long-term use of oral contraceptives containing both estrogen and progesterone in each pill has been found to offer protection against what type of cancer?
    (A)   vaginal cancer
    (B)   colorectal cancer
    (C)   breast cancer
    (D)   endometrial cancer

10. Each of the following is one of the primary purposes of cancer risk assessment **except**
    (A)   identifying the distribution and determinants of diseases and health problems in human populations.
    (B)   providing individuals with information about their health-related behaviors that may increase cancer risk.
    (C)   educating patients about the relationship between risk factors and the likelihood of cancer.
    (D)   stimulating individuals to participate in activities aimed at changing lifestyle and improving health.

11. One of the major purposes of a health history in cancer risk assessment is to
    (A)   provide objective data that complement and verify the subjective data supplied by a physical examination.
    (B)   teach people to deal with their emotions and to accept the importance of risk assessment.
    (C)   help physicians to develop health regimens that are tailored to each individual's risk and tolerance for living with that risk.
    (D)   help identify factors that may increase an individual's risk of specific cancers.

12. For patients identified as having a high risk of cancer, one of the outcomes of the evaluation stage of cancer risk assessment may be rigorous intervention involving a surgical procedure that reduces the risk of a cancer developing. Another outcome may be
    (A)   generating a health history that provides subjective data on the patient's health.
    (B)   screening the patient more frequently and in greater detail than in low-risk patients.
    (C)   asking the patient to undergo a thorough physical examination that provides objective data on the patient's health.
    (D)   educating patients about the relationship between risk factors and quality of life.

ANSWER EXPLANATIONS

1. **The answer is (A).** Risk models have been successful in distinguishing low-, medium-, and high-risk persons and in estimating relative risk but are much less successful in estimating absolute risk in individuals or across populations. Despite the value of HRA in "prospective health assessment," a major concern with HRA is the value of quantitative estimates of absolute risk. The text suggests that more qualitative measures may have more valuable purposes in risk assessment. (103)

2. **The answer is (D).** Risk is the potential realization of unwanted consequences of an event, and it involves both a probability of occurrence of an event (e.g., what are the chances of getting cancer) and the magnitude of its consequences (e.g., how life-threatening is it likely to be). (103)

3. **The answer is (D).** Choice (A) is individual but under the person's control; choice (B) is typically a group risk factor shared by persons from the same occupation; choice (C) is typically a group risk factor shared by persons from the same geographic residence. Only choice (D), an inherited condition, is both individual and outside the person's control. (104)

4. **The answer is (C).** A delay in diagnosis for any number of reasons, including lack of insurance, financial funds, denial of a problem, etc., is the most likely factor to contribute to the mortality differences among ethnic groups. (104–105)

5. **The answer is (A).** One of the strongest risk factors for bladder cancer involves occupational exposure to aromatic amines, including benzidine and aniline dyes. Workers exposed to aromatic amines have a fourfold greater risk of bladder cancer. (108)

6. **The answer is (A).** Both race and personal factors, including sexual habits, are major risk factors in cervical cancer. African-American women in the United States have a twofold greater risk than white women. (108–109)

7. **The answer is (B).** Chronic hepatitis B virus infection is the leading cause of hepatocellular carcinoma throughout the world. (110)

8. **The answer is (C).** Occupations related to long-term exposure to the sun (e.g., farmers, ranchers) have been associated with cancer of the lip, an oral cancer. (110–111)

9. **The answer is (D).** The long-term use of combination oral contraceptives has been found to offer some protection against both ovarian and endometrial cancer. Long-term use of conjugated estrogens, on the other hand, is an iatrogenic risk factor for endometrial cancer. (111)

10. **The answer is (A).** Choice (A) is the definition of epidemiology, a study related to but distinct from cancer risk assessment. Categorizing risk factors is an important preliminary step in risk assessment. From this data base of risk factors an individual's cancer risk profile can be developed and specific interventions for risk reduction can be planned. Choices (B) through (D), however, are the primary objectives of cancer risk assessment. (112)

11. **The answer is (D).** An example of such a risk factor that might be identified in the health history is a family history of genetic susceptibility. Another objective of the health history is to help detect both early symptoms and symptoms that a patient might deny if asked outright. Although data in a health history are typically recorded on a questionnaire, the data are largely subjective. Objective data are gathered in the physical examination. (112)

12. **The answer is (B).** The patient will also be given advice about avoiding additional exposure to carcinogens, even when surgical intervention or more frequent screening are not called for. Note that choices (C) and (D) are the initial stages of the evaluation process. It is on the basis of data generated by the health history and physical examination that recommendations are made. (113, 119)

8 Assessment and Intervention for Cancer Prevention and Detection

STUDY OUTLINE

I. INTRODUCTION

1. Cancer was among the first chronic diseases recognized as potentially "controllable."
2. The establishment of the **National Cancer Institute** in 1937 and passage of the **National Cancer Act of 1971** gave clear expressions of congressional intent regarding cancer control.
3. **Emphasis, however, has tended to be more on cancer research than on cancer control.**
4. Obstacles to a broadscale program of cancer control included the following:
   a. Physicians generally did not view cancer as epidemic in nature.
   b. Physicians viewed governmental action in the area of cancer control to be an intrusion into physicians' right to practice.
   c. Economic resistance by lobbies such as the tobacco industry was aided by cancer's long latency period, which made identifying etiologic factors more difficult.
   d. Special interests in cancer research held onto money that might have gone into cancer control.
5. Organized cancer control has thus had three strong adversaries: the **private medical world,** the **private industrial world,** and the **biomedical research establishment.**

A. CAN WE PREVENT CANCER?

1. To effectively conquer most common cancers, preventive measures must reach the individual and seek to **modify personal habits and lifestyles.**
   a. But resistance to changing lifestyle can be strong (e.g., giving up tobacco, alcohol, fat, or sunbathing).
   b. And it is easier to blame industry and the environment for most of our ills, despite the fact that, with the exception of lung cancer, **most of the major cancers are no more common today than they were 50 years ago.**
2. The question is, are people willing to give up certain immediate desires in return for health and prolonged life?

II. LEVELS OF PREVENTION

1. **Prevention** consists of all measures, including definitive therapy, that limit the progression of disease **at any point of its course.**
2. Preventive strategies can therefore be adopted **before cancer is diagnosed (primary prevention), during diagnosis (secondary prevention),** or **after it has been diagnosed (tertiary prevention).**

A. PRIMARY PREVENTION

1. **Primary prevention** precedes disease or dysfunction and is applied to a healthy population. Its purpose is to decrease the vulnerability of the individual or the population to illness or dysfunction through health-promoting strategies, as well as to provide special protection.

2. Refer to **text page 126,** columns 1 and 2, for seven activities directed at promoting health and primary cancer prevention.
3. **Patient education** regarding good health behaviors is vital to successful primary prevention. It involves appropriate teaching levels and receiving information before disease diagnosis, during regular health maintenance visits.
4. Nursing roles in primary prevention have been increasing and expanding to new settings. **Occupational health and community health** nurses carry out primary prevention activities while educational programs stressing prevention are increasing in number.
5. **Knowledge regarding risk factors, health behaviors, cancer screening and detection methods, teaching methods, and counseling skills are required by nurses for successful primary and secondary prevention.**

A1. Health Promotion

1. **Health promotion** efforts focus on **maintaining or improving the general health of individuals, families, and communities.** It is carried out on both the **public level** (e.g., adequate housing) and the **personal level.**
2. Its strategies may be either **passive** (e.g., maintaining clean water) or **active** (e.g., changing eating or exercise habits).
3. Health promotion lacks the demanding element of immediacy and thus tends to be relegated to lower levels of importance.
4. Personal health promotion most commonly is provided by **health education.**
5. The goal of the health educator, including nurses, is to assist individuals to develop a **sense of responsibility for their own health** and a **shared sense of responsibility for avoiding injury to the health of others.**

A2. Specific Protection

1. **Specific protection** focuses on protecting persons from disease by **providing immunization** and **reducing exposure to environmental health risks.**
2. See **text page 127,** column 2, for a list of specific protection strategies.
3. Certain preventive measures will create enormous benefits but will also increase medical expenditures.
    a. Society must decide whether better health is worth the higher cost.
    b. Individuals must determine what best meets their own personal needs.

B. SECONDARY PREVENTION

1. **Secondary prevention** activities include defining and identifying high-risk groups and groups with precursor stages of disease. It includes **early detection and screening, prompt treatment, and limiting disability.**
2. **Early detection** refers to the early identification of disease in an individual, who may or may not have symptoms, through the use of tests, examinations, and observations.
3. Preventive measures in the category of limiting disability are directed at arresting disease, preventing further complications and death.
    a. **Screening** refers to an organized effort to find cancer in its early stages in a defined population.
    b. See **text page 128,** column 1, for activities carried out to ensure early diagnosis and prompt treatment.

C. TERTIARY PREVENTION

1. **Tertiary prevention** takes place when a disability is permanent and irreversible. It focuses on **rehabilitation** to help persons attain and retain optimal level of functioning regardless of their disabling condition.

III.   **ROLE OF THE NURSE IN PRIMARY AND SECONDARY CANCER PREVENTION**

     1.   Among the nurse's activities in promoting primary and secondary cancer prevention are **assessment, counseling, teaching, screening, planning,** and **acting as an advocate for healthier living.**

IV.   **CHEMOPREVENTION**

     1.   **Chemoprevention is the use of "defined chemicals or micronutrients to inhibit or reverse the process of carcinogenesis."**
     2.   Agents being studied in clinical trials include **vitamins A, C, D, and E; folic acid; calcium; and selenium.**

  A.   **VITAMIN A**

     1.   **Retinoids**
       a.   **Retinoids** are natural derivatives and synthetic analogs of vitamin A and are believed to be active in the prevention of ephithelial carcinogenesis.
       b.   Retinoids can suppress carcinogenesis in the ephithelial tissues of the skin, trachea, lungs, and oral mucosa.
       c.   **Dietary sources** of retinol include **butter, whole milk, egg yolk, and liver.**
       d.   Long-term use of retinoids is limited by hepatic toxicity.
     2.   **Beta-carotene**
       a.   **Beta-carotene** is a carotenoid with pro-vitamin A (retinol) activity. It is a precursor of vitamin A.
       b.   Dietary sources include leafy green and yellow vegetables converted to vitamin A in the gastrointestinal tract.

  B.   **VITAMIN C**

     1.   Dietary sources are citrus fruits, fruit juices, and vegetables.
     2.   Vitamin C prevents the formation of nitrosamines that result from ingesting nitrates and nitrites.
     3.   **Nitrosamines** are a potent carcinogenic agent associated with stomach cancer.

  C.   **VITAMIN E**

     1.   Dietary sources include vegetable oils, margarines, shortening, eggs, whole grains, and cereals.
     2.   Vitamin B appears to prevent nitrosamine formation.

  D.   **SELENIUM**

     1.   Dietary sources include seafood, meats, vegetables, whole grains, and milk.
     2.   Epidemiologic studies have shown an inverse relationship between selenium intake and cancer.

V.   **DETECTION OF MAJOR CANCER SITES**

     1.   The expectation is that all nursing students will incorporate the four cardinal techniques of physical assessment (**inspection, palpation, percussion, and auscultation**) into their daily clinical practice. These techniques enable the nurse to assume an active role in the early detection of cancer.

  A.   **LUNG CANCER**

     1.   **Lung cancer is the leading cause of death from cancer in men and women over 35 years old.** Within the last 5 years it has replaced breast cancer as the chief cause of cancer death among women.
     2.   The most important environmental carcinogen related to the increased incidence of lung cancer is **cigarette smoking,** which is also the major single cause of cancer mortality.

3. **History assessment**
   a. What to cover:
      (1) **Smoking habits,** including marijuana use.
      (2) **Occupational history,** including shipyard work and exposure to asbestos. Certain occupations require special scrutiny because of possible exposure of workers to suspected carcinogens (e.g., clothing and textiles).
      (3) **The general respiratory environment of both the workplace and home,** including exposure to a smoke environment.
   b. See **Figure 8-1, text page 132,** for a systematic approach to the occupational and environmental health history.
   c. See **text pages 131 and 133** for questions that should be included in the history.
   d. The first symptoms are usually not alarming and can easily be overlooked or attributed to other causes.
      (1) The most common symptom is a **cough that is productive** and often associated with **hemoptysis and chest pain.** A non-productive cough may indicate a cancer that is **centrally located** or that **involves the main carina only.**
      (2) Later symptoms include a combination of coughing, wheezing, pleuritic pain, hoarseness, local nerve disorders, edema of head, neck, or arms, dysphagia, and persistent pneumonitis.
4. **Physical examination**
   a. See **Figure 8-5, text page 136,** for a synopsis of physical findings commonly seen with tumors of different anatomic sites in the lungs.
   b. The only early physical finding is wheezing localized to a single lobe of the lung in an elderly person with a long history of smoking.
   c. Later findings may include **finger clubbing (Figure 8-2, text page 134), barrel chest** (associated with emphysema), **abnormal breathing, bulges of the thorax, breathlessness,** and **superior vena cava obstruction.**
   d. **Palpation of the thorax** includes testing for vocal fremitus, respiratory excursion, and compression and determining the position and moveability of the trachea. Symptoms to look for include
      (1) **A deviated or fixed trachea.**
      (2) **Decreased or absent vocal fremitus.**
   e. **Percussion and auscultation** may provide final clues to assessment of the individual who is at high risk for lung cancer. Physical signs to look for include
      (1) **Dullness, indicating pleural effusion (text page 135, Figure 8-4).**
      (2) **Decreased or absent breath sounds.**
      (3) **Unilateral wheezing and the bagpipe sign.**
      (4) **Presence of whispered pectoriloquy, bronchophony, and egophony.**
5. **Screening tests for asymptomatic individuals**
   a. No screening programs or tests for lung cancer have been shown to reduce mortality significantly.
6. **Smoking cessation**
   a. The greatest reduction in mortality can be achieved by **cessation of smoking.**
      (1) Smoking prevalence is decreasing across all race-gender groups, although more slowly among women.
      (2) **Educational level** is the major demographic predictor of both smoking and cessation of smoking.
      (3) Blue-collar workers, minorities, and women are the main targets of cigarette advertising. This information should assist health professionals in identifying and educating these high-risk groups.
   b. The role of the nurse is to
      (1) **Monitor** aggressively those who smoke, who have had a history of heavy smoking, or who were employed in high-risk occupations. These individuals should undergo a complete respiratory assessment.
      (2) **Assist** smokers in their efforts to stop smoking. See **Table 8-1, text page 137,** for a list of specific steps the nurse should follow.
      (3) **Remind** smokers that smoking cessation results in improved sensory, respiratory, and cardiovascular status. The effects of smoking **are** partially reversible.
      (4) **Remain nonjudgmental** in dealing with those who refuse or are unable to stop smoking. Nicotine is addictive, and the smoker may need repeated attempts before he or she is successful.

   (5) **Disseminate information** on the disease potential of smoking whenever possible.
   (6) **Serve as a positive role model** by not smoking.
   (7) **Take advantage of opportunities to advise smokers to quit** both in health care settings and in the community.
   (8) **Work with physicians and others** on a team approach to delivering individualized advice on multiple occasions and using multiple smoking cessation interventions.
  c. A reduction in the public's tolerance for smoking has made smokers more responsive to the antismoking message of health professionals.
  d. The **nicotine patch** is a new development in assisting people to stop smoking. The nicotine is released directly through the skin or through a membrane system in contact with the skin. Side effects are minimal.

B. GASTROINTESTINAL CANCER

1. **Colorectal cancer** incidence and mortality in the United States are second only to lung cancer.
2. **History assessment**
  a. What general signs or factors to look for:
   (1) **Rectal bleeding from diverticulosis.**
   (2) **Depression** as evidenced by anorexia, constipation, and somatic pains.
   (3) **Nutritional disturbances** that may account for weight loss.
   (4) **Unusual drug intake,** especially laxatives.
  b. See **text page 138,** column 2, for a list of specific questions to ask in preparing the history and review of systems.
  c. **Figure 8-6, text page 139,** identifies the most frequent presenting signs and symptoms of each area of the intestinal tract affected by cancer.
3. **Physical examination**
  a. The findings that most strongly suggest cancer of the colorectal area are
   (1) **A mass palpated in the rectum.**
   (2) **A palpable mass in the abdomen.**
   (3) **Evidence of blood in the feces.**
  b. **Inspection**
   (1) Signs to look for include
    (a) **Nodular umbilicus.**
    (b) **Masses that distort the abdominal profile.**
    (c) **Subcutaneous nodules under the skin.**
    (d) **Distention of the abdominal profile.**
    (e) **Venous distention** caused by blockage of the inferior vena cava.
    (f) **Visible peristaltic waves** associated with intestinal blockage.
    (g) **Bulging of the flanks.**
  c. **Auscultation**
   (1) Various **bowel sounds** heard with the stethoscope bell should be analyzed for abnormality. See **text page 140,** column 1.
   (2) Some **abdominal circulatory sounds** also signal cancer and should be listened for with the stethoscope bell. See **Figure 8-7, text page 140.**
  d. **Palpation and percussion**
   (1) The following findings on palpation merit further attention and may signal colorectal cancer:
    (a) **Hepatomegaly** (enlarged liver).
    (b) **Splenomegaly** (enlarged spleen).
    (c) **Enlargement of the colon.**
    (d) **Free fluid in the abdomen,** as determined by the shifting dullness, fluid wave, or puddle sign tests.
    (e) **Presence of lesions or rectal shelf** during digital rectal examination.
  e. Physical findings from other parts of the body are typical in abdominal carcinoma, including
   (1) **Enlargement of Virchow's node,** found frequently behind the clavicular head of the left supraclavicular group.
   (2) **Acanthosis nigricans,** a skin lesion that strongly suggests an intestinal malignancy.
   (3) **Jaundice,** which may indicate hepatic or pancreatic lesions.

4. **Screening tests for asymptomatic individuals**
   a. The two most important screen tests are **examination of the feces for occult blood** and the **digital rectal examination.**
   b. The role of fecal occult blood tests in early detection is still being evaluated.
   c. See **Figure 8-8, text page 143,** for the American Cancer Society's recommendations for screening asymptomatic individuals for colorectal cancer.
5. **Additional nursing interventions**
   a. The public is generally ignorant about the risk factors and nature of colorectal cancer and its diagnosis and treatment.
   b. The role of the nurse is to
      (1) **Inform the general public** about colon and rectum cancer, with special attention given to the elderly and other high-risk groups.
      (2) **Encourage the public** and especially these high-risk groups to participate in early detection and screening programs.
      (3) **Educate the general public** on the dietary recommendations for lowering overall cancer risk, including colorectal cancer. See **text page 144,** column 1, for these recommendations.
      (4) **Review and evaluate new research findings** relevant to diet, early detection, and other aspects of colorectal cancer.
   c. The nurse is in the ideal position to detect colorectal cancer in its initial stages in geriatric patients.

C. PROSTATE CANCER

1. **Prostate cancer** is currently the second most common cancer in American men.
   a. African-American men have the highest incidence in the world.
2. Prostate cancer increases in incidence with **age** more rapidly than any other cancer.
3. **A large percentage of men have advanced disease at the time of diagnosis.**
4. **History assessment**
   a. There are no real symptoms of early, probably curable, disease.
   b. Initial symptoms are related to **urinary difficulty** manifested by a **decrease in urinary stream** and a **frequency and urgency to urinate,** often associated with **pain.**
      (1) These symptoms may also be caused by enlargement of the prostate.
   c. Inquiries made during the history should be about nonspecific urinary symptoms. See **text page 145,** column 1, for a list of questions to use.
5. **Physical examination**
   a. An early diagnosis of prostate cancer can be done only by **rectal palpation of the prostate.**
   b. Early prostatic carcinoma usually appears as a **stony-hard nodule located within, not on, the posterior part of the prostate gland.** As the cancer progresses the entire prostate may become stony-hard.
   c. With **benign prostate hypertrophy,** found commonly in older men, the prostate is enlarged and diffuse but without masses.
6. **Screening tests for asymptomatic individuals**
   a. The **digital rectal examination** is currently the most efficient test for the diagnosis of prostate cancer.
   b. **Transrectal ultrasound,** used commonly in Japan, holds promise of even greater sensitivity.
   c. Two biochemical indicators, or **tumor markers,** used to detect prostate cancer are **prostate-specific antigen** and **prostatic acid phosphatase.**
   d. The most effective screening technique for prostate cancer is the **prostate-specific antigen (PSA)** combined with a **digital rectal examination.**
   e. The nurse can assume an important role in educating especially older men and African-American men on the importance of regular rectal examinations.
   f. The nurse may also be called on to perform rectal examinations in some communities or to arrange for a male physician or nurse practitioner to complete this examination.
   g. Special attention should be given to **hospitalized elderly men.**

D. BREAST CANCER

1. **Breast cancer is the most common cancer in women in the Western World.** It is the leading cause of cancer deaths in women 15 to 54 years of age and the second cause of cancer deaths in women older than 55.

2. **History assessment**
    a. See **text page 147,** column 1, for a list of questions to ask.
    b. The most common presenting complaint of women with breast cancer is a **painless lump or mass in the breast.** Most tumors are discovered by **women themselves.**
3. **Physical examination**
    a. Breasts should be examined from several positions. See **Figure 8-12, text page 148.**
    b. Signs to look for include
        (1) **Dimpling of the breast.**
        (2) **Unilateral flattening of the nipple** caused by fibrosis and contraction of this fibrotic tissue.
        (3) **Abnormal contours or flattening** as the woman changes position.
        (4) **Peau d'orange,** or orange peel skin, caused by interference with the lymphatic drainage of the skin.
        (5) **Increased venous prominence,** usually unilateral.
        (6) **Scaling or eczematoid lesions of the nipple** indicating Paget's disease.
    c. **Palpation**
        (1) After inspection, the entire breast should first be lightly palpated for thickening, using the pads of the fingers. Cancer occurs as a **hard, poorly circumscribed nodule.**
        (2) If cancer is suspected, the breast should be gently **moved or compressed for dimpling.** A malignant lump attached to the deep fascia will limit mobility of the breast.
        (3) The breast should then be **thoroughly palpated** while the woman is supine and her arms above her head. Any mass that is felt should be charted. Special attention should be paid to the **breast tissue along the inframammary crease.**
        (4) The breast should next be examined in the **right and left semilateral decubitus positions.** See **Figure 8-16, text page 150.**
        (5) The **nipple should be checked for discharge.** Smears should be taken for cytologic examination of any suspicious discharge.
        (6) The **axillae and supraclavicular regions should be carefully palpated** to check for metastasis to the lymph nodes. Hard, fixed nodes raise the suspicion of cancer.
        (7) Physiologic changes in the breasts of older women may simulate cancer of the breast. **It is best to refer all suspicious signs rather than assume they are due to aging.**
    d. **Screening tests for asymptomatic individuals**
        (1) Three methods used in screening for breast cancer are **physical examination of the breast by the health professional; teaching the woman breast self-examination (BSE); and mammography.**
        (2) See **text page 150,** column 1, for the American Cancer Society's revised recommendations for screening.
        (3) BSE should be encouraged as part of a woman's regular medical care.
        (4) **Lack of knowledge and confidence in their ability** are the usual reasons women give for not practicing BSE.
        (5) Because personal instruction results in more frequent BSE than any other method, nurses should include one-on-one instruction in BSE techniques whenever possible.
        (6) Self-instruction includes teaching a woman to do BSE by **using her own hand on her breast** under the direct guidance of the individual.

E. **TESTICULAR CANCER**

1. **Testicular cancer** is the most common solid tumor in young men between 20 and 35 years of age. It affects Caucasian men more than African-American men.
2. **History assessment**
    a. See **text page 152,** column 1, for a list of questions to ask.
    b. The most common presenting complaint is a **painless enlargement of the testis, or "heaviness."**
    c. Nodules in the testes are typically **small, hard, and usually painless,** and they are slightly more common in the **right testis.**
    d. The major obstacle to early detection is avoidable delay.
        (1) Most men are uninformed about testicular cancer and about testicular examination, and most ignore the unilateral enlargement of a testis for some time.

3. **Physical examination**
   a. The testes will normally appear somewhat **rubbery and spongy,** and will have a **uniform consistency throughout** with a **surface free of lumps or indurations.**
   b. Cancer of the testes may be manifested by **asymmetry of the scrotum,** and the scrotal skin may appear **stretched and thin** over the tumor. The most common sites for tumors are on the **testicular anterior and lateral surfaces.**
   c. Testes should be **transilluminated** in a darkened room to check for a **hydrocele,** which may develop as a result of a tumor. A testicular tumor occurs as a **painless mass that does not transilluminate.**
   d. Other areas should be checked to ascertain if there has been metastasis, including the **epigastrium, Virchow's node,** and **abdomen.**
4. **Education: testicular self-examination (TSE)**
   a. Nurses must participate in the vital job of educating the public about early detection and treatment, including TSE.
   b. Teaching TSE should be incorporated into routine physical examinations.
   c. A nursing assessment of any male younger than 40 years of age should include a **health history** to elicit any subjective symptoms and established risk factors for testicular cancer.
   d. **Parents of boys with undescended testes** should be taught how to palpate the testes and what physical findings are significant. These children should be instructed in TSE as they mature.
   e. See **text page 154,** column 1, for a list of methods to disseminate information about testicular cancer and TSE.

F. **SKIN CANCER**

1. **Cancers of the skin are the most common cancers in humans.** Approximately one in three newly diagnosed cancers is a malignancy of the skin.
2. **Malignant melanoma accounts for almost three-fourths of all skin cancer deaths.** The median age at diagnosis of persons with malignant melanoma is 45 years.
3. **History assessment**
   a. See **text page 155,** column 2, for a list of questions to ask.
   b. A **change in a preexisting mole** or the **development of a new mole** in an adult is of great importance and requires inspection.
4. **Physical examination**
   a. The **entire integument** must be inspected; all areas exposed to the sun should be meticulously assessed.
   b. The surface distribution of melanomas in black-skinned persons differs from that in white-skinned persons, with **relatively unpigmented areas** (e.g., palms) being primary sites.
   c. Location of moles should be **mapped** to serve as a baseline for future skin assessments.
   d. If a lesion is detected, the nurse should
      (1) Document the size, location, and description of the lesion.
      (2) Refer the patient to a physician for diagnosis.
      (3) Follow up with the patient for recurrent disease.
   e. The three types of skin cancers are **basal cell carcinoma, squamous cell carcinoma,** and **melanoma;** the three precancerous skin conditions are **leukoplakia, senile and actinic keratoses,** and **dysplastic nevi.** See **Table 8-6, text page 156,** and **Table 8-7, text page 157,** for further information about these conditions.
5. **Education**
   a. **Ultraviolet radiation from the sun** is the leading cause of skin cancer.
   b. The most carcinogenic of the ultraviolet wavelengths can be blocked by **sunscreening agents.**
      (1) Screening agents are rated according to **sun protection factor (SPF)** (e.g., 2 to 29).
      (2) An SPF of 2 means that proper application allows users to stay in the sun **twice as long** as they could without protection.
   c. Skin types are rated **from 1 to 6,** with **1 burning most easily** and **6 least easily.**
   d. See **text page 157,** column 1, for information that should be shared with patients about decreasing skin cancer risks.
   e. Routine self-examination of the skin is the best defense against skin cancer, especially malignant melanoma.
   f. High-risk individuals should be examined regularly, and a chart should be kept of their lesions.

g. Patients should also be instructed about the **changes in moles** that merit immediate attention: **size, color, elevation, surface characteristics,** and **sensation.**

h. Individuals with **familial DNS (dysplastic nevus syndrome)** should visit their clinician or dermatologist twice a year for assessment and follow-up.

i. Elderly persons should be singled out for instruction in self-assessment.

G. ORAL CANCER

1. The majority of **oral cancers** are cancers of the **mouth;** approximately 95% begin in the **surface mucosa.**

2. Success in treatment has not made significant headway during the past decade.

3. **History assessment**
    a. See **text page 159,** column 1, for a list of questions to ask.
    b. The majority of oral cancers cause no symptoms in their early stages. A "sore" in the mouth is usually attributed to other causes.
    c. Physical examination of the mouth includes **inspection, digital palpation,** and **olfaction of the oral cavity.**
    d. See **text page 159,** column 2, for a list of maneuvers that should be performed during the oral examination.
    e. Lesions of the **base of the tongue** are most often overlooked and must be both inspected and palpated.
    f. Squamous cell carcinomas frequently are found on the **floor of the mouth.**
    g. Individuals who use smokeless tobacco may develop **leukoplakias** and sometimes **keratoses** where they hold the quid; white lesions that adhere to the surface are classified as **keratotic** and have a greater probability of malignancy.
    h. **Solar keratoses** occur on sun-exposed surfaces and are flat, reddish-to-tan plaques that are usually scaly. The lip should be palpated to determine malignancy.
    i. All large, fungating oral cancers produce a **marked halitosis.**

4. **Screening**
    a. **Alcoholics who smoke** constitute the largest risk group for oral cancers. Screening should be geared to this population.
    b. Screening programs directed at alcoholics should be conducted in settings in which they can be approached as a group (e.g., shelters for the homeless).
    c. The role of the nurse is to
        (1) Encourage individuals over the age of 40 to have periodic oral and dental examinations.
        (2) Stress to young people the dangers of smokeless tobacco.

H. GYNECOLOGIC CANCER

1. **Cervical cancers** are less prevalent but more fatal than **endometrial cancers.** The risk of endometrial cancer is age-related.

2. **Ovarian cancer has a much higher mortality rate than either cervical or endometrial cancer.** It accounts for about 52% of all gynecologic cancer deaths.

3. **History assessment**
    a. The majority of women at risk for cancer of the reproductive organs can be identified only **after a thorough gynecologic history** has been obtained.
    b. See **text page 161,** column 1, for questions to ask.

4. **Physical examination**
    a. The early signs and symptoms of the different gynecologic cancers vary.
        (1) Ovarian cancer usually has **no early manifestations.**
        (2) An early sign of endometrial cancer may be **unexplained bleeding** or a **malodorous watery discharge.**
        (3) Symptoms of cervical cancer typically are **abnormal vaginal discharge, irregular bleeding, elongation of menstrual period,** or **bleeding that occurs after douching or intercourse.**
    b. The gynecologic examination includes **inspection and palpation of the abdomen, vulva, vagina, cervix, uterus and adnexa, ovaries, and rectovaginal area.**
    c. In general the findings on the pelvic examination that can alert the nurse to possible ovarian cancer are **adnexal enlargement, fixation or immobility, bilateral irregularity or nodulation and masses, relative insensitivity of the mass,** and **bilaterality of the mass.**

(1) A mass in the upper portion of the abdomen may suggest the presence of **omental cake,** a sign of advanced disease.

   d. Infection with **human papillomavirus (HPV)** may produce vulvar warts and may infect the entire lower female genital tract.

     (1) Warts can be observed by simple observation or by **staining by acetic acid** (the acetowhite reaction).

     (2) **Colposcopic examination** can then be used to inspect the lesions.

   e. **Induration** and **nodulation** may indicate submucosal vaginal lesions. Most squamous cell carcinomas are found in the **posterior vaginal wall** and in the **upper third of the vagina.**

   f. A **Pap smear** should be taken for cytologic examination of the cervix. The sample should include cells from the squamous epithelium of the vaginal portion of the cervix, the transformation zone, and the endocervical epithelium.

   g. The cervix is freely movable, firm, and smooth; if it has been invaded with cancer it becomes **hard and immobile** and develops a **rough, granular surface.**

   h. **Suction curettage** is preferred over the conventional Pap smear for detection of endometrial cancer. It is recommended for **menopausal women** and women who have received **long-term estrogen therapy.**

   i. **Uterine tenderness, immobility, or enlargement** merits further investigation. An enlarged boggy uterus is an indication of advanced disease.

   j. Palpation of the anterior rectal wall in the region of the peritoneal rectovaginal pouch is important in the detection of the spread of cervical and ovarian cancer.

5. **Screening of asymptomatic individuals**

   a. The ACS recommends that all women who are, or who have been, **sexually active** or have **reached 18 years of age,** have an annual Pap test and pelvic examination.

   b. False-negative results from Pap smears and other errors can be made by the patient, physician, or laboratory. Nurses can play a significant role in decreasing patient and physician error by

     (1) Educating women about the **early symptoms of gynecologic cancer** and the necessity of seeking medical advice with these early symptoms.

     (2) Educating women about the **recommended intervals for Pap tests** and about the necessity of **asking for a Pap test** when they have a physical examination.

     (3) Educating women about **how Pap tests are reported** and about **how to discuss results with the physician.**

     (4) Educating women about the importance of receiving **additional medical care with an abnormal or questionable Pap smear finding.**

     (5) **Performing Pap smears** only after they are thoroughly versed in the proper procedures for obtaining a smear.

   c. Two classification methods are used to identify abnormal changes in the Pap smear.

     (1) The World Health Organization identifies two types of lesions, **dysplasia** and **cancer in situ,** and distinguishes among **grades of dysplasia.**

     (2) The **CIN (cervical intraepithelial neoplasia) nomenclature** is a continuum of change and passes through phases **CIN 1, CIN 2,** and **CIN 3,** corresponding to mild, moderate, and severe dysplasia/carcinoma in situ.

     (3) See **Table 8-8, text page 163,** for a comparison of Pap terminology to the CIN classification.

   d. **Colposcopic examination** is used to evaluate the cervix and vagina of a woman with an abnormal Pap smear. It provides both **visualization** of the cervical transformation zone and a **biopsy** of specific areas of the epithelium.

6. **Additional nursing interventions**

   a. Nurses are urged to seek out, screen, and if necessary refer to physicians women who are at high risk for gynecologic cancer, including

     (1) **Postmenopausal women** who are at risk for ovarian and endometrial cancers, including those who are taking estrogens.

     (2) Women who are being followed routinely for **chronic problems.**

     (3) **Older women** who are at high risk for endometrial, vulvar, vaginal, and ovarian cancer.

     (4) Young women who have had **venereal disease** or who have **vulvar condyloma acuminatum and warty infections** such as koilocytotic cells or who show cells consistent with squamous papilloma or warty atypia.

   b. Nurses are urged to help overcome the barriers to early detection in older women, including

     (1) The mistaken belief that women do not need pelvic examinations after menopause.

        (2)   Fear of physical examinations associated with physical changes in the bodies of older women.

        (3)   Misattribution of cancer symptoms to normal signs of aging of the reproductive system.

    c.   Nurses are urged to acquire physical assessment skills that will enable them to perform pelvic examinations.

        (1)   This will allow them to reach those women who are at highest risk but who are least likely to use conventional screening programs or have routine health examinations, including older and poorer women.

        (2)   It will also expand the total number of screening programs available to women.

PRACTICE QUESTIONS

1. Which of the following statements about prevention and its three levels is correct?
   - (A) One purpose of secondary prevention is to decrease the vulnerability of the individual to illness through health-promoting strategies.
   - (B) Prevention can occur long after a disease has been diagnosed.
   - (C) Tertiary prevention focuses on protecting persons from disease by providing reduced exposure to environmental health risks.
   - (D) An ounce of prevention is always worth a pound of cure.

2. An example of a health promotion program that is both **active** and **public** would be a
   - (A) government-sponsored fitness program.
   - (B) weight-control clinic sponsored by a health club.
   - (C) government program to clean up polluted rivers.
   - (D) plan by power companies to reduce acid rain.

3. Chemoprevention is **best** defined by which of the following definitions?
   - (A) It is the use of natural body immune mechanisms to bolster the body's response to cancer in order to avoid use of chemotherapy.
   - (B) It is the use of chemicals or micronutrients to inhibit or reverse the process of carcinogenesis.
   - (C) It is the use of radiotherapy alone as the primary treatment modality for a specific cancer.
   - (D) It is the use of high doses of vitamins as the primary treatment modality for fighting cancer.

4. Which of the following questions would a nurse be **least** likely to ask in preparing a history and review of systems for lung cancer?
   - (A) Does your spouse smoke?
   - (B) Did you ever work in a shipyard?
   - (C) Have you ever been told you have emphysema?
   - (D) How often do you eat red meat?

5. Which of the following signs would be **most** indicative of lung cancer?
   - (A) occult blood
   - (B) peau d'orange
   - (C) finger clubbing
   - (D) actinic keratoses

6. Percussion and auscultation may provide final clues to assessment of the individual who is at high risk for lung cancer. Physical signs to look for include all of the following **except**
   - (A) dullness, indicating pleural effusion.
   - (B) decreased or absent breath sounds.
   - (C) the bagpipe sign.
   - (D) deep, sustained borborygmi.

7. The major demographic predictor of both smoking and the cessation of smoking is
   - (A) income.
   - (B) education level.
   - (C) gender.
   - (D) race.

8.   Three findings during the physical examination strongly suggest cancer of the colorectal area. These include all of the following **except**
     (A)   a mass palpated in the rectum.
     (B)   a hydrocele mass in the colon.
     (C)   a palpable mass in the abdomen.
     (D)   evidence of blood in the feces.

9.   A dietary regimen that might be suggested by a nurse educator as a means of lowering overall cancer risk, including risk of colorectal cancer, would likely include all of the following recommendations **except**
     (A)   Consume more high-fiber foods.
     (B)   Decrease total fat intake.
     (C)   Decrease vitamin A and C intake.
     (D)   Consume moderate amounts of alcoholic beverages.

10.   Early prostate cancer can usually be distinguished from benign prostate hypertrophy by the
      (A)   presence of hard nodules located within the posterior part of the prostate.
      (B)   enlargement of the prostate and the presence of spongy masses on the anterior side of the gland.
      (C)   existence of specific and sensitive tumor markers, including prostate-specific antigen.
      (D)   enlargement of the prostate and the diffusion of tissue into an undifferentiated mass.

11.   The **most** effective screening technique for prostate cancer is a(n)
      (A)   PSA level combined with a digital rectal examination.
      (B)   abdominal CT scan.
      (C)   ultrasound and abdominal CT scan.
      (D)   PSA level, CT scan, and ultrasound.

12.   Most palpable breast tumors are discovered by
      (A)   mammography.
      (B)   palpation by the examining clinician.
      (C)   women themselves.
      (D)   ultrasound.

13.   In a physical examination of a woman at high risk for breast cancer, which of the following signs would be visible evidence of a tumor?
      (A)   spoke wheel-like ducts on the nipple
      (B)   a soft, round mass in the deep tissue of the breast
      (C)   an absence of typical unilateral venous prominence
      (D)   unilateral flattening of the nipple

14.   Which of the following statements about breast self-examination (BSE) is correct?
      (A)   The U.S. Preventive Services Task Force recommends including BSE instruction as part of the periodic health examination.
      (B)   To date there have been no prospective randomized studies testing the benefits of BSE.
      (C)   Authorities are in agreement that there is sufficient evidence to justify BSE as a large-scale, community-based intervention.
      (D)   Nurses instructing women on BSE should demonstrate the procedure using their hands and the patient's breast.

15.   Physical examination of a patient at risk for testicular cancer reveals testes that are symmetric and somewhat rubbery and spongy, and with small indurations on the surface of one testis. Scrotal skin is loose and thick. Transillumination in a darkened room indicates the presence of a hydrocele. Which of these signs is indicative of possible malignancy?
      (A)   the indurations and the hydrocele
      (B)   the smooth surface and the rubbery composition of one testis
      (C)   the hydrocele and the loose, thick scrotum
      (D)   the symmetry of the testes and the smooth surface of one testis

16. Physical examination of the integument of a patient reveals the presence on the forearm of a flat plaque with defined margins and a crusted and erythematous center. The **most** likely diagnosis is
    (A) dysplastic nevi.
    (B) squamous cell carcinoma.
    (C) malignant melanoma.
    (D) basal cell carcinoma.

17. Individuals who use smokeless tobacco are most likely to develop which of the following?
    (A) dysplastic nevi on the tongue
    (B) leukoplakias between the cheek and gums
    (C) squamous cell carcinomas on the floor of the mouth
    (D) large, fungating cancers in the upper throat

18. Which of the following factors is **most** likely to be associated with oral cancer?
    (A) alcohol use
    (B) a diet high in fat
    (C) overexposure to sun
    (D) exposure to asbestos

19. The most fatal of the various gynecologic cancers is
    (A) cervical cancer.
    (B) endometrial cancer.
    (C) ovarian cancer.
    (D) vaginal cancer.

20. The Pap smear is used commonly to detect cervical endometrial cancers. Another diagnostic method, suction curettage, is preferable to the Pap smear under what conditions?
    (A) for diagnosing endometrial cancer in postmenopausal women
    (B) for detecting cervical cancer in women infected with HPV
    (C) for reducing false-negative results in women at high risk for ovarian cancer
    (D) for detecting tumors in the region of the peritoneal rectovaginal pouch

21. Abnormal changes in a woman's Pap smear are classified as CIN 3 in the cervical intraepithelial (CIN) nomenclature. The CIN 3 classification corresponds with what class in the World Health Organization's classification of cervical abnormality?
    (A) Class II: atypical cells below the level of neoplasia
    (B) Class III: moderate dysplasia
    (C) Class III: mild dysplasia
    (D) Class IV: severe dysplasia and carcinoma in situ

22. All of the following are responsibilities of nurses in educating women about gynecologic cancers **except**
    (A) helping older women overcome their anxieties about pelvic examinations.
    (B) reminding postmenopausal women that they no longer need regular pelvic examinations.
    (C) alerting younger women who have had venereal disease to the necessity of having regular Pap smears.
    (D) referring women with vulvar condyloma acuminatum for a thorough gynecologic examination that includes acetic acid compress application.

ANSWER EXPLANATIONS

1. **The answer is (B).** Prevention consists of all measures, including definitive therapy, that limit the progression of disease **at any point of its course.** Preventive strategies can therefore be adopted while one is healthy, during the phase of determining whether one has the disease, or during the phase of dealing with a disease already contracted. Despite the old saying about prevention and cure, prevention **can** at times be more expensive than a cure. Society and the individual must look at relatives costs and benefits of preventive measures. (126)

2. **The answer is (A).** The program is government-sponsored and is therefore public. And because it depends on individuals to adopt the fitness program, it is active. Choice (B) is private and active; (C) is public and passive; (D) is private and passive. (127)

3.　**The answer is (B).**　Chemoprevention is the use of defined chemicals or micronutrients to inhibit or reverse the process of carcinogenesis. The agents being commonly studied in clinical trials include vitamins A, C, D, and E; folic acid; calcium; and selenium. (129)

4.　**The answer is (D).**　The first three questions all address major risk factors in lung cancer; the fourth is more appropriate for a history of someone at risk for colorectal cancer. Choice (A) deals with the risks of passive smoking and would be especially appropriate if the patient was not a smoker himself or herself. (131)

5.　**The answer is (C).**　Finger clubbing may be either an early or a late sign of thoracic disease, and it may be absent even in the presence of advanced disease. Choice (A) would apply to colorectal cancer if the blood were in the feces; choice (B) is a sign of breast cancer; choice (D) is a sign of skin cancer particularly. (133)

6.　**The answer is (D).**　Borborygmi are bowel sounds that are heard without the use of a stethoscope. The other signs, along with whispered pectoriloquy, bronchophony, and egophony, are all associated with lung cancer. (133–135)

7.　**The answer is (B).**　A person who does not attend college is more than twice as likely to start smoking than the person who does. In addition, smoking cessation occurs more frequently in groups with higher levels of education than in groups with less education, and the gap is widening over time. (133)

8.　**The answer is (B).**　Hydroceles may develop as a result of a tumor, but a hydrocele would be unlikely to show up in a physical examination for colorectal cancer. The other signs are all strongly suggestive of colorectal cancer. (141)

9.　**The answer is (C).**　The ACS and NCI recommendations call for including foods rich in vitamins A and C, such as carrots, tomatoes, spinach, and peaches, as well as foods low in fat and high in fiber. Other recommendations include avoiding obesity, eating moderate amounts of salt-cured, smoked, and nitrite-cured foods, and including cruciferous vegetables in the diet. (144)

10.　**The answer is (A).**　Enlargement of the prostate is a sign of benign prostate hypertrophy. Neither prostate-specific antigen nor prostatic acid phosphatase, two biochemical indicators (or tumor markers) used to detect prostate cancer, has been shown to be specific or sensitive enough to use in early detection. (145–146)

11.　**The answer is (A).**　Screening techniques for prostate cancer require both a prostate-specific antigen (PSA) level and a digital rectal examination since each one by itself is inadequate in finding cancer. Ultrasounds and CT scans are more costly and require time availability, neither of which enhances routine screening. (146–147)

12.　**The answer is (C).**　The most common presenting complaint of women with breast cancer is a painless lump or mass in the breast. An estimated 90% of all palpable breast tumors are discovered by women themselves either accidentally or through planned self-examination. Both mammography and palpation of the breast by the health professional are also important means of tumor detection. (148)

13.　**The answer is (D).**　Spoke wheel-like ducts on the nipple and an absence of venous prominence on the breast are both normal. Breast tumors are typically hard, poorly circumscribed nodules fixed to the skin. Unilateral flattening of the nipple is caused by fibrosis and contraction of fibrotic tissue, which indicate a breast tumor. (148)

14.　**The answer is (B).**　Although many authorities believe BSE should be encouraged as part of a woman's regular medical care, there probably is not sufficient evidence to justify BSE as a large-scale, community-based intervention. Part of the problem is that to date there have been no prospective randomized studies testing the benefits of BSE. There is therefore considerable debate about the value of BSE in reducing mortality and increasing survival rates. (151)

15.　**The answer is (A).**　The testes should be smooth, fairly symmetric (with the left testis often slightly lower), and spongy and rubbery to the feel. Lumps and indurations are abnormal, as is the presence of a hydrocele, which may develop as a result of tumor. Scrotal skin should not appear stretched and thin. (153)

16.   **The answer is (D).**   Squamous cell carcinomas are opaque and appear as either elevated nodules, punched-out ulcerative lesions, or large fungating masses. Both dysplastic nevi and malignant melanoma have irregular borders and are more deeply pigmented. Malignant melanomas also appear mainly on covered parts of the body. Superficial basal cell carcinomas fit the description in choice (D). (pp. 156–157, Tables 8-6, 8-7)

17.   **The answer is (B).**   Tobacco chewers often develop leukoplakias and sometimes keratoses where they hold their quid (tobacco). White lesions that adhere to the surface are classified as keratotic and have a greater probability of malignancy. Other precancerous and cancerous conditions may also develop. (160)

18.   **The answer is (A).**   Exposure to sun may cause solar keratoses and cancer of the lip, but alcoholics who smoke constitute the largest risk group for oral cancers. (160)

19.   **The answer is (C).**   Ovarian cancer has a far higher mortality rate than the other gynecologic cancers. Its incidence rate, however, is lower than that of endometrial cancer though higher than that of cervical cancer. (161)

20.   **The answer is (A).**   The conventional Pap smear is inaccurate for a diagnosis of endometrial lesions. For this reason suction curettage is recommended for menopausal women and women who have received long-term estrogen therapy. Suction curettage can provide an excellent sample and in most cases can be done in the office without need for anesthesia. (162)

21.   **The answer is (D).**   The results of the Pap smear indicate that the smear contains abnormal cells consistent with carcinoma in situ, Class IV of the World Health Organization's classification. (163 and Table 8-8)

22.   **The answer is (B).**   This should be obvious. Many postmenopausal women mistakenly believe that once they are past child-bearing years and/or are sexually inactive, they no longer need pelvic examinations. When appropriate, nurses should discuss the myths of menopause with both pre- and postmenopausal women, including the myth that sexual inactivity or menopause means the end of risk for gynecologic cancers. (164)

9   Diagnostic Evaluation, Classification, and Staging

STUDY OUTLINE

I.   **DIAGNOSTIC EVALUATION**

    A.   **FACTORS THAT AFFECT THE DIAGNOSTIC APPROACH**

       1.   **Early diagnosis of a precancerous lesion or a malignant neoplasm affords the best opportunity for treatment and survival.**
       2.   The nurse can intervene in the diagnostic process by
          a.   Alerting the public to the seven warning signals of cancer.
          b.   Developing detection programs that are accessible, affordable, and ethnically relevant.
       3.   The major goals of the diagnostic evaluation for suspected cancer are to determine
          a.   **Whether the tumor is benign or malignant.**
          b.   **The tissue type of the malignancy.**
          c.   **The primary site of the malignancy** (or **site of origin**).
          d.   **The extent of disease within the body** (or **metastatic sites**).
       4.   Diagnoses begins with an effective clinical evaluation of the patient, including
          a.   **A comprehensive history with the identification of known risk factors.**
          b.   **A thorough physical examination.**
          c.   **Histologic verification of the malignancy.**
          d.   **Appropriate laboratory and imaging tests based on results of biopsy.**
       5.   The diagnostic approach used for an individual with a suspected malignancy depends on
          a.   **The patient's presenting signs and symptoms.**
          b.   **The biologic characteristics of the suspected malignancy.**
          c.   **The patient's clinical status and ability to tolerate invasive procedures.**
          d.   **The diagnostic equipment in the patient's community.**
          e.   **The anticipated goal of treatment when the diagnosis is made.**
       6.   The proper test is one that **yields information on the suspicious site of malignancy** and **complements known information.**
       7.   One danger is **overinvestigation** by the physician. This may be caused by several factors, including
          a.   The increased availability of sophisticated equipment.
          b.   The fear of litigation if tests are not conducted.
          c.   Pressure from patients and families.
       8.   Third party payers and health maintenance organizations will play an important role in the diagnostic evaluation.

    B.   **NURSING IMPLICATIONS IN DIAGNOSTIC EVALUATION**

       1.   A major function of the nurse is to **provide accurate information through patient/family education.** The first step is to **assess the patient's and family's desire to know and ability to understand.**
       2.   The nurse should prepare the patient for the examination by
          a.   **Explaining the procedure to be followed.**
          b.   **Describing any physical sensations that might be expected, including pain or discomfort, as well as any potential complications that may arise from the procedure.**

    c.   **Identifying the purpose of the examination, when the results can be expected, and from whom to expect them.**

    d.   **Providing more specific nursing interventions as called for by the diagnosis.**

3.   Many opportunities exist for a nurse to promote the **early detection and diagnosis** of cancer. Nurses need to realize the **meaning of clinical signs** of cancer, be able to **assess** an **individual's risk** for cancer, and **take responsibility** for **encouraging investigation** and **intervention.**

4.   See **Table 9-1, text page 172,** for **seven warning signals** of cancer and their significance.

5.   In addition to nurses being proficient in **physical assessment and screening techniques,** they can integrate **instruction** on **breast self-examination** or **testicular self-examination** in most practice settings.

6.   Nurses are involved in **providing support** to patients facing the potential threat of cancer during the **prediagnostic period** when patients are attaching meaning to a suspicious symptom through the diagnostic evaluation when they are experiencing tests.

7.   See **text page 173** for **specific nursing interventions.**

C. **LABORATORY TECHNIQUES**

1.   **Laboratory studies are performed to help formulate a clinical diagnosis and to monitor the patient's response to a specific therapy.** The data provide information on the functioning of specific organs and metabolic processes that may be altered by disease and treatment.

2.   **Biochemical analysis** of blood, serum, urine, and other body fluids identifies chemical and hematologic **values outside the narrow, homeostatic range.** Specific malignancies characteristically alter chemical composition of the blood, but there is no single value diagnostic for a malignancy.

3.   The value of a laboratory study or imaging technique is measured in terms of **sensitivity** and **specificity.**

    a.   **Sensitivity** establishes the percentage of patients with cancer who will have positive (abnormal) test results, known as **true positive** results. Negative results on a patient with cancer—whose results **should** be positive—are termed **false negative** findings.

    b.   **Specificity** establishes the percentage of patients without cancer who will have negative (normal) test results, known as **true negative** results. Positive results on a patient free of cancer—whose results **should** be negative—are termed **false positive** results.

    c.   The most clinically useful tests are those with **both high sensitivity and high specificity.**

4.   Among the most common laboratory tests are **biochemical analyses of blood, serum, urine, and other body fluids.** Chemical values outside the normal, narrow range may indicate malignancy, e.g., immature blast cells in complete blood count indicative of leukemia.

5.   **Tumor markers** (discussed in Chapter 8) are biochemical molecules released from the tumor into the blood or produced by normal tissue in response to the tumor.

    a.   Most tumor markers **lack specificity,** however, and are more useful in monitoring disease than in detecting it.

    b.   One tumor marker with both high specificity and high sensitivity is **human chorionic gonadotropin,** used to detect gestational trophoblastic tumors.

    c.   **Radioimmunoassay** is used to measure tumor markers. It determines the **amount of tumor antigen in a serum sample.**

    d.   See **Table 9-2, text pages 174–175,** for a discussion of **tumor markers** in the diagnosis and monitoring of malignant disease.

6.   All laboratory studies must be evaluated in conjunction with the results of other clinical data.

7.   **Flow cytometry describes DNA characteristics** and **cell surface markers** that correlate with patient prognosis and are useful in diagnosing malignancy and monitoring therapy response.

D. **TUMOR IMAGING**

1.   **Tumor imaging is used to ascertain the presence of a tumor mass, localize the mass for biopsy, provide tissue characterization, and further assess or stage the anatomic extent of disease.**

2.   **Table 9-3, text page 177,** identifies preferred imaging procedures for tumor definition and staging in several organ sites.

3.   **Radiographic techniques**

    a.   **Radiographic studies,** or **X-ray films,** distinguish between normal and abnormal internal structures of the body. They may be **site specific** (e.g., a chest X ray) or they may view the **dynamic function of an entire organ system** (e.g., a series of X-ray films of the gastrointestinal system).

b. **Screen-film mammography** and **xeromammography** are used to detect breast tumors. The latter may be preferred for diagnostic imaging because it **penetrates deeper into tissue and is better able to image the retromammary space.**

c. **Tomography** provides a radiographic image of a **selected layer or plane of the body that would otherwise be obscured by shadows of other structures.** It is particularly helpful in evaluating small calcified or cavitated lesions in the chest, hilar adenopathy, and mediastinal abnormalities.

d. **Computerized axial tomography (CT or CAT)** also provides sectional views of structures in the body.
   (1) A computer analyzes **serial X-ray exposures through different angles of the body.**
   (2) It is used to detect **minor differences between tissue densities** in any area of the body.
   (3) Its major drawback is its production of **artifact** in areas of cortical bone content.
   (4) CT frequently is used to direct a needle to the tumor site for percutaneous biopsy.

e. Several radiographic examinations rely on **contrast materials** to enhance the outline structures to be visualized, e.g., an excretory radiograph that uses **iodinated contrast agents.**
   (1) Iodinated contrast agents can produce adverse reactions, including **nausea, localized pain at the injection site, a metallic or bitter taste, and flushing,** lasting from 1 to 3 minutes.
   (2) Severe reaction is uncommon, but any patient with a history of allergic response should be closely monitored.

f. **Lymphangiography** involves injection of an oily iodinated contrast agent to allow **visualization of the lymphatic tissues and nodes.**
   (1) This is indicated in the diagnosis and staging of **Hodgkin's and other lymphomas** and in some **pelvic cancers.**
   (2) Nurses should be aware of the potential reaction of **pulmonary microembolization.**

g. **Intrathecal contrast agents** are used in myelography and in computerized tomography.

h. **Barium sulfate,** a nonabsorbable, radiopaque contrast agent that coats the intraluminal surface, is used in the examination of the gastrointestinal tract.
   (1) **Combined with air** in a double contrast study, it gives a more sensitive method of detecting gastrointestinal tumors than if it is used alone.
   (2) A laxative or enema may be administered to counteract fecal retention that may occur.

4. **Nuclear medicine techniques**
   a. **Nuclear medicine imaging** involves the intravenous injection or the ingestion of radioisotope compounds, followed by the sensitive camera imaging of those organs or tissues that have concentrated the radioisotopes.
      (1) These studies are very sensitive and will often detect malignancies or sites of abnormal metabolism months before they are seen on a radiograph.
      (2) Computerized tomography, however, has replaced many radioisotope examinations.
   b. **Positive emission tomography** provides information on the biochemical and metabolic activity of tissue.
      (1) Compounds such as glucose are tagged with **radioactive particles that emit positrons.** The image in tissues is then detected by **gamma camera tomography.**
      (2) It has proved most useful in **brain imaging.**
   c. Nuclear imaging with **radiolabeled monoclonal antibodies,** which bind to antigens on the tumor, are also being used investigationally to visualize microscopic sites of metastasis or suspected malignancy.
      (1) Sensitivity and specificity are high in some tumor types (e.g., the colon, breast, and ovaries).
      (2) There are no apparent side effects.

5. **Ultrasonography**
   a. **Ultrasonography** is a nonradiographic and noninvasive technique of imaging deep structures within the body.
      (1) **High-frequency sound waves** are directed into specific tissue and their **reflecting echoes are recorded on an imaging screen.**
      (2) It is most useful for **tumors larger than 2 cm in diameter in the pelvis, retroperitoneum, and the peritoneum.**

6. **Magnetic resonance imaging**
   a. **Magnetic resonance imaging** creates sectional images of the body, similar to computerized tomography, without exposing the patient to radiation.
   b. A powerful **magnetic field** is used to align the body's hydrogen nuclei in one direction. Radiofrequency pulses are then used to **excite the magnetized nuclei and change their alignment.**
   c. Between pulses nuclei return to their relaxed state, and various signals are transmitted on the basis of tissue characteristics.
   d. These signals are **analyzed by the computer,** and **multiplaner images are generated.**
   e. Images can be enhanced with the intravenous paramagnetic contrast agent **DTPA.** Adverse reactions are rare.
   f. MRI imaging is most applicable in the detection, localization, and staging of tumors in the central nervous system, spine, head and neck, and musculoskeletal system. DTPA-enhanced imaging is the preferred imaging modality in **brain tumors.**
   g. Patients with **any metallic implant** are excluded from MRI imaging.

E. **INVASIVE DIAGNOSTIC TECHNIQUES**

1. **Endoscopy**
   a. **Endoscopy** is a method of directly visualizing the interior of a hollow viscus by the insertion of an **endoscope** into a body cavity or opening. The scope can be rigid or flexible.
   b. Various types of endoscopes allow visualization of the GI tract, respiratory system, reproductive system, peritoneum, pleura, mediastinum, and diaphragm.
2. **Biopsy**
   a. **Histologic or cytologic proof of malignancy is vital.** For example, treatment decisions for cancers arising within the same organ may differ on the basis of the histopathology report.
   b. **Cytologic examination of aspirated fluids, scrapings, or washings of body cavities** is useful in revealing malignant cells that have exfoliated from a primary or metastatic tumor, e.g., a Pap smear.
      (1) Tissue will not be obtained in this manner, however, which limits the ability to establish the primary site of a tumor.
   c. A **biopsy** provides tissue for histologic examination. Specimens must be adequate for diagnostic evaluation.
   d. What tissue is to be biopsied depends on the **clinical status of the patient, the patient's willingness to undergo invasive procedures, the size and location of the identified tumor,** and **amount of tissue needed for analysis.**

II. **CLASSIFICATION AND NOMENCLATURE**

A. **BASIC TERMINOLOGY**

1. **Tumor** is a swelling or mass of tissue that may be malign or malignant.
2. **Cancer,** or **malignant neoplasm,** is an uncontrolled "new growth" capable of metastasis and invasion that threatens host survival.
3. **Primary site** is used to describe the original histologic site of tumorigenesis.
   a. A **secondary** or **metastatic tumor** resembles the primary tumor histologically but sometimes may be so anaplastic as to obscure the cell of origin.
   b. A **second primary lesion** refers to an additional, histologically separate cancer in the same patient.

B. **BENIGN AND MALIGNANT TUMOR CHARACTERISTICS**

1. With the exception of the properties of invasion and metastasis, the differences between a benign process and malignant process are **relative.** Some cancers appear benign; some benign tumors become malignant over time.

C. **TUMOR CLASSIFICATION SYSTEM**

1. See **Table 9-6, text page 187,** for selected benign and malignant neoplasms listed by histogenetic classification.

2. Tumors may be classified by their **biologic behavior** (benign or malignant) or by their **tissue of origin.** Virtually every cell (and therefore tissue) in the body is capable of forming into a malignant cell.
   a. Normal tissue arises from the **ectoderm, mesoderm, or endoderm** of embryonic tissue.
3. Some common suffixes and prefixes that identify types of growths are
   a. **-oma** = a benign tumor usually. Exceptions are **lymphoma, melanoma,** and **hepatoma.**
   b. **Sarcoma** = a malignant tumor of the **connective tissues.**
   c. **Carcinoma** = a malignant tumor arising from **epithelial tissues.** These generally are of 2 types depending on the tissue of origin.
      (1) **Adeno** = a carcinoma that arises from **glandular epithelial tissue.**
      (2) **Squamous** = a carcinoma that arises from **squamous epithelial tissues.**
   d. **Blastoma** = malignant tumor that resembles the **primitive blastula stage in embryonic development,** e.g., neuroblastoma.
   e. **Mixed tumor** = a tumor with mixed elements but arising from the **same germ layer and tissue,** e.g., adenosquamous tumor.
   f. **Teratoma** or **tetracarcinoma** = a tumor that arises from tissues of **all three germ layers** and with **no relationship to the site of origin.**
   g. A few malignancies are named after the person who characterized them, e.g., **Hodgkin's disease, Ewing's sarcoma,** and **Wilms' tumor.**
   h. **Hematopoietic tumors** are classified separately by **predominant cell type** and their **acute or chronic nature.**

D. TUMORS OF UNKNOWN ORIGIN

1. The site of origin of some cancers may never be determined, however, even on autopsy. Most frequently the classification will be adenocarcinoma.
2. Prognosis with an **unknown primary** is **poor,** with an overall median survival of 5 months.
3. **Treatment** is based on the histology and is usually systemic (chemotherapy or hormone therapy).
4. Surgery or radiation therapy is used to **relieve the symptoms** of disease.

III. STAGING AND GRADING CLASSIFICATIONS

A. STAGING AND THE EXTENT OF THE DISEASE

1. **The staging process is a method of classifying a malignancy by the extent of spread within the body. It is based on the premise that cancers of similar histologic features and site of origin will extend and metastasize in a predictable manner.**
2. The objectives of solid tumor staging are to
   a. **Aid in treatment planning.**
   b. **Give prognostic information.**
   c. **Facilitate the exchange of information and comparative statistics between treatment centers.**
3. The TNM staging system classifies solid tumors by the **anatomic extent of the disease,** as determined clinically and histologically. Three categories are quantified: **T (primary tumor), N (regional lymph node metastasis),** and **M (distant metastasis).**
   a. The extent of the **primary tumor (T)** is evaluated on the basis of **depth of invasion, surface spread,** and **tumor size.**
      (1) T_0 signifies no evidence of a primary tumor.
      (2) T_1 **through** T_4 indicates gradations of progressive tumor size or extent.
      (3) **Tis** signifies carcinoma in situ.
   b. The extent of **regional lymph node metastasis (N)** is evaluated on the basis of **size and location of the nodes.**
      (1) N_0 signifies no regional involvement.
      (2) N_1 **through** N_3 signify gradations of progressive involvement of regional lymph nodes.
   c. The extent of **distant metastasis (M)** is evaluated on the basis of **single versus multiple sites,** and **degree of organ involvement.**
      (1) M_0 signifies **no distant metastasis.**
      (2) M_1 **through** M_3 signify gradations of **progressive metastases.**
      (3) A **subscript** may also specify the **site of the metastasis,** e.g., M_1PUL denotes pulmonary metastasis.

d. The TNM classification is based on **clinical** and **pathologic analyses.**
   (1) **cTNM or TNM refers to the clinical classification.** It accounts for information obtained from all clinical studies, from physical examination, and through surgical exploration.
   (2) **pTNM** includes all information from the clinical TNM staging plus information from pathologic examination of a resected specimen. This includes **resected tumor (pT), lymph nodes (pN),** and **distant metastasis (pM)** if they are evident on clinical staging.
   (3) **Retreatment TNM (rTNM)** and **autopsy TNM (aTNM)** are other classifications used less frequently.
e. After numerical values are assigned to the T, N, and M categories, they are **clustered into one of four stages (I through IV), or stage 0 for carcinoma in situ.**
   (1) All tumor sites are grouped differently on the basis of characteristics of the disease.
   (2) See **Table 9-8, text page 189,** for a description of staging criteria and percent 5-year survival.
f. Some malignant tumors are classified differently according to **depth of invasion into neighboring tissues** (e.g., melanomas, colorectal cancer, cervical and endometrial cancers) or by **symptomatology** (e.g., Hodgkin's disease).
g. The nonsolid tumors do not conform to solid tumor staging principles because of their disseminated nature, e.g., **leukemias and myelomas.** Different factors are used to classify these, including, for leukemias, **cell types, cell maturation,** and **acute or chronic nature.**
h. **Staging systems** for malignancies not yet classified by the TNM system are presently being **developed.** These include cancers of the **small intestine, mesothelioma, spinal cord, carcinoid,** and **Kaposi's sarcoma.**
i. The **staging system** of the **future** will be an **estimation of risk** based on the sum of risks associated with anatomic stage, morphologic grade, biologic grade, and genetic potential.

B. **PATIENT PERFORMANCE CLASSIFICATION**

1. The patient's **physical performance at the time of diagnosis and staging** will often influence the type of treatment selected and provide prognostic information.
2. **Host performance scales** (see **Table 9-9, text page 190**) are often used to evaluate the effects of treatment and disease on the ability of the patient to perform the normal activities of daily living.

C. **GRADING**

1. **Grading a malignant neoplasm is a method of classification based on histopathologic characteristics of the tissue.**
2. It assesses the **aggressiveness or degree of malignancy** by comparing the cellular anaplasia, differentiation, and mitotic activity with normal counterparts. Characteristics vary with each type of cancer.
3. Depending on the type of tumor, grading may have more or less prognostic value than staging does.
4. Grading systems may be **descriptive** or **numeric.** Each identifies the degree that normal differentiation has been lost in cells.

PRACTICE QUESTIONS

1. Each of the following is a major goal of the diagnostic evaluation of suspected cancer **except**
   (A) to determine the primary site of the malignancy.
   (B) to determine the risk factors of the malignancy.
   (C) to determine the extent of disease within the body.
   (D) to determine the tissue type of the malignancy.

2. Before a diagnostic evaluation is performed, the nurse should prepare the patient for the examination by doing all of the following **except**
   (A) explaining the procedure to be followed.
   (B) describing any physical sensations the patient may experience.
   (C) identifying the purpose of the examination.
   (D) reviewing the treatments that will follow.

3. A particular diagnostic test for cancer correctly identifies a high percentage of patients tested who have cancer. It also incorrectly identifies a large number of patients who do not have cancer as having the disease. This test has
   (A) high specificity and high sensitivity.
   (B) high specificity and low sensitivity.
   (C) low specificity and high sensitivity.
   (D) low specificity and low sensitivity.

4. The preferred imaging procedure for detection of tumors in the deep tissue of the breast is
   (A) xeromammography.
   (B) screen-film mammography.
   (C) computerized axial tomography.
   (D) lymphangiography.

5. The sensitivity of barium sulfate as an imaging agent in examination of the gastrointestinal tract is enhanced by combination with
   (A) DTPA.
   (B) an oily iodinated contrast agent.
   (C) a water-soluble iodinated contrast agent.
   (D) air.

6. Nuclear imaging with radiolabeled monoclonal antibodies has been very useful for visualizing microscopic sites of metastases or suspected malignancy. These antibodies work by
   (A) binding to antigens on the tumor surface.
   (B) concentrating in the cortical areas of small tumors.
   (C) penetrating the blood-brain barrier to reach the central nervous system.
   (D) emitting positrons that can then be detected by gamma camera tomography.

7. Ultrasonography is preferred to magnetic resonance imaging for detection of tumors in which of the following patients?
   (A) a patient with a pacemaker
   (B) a patient who is allergic to iodinated contrast agents
   (C) a patient who cannot be exposed to ionizing radiation
   (D) a patient with a tumor smaller than 2 cm

8. A flexible tube is passed through the mouth and stomach to the upper duodenum, where it is used to visualize and biopsy a lesion on the surface of the duodenum. The diagnostic device being used is the
   (A) thoracoscope.
   (B) peritoneoscope.
   (C) colposcope.
   (D) endoscope.

9. Cytologic examination of aspirated fluids, scrapings, or washings of body cavities is **most** useful in
   (A) establishing the primary site of a tumor.
   (B) revealing malignant cells that have exfoliated from a metastatic tumor.
   (C) supplying tissue that may be used for histologic examination of a tumor.
   (D) establishing the size and type of a primary tumor.

10. A malignancy is diagnosed as an adenosquamous carcinoma. What do we know about the tumor on the basis of this diagnosis?
    (A) that it resembles the primitive blastula stage in embryonic development
    (B) that it is a tumor with mixed elements that arose from the same germ layer and tissue
    (C) that it arose from the tissues of all three germ layers and has no relation to the site of origin
    (D) that it arose from a combination of glandular epithelial and connective tissues

11. A method of classifying a malignancy by the extent of spread within the body is **most** accurately called
    (A) grading.
    (B) staging.
    (C) imaging.
    (D) testing.

12. A TNM classification of a tumor identifies it as Stage II, T_2, N_1, M_0. What can we state with **greatest** certainty about this tumor?
    (A) that it has metastasized to multiple sites
    (B) that it is a carcinoma in situ
    (C) that it has metastasized to the lymph nodes
    (D) that it is operable but not resectable

13. A pTNM differs from a cTNM in that it includes information from
    (A) pathological studies only.
    (B) both clinical and pathological studies.
    (C) imaging studies, biopsy, and surgical exploration.
    (D) biopsy and surgical exploration only.

14. A method of classifying a malignant neoplasm based on histopathologic characteristics of the tissue is called
    (A) imaging.
    (B) performance classification.
    (C) testing.
    (D) grading.

ANSWER EXPLANATIONS

1. **The answer is (B).** Determination of risk factors in cancer is part of the process of assessment and detection primarily and is not a major goal of diagnostic evaluation. Some overlap exists, of course, in that diagnosis begins with a comprehensive history and the identification of known risk factors. (171)

2. **The answer is (D).** The nurse may also provide more specific nursing interventions as called for by the nursing diagnosis, including those related to knowledge deficits, grieving, ineffective coping, spiritual deficit, fear of death, and self-care deficit. (172–173)

3. **The answer is (C).** Sensitivity establishes the percentage of patients with cancer who will have positive (abnormal) test results, known as true positive results. Specificity establishes the percentage of patients without cancer who will have negative (normal) test results, known as true negative results. Positive results on a patient free of cancer—whose results should be negative—are termed false positive results. (174)

4. **The answer is (A).** The xeromammographic process penetrates deeper into the tissue than screen-film mammography. It is better able to image the retromammary space. (176)

5. **The answer is (D).** By combining barium with air, a double contrast study is performed, using radiography, that is more sensitive than barium alone in detecting primary gastrointestinal tumors. (181–182)

6. **The answer is (A).** Nuclear medicine imaging involves the intravenous injection or the ingestion of radioisotope compounds, followed by the sensitive camera imaging of those organs or tissues that have concentrated the radioisotopes. In the case of nuclear medicine with radiolabeled monoclonal antibodies, antibodies selectively bind to antigens on the tumor surface, even that of microscopic tumors, where they can be detected by camera imaging. Sensitivity and specificity are high in some tumor types (e.g., the colon, breast, and ovaries), and there are no apparent side effects. (182)

7. **The answer is (A).** Neither ultrasonography nor MRI uses ionizing radiation; MRI uses DPTA, a noniodinated contrast agent. Ultrasonography is largely ineffective in detecting tumors smaller than 2 cm. However, MRI has the drawback of not being available to patients with any type of metallic implant, including pacemakers, which might be removed from the patient's body by the powerful magnetic force used in MRI. (182)

8. **The answer is (D).** All of the others are specific types of endoscopes that may be inserted into other body cavities or openings and used to detect, diagnose, and remove tumors. The endoscope contains fiberoptic glass bundles that transmit light and then return an image to the optical head of the endoscope. Visual inspection, tissue biopsy, staging the extent of the disease, and the excision of pathologic processes are all possible through the endoscope. (184)

9. **The answer is (B).** Tissue will not be obtained in this manner, which limits the ability to establish the primary site of a tumor. A biopsy provides tissue for histologic examination. (184)

10. **The answer is (B).** A mixed tumor such as an adenosquamous carcinoma is a tumor with mixed elements that arise from the same germ layer and tissue. "Adeno" signifies that it arises from glandular epithelial tissue; "squamous" that it arises from squamous epithelial tissues. A malignant tumor of the connective tissues is a sarcoma and not a carcinoma. A tumor that arises from tissues of all three germ layers and with no relationship to the site of origin is a tetracarcinoma. A tumor that resembles the primitive blastula stage in embryonic development is a blastoma. (185)

11. **The answer is (B).** The staging process is a method of classifying a malignancy by the extent of spread within the body. It is based on the premise that cancers of similar histologic features and site of origin will extend and metastasize in a predictable manner. Its objectives are to aid in treatment planning, give prognostic information, and facilitate the exchange of information and comparative statistics between treatment centers. (185–186)

12. **The answer is (C).** T_2 indicates that it is a growing primary tumor; N_1 that it has invaded surrounding tissue and first-station lymph nodes; and M_0 that it has not metastasized any farther. The lesion is operable and resectable, but because of greater local extent, there is uncertainty as to completeness of removal. The stage indicates a good chance of survival (50% ± 5%). (Table 9-8, 189)

13. **The answer is (B).** pTNM, or pathological classification, includes all information from the clinical TNM staging (cTNM), including physical examination, imaging studies, biopsy, and surgical exploration, plus information from pathologic examination of a resected specimen. (188)

14. **The answer is (D).** Grading assesses the aggressiveness or degree of malignancy by comparing the cellular anaplasia, differentiation, and mitotic activity of tumor cells with normal counterparts. Characteristics vary with each type of cancer. (189–190)

10 Quality of Life as an Outcome of Cancer Treatment

STUDY OUTLINE

I. **INTRODUCTION**

1. Over the past two decades, the evaluation of **quality of life,** or **health-related quality of life (HQL),** has emerged as a key aspect of outcome evaluation of cancer treatment.
   a. Prior to this, length of survival was the primary outcome evaluated in oncology treatment research.
   b. It is now widely accepted that in most circumstances, **quality** of survival is as important as **quantity** of survival, and that severely toxic treatment must be evaluated for its detrimental impact as well as its survival benefit.
2. HQL evaluation entails a multidimensional quantification of patient functional status, usually as perceived by the patient.
3. Given the advent of hematopoietic growth factors and improved antiemetic regimens, the trend toward the application of treatment intensification strategies that can result in increased toxicity is likely to continue. This further increases the importance of evaluating toxicity, patient function, and patient preferences for treatment.
4. **HQL evaluation differs from classic toxicity ratings** in two important ways.
   a. HQL incorporates more aspects of function (such as mood, affect, social well-being) than those addressed by typical toxicity rating scales.
   b. HQL evaluation focuses on eliciting the patient's perspective.

II. **THE ROLE OF NURSING**

1. The **assessment of disease symptoms and treatment side effects** is a major component of HQL as it is understood today. Nursing is well positioned to play a leadership role in the HQL evaluation of clinical trials, since assessing and managing symptoms and side effects of treatment has been a primary domain of nurses caring for people with cancer.
2. Cooperative clinical trial organizations have exhibited a rapid growth of interest in including HQL in selected trials. In fact, every large cooperative clinical trial organization in Europe and North America is actively examining quality of life in some of its trials, and nursing has played a leadership role in a number of these initiatives.

III. **EVALUATING METHODS OF ASSESSMENT**

1. A number of validated HQL measures have become accepted for use in oncology in particular and chronic illness in general. The diversity of available measures is potentially valuable in that it provides the user with choices based on specific characteristics of the disease site, clinical trial, or HQL domain of interest.
2. Since there is no "gold standard" when selecting a measure, the **development, initial testing,** and **field performance** of a given measure should be critically evaluated.

A. **CONSTRUCT DEFINITION AS A FRAME FOR MEASUREMENT**

   1. A construct must be defined before it can be measured. The many different definitions of HQL found in the literature suggest that **all measures** of this concept are not conceptually equivalent.
   2. In evaluating a measure of HQL, one must consider the definition of HQL used to design the measure.
   3. Definitions of HQL may differ across studies, and the instrument may still measure reliably and validly within the parameters of the definition adopted and within the range of the instrument's item content.

IV. **APPROACHES TO MEASURING HEALTH-RELATED QUALITY OF LIFE**

   1. Two approaches to measuring HQL have evolved: **psychometric** and **utility.** Integrating these two approaches is a critical challenge in HQL assessment.

A. **PSYCHOMETRIC APPROACH**

   1. The **psychometric approach** includes both generic health profile instruments and instruments intended to measure the multidimensional impact of a specific disease, treatment, or condition.
       a. An advantage of the psychometric approach is that it measures individual responses and **subjective** or **perceived** well-being and thus captures the variability in HQL across individuals.
       b. Studies have not connected these individual responses and perceptions to patients' values and preferences regarding their current health status. Without a rating of patient preference, one cannot appropriately make a decision about the value of a given treatment to a given patient.
       c. This poses a problem in a clinical trial where the primary purpose for integrating HQL measurement is to incorporate data on the impact of treatment on both length of life and quality of life into conclusions about treatment efficacy.

B. **UTILITY APPROACH**

   1. The utility approach is concerned with evaluating treatments as to their benefit compared in some way to their cost.
   2. There are two general utility methods.
       a. In the **standard gamble approach,** people are asked to imagine a particular state of health and then to choose between that state of health and a "gamble" in which they have various probabilities for death or perfect health (cure).
       b. In the **time trade-off method,** people are asked how much time they would be willing to give up in order to live out their remaining life expectancy in perfect health. All utility approaches use a 0–1 scale in which 0 = death and 1 = perfect health.
   3. Most utility analyses have employed expert estimates of weights or weights provided by healthy members of the general public. Studies have suggested that these surrogates may not provide accurate approximations of the perceptions of actual patients.
   4. Practical barriers to the collection of utilities directly from patients include the complexity of the concepts involved and the requirement for an interviewer-administered questionnaire.
   5. The usefulness of utility assessments of HQL may also be limited since they do not provide information about important disease- and treatment-related problems, may be less sensitive than psychometric approaches to changes in HQL over time, and may not be independent of mood and depression.
   6. A modified utility approach Q-TWiST (Quality-Adjusted Time Without Symptoms and Toxicity) is used to evaluate the effectiveness of adjuvant chemotherapy for early-stage breast cancer. The Q-TWiST discounts survival time spent with toxicity or symptoms relative to disease-free survival off therapy. However, the utility estimates of Q-TWiST are based on the patient preferences hypothesized by investigators.
   7. **Integrating** psychometric and utility approaches to the assessment of HQL is a key challenge since neither approach alone is sufficient.

V.   **EVALUATING PSYCHOMETRIC MEASURES**

1.   When selecting a measure to evaluate HQL, the investigator must carefully consider several factors, including the **purpose of the investigation,** the **psychometric properties** and **known performance** of available HQL measures, and the **relevance and appropriateness** of the instrument items. Evaluation of the measure for relevance and appropriateness is critical since it prevents selection of an otherwise valid measure that will not be sensitive for the application selected.

A.   **RELIABILITY**

1.   Reliability is the degree to which a measure will always produce the same score when applied in a particular situation, whether the measure is done by the same person or two different people.
2.   Reliability has two dimensions: **repeatability** and **consistency.**
   a.   Repeatability refers to the extent to which a measure applied at two different times (**test-retest reliability**) or in two different ways (**alternate form reliability and interrater reliability**) produces the same score.
   b.   **Consistency** refers to the degree to which all the items of a scale measure are **homogeneous** with respect to the concept or trait being measured. A measure's internal consistency is usually expressed in terms of Cronbach's coefficient alpha, because it is the most comprehensive strategy among those available and can be easily done with most computer statistical packages.
3.   Reliability is expressed as a **correlation coefficient** ranging between 0.0 and 1.0. The closer the correlation coefficient is to 1.00, the more reliable is the measure.
4.   Reliability is a matter of degree.
   a.   Reliability is not a fixed property of a measure but rather a property of a measure when used with certain people under certain conditions.
   b.   Reliability is not generalizeable; it must be reevaluated each time an instrument is used.
5.   Reliability depends on the number of items.
   a.   As the number of items goes up, so too does the reliability coefficient.
   b.   Subtests will usually have lower reliability than the total score, because they have fewer items.
6.   Reliability is increased by **heterogeneous samples.**

B.   **VALIDITY**

1.   Validity refers to a scale's ability to measure what it purports to measure. A scale must be reliable in order to be valid, but it does not need to be valid in order to be judged reliable.
2.   Validity can be divided into three types: **content, criterion, and construct.**
   a.   **Content validity** can be further divided into **face validity** and **true content validity.**
      (1)   **Face validity** is the degree to which the scale superficially appears to measure the construct.
      (2)   **True content validity** is the degree to which the items accurately represent the range of attributes covered by the construct.
      (3)   Content validity is not a statistical test but rather a judgment about a measure made by examining the strategy used to develop the measure, as well as the actual content of the items themselves.
      (4)   To be judged to have content validity, an HQL measure should contain items that address physical, psychological, and social functioning.
   b.   **Criterion validity** can be divided into **concurrent validity** and **predictive validity.** The distinction between the two is a function of when the criterion data are collected.
      (1)   Criterion data that are collected simultaneously with the scale data provide evidence of **concurrent validity.**
      (2)   Data that are collected some time after the scale data provide evidence of **predictive validity.**
   c.   Assessing a measure's **construct validity** involves testing the scale against a theoretical model or a set of statements about the relationships between variables.
   d.   There are many different **approaches** to construct validation.
      (1)   The **multitrait-multimethod matrix** is a method of assessing construct validity by

examining the correlations between the measure in question and other measures of the same construct, measures of both related and unrelated concepts, and different methods of data collection (e.g., self-report, observer rating).

    (2) **Multidimensional scaling** and **factor analysis** can also be used to evaluate the construct validity of a scale.

  e. The **sensitivity** of an instrument is another aspect of its validity. Instruments that have sensitivity are able to demonstrate responsiveness to change over time, parallel to changes in clinical status, and are able to differentiate groups of patients expected to differ in HQL.

  f. Validity is not absolute.

    (1) Validity data are cumulative and are relative to the setting and sample in which they are collected.

  g. **An HQL measure should assess well-being in addition to impairment.**

    (1) The concept of HQL includes positive aspects of health status (well-being) as well as negative changes in health status (functional limitations), so measures of HQL should address both.

  h. Statistical significance is not always clinically meaningful.

C. ACCEPTABILITY OF MEASURES

1. The **acceptability** of an instrument to patients and staff is also very important. Intrusive or inappropriate items can damage the integrity of an otherwise sound HQL measure.

VI. QUALITY-OF-LIFE MEASURES FOR USE IN ONCOLOGY

1. The large number of available measures of HQL has both advantages and disadvantages.

  a. The user can choose an instrument that best addresses the specific characteristics of a given disease site or clinical trial.

  b. The large number of available measures may also fragment the field of HQL measurement and can make it difficult to make comparisons across studies and measures.

A. PSYCHOMETRIC MEASURES

1. **Quality-of-Life Index (QLI)**

  a. Originally developed as a 10-point physician rating of five areas of functioning (activity, daily living, health, support, outlook), this observer rating scale has also been used as a patient-rated scale with reasonable success. It was constructed using expert panels of both patients and professionals.

  b. Reliability data for the subscales of activity, daily living, and health are more robust than those for support and outlook. The instrument has demonstrated a degree of both construct validity and sensitivity.

2. **European Organization for Research and Treatment of Cancer Quality-of-Life Questionnaire—Core (EORTC-QLQ)**

  a. This 36-item instrument consists of both dichotomous responses (yes/no) and responses on a 4-point rating scale. The instrument has a number of subscales, and it measures physical, role, emotional, and social functioning, along with disease symptoms, financial impact, and global quality of life.

  b. Reliability and validity have been evaluated, and the instrument has demonstrated sensitivity in different clinical situations.

3. **Functional Living Index—Cancer (FLIC)**

  a. This 22-item scale uses a 7-point rating scale to measure the impact of cancer on "day-to-day" living.

  b. There is evidence of construct validity, and the FLIC has been used extensively in oncology with predominantly positive results.

4. **Functional Assessment of Cancer Therapy (FACT) Scales**

  a. This instrument consists of 28 core items (yielding subscales for physical well-being, social/family well-being, relationship with doctor, emotional well-being, and functional well-being) and a disease-specific subscale, which reflect symptoms or problems associated with specific types of cancer or HIV infection. The scale was constructed using expert panels of patients and professionals.

    b. Concurrent validity is supported, and there is evidence for both construct validity and sensitivity in differentiating groups of patients. A unique feature of the FACT scales is that they provide supplemental valuative ratings that allow patients to specify how much each dimension of the scale affects HQL.

5. **Cancer Rehabilitation Evaluation System—Short Form (CARES—SF)**
    a. This 59-item self-administered instrument is comprised of a list of statements reflecting problems encountered by patients with cancer. The measures yield a global score, five summary scores (reflecting physical, psychosocial, medication interaction, marital, and sexual dimensions), and 31 subscales.
    b. The instrument appears to be sensitive in several oncology populations, and it has adequate test-retest reliability, internal consistency, and evidence of concurrent validity.

6. **Linear Analogue Self-Assessment (LASA) Scales**
    a. LASA scales use a 100-mm line with descriptors at each extreme. Respondents are required to mark their current state somewhere along that line, which is then measured as a score in centimeters or millimeters from the 0 point.
    b. Reliability and validity assessments have been conducted on all three of the main LASA scales that have been developed for cancer patients.
    c. Linear analogue scales are appealing because they are easy to administer and have good sensitivity. They have been criticized on the basis that it can be difficult to know the minimal clinically significant difference. Their use may also be limited by the fact that they cannot be administered over the telephone. However, they have performed well in studying the patterns of HQL in women with metastatic breast cancer receiving various regimens of chemotherapy.

7. **Medical Outcomes Study 36-Item Short-Form Status Health Survey (SF-36)**
    a. This instrument is a 36-item measure of eight health concepts: physical functioning, limitations in role functioning due to physical health problems, social functioning, bodily pain, general mental health, limitations in role functioning due to emotional problems, vitality, and general health perceptions.
    b. Reliability is reported as satisfactory; validity studies have demonstrated the instrument's ability to differentiate groups of patients expected to differ in HQL.

B. **UTILITY MEASURES**

1. **Quality of Well-Being (QWB) Scale**
    a. The Quality of Well-Being Scale is a 25-item list of symptom/problem complexes (CPX) covering the domains of mobility, physical activity, and social activity, each representing related but distinct aspects of daily functioning. Community weights for each CPX control for its relative desirability, with higher weights reflecting more desirable states.
    b. The instrument has demonstrated good reliability and adequate content, convergent, and discriminant validity.

2. **Quality-Adjusted Time Without Symptoms and Toxicity (Q-TWiST)**
    a. The Q-TWiST is the only utility approach that was developed to be cancer-specific. Like other utility methods, it has not yet been used to generate utility weights from patients themselves, but rather it depends on the weights provided by surrogates.
    b. It is conceptually distinct from patient-related HQL in that it infers rather than measures patient preferences.

PRACTICE QUESTIONS

1. Which of the following is the **least** important element in the definition of HQL?
    (A) physical and emotional function and well-being
    (B) social function and well-being
    (C) the relative value a patient assigns to various health states
    (D) objective evaluation of disease- and treatment-related symptomatology

2. An HQL measure that is based on the psychometric approach is **most** likely to emphasize
    (A) asking respondents how much time they would be willing to give up in order to live out their remaining life expectancy in perfect health.
    (B) surrogate perceptions and ratings of the importance of various symptoms.

(C)   an individual's subjective or perceived responses and well-being.

(D)   items that reflect physical, mental, and social dimensions of the cancer experience.

3.   Which of the following statements about utility analyses is correct?

(A)   Studies have demonstrated that the treatment utilities obtained from health professionals are generally more accurate than those provided by patients.

(B)   The standard gamble approach and the time trade-off method are two utility-based approaches to assessing the patient's perspective on HQL.

(C)   Utility analyses are more objective, and thus detect statistically significant differences in HQL more sensitively, than psychometric instruments.

(D)   Utility analyses are concerned with evaluating the HQL benefit produced by the clinical effects of a treatment.

4.   An example of an approach to assessing reliability is

(A)   assessment of repeatability.

(B)   assessment of sensitivity.

(C)   factor analysis.

(D)   the multitrait-multimethod matrix.

5.   Which of the following statements about validity is true?

(A)   Validity refers to a scale's ability to measure a construct consistently when it is applied at two different times or in two different ways.

(B)   A scale must be valid if it is to be considered reliable.

(C)   A scale is either valid or it is not.

(D)   Face or content validity is assessed by examining the strategy used to develop the scale, as well as the actual content of the items themselves.

6.   In selecting a measure to evaluate HQL for breast cancer patients on adjuvant chemotherapy, you would give **strongest** consideration to

(A)   a measure that allows family members to be used as surrogate raters if the patient is unable to the complete the measure.

(B)   a measure that has good psychometric properties and evaluates factors such as mobility and physical function.

(C)   a measure that has been used and evaluated in a population of patients with stage II cancer of the cervix.

(D)   a measure that has been shown to be extremely valid and reliable in the bone marrow transplant population.

7.   Which of the following is **not** an important future challenge in the assessment of HQL?

(A)   development of a "gold standard" measure by which to assess the HQL of patients with cancer

(B)   understanding the diverse costs and benefits of intensive experimental therapies that have severe toxicity and uncertain benefit

(C)   integrating psychometric and utility approaches to HQL assessment

(D)   identifying streamlined methods to elicit HQL data from patients who may have less energy or ability to participate in complex HQL assessment methods

ANSWER EXPLANATIONS

1.   **The answer is (D).**   HQL definitions place heavy emphasis on the subjective (from the patient's perspective) evaluation of disease- and treatment-related symptoms. (199)

2.   **The answer is (C).**   An important contribution of the psychometric approach is that it measures subjective or perceived responses and well-being. Any instrument to assess HQL should, by definition, include items that reflect physical, mental, and social domains. (198–199)

3.   **The answer is (D).**   The standard gamble approach and the time trade-off method **do not** elicit the patient's perspective on HQL. (199)

4.   **The answer is (A).**   Repeatability is the extent to which a measure applied two different times (test-retest) or in two different ways (alternate form and interrater) produces the same score. (200)

5.   **The answer is (D).**   Validity refers to a scale's ability to measure what it purports to measure. An instrument can be reliable without necessarily being valid. (200)

6.   **The answer is (C).**   In selecting a measure to evaluate HQL, it is important to consider the purpose of the investigation, a critical evaluation of the psychometric properties and field performance of available measures, and a review of the item content for relevance, appropriateness, and acceptability to the patient population to be studied. Since patients on adjuvant chemotherapy are most likely to remain physically and functionally competent, measures that focus on mobility and physical function (as in choice B) and measures that use a surrogate rater (as in choice A) would not seem to be well suited to the purposes of the investigation. Similarly, since the expected toxicities and effects of an adjuvant regimen are not likely to be similar to those of a high-dose chemotherapy regimen such as bone marrow transplantation, the measure described in choice (D), although valid and reliable in the BMT patient population, would not provide the best fit. The measure described in choice (C) would hold promise in measuring HQL in the breast cancer population since it has been used in a population of women with modest disease, who may be presumed to be of similar physical and psychological functioning. (200)

7.   **The answer is (A).**   There are so many HQL measures with established psychometric properties available for use that it is unlikely that a single "gold standard" will ever emerge. (198)

11   Principles of Treatment Planning

STUDY OUTLINE

I. **INTRODUCTION**

    1. Therapeutic decisions in oncology are based on the **location, cell type,** and **extent of the malignancy,** with established modes of therapy directed toward the particular disease presentation.

    2. **The aim of treatment is to cure or to palliate, causing minimal structural or functional impairment of the individual.**

    3. The sequence in treatment planning consists of **gathering information, planning, executing the plan, and evaluating.**

    4. The recipient of cancer treatment is a unique human being; every aspect of the design and evaluation of therapeutic activities must take the **individual's** unique needs into consideration.

II. **IIISTORICAL PERSPECTIVES ON CANCER TREATMENT**

    1. The early history of cancer treatment is summarized on **text pages 209–211.** Students with a particular interest in this topic, and students whose class assignment covers historical perspectives, are urged to review this material.

    2. Survival rates for cancer during the first 50 years of this century improved dramatically as methods for detecting and surgically removing primary tumors improved and morbidity from treatment decreased. However, by the 1950s cancer survival plateaued as cancers believed to be localized were shown to have micrometastases at diagnosis.

    3. Traditionally, surgeons managed the treatment of most cancer patients. Over the past 30 years a number of developments have marked a new approach to cancer therapy.

       a. Treatment involving a combination of surgery, radiotherapy, and chemotherapy began to emerge.

       b. Medical oncology became a specialty.

       c. Oncology nursing became more sophisticated and carried greater responsibility for all aspects of patient management.

       d. Consultation by oncology specialists became freely available.

       e. Patients could often be treated in the community.

       f. Care became increasingly palliative and research-oriented.

       g. Special oncology units and cancer rehabilitation programs in local hospitals and hospice development in local communities became common.

    4. **Control** has joined cure and palliation as a part of cancer treatment. Control refers to keeping cancer within bounds for increasingly longer periods through a combination of therapies.

III. **FACTORS INVOLVED IN TREATMENT PLANNING**

    A. **THE PATIENT PRESENTS**

    B. **A DIAGNOSTIC WORKUP IS BEGUN**

C. **A BIOPSY IS DONE**

1. Biopsy allows full investigation of the person and prevents hasty local treatment measures that might jeopardize later plans.

D. **THE BIOPSY ESTABLISHES THE DIAGNOSIS**

E. **CLASSIFYING THE TUMOR**

1. **Table 11-1, text page 213,** displays how cancers are classified.
    a. **Pathological classification** is based on information about the tumor, while **clinical classification** is based upon information concerning the host.
2. **Pathological classification**
    a. A **benign** tumor is well circumscribed or encapsulated, appears orderly and is cellularly characteristic of the host tissue.
    b. A **malignant** tumor varies in size and shape, invades the organs from which it grew, and can eventually spread into neighboring tissue.
    c. Benign tumors are named by adding the **suffix -oma** to the tissue type from which it originated.
    d. **Carcinoma** refers to malignant tumors arising in epithelial tissues.
        (1) **Squamous cell carcinomas** are tumors of the squamous epithelium.
        (2) **Transitional cell carcinomas** refer to neoplasms of transitional epithelium.
        (3) **Adenocarcinomas** are neoplasms of glandular epithelium.
    e. **Sarcoma** refers to malignant tumors involving mesenchymal tissues.
    f. **Histopathologic** type describes the neoplasm by the tissue or cell type from which it originated. The tissue of origin is important because it determines the behavior of the tumor.
    g. A **metastatic** tumor is a tumor with the same cell type at a site different from the original or primary site.
    h. A second primary cancer is a tumor with a different cell type from a previous tumor cell type.
    i. **Histopathologic grade** is a quantitative assessment of the extent the tumor cells resemble the tissue cells of origin.
    j. Grading can be done **numerically.**
        (1) **Grade I** indicates that tumor cells are well differentiated and resemble the normal parent cells.
        (2) **Grade IV** tumor cells are so anaplastic that it is often difficult for the pathologist to determine their cell of origin.
        (3) **Grades II and III** are intermediate designations.
    k. Grading can also be done **descriptively: well differentiated** (grade I), **moderately well differentiated** (grade II), **poorly differentiated** (grade III), or **undifferentiated** (grade IV).
    l. The prognostic value of grading varies with different types of tumors, e.g., bladder cancer (good) versus melanoma (poor).
    m. Different tumors tend to behave in different but often predictable ways. This knowledge helps the medical team plan its treatment of an individual with a particular tumor.
3. **Clinical classification**
    a. Once the diagnosis is established, further definitive testing is needed to assess the anatomic extent of the disease.
    b. The TNM classification system is considered by many to be too complex and by others to be too simple. It is also not relevant to types of malignancies that
        (1) Do not metastasize, e.g., brain tumors.
        (2) Metastasize primarily by vascular routes, e.g., bone and renal and hepatic carcinomas.
        (3) Have a lymph node as the primary site, e.g., Hodgkin's disease and lymphomas.
    c. The Ann Arbor classification is used for lymphomas; Duke's staging of rectal and colonic cancer is also widely used.
    d. Clinical staging systems estimate chances of survival for the individual and assist physicians in selecting appropriate treatment. They also facilitate comparisons among institutions.
    e. **A major weakness is that they do not use histologic criteria.**
    f. **There are two main staging periods:**
        (1) Before treatment staging
            (a) **Pretreatment** staging occurs before the first treatment is started and is based on tests and gathered data.

(b) **Clinical-diagnostic staging** is an aspect of pretreatment staging used for patients who have had a biopsy.

(c) **Postsurgical resection-pathologic staging** is also an aspect to pretreatment staging and includes a complete evaluation of the surgical specimen by a pathologist.

(2) Retreatment staging

(a) **Retreatment staging** is the second main staging period following a disease-free interval and needs further treatment.

(b) **Autopsy staging** may occur if the extent of disease at the time of disease needs to be assessed.

g. The **Duke's classification for colorectal cancer** and the **Ann Arbor classification system** for lymphomas are other staging systems developed.

(1) An attempt has been made to have the now universally accepted TNM system consistent with other classifications.

(2) **TNM staging** of all cancer patients is required for approval of cancer programs by the Commission on Cancer.

IV.   DETERMINING THE TREATMENT PLAN

1. Decisions concerning treatment method involve integration of the extent of the disease and the individual's condition with knowledge relating to
   a. **Prognosis.**
   b. **Anticipated response to various forms of therapy.**
   c. **Anticipated complication rates.**
   d. **Other relevant clinical considerations.**
2. Primary therapy is the name given to the most definitive treatment aimed at cure for a given cancer.

A.   SHOULD TREATMENT BE AIMED AT CURE?

1. Generally, oncologists tend to think of tumors with 5-year **survival probabilities** in the range of 1%–5% as having no or minimal chance for cure.
2. The risks involved with any method must then be related to the person's age and condition.
3. A correct decision on whether to treat for cure is one of the **most important** decisions that the oncologist must make.

B.   WHICH MODALITY SHOULD BE USED?

1. After the decision to treat for cure, the next decision involves choosing the optimal modality or combination thereof. **Multimodality therapy** is the treatment strategy most often utilized.
2. Some basic principles that have evolved for treatment selection include the following:
   a. **Radiotherapy** might be given prior to surgery to cause tumor shrinkage and thus make surgical resection easier, while intraoperative radiation may also be given during a surgical procedure.
   b. **Radiotherapy** is usually indicated if the tumor is invading nearby tissues and cannot be surgically resected.
   c. **Chemotherapy** may be given after surgery to eliminate micrometastasis. It is sometimes used prior to therapy to shrink a lesion.
   d. The **combination** of radiation and chemotherapy produce a more powerful antitumor effect than either treatment alone. Both may be given after surgery.
   e. **Biological therapies** are being blended with radiotherapy and chemotherapy in research studies.
   f. See **Table 11-4, text page 218,** for the advantages and disadvantages of treatment modalities.
3. The patient's best interests are usually served by a multidisciplinary approach that includes
   a. The **surgeon,** who specifies the therapeutic potential and operability of the tumor.
   b. The **radiotherapist,** who tells the expectation of curability by primary radiotherapy or the augmentation effect that radiotherapy might have before or following surgery.
   c. The **chemotherapist,** who specifies the contribution that chemotherapy can make to cure the particular tumor and the potential for chemotherapeutic or hormonal palliation should cure be impossible.

     d. The **pathologist,** who explains the details of the biopsy and the microscopic appearance of the tumor.

     e. The **radiologist,** who reviews the various radiographs and scans.

     f. The **nurse practitioner,** who is the primary care provider and who may present the person's case to the board.

     g. The **enterostomy nurse,** who may make contributions regarding postoperative care feasibility and rehabilitation.

     h. A **research assistant nurse,** who may explain details of a chemotherapy protocol under consideration.

     i. A **primary nurse,** who may make contributions to the patient's hospital care based on his or her knowledge of the patient's pain, vocational incapacitation, familial problems, emotional reactions, financial burdens, geographic location, or other aspects of the patient's life.

4. How radical the treatment should be is based on several factors, including
     a. **The aggressiveness of the cancer.**
     b. **The predictability of its spread.**
     c. **The morbidity and mortality expected in the patient from the therapeutic procedure being considered.**
     d. **The cure rate that can be expected from it.**
     e. **The patient's desires.**

5. Patients generally benefit from the highly individualized prescription that a tumor board consultation affords. Each member of the board brings a fresh approach to the question at hand.

C. THE BENEFIT OF CLINICAL TRIALS

1. Clinicians turn to **clinical trials** for guidance in making therapeutic decisions. These constitute the only sure foundation for therapeutic progress.

2. **A clinical trial is defined as a carefully and ethically designed experiment with the aim of answering a precisely framed question. A valid protocol** should cover all foreseeable eventualities and ambiguities in the trial.

3. The **publication of results** of clinical trials allows clinicians from around the world to build on treatment successes. **Replication** of the experiment at other institutions ensures that treatment outcomes are not serendipitous.

4. However, no clinical trial can absolutely guarantee the best treatment for an individual.

D. SELECTING A TREATMENT PLAN

1. For cases in which a patient cannot be entered into an existing clinical trial, the physician can choose to
     a. Use a "conventional" treatment program based on a regimen that has been **studied extensively** and **used for a long time** and is **widely accepted** for common cancers.
     b. Rely on a study in a **journal article** or **abstract publication.**
     c. Put together a protocol specific to the situation.

2. A treatment plan may involve a **single modality** or **multiple modalities.**
     a. **Primary therapy,** usually surgery, chemotherapy, or radiotherapy, indicates the best, most definitive treatment aimed at cure for a given cancer.
     b. **Adjuvant (assisting) therapy** refers to a situation where other modalities are used after the primary treatment, usually surgery. These modalities may include chemotherapy, radiotherapy, immunotherapy, or some combination thereof used in an attempt to eradicate any tumor cells left behind.
     c. **Neoadjuvant therapy** uses adjuvant modalities to treat micrometastatic disease before the primary, definitive treatment. It is not concerned with the primary tumor itself.
     d. With chemotherapy, use of **first-line drugs**—those most likely to lead to cure or remission—may be followed by use of **second-line drugs** if the tumor recurs.
     e. See **Table 11-5, text page 219.**

V. ASSESSING RESPONSE TO TREATMENT

1. Responses to treatment may be **objective** or **subjective.**
2. Objective responses include

a. **Complete response:** Complete disappearance of signs and symptoms of cancer, lasting at least 1 month.
b. **Partial response:** A 50% or more reduction in the sum of the products of the greater and lesser diameters of all measured lesions, lasting at least 1 month, without the development of any new lesions during therapy.
c. **Progression:** A 25% or more increase in the sum of the products of the greater and lesser diameters of all measured lesions, or the emergence of new lesions.
3. A baseline for evaluation is established by **objective parameters** measured before initiating therapy. Common parameters include **pulmonary lesions, liver involvement,** and **enlarged lymph nodes.**
4. With some tumors, response to treatment is assessed by **restaging,** which involves reestablishing the clinical extent of the disease at the completion of a prescribed course of therapy or at the time of relapse.
    a. Restaging does not imply that a person who goes through remission reverts to a lesser stage. **The stage at the time of diagnosis is the one that characterizes the illness throughout, even if there is no clinical evidence of disease after treatment.**
5. **Subjective response** represents improvement from the patient's point of view.

A. SURVIVAL STATISTICS

1. The only precise definition of "cure" is if there is no evidence of tumor at autopsy. However, most clinicians accept **freedom from clinical evidence of recurrent metastatic disease during the person's lifetime** as a reasonably reliable estimate.
2. Cure is also assessed by **survival statistics.**
    a. A **time interval** is selected that must elapse without evidence of recurrence.
        (1) This interval depends on how long after the primary treatment residual disease can be expected to become evident. This may be up to 15 or 20 years for many tumors or as little as 5 years for more aggressive tumors.
        (2) The time interval is best understood to be the **time after treatment at which the annual death rate of the treated person is no longer greater than that of the normal population.**
        (3) It must be clear whether "cure" means survival with evidence of tumor or without.
        (4) Survival times must also be **corrected for age** by comparison with healthy groups of comparable age distribution.

B. PATIENT FOLLOW-UP

a. A hospital's **tumor registry** contains data compiled over time on each person diagnosed with cancer at that institution.
b. These data aid in systematic follow-up of individuals with cancer and facilitate the hospital's evaluation of therapy.
c. Many states or regions also have cancer data registry programs in which the information from each individual tumor registry is fed into a larger program.
    (1) Such a **regional database** is helpful in examining trends in cancer therapy and patient survival.

VI. WHEN CURE IS NOT ACHIEVED

1. Failure to "cure" and recurrence of disease may mean a long period during which treatment is aimed at **"control."** For this reason, cancer is viewed as a chronic disease.
2. The principles of treatment of advanced disease take into consideration
    a. **The specific diagnosis and site or sites of the disease.**
    b. **The status of the bone marrow.**
    c. **The status of the liver and renal function.**
    d. **The presence of complications due to the tumor.**
    e. **The patient's immunologic status.**
    f. **The patient's general condition.**
3. For incurable cancers, e.g., myeloma, therapy is aimed at control from the onset. Survival can be prolonged and improved with proper treatment.

4. If neither cure nor control is an option, treatment turns to **palliation.** This may consist of
    a. **Radiation or chemotherapy** to relieve disease symptoms.
    b. A **palliative surgical procedure** to provide relief from a bulky tumor.
    c. **Palliative measures for asymptomatic people** in whom the impending catastrophic problem can be predicted, e.g., obstruction of the superior vena cava.
    d. **Palliative measures aimed at the person's emotional well-being.** Hope may be maintained though continued chemotherapy, even though there are no physical benefits to the therapy.
5. Palliation is normally deferred until specific problems appear. Thereafter palliation should be matched with need, including the use of aggressive palliative measures and emotional support for those whose problems cannot be relieved by simple medication.

VII.   **FUTURE PROSPECTS**

1. The rate of treatment progress will depend on developments in molecular biology, immunology, and genetics.

PRACTICE QUESTIONS

1. The term **cancer control** refers most accurately to the process of
    (A)   identifying those factors in the environment that are most likely to place the population at risk of cancer.
    (B)   classifying malignant neoplasms on the basis of histopathologic characteristics of the tissue.
    (C)   performing studies to help formulate a clinical diagnosis and monitoring the patient's response to a particular therapy.
    (D)   keeping an individual's cancer within bounds for increasingly longer periods through a combination of therapies.

2. Which of the following statements **best** describes the requirements of the language used by clinicians to communicate information about cancer?
    (A)   It is highly technical and specialized.
    (B)   It is quantitative rather than qualitative in nature.
    (C)   It is simple, succinct, and standardized.
    (D)   It varies with clinic and country depending on local standards.

3. In establishing the degree of malignancy in tumor cells, the numerical Grade IV corresponds with the description
    (A)   well-differentiated.
    (B)   moderately well-differentiated.
    (C)   poorly differentiated.
    (D)   undifferentiated.

4. Which of the following factors will a physician generally **not** take into account in the decision to attempt a cure of a patient's malignancy?
    (A)   the chances for a cure
    (B)   the patient's feeling and values
    (C)   any previous treatment that might limit tissue tolerance
    (D)   the palliative procedures used in testing

5. In treating a malignancy, a physician would be **most** likely to use surgery coupled with radiotherapy if the malignancy is
    (A)   widespread.
    (B)   localized.
    (C)   metastasized.
    (D)   invasive.

6. How radical the treatment for a malignancy should be is typically based on several factors, including all of the following **except**
    (A)   the aggressiveness of the cancer.

     (B)   the clinical trial involved.
     (C)   the cure rate that can be expected from the treatment.
     (D)   the patient's desires.

7.   Within the framework of therapy, an important objective of a well-conceived clinical trial is to
     (A)   identify risk factors that may apply to the general population.
     (B)   assess the toxicities of the treatment.
     (C)   reveal the clinical extent of disease within an individual patient.
     (D)   design staging procedures that apply to a particular malignancy.

8.   The use of immunotherapy as a follow-up to surgical treatment of a malignancy would constitute
     (A)   adjuvant therapy.
     (B)   neoadjuvant therapy.
     (C)   primary therapy.
     (D)   single-modality therapy.

9.   In order for a response to therapy to be called **complete,** how long must there be a complete disappearance of signs and symptoms of cancer?
     (A)   at least 1 month
     (B)   at least 5 years
     (C)   at least 15 years
     (D)   until the person dies and the response is confirmed by autopsy

10.   For cure to be assessed by survival statistics, a time interval is selected that must elapse without evidence of recurrence of the tumor. Which of the following statements about this time interval is **correct?**
     (A)   It is age-independent.
     (B)   It is set at 5 years for most types of cancers.
     (C)   It varies depending on the aggressiveness of the cancer.
     (D)   It refers to the time after treatment at which the annual death rate of the treated person is greater than that of the normal population.

11.   Which of the following is an example of a **palliative measure** used in cancer treatment?
     (A)   the use of radiotherapy to destroy all cancer tissue in the body
     (B)   the use of the TNM staging classification
     (C)   the use of barium sulfate to detect a malignancy in the duodenum
     (D)   the use of chemotherapy to relieve disease symptoms

ANSWER EXPLANATIONS

1.   **The answer is (D).**   Control has joined cure and palliation as a part of cancer treatment. Control refers to keeping cancer within bounds for increasingly longer periods through a combination of therapies. Choice (B) is the definition of grading; choice (C) is the purpose of laboratory studies. (209)

2.   **The answer is (C).**   A widely understood, standardized, and simple shorthand language is used by pathologists to assist clinicians in planning treatment, determining patients' prognoses, and helping clinicians around the world to share the results of their treatment regimens. (212–214)

3.   **The answer is (D).**   Grade I corresponds with the description of cells that are so well-differentiated that they closely resemble normal parent cells. Grade IV tumor cells are so anaplastic that it is often difficult for the pathologist to determine their cell of origin. Grades II and III are intermediate designations. (214)

4.   **The answer is (D).**   The person's age and general physical condition will also be considered. (216)

5.   **The answer is (B).**   Modern treatment programs use the appropriate treatment methods to exploit the different biologic characteristics of a variety of cancers. Surgery and radiotherapy may be curative if the disease is truly localized, but they may leave behind viable malignant cells. Chemotherapy may be curative when widespread disease is present, but it may leave behind cancer cells if a bulky tumor mass is present. (217–218)

6.   **The answer is (B).**   The treatment may or may not be part of a clinical trial. The remaining factors are all part of the interdisciplinary decision concerning treatment approach. Cancer treatment is by nature radical because extraordinary measures are needed to control the disease. The basic principle is to choose the treatment method that offers the best chance for cure with the least structural and physical impairment. (218–219)

7.   **The answer is (B).**   A clinical trial is a carefully and ethically designed experiment with the aim of answering a precisely framed question. Clinical trials constitute the only sure foundation for therapeutic progress. One of its objectives is to assess the toxicities of the treatment. Another major objective is to demonstrate the effectiveness or ineffectiveness of a particular form of treatment and to compare two or more treatment regimens. (218–219)

8.   **The answer is (A).**   Adjuvant therapy refers to a situation where other modalities are used after the primary treatment, in this case surgery. Adjuvant modalities may include chemotherapy, radiotherapy, immunotherapy, or some combination thereof used in an attempt to eradicate any tumor cells left behind. Primary therapy indicates the best, most definitive treatment aimed at cure for a given cancer. Neoadjuvant therapy uses adjuvant modalities to treat micrometastatic disease before the primary, definitive treatment. It is not concerned with the primary tumor itself. (217)

9.   **The answer is (A).**   There must be a complete disappearance of signs and symptoms of cancer for at least 1 month. For a partial response, there must be a 50% or more reduction in the sum of the products of the greater and lesser diameters of all measured lesions, lasting at least 1 month, without the development of any new lesions during therapy. For progression, there must be a 25% or more increase in the sum of the products of the greater and lesser diameters of all measured lesions, or the emergence of new lesions. (220)

10.   **The answer is (C).**   It may be as little as 5 years for more aggressive tumors or up to 15 or 20 years for slower-growing tumors. Survival times must be corrected for age by comparison with healthy groups of comparable age distribution. Choice (D) would be correct if it read "... no greater than ..." (220)

11.   **The answer is (D).**   If neither cure nor control is an option, treatment turns to palliation. This may consist of radiation or chemotherapy to relieve disease symptoms, a surgical procedure to provide relief from a bulky tumor, a measure for asymptomatic people in whom the impending catastrophic problem can be predicted, e.g., obstruction of the superior vena cava, or a measure aimed at the person's emotional well-being. Palliation is normally deferred until specific problems appear. Thereafter palliation is matched to the patient's needs and includes the use of aggressive palliative measures and emotional support for those whose problems cannot be relieved by simple medication. (220–221)

12 Surgical Therapy

STUDY OUTLINE

I. INTRODUCTION

1. Approximately 55% of all individuals with cancer are treated with surgical intervention. Of the 40% that are treated by surgery alone, **one-third** are cured.
2. Combining surgery with other therapies has significantly lengthened disease-free intervals.
3. **Surgery can be used for prevention, diagnosis, definitive treatment, rehabilitation, or palliation.**

II. FACTORS INFLUENCING TREATMENT DECISIONS

A. TUMOR CELL KINETICS

1. The biologic characteristics of tumor cells affect the treatment decision. These characteristics include **growth rate, differentiation, invasiveness,** and **metastatic potential and pattern.**
2. See Chapter 3 and especially Chapter 4 of the text and guide for a review of these cell kinetics processes.

B. TUMOR LOCATION

1. After diagnosis and staging to determine tumor location and extent, the clinician can assess the structural and functional changes that can be anticipated with surgery.
2. Tumors are more easily resected if they are **superficial** (e.g., a skin carcinoma) or **encapsulated** rather than embedded in delicate or inaccessible tissue, including vital structures, or if they have invaded tissues in multiple directions.

C. PHYSICAL STATUS

1. Preoperative assessment of the patient's **physical status** is critical for evaluating the factors that might increase surgical morbidity and mortality.
2. Among the other factors that are weighed prior to surgery are the **severity of the disease and comorbid conditions;** the **age** and **rehabilitation potential** of the patient; and the possible **effects of surgery** on the physical and physiologic functioning of the patient, including effects on their quality of life.

D. QUALITY OF LIFE

1. Selection of treatment includes consideration of the quality of life when the treatment is complete.
2. Some radical surgical procedures are not warranted because they do not improve the outcome or because they interfere with the person's functional or psychological well-being.
3. Multidisciplinary planning with the patient and family helps tailor the treatment plan to individual needs.

III. PREVENTING CANCER USING SURGICAL PROCEDURES

1. Certain conditions or traits are associated with a higher risk of developing cancer.
2. A good example of the use of surgery for prevention of cancer is the surgical excision of colon polyps, which reduces the risk of colon cancer.

IV. **DIAGNOSING CANCER USING SURGICAL TECHNIQUES**

1. In selecting the most appropriate **biopsy technique** and performing the biopsy, the surgeon should
   a. Consider the possible treatment regimens that will be used if cancer is diagnosed.
   b. Place the biopsy site so that it will be removed at surgery if the biopsy is not used to remove the whole tumor.
   c. Use different biopsy equipment for each biopsy site, if multiple biopsies are to be taken.
   d. Consider aesthetic results (e.g., scars) when selecting a biopsy site and performing the procedure.
   e. Include both normal and tumor cells in the biopsy specimen for comparison.
   f. Take care not to crush or contaminate the specimen.
   g. Label and preserve the specimen properly.
2. **Only positive biopsy results are definitive; a negative result can mean either no cancer or that the specimen was not representative of the tumor.**
3. Different types of biopsies are used, depending on tumor size, location, and growth characteristics.

A. **NEEDLE BIOPSY**

1. **Needle biopsy** is performed in an outpatient or office setting. A needle is inserted through the skin into the tumor site, where a core of tissue is removed. Local or topical anesthesia is used.

B. **SURGICAL BIOPSY**

1. **Incisional biopsy** is generally used to diagnose a large tumor that will require major surgery for complete removal.
2. **Excisional biopsy** is performed on small, accessible tumors to remove the entire mass and little or no margin of surrounding tissue. Often it will be used alone as definitive therapy, e.g., a skin cancer.
3. **Endoscopy** can be used for diagnosis of tumors in accessible lumen. See **text pages 183–184** for further review.
4. Possible complications following any biopsy are pain, bleeding, hematoma, infection, dehiscence, and tumor cell seeding. See **Table 12-1, text page 226**—Approaches for Biopsy.

V. **STAGING CANCER USING SURGICAL PROCEDURES**

1. **Surgical procedures have a significant role in diagnosing cancer and in defining the extent of tumor involvement.**
   a. Examples include **laparotomy** for staging lymphomas and **exploratory surgical procedures** that are done to diagnose or stage intracavitary tumors.
2. In addition to the cTNM and pTNM staging classifications discussed on **text page 188, surgical evaluative staging (sTNM)** is reserved for tumors that are inaccessible, difficult to evaluate, or inadequately staged by other means.

VI. **SURGERY FOR TREATMENT OF CANCER**

1. The goal of therapy will be based on a collation of the **patient's desires, general condition,** and **tumor stage and classification.** The sequence methods used will be guided by the most effective protocol available.
2. See **Table 12-2, text page 228,** for a prepoerative assessment and teaching guide.

A. **SURGERY AIMED AT CURE**

1. Surgical approaches rely often on effective use of radiotherapy, chemotherapy, or biotherapy.
2. **Excision of primary tumors**
   a. The type of surgical procedure selected depends on specific tumor cell characteristics and site of involvement.
   b. **Local incision** is used to resect small lesions if the entire tumor and a margin of safety can be encompassed, e.g., tumors of the ear, skin, or lip.

      c.   **Major surgical resections** are performed when the tumor is surgically accessible, and there is hope that the tumor can be removed as a whole along with the necessary local or regional tissues and lymphatics.

   3.   **Surgery and adjuvant therapies**
      a.   Adjuvant therapy may be given preoperatively, interoperatively, or postoperatively.
      b.   Surgery is sometimes used to reduce a tumor to a size where radiation therapy and chemotherapy can be most effective, e.g., ovarian cancer.
         (1)   Definitive therapy then may follow.

   4.   **Excision of metastatic lesions**
      a.   Surgery may also be done to resect a metastatic lesion if
         (1)   The primary tumor is believed to be eradicated.
         (2)   The metastatic site is solitary.
         (3)   The patient can undergo surgery without major morbidity.
      b.   Excision is not indicated if there is evidence of advanced metastatic disease or if the metastatic lesion is particularly aggressive or inaccessible.

B.   SURGERY AIMED AT PALLIATION

   1.   The goals of palliative surgery are to
      a.   Relieve suffering and minimize symptoms of the disease.
      b.   Control the cancer.
      c.   Improve the quality of life.
   2.   Procedures include
      a.   **Alleviation of obstruction,** e.g., a tracheostomy to restore airway patency in a patient with a tumor of the hypopharynx.
      b.   **Decompression of vital structures,** e.g., resection of a tumor to relieve pressure and allow adjuvant therapy with radiation or drugs.
      c.   **Control of pain,** e.g., a nerve block or other surgical procedure on the nervous system to interrupt the nerve pathways.

C.   SURGERY FOR REHABILITATION

   1.   Examples of surgical rehabilitation include **breast reconstruction** following mastectomy, **facial reconstruction** after head and neck surgery, and **skin grafting.** These procedures are intended to improve the cancer patient's quality of life.
   2.   Rehabilitation potential is considered before initiation of primary therapy; rehabilitation teaching and counseling also take place at this stage.
   3.   Success is measured both by improvements in function and self-esteem and by cosmetic improvement.

VII.   CARING FOR THE INDIVIDUAL WITH CANCER WHO IS UNDERGOING SURGERY: SPECIAL CONSIDERATIONS FOR NURSING CARE

A.   SURGICAL SETTING

   1.   Many surgical procedures are moving to the ambulatory area with predictions that 60% of all hospital-based surgeries will be on an ambulatory basis by 1995.
   2.   Change in the delivery system to ambulatory necessitates changes in the way care is provided. Nurses rely more on the telephone for communication via follow-up or in writing.
   3.   **Support systems must be identified before the surgery takes place.**

B.   PREOPERATIVE CONCERNS/PREVENTIVE STRATEGIES

   1.   **Autologous blood donation**
      a.   Blood donation in preparation for surgery can be done 42 days to 72 hours prior to surgery.
   2.   **Anxiety/pain control**
      a.   In the preoperative period discussions about pain and anxiety as a result of surgical procedures will facilitate patient verbalization of fears, decrease anxiety, and allow the patient to become aware of advances in pain control.

    b.   Patient-controlled analgesia, meditation, relaxation, etc., are means of managing pain after surgical procedures. See **Table 12-3, text page 231,** on nonpharmacologic interventions for pain control.

3. **Nutrition**
    a.   The nutritionally debilitated person with cancer is a poor surgical risk and often requires preoperative correction of the underlying nutritional deficit.
       (1)   The undernourished person may be unable to adapt to surgical trauma with preservation of lean mass. A negative nitrogen balance may develop.
       (2)   Risks include **poor wound healing, infection, pneumonia,** and **increased morbidity.**
    b.   Nutritional management should be aimed at reversing protein calorie malnutrition and preventing weight loss.
    c.   People who are nutritionally compromised should receive preoperative enteral or parental support to reduce complications and surgical mortality.

4. **Hemostasis**
    a.   **Thrombosis** and **hypercoagulability** associated with abnormal clotting factors are particular problems in cancer patients.

C. COMPLICATIONS OF MULTIMODAL THERAPY

1. Chemotherapy, radiotherapy, and immunotherapy are now used in various sequences before, during, and after surgery for certain tumors.
2. The interactive and compounding effect of these therapies may produce difficult problems and side effects for the cancer nurse to manage, including
    a.   **Postoperative wound healing** in the person who has previously received **radiation** to the surgical site.
       (1)   This may cause postoperative wound dehiscence, infection, and tissue and bone necrosis.
    b.   **Postoperative wound healing** in the person who receives **chemotherapy** early in the postoperative period.
       (1)   Bleomycin, doxorubicin, and corticosteroids have all been shown to modify the process of wound healing at specific times during the postoperative period.
    c.   The **toxic effects** of certain chemotherapeutic agents to specific organ systems.
       (1)   Bleomycin therapy given before surgery may predispose the person to postoperative respiratory distress.
       (2)   Methotrexate and busulfan can produce a diffuse interstitial and alveolar pneumonitis.
       (3)   Cis-platinum, streptozocin, and methotrexate can result in a persistent decrease in glomerular filtration rate (GFR) due to renal tubular damage.
       (4)   A cumulative dose of 500 mg/m^2 or more of anthracyclines, doxorubicin, and daunorubicin increases the risk of intraoperative and postoperative congestive heart failure and pulmonary edema.
3. **Intraoperative radiotherapy and chemotherapy** is a method used to deliver a single, high dose directly to the surgically exposed tumor or tumor bed.
    a.   These treatments are administered for locally advanced abdominal and pelvic malignancies.
    b.   They require extensive multidisciplinary collaboration.
    c.   Potential side effects appear to be similar to traditional delivery methods.
4. See **Tables 12-4 and 12-5, text page 232,** for effects of chemotherapy on specific organs and possible effects of chemotherapy on wound healing.

PRACTICE QUESTIONS

1. A surgical procedure is **least** likely to be called for under which of the following conditions?
    (A)   The tumor is encapsulated.
    (B)   The tumor involves a vital structure.
    (C)   The tumor is invasive.
    (D)   The tumor is superficial.

2. Many factors are weighed prior to a decision to perform surgery on a cancer patient. Among the following, the factor **least** likely to be considered is the
    (A)   age of the patient.
    (B)   rehabilitation potential of the patient.

    (C)   severity of the disease.

    (D)   cell kinetics of the tumor.

3.   A commonly performed surgical procedure that is **preventive** in nature is a

    (A)   biopsy.

    (B)   polypectomy.

    (C)   laparotomy.

    (D)   tracheostomy.

4.   An excisional biopsy is **most** likely to be performed when a tumor

    (A)   is located in the peritoneum.

    (B)   is small and accessible.

    (C)   has metastasized.

    (D)   is large and encapsulated.

5.   Under which of the following conditions is a major surgical resection **most** likely to be performed?

    (A)   when the tumor is on the surface of the body

    (B)   when the tumor is deeply imbedded

    (C)   when the tumor is surgically accessible

    (D)   when the tumor is metastatic

6.   Under which of the following conditions is a metastatic lesion **most** likely to be surgically excised?

    (A)   if the primary tumor is growing

    (B)   if the lesion is one of many secondary lesions

    (C)   if the patient is unlikely to undergo surgery without morbidity

    (D)   if the primary tumor is of unknown origin

7.   Different surgical procedures are used palliatively to relieve suffering and minimize symptoms of cancer. These procedures include all of the following **except**

    (A)   alleviation of an obstruction.

    (B)   decompression of a vital structure.

    (C)   interruption of the nerve pathways.

    (D)   reconstruction of a tissue.

8.   At which stage in the process of treating cancer is rehabilitation potential normally considered?

    (A)   during diagnosis and staging

    (B)   before initiation of primary therapy

    (C)   during the postoperative stage of therapy

    (D)   as part of palliation

9.   The primary aim of the nutritional management of cancer patients is

    (A)   preventing weight loss.

    (B)   limiting hemostatic problems.

    (C)   slowing metastasis.

    (D)   assuring accurate staging.

10.   Surgery at previously radiated sites is an example of multimodality therapy. What will be a major challenge in caring for the postoperative patient?

    (A)   infection

    (B)   wound healing

    (C)   myelosuppression

    (D)   gastrointestinal toxicity

ANSWER EXPLANATIONS

1.   **The answer is (C).**   Tumors that are encapsulated or superficial (such as a skin cancer) are more likely candidates for surgical intervention than are tumors that involve a vital organ (such as the brain). If a tumor is embedded in delicate or inaccessible tissue, or if it has invaded tissues in multiple directions, other therapies will be called for. (227–228)

2. **The answer is (D).**   Other factors that are considered are the location of the tumor, the comorbid conditions of the disease, and the possible effects of surgery on physiologic and physical functioning of the patient. (223–224)

3. **The answer is (B).**   Biopsy is diagnostic; laparotomy is often used in staging; tracheostomy is usually palliative. Only polypectomy, the excision of colon polyps in order to prevent colon cancer, is preventive. (224)

4. **The answer is (B).**   Excisional biopsy is performed on small, accessible tumors to remove the entire mass and little or no margin of surrounding tissue. Often it will be used alone as definitive therapy, e.g., a skin cancer. Incisional biopsy is generally used to diagnose a large tumor that will require major surgery for complete removal. (225–226)

5. **The answer is (C).**   A major surgical resection is most likely to be performed when the tumor is surgically accessible, and there is hope that the tumor can be removed en bloc along with local or regional tissues and lymphatics. Local incision is used to resect small lesions where the entire tumor and a margin of safety can be encompassed, e.g., tumors of the ear, skin, or lip. (227–228)

6. **The answer is (D).**   Metastasis from primary tumors of unknown origin are an example of how surgery may be employed. When the only identifiable site of the disease is the metastasis, it is reasonable to manage the person's disease in an aggressive manner, particularly if the metastatic disease is life-threatening. (228–229)

7. **The answer is (D).**   Tissue reconstruction, including breast or facial reconstruction, falls more accurately under the heading of surgical rehabilitation, although some palliative function is no doubt served. The other three procedures are all basic palliative procedures. (229)

8. **The answer is (B).**   Careful interdisciplinary planning will assist the clinician to prepare the person emotionally and physically for both the primary treatment and subsequent rehabilitation. Nurses can assist the patient to see that rehabilitation is desirable and sometimes necessary for achieving a high level of functioning. (229)

9. **The answer is (A).**   Nutritional management first should be aimed at reversing protein calorie malnutrition and reversing weight loss. Other therapeutic outcomes of good nutritional management, including proper wound healing, limited infection, and decreased morbidity, proceed from fulfillment of this primary goal. (230–231)

10. **The answer is (B).**   A major challenge in multimodality therapy is the problem of postoperative wound healing in the person who has previously received radiation to the surgical site. Radiation may cause long-term damage to the underlying tissues, such as fibrosis and obliteration of lymphatic and vascular channels. Once the integrity of the tissue is damaged by radiation, additional traumas, such as surgery are not well tolerated. (231–232)

13   Radiotherapy

STUDY OUTLINE

I. **THE CURRENT APPLICATION OF RADIOTHERAPY IN THE MANAGEMENT OF THE PERSON DIAGNOSED WITH CANCER**

1. Radiation therapy is often combined with surgery or chemotherapy or immunotherapy. It is also used as the sole treatment of cancer in some instances, e.g., in treatment of stage IIB squamous cell carcinoma of the cervix.
2. Like surgical therapy, radiation therapy may be used for **cure** (e.g., skin cancer, cervical carcinoma, Hodgkin's disease), **control** (e.g., lung cancer), or **palliation.**
    a. Curative treatment is vigorous and often lengthy.
    b. Palliative radiotherapy may be used for **pain relief, prevention of pathologic fractures,** or to **reduce hemorrhage, ulceration, and fungating lesions.**
    c. **"Anticipatory" palliation** treats potentially symptomatic lesions before they become a problem (e.g., obstruction of the superior vena cava by a mediastinal mass).

II. **APPLIED RADIATION PHYSICS**

1. The use of **ionizing radiation** in the treatment of cancer is based on the ability of radiation to interact with the atoms and molecules of tumor cells to produce specific harmful biologic effects.
2. See **Figure 13-2, text page 237,** for a classification system of ionizing radiations. Among the types of ionizing radiations used in radiation therapy are electromagnetic **X rays** and **gamma rays** and **alpha** and **beta particles.**
    a. **X rays** and **gamma rays** are packets of energy released upon collision with a substance. Both have no mass and can therefore penetrate deeply into tissue.
    b. **Alpha** and **beta particles** have a mass and penetrate less deeply. Beta particles are smaller than alpha particles and penetrate more deeply.
    c. X rays are produced within a tube when a stream of fast-moving electrons strikes a target (usually tungsten) and the electrons give up their energy. X-ray machines focus this energy on selected tissue.
    d. Some treatment machines produce particles in the form of **electrons** (see **Figure 13-3, text page 238),** which are suitable for treating surface lesions and lesions located just below the skin.
    e. Ionizing radiations are also produced through the process of **decay of radioactive elements and isotopes.**
        (1) Because most isotopes are produced by neutron bombardment of stable elements (e.g., cobalt or gold) or nuclear fission of uranium in a nuclear reactor, they are referred to as **artificial isotopes.**
    f. See **Table 13-1, text page 239,** for a list of common radioactive isotopes used in radiotherapy.

III. **EQUIPMENT AND BEAMS USED IN RADIOTHERAPY**

1. The radiation used in radiotherapy can come from a source at a distance from the body **(teletherapy)** or from a source placed within the body or body cavity **(brachytherapy).** See **Figures 13-4** and **13-5, text pages 239–240,** for a classification of these two approaches.
2. In addition to teletherapy and brachytherapy, radiotherapy may be administered systemically using **radioisotopes.**

A. **TELETHERAPY EQUIPMENT**

1. **Conventional or orthovoltage equipment**
    a. **Conventional** or **orthovoltage** equipment produces X rays of varying energies depending on the voltage used. The higher the voltage, the greater the depth of penetration of the X-ray beam.
    b. In selecting the proper beam for treatment of a particular lesion, both the **percentage depth dose of the beam** and the **depth within the body of the lesion** must be known.
        (1) **Percentage depth dose** is defined as the percentage of the intensity of any given beam at a given depth in tissue compared with the presumed 100% dose level.
    c. Orthovoltage equipment, with voltage in the range of 250–400 kilovolts (kV), has been used for many years but has the disadvantages of
        (1) Poor depth of penetration.
        (2) Severe skin reactions, because most of the dose is at the skin level.
        (3) Bone necrosis, because bone absorbs more orthovoltage radiation than does soft tissue.

2. **Megavoltage equipment**
    a. **Megavoltage equipment** operates at 2 to 40 million electron volts (MeV). Compared with orthovoltage, it has significant advantages of
        (1) Deeper beam penetration.
        (2) More homogeneous absorption of radiation, minimizing bone absorption.
        (3) Greater skin sparing.
    b. Equipment includes the **cobalt** and **cesium unit,** the **linear accelerator,** and the **betatron.**
    c. **Cobalt-60 radiotherapy units** are easy to operate and maintain.
        (1) Because cobalt atoms are decaying as they release gamma rays, the cobalt source must be replaced every 5 or 6 years.
        (2) Cobalt units are characterized by lower dose rates and a lower percentage depth dose compared with a linear accelerator.
    d. **Cesium units** are used widely outside the United States. Because of the low specific activity of cesium, the source must be placed closer to the skin (35 cm) than with cobalt units (80 cm).
    e. **Linear accelerators,** although more complex to operate and maintain than cobalt units, are widely used in a variety of treatment settings.
        (1) They are **fast** and produce a **sharply defined field of irradiation** for treating only the desired tissue volume.
    f. Some linear accelerators are also equipped to allow use of the electron beam itself (particle radiation).
        (1) **Electron beam therapy** is particularly useful in superficial lesions, e.g., skin cancers and chest wall recurrence of breast cancer.
        (2) Electrons, being particles, have the advantage over X or gamma rays in that almost all energy is expended at a particular tissue depth, sparing whatever structures lie beyond the tumor site.
    g. The **betatron** uses higher-velocity electrons and is especially useful for deep-seated lesions.

3. **High-energy radiation**
    a. With **high LET radiation,** such as **neutron beam therapy, heavy ion therapy,** and **negative pi-meson therapy,** the number of ionizing events produced in molecules is much greater than with **low LET radiation,** such as gamma rays, X rays, and electrons.
    b. Compared with low LET, high LET radiation produces **more biologic effectiveness, reduced radioresistance,** and **less intertreatment recovery of tumor cells.**
    c. Also, a beam can be shaped to fit the tumor precisely, thus minimizing the amount of radiation damage to surrounding normal tissue.
    d. The cost and sophistication of high energy radiation facilities limit their use to referral centers for carefully selected individuals with cancer.

B. **BRACHYTHERAPY EQUIPMENT**

1. **Brachytherapy** uses sealed sources of radioactive material placed within or near a tumor. It is frequently combined with teletherapy and also may be used preoperatively and postoperatively.

2. Radioisotopes may be in the form of **wires, ribbons, tubes, needles, grains or seeds,** and **capsules.** The decision of what form to use depends on
    a. The **site** to be treated.
    b. The **size** of the lesion.
    c. Whether the implant is to be **temporary or permanent.**
3. Delivery of the radioisotope may be handled in several ways.
    a. Needles, wires, and ribbons are particularly useful for treating head and neck lesions.
    b. Gold or iodine seeds introduced through needles, tubes, or a "seed gun" are used for intra-abdominal and intrathoracic lesions.
    c. Intracavity radiotherapy is often used for gynecologic cancers. A radioactive source is contained in two vaginal ovoids separated by a spacer, with a central uterine tandem added when the corpus and cervix are to be treated.
        (1) Applicators are typically "afterloaded," with the isotope added after the applicator is positioned correctly.
4. **High-dose-rate (HDR)** sources for brachytherapy produce the same radiobiologic effect in shorter time periods than low-dose-rate (LDR) sources.
    a. The total dose and number of fractions is decided based on the body site, desired tumor effect, and potential to minimize the effect on early and late responding normal tissues.
5. **HDR brachytherapy** can be used for intraluminal, interstitial, intracavitary, and surface lesions.
    a. **Remote** afterloading HDR decreases personnel exposure, enables flexible techniques, results in both shorter treatment time and the potential for completion on an outpatient basis.
6. **Nursing implications** include pretreatment education, assessment, treatment phase support, and posttreatment education and follow-up.

IV. SIMULATION AND TREATMENT PLANNING

1. Treatment of cancer with radiotherapy involves three stages: **staging and assessment, treatment planning,** and the treatment itself.
2. The decision to employ radiotherapy is made after consideration of a number of factors, including
    a. **Histologic confirmation of the diagnosis and staging of the disease.**
    b. **The person's age and general condition.**
    c. **The site of the tumor.**
    d. **The radioresponsiveness of the tumor.**
    e. **Risk versus benefit.**
    f. **Patient consent.**
    g. **Availability of treatment facilities.**
3. Treatment planning involves
    a. **Localizing the tumor** and **defining the volume** to be treated. This is often done through sophisticated **simulator** machinery and may involve the use of
        (1) **Diagnostic X rays.**
        (2) **Fluoroscopic examination.**
        (3) **Tattooing of the treatment area.**
        (4) **Transverse axial tomography or a CT scan.**
        (5) **Ultrasound.**
    b. Designing various **restraining** and **positioning devices** to immobilize the person and assure proper position.
    c. **Shaping the field** and **determining what structures are to be blocked and protected** from radiation.
        (1) Tracing the contours of the person's body on paper is a method used to produce an isodose plot.
    d. Consultation between the physician and the radiotherapist on such issues as
        (1) Field arrangement.
        (2) Dose calculations.
        (3) Monitoring of tumor response.
        (4) Accuracy of technical aspects.
4. If the patient can be helped to understand the importance of careful planning, the necessary steps will be accepted or at least tolerated better.

V.   **RADIOBIOLOGY**

    1.   The biologic effects of radiation on humans are the result of a sequence of events that follows the **absorption of energy from ionizing radiation** and the **organism's attempt to compensate for this assault.**

    2.   Radiation effect takes place at the **cellular level,** with consequences in tissues, organs, and the entire body.

A.   **CELLULAR RESPONSE TO RADIATION**

    1.   A **direct hit** effect accounts for most effective and lethal injury produced by ionizing radiation. It occurs when any of the key molecules within the cell, such as DNA or RNA, are damaged.

    2.   Damage from an **indirect hit** is more probable, however, because of the relative proportion of water to DNA in a cell. An indirect hit occurs when ionization of cellular water results in free radicals, triggering toxic chemical reactions within the cell.

    3.   **Cell cycle and radiosensitivity**

        a.   Bergonie and Tribondeau's law states that the **sensitivity of cells to irradiation is in direct proportion to their reproductive activity (how rapidly they are dividing) and inversely proportional to their degree of differentiation.**

            (1)   The effect of radiation is **greatest during mitosis.**

            (2)   The maximum effect of radiation occurs **just before the M and G_2 phases of the cell cycle.** (See **Figure 13-11, text page 245.**)

            (3)   **Undifferentiated** cell populations (e.g., stem cells) are generally most sensitive to radiation. In contrast, **well-differentiated** cells (e.g., erythrocytes) are relatively radioresistant.

        b.   Radiation can produce changes in mitotic activity. **Complete inhibition** of mitosis renders the cell incapable of division; **delayed onset** of mitosis indicates that repair was accomplished and division takes place.

    4.   **Cell death**

        a.   **Mitotic death** occurs after one or more divisions and with relatively small radiation doses.

        b.   **Interphase death** takes place many hours after irradiation and before the cell begins the mitotic process.

        c.   **Instant death** occurs rarely and following extremely high doses of radiation.

    5.   **Other factors**

        a.   **Oxygen effect**

            (1)   **Well-oxygenated tumors show a much greater response to radiation than poorly oxygenated tumors.**

            (2)   The presence of oxygen modifies the dose of radiation needed to produce biologic damage.

            (3)   The magnitude of oxygen effect is expressed as the **oxygen enhancement ratio (OER),** which is the ratio of radiation dose in the absence of oxygen to the radiation dose in the presence of oxygen required for the same effect.

        b.   **Linear energy transfer**

            (1)   **Linear energy transfer** describes the rate at which energy is lost from different types of radiation while traveling through matter.

            (2)   Radiation from **higher LET** (alpha particles, neutrons, and negative pi-mesons) has a greater probability of interacting with matter and producing more direct hits.

        c.   **Relative biologic effectiveness**

            (1)   Because different radiations have varying rates of energy loss, their biologic responses will be different.

            (2)   **Relative biologic effectiveness (RBE)** compares the dose of test radiation with a dose of standard radiation that produces the same biologic response.

        d.   **Dose rate**

            (1)   **Dose rate** refers to the rate at which a given dose is delivered by a treatment machine.

            (2)   Low dose rates are much **less** effective in producing lethal cell damage than high dose rates.

        e.   **Radiosensitivity**

            (1)   According to Bergonie and Tribondeau's law, ionizing radiation is most effective on cells that are **undifferentiated** and **undergoing active mitosis.**

    f.   **Fractionation**
- (1) **Fractionation** means dividing a total dose of radiation into a number of equal fractions. It is based on four important factors: **repair, redistribution, repopulation,** and **reoxygenation.**
- (2) One goal of fractionation is to deliver a dose sufficient to prevent tumor cells from being **repaired** while allowing normal cells to recover before the next dose is given.
- (3) A second goal is to **redistribute cell age** within the cell cycle, making more tumor cells radiosensitive.
- (4) A third goal is to allow normal cells to **repopulate,** sparing them from some of the late consequences that might occur if new growth was inhibited.
- (5) A fourth goal is to allow time between treatments for the tumor to **reoxygenate,** thus becoming more radiosensitive.

    g. Tissue and organ response to radiation can be understood on the basis of sensitivity of cellular components.
- (1) Tissues and organs are composed of more than one cell category, each cell category having different degrees of radiosensitivity.
- (2) Radioresistance of **parenchymal tissue** in an organ will determine if radioactivity will have its greatest effect on the parenchyma or on **stromal** components that support the parenchyma.

VI.   CHEMICAL AND THERMAL MODIFIERS OF RADIATION

A.   RADIOSENSITIZERS AND RADIOPROTECTORS

1. **The goal of radiotherapy is to achieve maximum tumor cell kill while minimizing injury to normal tissues.** This is referred to as the **therapeutic ratio.** One way to improve the therapeutic ratio is through the use of **radiosensitizers** and **radioprotectors.**
2. **Radiosensitizers** enhance or potentiate the effects of radiation.
    a. They are compounds that apparently promote **fixation of free radicals** produced by radiation damage at the molecular level. These biochemical reactions render the molecules incapable of repair.
    b. The most promising radiosensitizer at the present time is SR-2508 **(etanidazole).**
    c. Others, including metronidazole (Flagyl) and misonidazole, were found to be ineffective and overly toxic.
3. **Radioprotectors** are compounds that can protect aerated (nontumor) cells while having a limited effect on hypoxic (tumor) cells.
    a. This action serves to increase the therapeutic ratio by **promoting the repair of irradiated normal tissue.**
    b. Repair or return to a nondamaged state takes place through the chemical process of **reduction,** which can be viewed as the opposite of what occurs when radiosensitizers are used.
    c. Thiophosphate compounds, containing sulfhydryl and aminopropyl groups, were among the earliest radioprotectors synthesized. The compound that appears to be most useful at present is designated **WR-2721.**
4. See **text page 248,** column 1, for a list of some nursing responsibilities in the use of radiosensitizers and radioprotectors.

B.   COMBINED MODALITY THERAPY

1. Since both chemotherapy and radiotherapy have dose-limiting toxicities, greater tumor control with minimal tissue damage (therapeutic index) can be achieved with a **combination** of both.
2. Chemotherapy can
    a. Shrink a tumor when given **prior** to local radiation.
    b. Increase cell kill when given **during** radiation therapy.
    c. **Control** micrometastasis or subclinical disease after radiation therapy.
3. The **sandwich technique** involves radiation and chemotherapy on a planned, alternating schedule.
4. **Combined modality therapy** is being utilized for many cancers, with organ preservation occurring in some individuals with carcinoma of the bladder, larynx, or anus.

5. Examples of **radiosensitizing chemotherapeutic agents** include: cisplatin, methotrexate, doxorubicin, vinblastine, VP-16, mitomycin-C, 5-fluorouracil, actinomycin-D, and bleomycin.
6. Combined modality therapy has the potential for enhanced side effects as well as enhanced tumor effect.
7. The gastrointestinal, integumentary, and myeloproliferative systems are at greatest risk for toxicity with combined modality therapy.

C. **HYPERTHERMIA**

1. Controlled **hyperthermia** combined with radiation achieves tumor cell kill without excess toxicity.
   a. Tumor cells are normally **least** radiosensitive during S-phase, the same phase during which hyperthermia is **most** effective.
   b. The combined effect of radiotherapy and hyperthermia therefore raises tumor cell radiosensitivity and produces greater cell kill than does either alone.
   c. Hypoxic cells, which are generally radioresistant, are also quite thermosensitive.
   d. Finally, heat inhibits the repair of radiation damage, thus increasing the therapeutic ratio.
2. Hyperthermia is achieved in several ways, including immersion of the local area in heated water, ultrasound, microwaves, interstitial implants, and perfusion techniques.
3. **Side effects** of combined hyperthermia and radiation include local skin reaction, pain, fever, gastrointestinal effects, and cardiac arrhythmias.
4. See **Figure 13-3, text page 249,** for an overview of the nursing responsibilities in hyperthermia treatment.

VII. **TISSUE AND ORGAN RESPONSE TO RADIATION**

1. Effects of radiation may be **acute and immediate,** seen within the first 6 months, or they may be **late,** seen after 6 months.
   a. Acute effects are due to **cell damage** in which mitotic activity is altered.
   b. If early effects are not reversible, late or permanent tissue changes occur. These late effects are due to the organism's attempt to heal or repair the damage inflicted by ionizing radiation.
2. The unit of radiation dose is called a **gray (Gy).** One gray equals 100 rad. One **cGy** equals 1 rad (1/100th of a gray).
3. Radiation response is seen mostly in tissues and organs that are within or adjacent to the treatment field. For example, an individual being treated in an abdominal field will not lose scalp hair from radiation.
4. Side effects are specific. Preparation, teaching, and care must be planned for each patient.
5. **Integumentary system**
   a. **Radiosensitivity:** high
   b. **Skin**
      (1) The skin is in a continuous state of reproductive activity.
      (2) The skin may be irradiated when other sites within the body are treated.
      (3) The skin in certain areas (e.g., groin, gluteal fold, axilla, and under the breasts) is usually more affected.
      (4) **Acute reactions:** erythema, dry skin, and changes in pigmentation.
      (5) **Late reactions** (rare): fibrosis, atrophy, ulceration, necrosis, and skin cancer.
   c. **Hair follicles** and **sweat and sebaceous glands** are also radiosensitive due to their high rate of growth and mitotic activity.
      (1) Inhibition of hair growth coupled with accelerated hair loss produces a net loss of hair **(alopecia),** which is usually temporary.
      (2) High doses may produce permanent alopecia.
6. **Hematopoietic system**
   a. **Radiosensitivity:** high (stem cells of red bone marrow, spleen, lymph nodes); low (mature, nondividing blood cells; lymphatic vessels).
   b. **Reactions:** reduced marrow activity; suppression of erythroblasts and myeloblasts; alteration of spleen functions in hemolysis, red blood cell and iron storage, and antibody production; shrinkage of spleen.
   c. Interference with lymphatic vessel function. Fibrotic changes and obstruction cause.

7. **Gastrointestinal system**
   a. **Radiosensitivity:** high (mucous membranes of the entire system, especially the **crypt cells** of the small intestine; glandular tissue). Severity of reactions is highly dose-dependent.
   b. **Reactions to lower doses:** mucositis and alteration of salivary function; alterations in the sense of taste; reduction of gastric secretions; nausea, dyspepsia, and pyloric spasm; anorexia; nausea; cramping; diarrhea; tenesmus.
   c. **Reactions to higher doses** and **late changes:** atrophy of salivary glands, esophagus, and stomach; loss of absorptive tissue in intestines and accompanying nutritional deficiencies; fibrosis, ulcerations, necrosis, and hemorrhage in intestines; intestinal obstruction (especially when combined with surgery).
8. **Liver**
   a. **Radiosensitivity:** moderate.
   b. **Reactions:** vascular injury; radiation hepatitis (high doses).
9. **Respiratory system**
   a. **Radiosensitivity:** high (mucous membranes).
   b. **Acute reactions:** hoarseness; pneumonitis.
   c. **Late reactions:** fibrosis in the lung tissue; thickening of pleura.
10. **Reproductive system**
    a. **Radiosensitivity:** high (vaginal mucous membrane; intermediate follicles; testes); moderate to low (mature graafian follicles, small follicles, cervix, uterine body).
    b. **Reactions:** mucositis and inflammation; temporary or permanent sterility in females, depending on dose and patient's age; sterility in males; damage to intermediate follicles; hormonal changes (especially loss of estrogen) and early menopause; genetic damage, especially at low doses.
11. **Urinary system**
    a. **Radiosensitivity:** moderate.
    b. **Reactions:** low doses (cystitis, urethritis); high doses (nephritis).
12. **Cardiovascular system**
    a. **Radiosensitivity:** low to moderate.
    b. **Reactions:** vascular damage; thrombosis; telangiectasia, petechiae, sclerosis (late); damage to heart vasculature (high doses).
13. **Nervous system**
    a. **Radiosensitivity:** low.
    b. **Reactions:** low doses (myelopathy); moderate to high doses (Lhermitte's syndrome, paralysis, paresis, transverse myelitis, vascular insufficiency to sense organs).
14. **Skeletal system**
    a. **Radiosensitivity:** low.
    b. **Late reactions:** high doses (avascular necrosis, damage to epiphyses and stunting in children).

A. **SYSTEMIC EFFECTS OF RADIATION**

1. The person receiving radiotherapy may experience certain subjective **systemic** effects, including nausea, anorexia, and malaise, in addition to the local effects described above.
   a. These effects can be linked to the **release of toxic wastes** into the bloodstream resulting from tumor destruction.
   b. The extent of the effects depends on the **volume of the irradiated area,** the **anatomic site,** and the **dose.**
2. **Whole body and hemibody radiation**
   a. In some treatments the whole body is irradiated.
   b. Delivery may be in the form of
      (1) **Small daily doses** fractionated over a 10-week period. Side effects are negligible.
      (2) A **large dose** (1000 Cgy) administered over 6 to 8 hours before bone marrow transplantation. Side effects are extensive and include both immediate reactions (e.g., nausea, alopecia, pancreatitis) and delayed reactions (e.g., cataracts, sterility, and major organ damage).
   c. **Hemibody radiation** is treatment of the upper, middle, or lower body in a single large fraction. This is used for patients with widespread bone metastasis to achieve rapid palliation of pain.

   d.   **Side effects** of hemibody radiation are significant as a result of the large dose. The effects are specific to the site treated, such as nausea, in the event of upper and mid-body treatment.

3.   **Altered fractionation schedules**
   a.   Standard treatment is single daily fractions, given 5 days per week in daily doses.
   b.   Fractionation **schedules** are guided by patient tolerance, convenience, staff availability, and tissue tolerance.
   c.   **Hyperfractionation** is increased numbers of fractions delivered over the same total treatment time as standard fractionation.
   d.   **Accelerated fractionation** uses three fractions per day to achieve the same total dose as hyperfractionation, while shortening the overall treatment time by about two weeks.
   e.   **Dynamic fractionation** occurs when doses are escalated over the length of the treatment course.

4.   **Chronic low-dose exposure**
   a.   Naturally occurring radioactive substances cause chronic low-dose radiation exposure, without producing ill effects.

5.   **Total body radiation syndrome**
   a.   **Total body radiation syndrome** refers to the effects of the acute exposure of the organism to doses of radiation in a matter of minutes rather than hours or days, e.g., a nuclear accident such as Chernobyl.

6.   **Radiation-induced malignancies in humans**
   a.   Acute high-dose exposure and chronic low-dose exposure are the exceptions, occurring principally in **radiation accidents** and **occupational exposure.**
   b.   The usually prescribed therapeutic doses (2500 to 6500 Cgy) are believed to be less carcinogenic than lower doses given over a much longer time period.
   c.   The most common carcinomas associated with radiation exposure are **skin carcinoma** and **leukemia.**
   d.   Radiation carcinogenesis depends on a number of factors, including a **long latent period** (1 to 30 years), **radiation dose, concomitant factors in the person's environment,** and the **actual fate of the cell** as it responds to radiation injury.

VIII.   **NURSING CARE OF THE PATIENT RECEIVING RADIOTHERAPY**

1.   **Nursing care should focus on all of the patient's needs and problems associated with a diagnosis of cancer, not just the specific disease site or treatment.** This includes consideration of long-term needs.
2.   Each person must be assessed and managed on an individual basis.
3.   The nurse's role in the care of the patient receiving radiotherapy encompasses a variety of specific issues, including
   a.   **Diagnosis and the person's acceptance of treatment.**
   b.   **Misconceptions the person may have about radiotherapy.**
   c.   **The potential side effects of the therapy.**
   d.   **The length of the treatment period (average = 5 weeks).**
   e.   **Preparation (both physical and psychological) for treatment.**
   f.   **Transportation arrangements that may need to be met.**
   g.   **Symptomatic relief of side effects and nutritional support.**
   h.   **Social and financial assistance.**
   i.   **Variations in the treatment plan.**
   j.   **Acceptance and continuation of treatment despite immediate discomforts.**

IX.   **SPECIFIC NURSING CARE MEASURES FOR PATIENTS RECEIVING RADIOTHERAPY**

1.   During a course of radiotherapy, certain treatment-related side effects can be expected to develop. Most of these are **site-specific,** as well as dependent on **volume, dose fractionation, total dose,** and **individual differences.**
2.   Many symptoms do not develop until approximately 10 to 14 days into treatment. Some do not subside until 2 or more weeks after treatments have ended.

A.   **FATIGUE**

1.   **Symptoms:** Fatigue is common among individuals during radiotherapy and for varying periods afterwards.

2. **Table 13-4, text page 257,** lists common factors that contribute to fatigue.
3. **Management:** Patients should be encouraged to rest frequently and alter their schedule. **Management** includes **pretreatment education** regarding the potential for treatment-induced fatigue, effective **pain** management, encouraging the patient to rest **frequently,** and reducing the normal activity level as needed.

B. **ANOREXIA**

1. **Symptoms:** Anorexia occurs frequently regardless of the treatment site. It is related to the presence in the person's system of waste products of tissue destruction.
2. **Management:** Utilize all the techniques known to encourage adequate intake (see **text Chapter 24).**

C. **MUCOSITIS**

1. **Symptoms:** Mucositis is a patchy, white membrane that becomes confluent and may bleed if disturbed. The reaction is most visible when radiation is given to the mouth and oropharynx.
2. **Management:**
   a. The patient should be encouraged to avoid alcohol and other oral irritants.
   b. One ounce of Benadryl elixir diluted in 1 quart of water provides an ideal mouthwash agent.
   c. Mouth care should be done every 3–4 hours. Care should be taken not to dislodge the plaquelike formations of mucositis, causing bleeding.
   d. Maalox and Lidocaine may be used to coat or soothe the mucosa.

D. **XEROSTOMIA**

1. **Symptoms:** Xerostomia is the dry mouth that results from radiation to the salivary glands. It is sometimes accompanied by alterations in taste.
2. **Management:** Frequent mouth care, saliva substitutes, and frequent sips of water are most useful.

E. **RADIATION CARIES**

1. **Symptoms:** Absence or decrease in saliva and the altered Ph produced by treatment promote decay.
2. **Management:** Proper preventive oral care before, during, and after treatment should include Benadryl mouth sprays, followed by a 5-minute application of fluoride gel, and brushing with a soft-bristled brush several times daily.
   a. If extensive decay and general poor dentition exist, full mouth extraction is usually the treatment of choice.
3. See **Table 13-5, text page 259,** for a patient information sheet on oral and dental care.

F. **ESOPHAGITIS AND DYSPHAGIA**

1. **Symptoms:** Treatment to the mediastinum may produce symptoms of transient esophagitis. It may interfere with the patient's swallowing and cause a decrease in intake of foods and fluids.
2. **Management:** See **text page 258,** column 2, for a mixture that gives temporary relief. The diet should consist of high-calorie, high-protein, high-carbohydrate liquids and soft, bland foods.

G. **NAUSEA AND VOMITING**

1. **Symptoms:** Although nausea and vomiting are not common, the fear that they will occur causes great stress in many individuals.
2. **Management:** Nausea can be controlled by antiemetics administered on a regular schedule and by adjusting the eating pattern so that treatment is given when the stomach is relatively empty.

H. **DIARRHEA**

1. **Symptoms:** Diarrhea occurs if the areas of the abdomen and pelvis are treated after about 2000 Cgy have been given.
2. **Management:** For most individuals, a low-residue diet (see **Table 13-6, text page 260)** and prescription of loperamide hydrochloride are usually sufficient.

I.   **TENESMUS, CYSTITIS, AND URETHRITIS**

1.   **Symptoms:** These symptoms occur in some individuals receiving pelvic irradiation.
2.   **Management:**
   a.   Relief can sometimes be obtained from gastrointestinal and urinary antispasmodics and anticholinergic preparations.
   b.   Antibiotics may be used for cystitis and urethritis if infection is found by culture.
   c.   High fluid intake is encouraged.
   d.   Sitz baths are contraindicated if the perineal area is being irradiated.

J.   **ALOPECIA**

1.   **Symptoms:** Alopecia will occur with treatment to the scalp area, as with a primary brain tumor. Hair loss typically occurs gradually over a 2- or 3-week period followed by a sudden loss of all hair. Hair loss may also occur regionally or in patches.
2.   **Management:**
   a.   The patient can prepare by procuring a wig, attractive scarf, or cap.
   b.   Gentle hair and scalp care is important, and harsh chemicals should be avoided.
   c.   The top of the head should be protected from sunburn with a cap.

K.   **SKIN REACTIONS**

1.   **Symptoms:** The response of normal skin to radiation varies from mild erythema to moist desquamation that leaves a raw surface similar to second degree burn. Healing and cosmesis are usually satisfactory. Some patients may have permanent tanning. Others will have fibrosclerotic changes in subcutaneous structures, and their skin will be smooth, taut, and shiny. Telangiectasia may also be present.
2.   **Management:**
   a.   The skin should be kept as dry as possible. (See **text page 261,** column 2, for guidelines.)
   b.   Cornstarch or A and D ointment followed by a Telfa dressing may be applied to specific skin reactions.
   c.   Exposure to sun should be minimized for treated areas.
   d.   See **Table 13-8, text page 263,** for skin care guidelines during sun exposure.

L.   **BONE MARROW DEPRESSION**

1.   **Symptoms:** When large volumes of active bone marrow are irradiated (especially the pelvis or spine in the adult), the effect on the marrow can be quite significant.
2.   **Management:**
   a.   Blood counts should be done 2 to 3 times weekly for patients also receiving chemotherapy (e.g., for Hodgkin's disease) and more often for patients receiving total body irradiation or splenic irradiation.
   b.   For significant effects, transfusions may be needed.
   c.   Nurses, patients, and family should look for signs of bleeding, anemia, and infection.

M.   **RADIATION SIDE EFFECTS: SPECIAL CONSIDERATIONS**

1.   Other less common side effects include **transient myelitis, parotitis, visual and olfactory disturbances,** and **radiation recall.**

X.   **NURSING CARE OF THE PATIENT WITH A RADIOACTIVE SOURCE**

1.   The nurse should develop a healthy respect for all that is implicit in working with radioactive isotopes.
2.   In addition to radioactive implantation (**Figure 13-5**), some radioactive isotopes are administered **orally, intravenously,** or by **installation.**
   a. ^{131}I, ^{32}P, ^{198}Au are all administered as **colloids** or **solutions** and are adsorbed or metabolized.
   b.   Liquid sources present a possibility of contamination of equipment, dressings, and linens, depending on the mode of administration and metabolism.

3. See **text page 264,** column 2, for information to provide safe and effective nursing care for individuals with a radioactive source.
   a. From this information, the nurse can plan and administer nursing care utilizing appropriate precautions, including disposal of wastes and care of linens and equipment.
4. The three primary factors in radiation protection in care of the patient with a radioactive source are **time, distance,** and **shielding.**

A. **TIME**

1. The exposure to radiation that personnel receive is directly proportional to the time spent within a specific distance from the source.
2. Nurses should limit the time spent in close contact with the patient.

B. **DISTANCE**

1. As radiation is emitted from a point source, the amount of radiation reaching a given area decreases according to the law of inverse square. **Figure 13-13, text page 265,** illustrates this principle.

C. **SHIELDING**

1. When planning nursing care for the person with a radioactive source, time and distance are the factors that can most easily be controlled.
2. Shielding is not always possible or practical.
   a. The **HVL (half-value layer,** or the thickness of shielding material that is required to reduce radiation to half of its original quantity) for ^{137}Cs is approximately 6 mm of lead or 10 cm of cement.
   b. Portable radiation shields are impractical for direct care.
   c. Lead aprons are insufficiently thick to provide protection.
3. See **Table 13-9, text page 266,** for a list of ways to reduce exposure to personnel caring for the individual with a radioactive source.

D. **PATIENT EDUCATION AND SUPPORT**

1. Planning and emotional support are major components of nursing care for individuals with a radioactive implant.
2. Patient education issues to discuss include:
   a. Description of the procedure.
   b. Possible change in appearance.
   c. Anticipated pain and discomfort and measures available for relief.
   d. Potential short-term and long-term side effects and complications.
   e. Restrictions on activity while the radioactive sources are in place.
   f. Visiting restrictions.
   g. Radiation precautions observed by hospital personnel.

XI. **ADVANCES IN RADIOTHERAPY**

1. **Radiolabeled antibody therapy** is perhaps the most exciting area of current investigation in radiotherapy. When perfected, it will allow clinicians to deliver radioisotopes to tumors directly, relying on specific tumor antigens and labeled tumor-specific antibodies.

PRACTICE QUESTIONS

1. An example of the use of radiotherapy for palliation is the treatment of
   (A) poorly oxygenated tumor cells with a radiosensitizer.
   (B) CNS symptoms caused by spinal cord compression with radiation.
   (C) postoperative esophagitis with a combination of soft food and a topical pain reliever.
   (D) a tumor embedded in neck tissue with brachytherapy.

2. An important advantage of megavoltage equipment over conventional or orthovoltage equipment used in radiotherapy is that it
    (A) is more effective in treating surface lesions.
    (B) reduces absorption of radiation by bone.
    (C) delivers radioisotopes to the site of the tumor.
    (D) limits release of dangerous heavy ions and negative pi-mesons.

3. An advantage that high LET (linear energy transfer) radiation has over low LET radiation is that
    (A) equipment used to produce high LET radiation is generally less costly.
    (B) high LET radiation produces fewer ionizing events in molecules.
    (C) a particle beam can be shaped to fit the tumor precisely.
    (D) high LET radiation increases the radioresistance of hypoxic cells in tumors.

4. For which of the following types of lesions would mould therapy **most** likely be used?
    (A) a skin carcinoma on the ear
    (B) a brain tumor
    (C) a metastatic abdominal tumor
    (D) Hodgkin's disease

5. Simulators are used in treatment planning for radiotherapy in order to localize a tumor and to
    (A) define the volume to be treated with radiotherapy.
    (B) remove a section of a tumor for laboratory evaluation.
    (C) reduce the size of a tumor prior to surgical resection.
    (D) prepare a histopathologic profile of a tumor.

6. Radiation effects take place **primarily** at the level of
    (A) cells.
    (B) tissues.
    (C) organs.
    (D) the whole body.

7. Which of the following cells is likely to be **most** radiosensitive?
    (A) a well-differentiated, nondividing, and well-oxygenated cell
    (B) an undifferentiated, dividing, and poorly oxygenated cell
    (C) a well-differentiated, nondividing, and poorly oxygenated cell
    (D) an undifferentiated, dividing, and well-oxygenated cell

8. One of the primary goals of dose fractionation is to
    (A) redistribute cell age within the cell cycle, making normal cells less radiosensitive.
    (B) allow tumor cells to repopulate, making them more vulnerable to the late consequences that occur if new growth was inhibited.
    (C) deliver a dose sufficient to prevent tumor cells from being repaired while allowing normal cells to recover before the next dose is given.
    (D) provide time between treatments for normal cells to reoxygenate, thus making them less radiosensitive.

9. The late effects of radiation that are often seen after 6 months or more following radiotherapy are the result of
    (A) cell damage in which mitotic activity is temporarily altered in some way.
    (B) acute damage that occurs to tissues and organs outside the treatment field.
    (C) the organism's attempt to repair the damage inflicted by ionizing radiation.
    (D) acute, site-specific reactions to treatment.

10. A patient being treated in an abdominal field is concerned about hair loss that she expects to experience following radiotherapy. You can **best** reassure her by telling her that
    (A) hair follicles are relatively radioresistant due to their low rate of growth and mitotic activity.
    (B) radiation response is seen mostly in tissues and organs that are within the treatment field.
    (C) alopecia is permanent only when radiation is administered in low doses over an extended period of time.
    (D) alopecia is more closely associated with brachytherapy than with teletherapy.

11. In tissues such as the liver or heart that are relatively radioresistant, damage from high doses of radiation is **most** likely to occur from damage to
     (A) parenchyma.
     (B) vascular tissue.
     (C) mucous membranes.
     (D) rapidly dividing cells.

12. Subjective systemic reactions to radiation, including fatigue, anorexia, and nausea, are **most** often caused by
     (A) acute exposure of the organism to doses of radiation in a matter of minutes rather than hours or days.
     (B) chronic exposure of the whole body to low doses of radiation.
     (C) acute, site-specific reactions that occur at the cellular and molecular levels.
     (D) the release of toxic wastes into the bloodstream resulting from tumor destruction.

13. A patient who has been treated with radiation to the mouth and oropharynx has developed mucositis. Effective management of this side effect would incorporate all of the following **except**
     (A) encouraging the patient to avoid alcohol and cigarettes.
     (B) administering a Benadryl solution as a mouthwash or spray.
     (C) removing the plaquelike tissue that forms with mucositis.
     (D) administering Maalox to coat and soothe mucosa.

14. Management of tenesmus, cystitis, and urethritis that may result when radiation is given to the pelvic area involves several nursing options, including all of the following **except**
     (A) administering gastrointestinal and urinary antispasmodics.
     (B) administering antibiotics if there is evidence of infection.
     (C) encouraging high fluid intake by the patient.
     (D) providing sitz baths if the perineal area is being irradiated.

15. Side effects of radiation to the skin are **least** likely to include which of the following?
     (A) mild erythema and moist desquamation
     (B) fibrosclerotic changes that make skin smooth, taut, and shiny
     (C) permanent tanning
     (D) complete or patchy alopecia

16. The possibility of contamination of equipment, dressings, and linens is greatest when radioactive isotopes are delivered in what form?
     (A) as implants
     (B) as colloids or solutions
     (C) as moulds
     (D) as ovoids separated by a spacer

17. The type of radiation that has the shortest wavelength and is capable of deep tissue penetration is:
     (A) infrared radiation
     (B) electrons
     (C) ionizing radiation
     (D) alpha particles

18. What is the term given to compounds that assist in maximizing the tumor cell kill achieved with radiation, while minimizing injury to normal tissues?
     (A) radioantagonists
     (B) radiosensitizers
     (C) oxygen enhancement ratio
     (D) linear energy transfer

19. Radiation therapy to the lower abdomen and pelvis of a woman leads to a number of potential side effects. Which of the following statements is **not** true?
     (A) older women are sterilized at lower doses than younger women
     (B) vaginal mucositis is a short-term side effect
     (C) vaginal stenosis can result from fibrosis
     (D) genetic damage becomes a potential problem only with higher doses of radiation

20. Nurses are often involved with managing the side effects that result from radiotherapy. Anticipating the occurrence of the side effects is crucial in order to assist the patient in self-care and to minimize the degree of the symptoms experienced. Which time frame is most appropriate for the nurse to schedule to see most patients in order to evaluate the symptoms being experienced from radiotherapy?
    (A) immediately after the first fractionated dose
    (B) upon completion of the scheduled 5-week course
    (C) at the end of the first week
    (D) 10–14 days after treatment has begun

ANSWER EXPLANATIONS

1. **The answer is (B).** Palliative radiation is used for a variety of treatment purposes, including pain relief, prevention of pathologic fractures, relief of central nervous system (CNS) symptoms caused by brain metastasis or spinal cord compression, and the reduction of hemorrhage, ulceration, and fungating lesions. (236)

2. **The answer is (B).** Megavoltage equipment operates at 2 to 40 **million** electron volts (MeV) compared to orthovoltage equipment's 40 to 400 **thousand** electron volts (Kv). It has the advantages of deeper beam penetration, more homogeneous absorption of radiation (minimizing bone absorption), and greater skin sparing. Megavoltage equipment includes cobalt and cesium units, the linear accelerator, the betatron, and such experimental units as those producing neutron beams, heavy ions, and negative pi-mesons. (239–240)

3. **The answer is (C).** With high LET radiation, including neutron beams, heavy ions, and negative pi-mesons, the number of ionizing events produced in molecules is much greater than with low LET radiation, such as gamma rays, X rays, and electrons. Because high LET beams consist of particles, a beam can be shaped to fit the tumor precisely, thus minimizing the amount of radiation damage to surrounding normal tissue. (246)

4. **The answer is (A).** Mould (or surface) therapy is a type of brachytherapy involving close contact of radio-active seeds, often of radon, encased in a plastic mould. The mould is placed in close contact with the lesion. This method is most useful for surface lesions in irregularly contoured areas such as the face. (238)

5. **The answer is (A).** Simulator machinery may involve the use of diagnostic X rays, fluoroscopic examination, transverse axial tomography, CT scans, and ultrasound, with the goal in mind of localizing a tumor and defining the volume to be treated with radiotherapy. Other aspects of treatment planning include the tattooing of the treatment area, installing various restraining and positioning devices to immobilize the person, shaping the field, and determining what structures are to be blocked and protected from radiation. (242–243)

6. **The answer is (A).** The biologic effects of radiation on humans are the result of a sequence of events that follows the absorption of energy from ionizing radiation and the organism's attempt to compensate for this assault. Radiation effect takes place at the cellular level, with consequences in tissues, organs, and the entire body. (244)

7. **The answer is (D).** According to Bergonie and Tribondeau's law, ionizing radiation is most effective on cells that are undifferentiated and undergoing active mitosis (dividing). In addition, well-oxygenated cells show a much greater response to radiation than poorly oxygenated (hypoxic) cells. Other factors that affect cellular response to radiation include the type, strength, and biologic effectiveness of the irradiation used, and the frequency at which a dose is administered (fractionation). (245–247)

8. **The answer is (C).** All of the other choices are opposites of the actual goals of fractionation. Fractionation redistributes cell age within the cell cycle, making tumor cells more radiosensitive. It allows normal cells to repopulate, sparing them from some of the late consequences that occur if new growth was inhibited. And it provides time between treatments for tumor cells to reoxygenate, thus making them more radiosensitive. (246–247)

9.   **The answer is (C).**   Effects of radiation may be acute and immediate, seen within the first 6 months, or they may be late, seen after 6 months. Acute effects are due to cell damage in which mitotic activity is altered. If early effects are not reversible, late or permanent tissue changes occur. These late effects are due to the organism's attempt to heal or repair the damage inflicted by ionizing radiation. (249)

10.   **The answer is (B).**   Radiation response is seen mostly in tissues and organs that are within or adjacent to the treatment field, i.e., they are site-specific. For example, an individual being treated in the mediastinum is unlikely to develop diarrhea, which is associated with pelvic treatment. (250)

11.   **The answer is (B).**   Many of the acute reactions to high doses of radiation occur as the result of indirect effects on the stromal components (especially the vasculature) that support the parenchyma of irradiated tissues and organs. This explains the damage that can occur to organs in which parenchymal tissue is relatively radioresistant. (247, 251)

12.   **The answer is (D).**   The presence of these toxins may account for the nausea and anorexia, whereas the increased metabolic rate required to dispose of the waste products might be partially responsible for the frequent complaint of fatigue. The extent of these effects depends on the volume of the irradiated area, the anatomic site, and the dose. (252–253)

13.   **The answer is (C).**   Gentle, frequent mouth care with soothing solutions can be helpful. Care should be taken, however, not to dislodge the plaquelike formations of mucositis, causing bleeding. (257)

14.   **The answer is (D).**   Sitz baths are contraindicated if the perineal area is being irradiated. (261–262)

15.   **The answer is (D).**   Except in cases of whole body irradiation or irradiation to the head, alopecia should not occur. (261)

16.   **The answer is (B).**   In addition to radioactive implantation, some radioactive isotopes are administered orally, intravenously, or by installation. Liquid sources administered as colloids or solutions are adsorbed or metabolized and present a possibility of contamination of equipment, dressings, and linens, depending on the mode of administration and metabolism. (264)

17.   **The answer is (C).**   X ray and gamma ray both describe ionizing electromagnetic radiation. Ionizing radiation has the shortest wavelength and the greatest energy of the electromagnetic spectrum and is therefore the form of energy used in radiotherapy. Both X rays and gamma rays have no mass, but are rather packets of available energy ready to be released on collision with a substance. Because they have no mass, X and gamma rays can penetrate much deeper into tissue before releasing their energy. (237)

18.   **The answer is (B).**   Efforts to improve the therapeutic ratio have resulted in the development of certain compounds that act to increase the radiosensitivity of tumor cells or to protect normal cells from radiation effect. Radiosensitizers are compounds that apparently promote fixation of the free radicals produced by radiation damage at the molecular level. (247)

19.   **The answer is (D).**   Chromosomal aberrations are a possibility that must be considered, especially at lower doses. The consequences of radiation to the gonads in both the male and female is the potential for genetic damage. The age of the person being treated and the dose of radiation to the ovaries determine whether a woman has temporary or permanent sterilization. Older women have fewer ova than younger women and therefore can become sterile at lower doses. (252)

20.   **The answer is (D).**   During a course of radiotherapy, certain treatment-related side effects can be expected to develop, most of which are site specific as well as dependent on volume, dose fractionation, total dose, and individual differences. Many symptoms do not develop until approximately 10–14 days into treatment, and some do not subside until 2 or more weeks after treatments have ended. (256)

14 Chemotherapy: Principles of Therapy

STUDY OUTLINE

I. **INTRODUCTION**

1. Advances in basic science have dramatically influenced drug development and clinical drug trials over the past 50 years.
2. Important examples of the relationship between basic science and clinical practice include our understanding about the behavior of tumors, the effect of tumor burden on therapy, metastatic processes and sensitivity, and resistance of tumor cells to chemotherapeutic drugs.
3. New knowledge in cancer biology has direct clinical application for the design of clinical trials, selection and administration of therapy, and the development of strategies to overcome drug resistance.

II. **FACTORS INFLUENCING CHEMOTHERAPY EFFECTIVENESS**

1. Responses to chemotherapy are influenced by the **biological characteristics of tumors, host factors, available chemotherapeutic drugs,** and **genetics.**
2. **Tumor factors** that influence response to chemotherapy include growth rate, growth fraction, tumor type, tumor cell heterogeneity, and tumor burden.
3. **Host factors** influencing response to chemotherapy include nutritional status, level of immune function, physical and psychological tolerance to specific drugs/regimens, and the availability and effectiveness of supportive therapies.
4. The **response to a specific drug regimen** is related to the sensitivity of the specific tumor type and tumor cells, the dose, the toxicity, and the route and schedule of administration.
5. **Genetic changes** in individual tumor cells that result in the emergence of drug resistance appear to be the most significant factors explaining the limitations to cure with chemotherapy.

III. **HISTORICAL PERSPECTIVE ON CHEMOTHERAPY AND RESISTANCE**

1. Despite significant advances, substantial limitations to the curability of various malignancies remain. The concept of **resistance** of tumor cells to drug therapy provides an explanation for our failures and our successes.
2. Views on the proposed mechanisms for drug resistance have evolved from **kinetic** to **biochemical** to **pharmacologic** to **genetic.**
3. The kinetic view of resistance is based on the cell cycle and on the hypothesis that drugs are most effective on actively dividing cells.
4. Clinical outcomes supported the kinetic hypotheses.
   a. Hematologic malignancies with highly proliferative cells were the focus of treatment.
   b. Solid tumors were observed as less responsive, which was explained by the kinetic factors of a long doubling time, low growth fraction, and a large percentage of cells in the resting phase.

A. **CELL CYCLE**

1. Knowledge of the cell cycle is important to understanding cell proliferation, tumor growth, and the rationale for chemotherapy.

2. There are three potential cell populations: those that are actively dividing, those that leave the cell cycle after a certain point and differentiate, and those that temporarily leave the cell cycle, remaining in a dormant state until reentry into the cycle.

3. The cell cycle consists of five phases: G_1, S, G_2, M, and G_0. See **Figure 14-3, text page 273.**
    a. Gap (represented by the capital letter G) is the term used for the time between mitosis and S phase.
    b. The G_1 phase is primarily directed at RNA and protein synthesis and can last anywhere from 2–3 hours to several days. Generally, a long G_1 phase reflects slow-growing cell populations, whereas a short G_1 phase reflects a rapidly proliferating cell population.
    c. The S phase is when DNA synthesis takes place.
    d. G_2 is a relatively brief phase after the cell completes DNA synthesis and is getting ready to begin mitosis.
    e. The M phase is mitosis, which results in cell division.
    f. The G_0, or resting, phase represents cells that are out of the cycle but have the potential to reenter.

4. **Cell cycle time** is the interval between mitosis for cycling cells.

5. **Growth fraction** is the fraction or percentage of cycling cells within the overall population of cells.

6. **Rate of cell loss** is the fraction or percentage of cells that die or go to other tissues.

7. **Doubling time** is the time it takes a tumor to double its size.

B. **CELL KILL HYPOTHESIS**

1. The basis of the cell kill hypothesis is **log kill.** See **Figure 14-4, text page 274.**

2. Each cycle of chemotherapy will kill a **constant proportion** of tumor cells, not a **constant number,** and thus there is a relationship among cell number, treatment, and tumor cell survival. The net tumor cell kill for a given treatment is the surviving tumor cells plus the cells that regrow before the next drug treatment.

3. This model assumes that the tumor cells remain sensitive to the chemotherapy drug(s) throughout the entire course of treatment.

4. The **Gompertzian model of tumor growth** proposes an exponential growth curve for a tumor in the early stages, followed by a decreasing growth rate and plateau as the tumor size increases.

5. According to this model, large tumors with **low growth fractions** would predictably fail to respond or have a poor response to the majority of antineoplastic drugs, which are directed at altering DNA metabolism. On the other hand, a large fraction of cells would be killed in smaller tumors that have high growth fractions (i.e., a large population of proliferating cells).

6. Kinetic, biochemical, and pharmacologic parameters alone fail to explain the observed variability of tumor responsiveness to chemotherapy and, in particular, fail to account for the development of unresponsiveness in tumors that were initially drug-sensitive.

IV. **DRUG RESISTANCE**

1. There are **two** major types of **drug resistance:** temporary and permanent.
    a. **Temporary** or **relative resistance** is related to factors such as variation in drug bioavailability, metabolism or elimination, the presence of tumor in sanctuary sites, limited drug diffusion, alteration in cell kinetics, host toxicity, and blood supply of the tumor.
    b. **Permanent** or **phenotypic** drug resistance is genetically based and is thought to be the major factor for chemotherapy drug failure.

2. **Somatic mutation theory** underlies the **Goldie-Coldman model** of the development of chemotherapy-resistant cancer cells. Somatic mutation theory proposes that **all biologic systems have an inherent probability of undergoing genetic variation as a consequence of random changes.**

3. The **Goldie-Coldman model** of drug resistance in cancer was proposed in the early 1980s to explain the development of cytotoxic drug resistance.
    a. The model contains several assumptions.
        (1) Somatic mutation theory.
        (2) Genetic changes in cells.
        (3) Random nature of changes.

      (4)   Genetic instability of neoplasms.
      (5)   Cure means zero resistant cells.
      (6)   Probability of resistant cells is a product of mutation rate and age of the tumor.
      (7)   Tumor cells have stem cell capacity.

    b.   According to this model, tumor burden, tumor cell heterogeneity, and the known genetic instability of tumor cells increase the risk of genetic changes and thus increase the potential for the development of mutant cells that are drug-resistant.

    c.   Genetic changes that may occur in cells include mutations, deletions, transposition of genetic elements, gene amplifications, chromosomal rearrangements, and translocations.

    d.   The development of even one resistant phenotype will decrease the ability to attain cure since it will be resistant to the chemotherapy drug(s) even at maximum doses. With increasing tumor size, there is an almost certain probability that at least one resistant mutation will have occurred. Thus the probability for cure decreases with a higher mutation rate or a greater tumor burden.

4.   Permanent drug resistance is either **intrinsic** or **acquired.**
    a.   **Intrinsic resistance** of tumor cells occurs without any prior drug exposure.
    b.   **Acquired resistance** develops after treatment and represents a permanent change in the nature of the tumor cells themselves.

5.   Several mechanisms of resistance to cytotoxic drugs have been identified. They include defective transport, defective drug metabolism, altered nucleotide pools, increased drug activation, altered DNA repair, gene amplification, altered target protein, and multidrug resistance.

6.   **Multidrug resistance (MDR)** or **pleiotropic drug resistance (PDR)** is a phenomenon in which exposure to a single drug is followed by **cross-resistance** to other drugs that are structurally unrelated and may have different mechanisms of action.
    a.   The initial drug involved appears to be a natural product such as doxorubicin, daunorubicin, vincristine, vinblastine, etoposide, taxol, mitomycin, or mitoxantrone.
    b.   While these natural products all vary in structure, they are presumed to use a similar transport system, and **drug transport** appears to be a critical component in multidrug resistance.

7.   Tumors that are drug resistant have reduced drug accumulation within the cell and within the nucleus of the cell. There are two proposed mechanisms for reduced drug accumulation.
    a.   Drugs enter the cell at normal rates but are removed by an efflux pump.
    b.   There is a barrier controlling entry of the drug into the cell.

8.   The causative factor in the development of chemotherapy resistance appears to be **P-glycoprotein.** It is thought that drugs bind to P-glycoprotein and are actively pumped out of the cell. **Overexpression of P-glycoprotein** is the **predominant gene alteration** responsible for multidrug resistance.

9.   Expression of P-glycoprotein and the MDR phenotypes have been documented in a substantial number of hematologic and solid tumors.

V.   THERAPEUTIC STRATEGIES

1.   Current understanding of **cell kinetics, pharmcokinetics, mechanisms of action, and mechanisms of resistance (intrinsic, acquired, and multidrug)** provides the rationale for many current treatment strategies, including combination drug regimens, scheduling, adjuvant therapy, sequencing, dose intensity, and agents to inhibit the function of P-glycoprotein in multidrug resistance.

A.   COMBINATION CHEMOTHERAPY

1.   Several principles underlie combination chemotherapy.
    a.   Maximum cell kill with tolerable toxicity.
    b.   Tumor cell sensitivity to each of the drugs in a regimen.
    c.   Broad coverage of resistant cell lines in a heterogeneous tumor population.
    d.   Minimizing or preventing the development of new resistant cell lines.

2.   Factors to be considered in designing a combination chemotherapy regimen include cell cycle specificity, different modes of action, varied toxicity, effectiveness of each single drug against a specific tumor type, drug synergy, maximum dose, and optimal schedule.

3.   For an example of how these principles have been applied to designing a combination chemotherapy regimen, review **text page 277** and see **Figure 14-7, text page 278.**

B. **DOSE**

1. In a sensitive tumor cell population, there is a relationship between drug dose and biological response.
2. Inadequate drug dosing (caused, e.g., by reductions in the prescribed dose) results in compromised therapeutic effect.
3. Intense dosing will have the greatest potential effect on sensitive cell populations.
4. There are three parameters to consider in discussing dose: size, total amount delivered, and rate.
   a. The **dose size** is the total amount delivered to the patient when corrections are made for creatinine clearance and body weight.
   b. The **total dose** is the sum of all doses of drug for an individual patient.
   c. The **dose rate** (or **dose intensity**) is the amount of drug delivered per unit of time.
5. **Dose intensity** is expressed as $mg/m^2/week$; dose-intensive treatments have been associated with improved outcome in several tumors. Optimal dose intensity should include both optimal **drug dose** and optimal **duration of treatment;** however, these are unknown for many of our current therapies.

C. **ADJUVANT THERAPY**

1. The rationale for adjuvant therapy is to achieve better cure rates by treating small tumor burdens (i.e., microscopic disease) following primary treatment (usually surgery). Approaches to adjuvant therapy include multidrug chemotherapy, hormonal agents, or chemoendocrine combinations.
2. Unfortunately, the degree of benefit of adjuvant therapy has been less than initially anticipated. Factors that may account for the observed limitations of adjuvant therapy include tumor cell burden, heterogeneous cell populations, and the development of drug resistance. It is also possible that drug doses, drug combinations, and the timing of adjuvant treatment have not yet been optimized.
3. Newer approaches to adjuvant therapy currently being explored (such as dose-intense regimens, with or without autologous bone marrow transplantation, and chemoendocrine combinations) represent attempts to address these factors.

D. **MODIFYING AGENTS**

1. The role of **modifying agents** that may enhance the efficacy of antineoplastic drugs is also being explored. See **Table 14-5, text page 279,** for examples of drugs that have been used as modifying agents.

E. **REVERSING MULTIDRUG RESISTANCE**

1. Major strategies to overcome drug resistance include
   a. Using high drug doses to increase intracellular drug concentrations.
   b. Alternating noncross-resistant chemotherapy regimens.
   c. Using monoclonal antibodies and drugs to inhibit P-glycoprotein.
2. The calcium channel blockers (e.g., verapamil) have demonstrated the capacity to function as **chemosensitizers.**
   a. They function to bind P-glycoprotein, thus increasing intracellular drug concentrations, resulting in greater cytotoxicity.
   b. The major limitation to the use of this therapy is the significant cardiac toxicity that develops as a side effect of the dosages required to reverse drug resistance.

F. **GLUTATHIONE**

1. Glutathione is a substance essential for the synthesis of DNA precursors. In addition, glutathione enzymes are responsible for detoxifying harmful substances, scavenging free radicals, and repairing damage to DNA.
2. Both glutathione and glutathione enzymes have been implicated in the formation of resistance to the alkylating agents.

3.   Drugs that inhibit the activity of glutathione and/or glutathione enzymes (e.g., buthionine sulfoxime) appear to enhance chemotherapy effectiveness in animal models and are entering clinical trials in humans.

VI.   **DRUG DEVELOPMENT**

A.   **PRECLINICAL EVALUATION**

1.   In the United States, drugs and biologic agents are made commercially available only after preclinical testing followed by clinical trials in the human.
2.   Drugs are screened from various sources, such as plant extracts, and then are produced in sufficient amounts for testing in animal models of a particular disease.
3.   Prospective anticancer drugs are tested against tumors implanted in mice and rats, as well as in a panel of tumor cell lines derived from human malignancies.
4.   Drugs found to have some level of activity in animal tumor models undergo toxicology studies in at least two animal species to examine toxic effects and to estimate a safe starting dose for human studies.

B.   **PHASE I STUDIES**

1.   Phase I studies are designed to evaluate acute toxicities, to establish the maximum tolerated dose for a particular schedule of administration, and to analyze pharmacologic data so the drug can be delivered in the most effective manner during future studies.
2.   Phase I studies are conducted in cancer patients who could potentially benefit from the drug.

C.   **PHASE II STUDIES**

1.   Phase II studies are designed to identify drugs that have anticancer activity and to identify the necessary administration techniques, precautions, acute toxicity, and supportive care.
2.   Since the chances of detecting an active drug are best when the phase II agent is administered before other treatments have been given, phase II studies are ideally done with patients who have not received previous treatment.

D.   **PHASE III STUDIES**

1.   Phase III studies aim at defining the role of a drug in a cancer treatment regimen, often by comparing the phase II drug with another treatment or by combining it with a standard treatment regimen.
2.   Extent and duration of response as well as toxicity and quality of life are the outcomes that are evaluated.
3.   The phase III study tries to determine if the new treatment is equal to or better than the standard therapy, whether it produces equivalent or less toxicity, and whether it has the potential for combination with other agents.

E.   **PHASE IV STUDIES**

1.   Phase IV studies occur after a drug is commercially available and seek to define new uses for the drug, newer dosing schedules, and additional information about risks and benefits.

VII.   **CLINICAL TRIALS**

1.   A clinical trial is a scientific study designed to answer important clinical and biologic questions.
2.   Clinical trials are carried out by **protocol,** a written guideline defining the essential elements of the study and how it will be carried out.
3.   The majority of the public and patients themselves have favorable views regarding the value of clinical research; however, only 2%–3% of patients with cancer are enrolled in clinical trials.
4.   Reasons for poor patient accrual into clinical trials include
    a.   Complex study protocols which require time to read and implement.
    b.   Time involvement in patient and family education and data collection.
    c.   Third-party payers' refusal to reimburse for the costs of a treatment that is offered as a part of a clinical trial.

5. In the field of oncology, almost all standard treatments arose from clinical trials. It is therefore important to be creative in the design and conduct of clinical trials and to provide the resources that will encourage patient recruitment and physician participation.

VIII.   CLASSIFICATIONS OF ANTINEOPLASTIC AGENTS

1. Cytotoxic drugs are classified by their chemical structure, cell cycle activity, and primary mode of action.
2. **Alkylating agents** are cell cycle nonspecific, and the primary mechanism of action is cross-linking strands of DNA, which prevents transcription of RNA and replication of DNA.
3. **Antitumor antibiotics** are cell cycle nonspecific. They interfere with DNA function, as well as altering the cell membrane and inhibiting certain enzymes.
4. **Plant alkaloids** include topoisomerase inhibitors which interfere with DNA replication by binding to DNA and the topoisomerase enzymes.
5. **Mitotic inhibitors** are cell cycle specific. They act in the mitosis phase, binding microtubule proteins and causing metaphase arrest.
6. **Antimetabolites** are cell cycle specific and act during the S phase, interfering with DNA and RNA synthesis.
7. While the primary mechanisms of action may be similar for drugs within a class, the pharmacokinetics, secondary mechanisms of action, spectrum of activity, and host toxicity may vary widely.

IX.   PRACTICE CONSIDERATIONS

1. Knowledge of the storage, reconstitution, stability, and compatibility of chemotherapy drugs is critical to professional practice and to patient and family teaching and support. Such knowledge may also influence the safety and effectiveness of therapy.
2. See **Table 14-7, text pages 282–286,** for a summary of the reconstitution, stability, and compatibility of the major injectable cancer chemotherapy drugs.
3. The pharmacokinetics and efficacy of a drug may be altered when it is administered in sequence or concurrently with another drug. The incidence of such **drug interactions** increases the more drugs a patient is taking.
4. **Table 14-8, text page 287,** lists the **proposed mechanisms of drug interactions.**
5. **Tables 14-9, 14-10,** and **14-11, text pages 287–289,** list the drug interactions with chemotherapy that have been reported.
6. Pretreatment and ongoing assessment of the patient's current medications can help to detect potential interactions and avert or minimize an adverse outcome.

PRACTICE QUESTIONS

1. Which of the following theories and models **best** explains the variability in responsiveness of tumors that both are small and demonstrate initial sensitivity to chemotherapy agents, such as etoposide, taxol, and doxorubicin?
   (A)   the Goldie-Coldman model
   (B)   the cell cycle theory
   (C)   the Gompertzian model
   (D)   multidrug resistance (MDR) or pleiotropic drug resistance (PDR)

2. Which of the following tumor cell populations is likely to be **most** sensitive and thus to exhibit the **best** response to chemotherapy?
   (A)   tumor cell populations with overexpression of P-glycoprotein
   (B)   large tumor cell populations with a low growth fraction
   (C)   small tumor cell populations with a high growth fraction
   (D)   a tumor with poor vascularity

3. An important advantage of combination chemotherapy over single-drug regimens is that it
   (A)   reduces the potential for nausea and vomiting.
   (B)   produces decreased tumor resistance.
   (C)   spares normal cells from severe toxicities.
   (D)   decreases the likelihood of drug-induced gonadal sterility.

4. Which of the following is **not** examined in phase I clinical trials?
    (A)   drug toxicities and their reversibility
    (B)   the effectiveness of new drugs on various common malignant diseases
    (C)   pharmacologic data on metabolism, tissue distribution, and excretion
    (D)   maximum dose

5. Reasons for poor patient accrual into clinical trials include all of the following **except**
    (A)   negative public perceptions regarding clinical research.
    (B)   complex study protocols which require additional time for clinicians to read and implement.
    (C)   reluctance of third-party payers to reimburse for the costs of a treatment that is offered as part of a clinical trial.
    (D)   time involved in patient and family education regarding the trial.

6. Chemotherapy drugs that are cell cycle specific act preferentially on cells that
    (A)   are differentiated.
    (B)   have entered G_0.
    (C)   are in the S or M phase.
    (D)   are no longer alive.

7. Which of the following statements about drug interactions with cytotoxic chemotherapy agents is true?
    (A)   Cytotoxic chemotherapy drugs should never be given concurrently with another drug.
    (B)   Drug interactions can result in additive toxicity, decreased effectiveness, or altered activity and outcome of nonchemotherapeutic drugs.
    (C)   Cytotoxic chemotherapy should never be administered in sequence with another drug.
    (D)   The incidence of drug interactions is not influenced by the number of drugs a patient is taking.

ANSWER EXPLANATIONS

1. **The answer is (D).**   Variability in responsiveness of tumors that are both small and demonstrate initial sensitivity to chemotherapy agents suggests the development of drug resistance. Neither the cell cycle theory nor the Gompertzian model of tumor growth explains these observations. The Goldie-Coldman model contains the basic assumptions and principles of the development of drug resistance, but the concept of multidrug resistance (MDR) or pleiotropic drug resistance (PDR) best explains the well-recognized phenomenon in which exposure to a single drug is followed by cross-resistance to other drugs. The initial drug involved appears to be a natural product such as etoposide, taxol, and doxorubicin. (275–276)

2. **The answer is (C).**   Small tumor cell populations with a high growth fraction are most likely to be sensitive to and have the best response to chemotherapy. Tumor cell populations with overexpression of P-glycoprotein may demonstrate initial sensitivity to chemotherapy but rapidly develop drug resistance. Large tumor cell populations with a low growth fraction could be expected to have a relatively poorer response to chemotherapy since the population of proliferating cells is relatively smaller than in large tumor cell populations with a high growth fraction. Tumors with poor vascularity may possess temporary or biochemical drug resistance since transport of the drug to the tumor may be inhibited. (274–275)

3. **The answer is (B).**   In most cancers, single-drug therapy has proved unsuccessful in achieving long-term remission and contributes to tumor drug resistance. Combination therapy has demonstrated long-term remissions, more effective prevention of drug resistance, and tolerable side effects with maximal doses. Improved therapeutic results from combination therapy are due to the synergistic and additive effects of the drugs. Decreased tumor resistance to drugs is another positive aspect of combination chemotherapy: few tumor cells are resistant to the total effect of all the drugs; therefore, few resistant cells can survive and continue dividing. Trials are also examining the role of alternating noncross-resistant chemotherapy regimens. (277)

4. **The answer is (B).**   After a new drug has been developed and tested in animals and has demonstrated antitumor activity, it enters clinical trials, which are organized into three phases. Phase I studies identify and describe drug toxicities, maximum dose, and pharmacologic data on metabolism, tissue distribution, and excretion. Phase II studies are designed to determine the effectiveness of the drug on various common malignant diseases. Phase III studies compare the effectiveness of the new drug or drug combination with that of the standard form of treatment. (280)

5.   **The answer is (A).**   The majority of patients and the public, when asked about clinical trials, have favorable views regarding the values of clinical research. The major reasons for poor patient accrual into clinical trials are issues involving the individual physician-patient relationship, time, and money. (281)

6.   **The answer is (C).**   Drugs that are cell cycle specific act preferentially on cells that are proliferating (dividing). Cells in the G_0 phase are in the resting or dormant phase and are out of the cell cycle. Cells that are differentiated are also out of the cell cycle. (273, 281–282)

7.   **The answer is (B).**   Contrary to choices (A) and (C), it is often necessary to administer chemotherapeutic drugs concurrently or in sequence with other drugs. Choice (D) is also untrue; the incidence of drug interactions increases the more drugs a patient is taking. Pretreatment and ongoing assessment are essential to detect potential interactions and avert or minimize an adverse outcome.

15 Chemotherapy: Principles of Administration

STUDY OUTLINE

I. **CHEMOTHERAPY ADMINISTRATION**

    A. **PROFESSIONAL QUALIFICATIONS**

        1. The Oncology Nursing Society's Cancer Chemotherapy Guidelines are guidelines for the administration of chemotherapy.

        2. See **text page 294,** column 1, for the basic qualifications required of nurses for antineoplastic agent administration.

        3. There are various types of training programs intended for chemotherapy certification. **Certification** provides proof of formalized training and demonstration of skill in the administration of antineoplastic agents.

    B. **HANDLING CYTOTOXIC DRUGS**

        1. Direct cytotoxic exposure can occur during **admixture, ingestion, or absorption.**

        2. Antineoplastic drugs are known to be **mutagenic, teratogenic, and carcinogenic,** with exposures resulting in rashes, skin discoloration, scarring, blurred vision, and dizziness.

        3. See **Table 15-2, text page 295,** for guidelines on handling cytotoxic drugs.

        4. The **Occupational Safety and Health Administration (OSHA)** requires employers to determine the exposure risk for each task performed by an employee.

        5. OSHA guidelines recommend **gowning and gloving** when handling excreta even beyond 48 hours after drug administration, since drugs and their metabolites continue to be excreted.

        6. It is important for patients and families to understand why gloves and gowns are being worn so that they do not feel alienated, and that they understand drug containment practices if treatment is planned in the home.

        7. The OSHA guidelines that must be followed at the minimum include **knowledge of the latest scientific information, established policies and procedures, and ongoing monitoring to ensure compliance and continuous improvement in quality.**

    C. **PATIENT AND FAMILY EDUCATION**

        1. A first step in education of patients and families is **clarifying information and dispelling misconceptions.**

        2. **Patient education** is an ongoing process, specific to the side effects and experiences patients are having. See **Table 15-3, text page 297,** for guidelines on patient education.

        3. Cancer chemotherapy patient education is very detailed and requires adjustment in order to meet the evolving needs of patients and families.

    D. **ADMINISTRATION PRINCIPLES**

        1. **Chemotherapy administration** is complex, requiring exact dose calculation, delivery determination, administration, problem solving, symptom management, and follow-up in order to avoid overdosing.

        2. **Vascular access devices and ambulatory pumps,** which have been developed in recent years, promote drug delivery in care settings other than traditional hospital settings.

3. **Reimbursement issues** have also received a great deal of attention since some third-party payers do not reimburse for certain treatments in certain settings.
4. See **Table 15-4, text page 299,** for chemotherapy administration guidelines.

E. VESICANT EXTRAVASATION ISSUES

1. A vesicant antineoplastic drug is a drug that can cause tissue necrosis if it infiltrates or extravasates out of the blood vessel and into the soft tissue.
2. See **Table 15-5, text page 300,** for a list of antineoplastic vesicants.
3. See **text pages 298–300** for guidelines to minimize the risk of extravasation.

II. ROUTES OF DRUG ADMINISTRATION

1. Regional drug delivery utilizes the following routes: **topical, intra-arterial, intraperitoneal, intrapleural, intravesical, intrathecal, and intraventricular.**

A. TOPICAL

1. **Cutaneous malignant lesions** can be treated topically with nitrogen mustard or with fluorouracil. Affected areas are treated once or twice daily until the lesions progress to the necrotic phase, which may be 1–3 weeks.
2. The expected result is usually a sloughing of the affected area with eventual regranulation of normal tissue.
3. See **text page 301** for special nursing considerations for patients receiving topical antineoplastic agent therapy.

B. ORAL

1. See **Table 15-6, text pages 302–303,** for a list of antineoplastic agents administered orally.
2. The oral route of administration is convenient, economical, noninvasive, and often less toxic.
3. Nursing responsibilities include **safe handling of the drug** and **monitoring for drug absorption and compliance** with the planned regimen. Additional recommendations for oral drug administration can be found on **text page 301,** columns 1 and 2.

C. INTRAMUSCULAR AND SUBCUTANEOUS

1. The development of biologic agents has increased the number of drugs administered intramuscularly or subcutaneously.
2. See **Figure 15-1, text page 304,** for a sample instruction sheet used by patients who are injecting subcutaneous medication.

D. INTRAVENOUS

1. Antineoplastic agents are most commonly administered through the intravenous route. Detailed nursing actions are included in **Table 15-4, text page 299.**
2. Drug sequencing can be controversial depending on the drugs being administered. Generally, antiemetics and pretreatments are given prior to intravenous push medications, short-term drip infusions, and long-term or continuous infusions.

E. INTRA-ARTERIAL

1. Administration of antineoplastic drugs directly to a tumor bed through the arterial catheter involves cannulation of the artery providing the tumor's blood supply.
2. **Fluorouracil, floxuridine, doxorubicin, and mitomycin C** are common antineoplastic drugs administered through the hepatic artery for liver metastasis from colon cancer, as well as hepatocellular carcinoma.
3. **External** intra-arterial drug delivery involves radiographic arterial catheter placement and attachment of the catheter to an external infusion pump for 3–7 days of drug delivery.

    a. Nursing care involves caring for the patient in a **supine position** with a pressure dressing over the catheter insertion site.

    b. Side effects are usually milder and possibly delayed as compared to intravenous drug delivery.

4. The **internal or implantable** method of intra-arterial drug delivery involves surgical placement of a totally implantable pump, with the catheter inserted into the appropriate artery and then attached to the pump located in a surgically created subcutaneous pocket in the abdomen. See **Figures 15-3 to 15-6, text pages 307–308.**

    a. A formalized educational program is required for the care and maintenance of the pump and the patient with the pump.

    b. Ongoing monitoring of pump functioning is required.

5. Patients have greater freedom with the implantable pump than with the external catheter.

F. INTRAPERITONEAL

1. **Cisplatinum, carboplatin, interferon, fluorouracil, and cytarabine** are antineoplastic agents used intraperitoneally for treatment of locally recurrent ovarian and colon cancers.

2. High concentrations of drugs can be achieved at tumor sites throughout the peritoneal space because of the **semipermeable nature of the peritoneal space.**

3. Side effects are mild or delayed in comparison to intravenous administration of the same drugs. Local side effects are due to the large volume of fluid filling the space.

4. Three methods of accessing the peritoneal space are **intermittent placement of temporary indwelling catheters, placement of a Tenckhoff external catheter, and placement of an implantable peritoneal port.**

5. Tenckhoff catheters or ports are placed when several months of therapy are planned.

    a. Tenckhoff catheters have the advantages of a very **rapid flow rate and the allowance of catheter manipulation** to dislodge fibrin deposits.

    b. The Tenckhoff is external, requiring care and maintenance by the patient and possibly resulting in an **increased incidence of infection or leakage around the catheter.**

    c. Advantages of the port are that it is internal and **does not require care when not accessed and that it has a potentially lower rate of infection.**

    d. Disadvantages of the port: it has a **slower flow rate, a needle stick is required every time access is needed, and a surgical procedure is necessary for removal** of the port.

6. Nursing care includes patient education, assessing patency, establishing access, administering systemic therapies instilling the drug, monitoring patient responses to the treatment, draining the infusate if ordered, management of side effects, and documentation. See **Table 15-7, text page 309,** for nursing considerations.

7. Regardless of the specific drug side effects, complications specific to the intraperitoneal route include **respiratory distress, abdominal pain, discomfort, and diarrhea.**

8. Mechanical difficulties include **inflow or outflow occlusions** caused by fibrin sheath formation over the catheter, other outflow occlusions, and **catheter migration.**

G. INTRAPLEURAL

1. Malignant effusions caused by malignant cells are recurrent, and treatment can include **sclerosis** with an antineoplastic agent.

2. The drugs are injected directly into the **chest tube** and clamped.

3. Severe **pleural pain** can accompany sclerosis and requires administration of a strong narcotic as a premedication and for 24–48 hours afterward.

4. Alternatives to traditional therapy include use of **different drugs, insertion of small-bore percutaneously placed catheters or implantable ports, and implantation of pleuroperitoneal shunts.**

H. INTRAVESICAL

1. **Instillation of chemotherapy into the bladder** is used for controlling superficial bladder cancer and carcinoma in situ.

    a. Instillation is usually weekly for 4–12 weeks and involves a **urinary catheter insertion, drug instillation, and retention of the drug for 1–2 hours** prior to unclamping the catheter or voiding.

    b. Fluid that is removed or drained should be treated as **cytotoxic waste.**

2. Local side effects include **bladder irritation and external genitalia dermatitis.**
3. Nursing care includes **drug administration, side effect monitoring, safe drug handling, and patient education with emphasis on hand washing and personal hygiene.**

I.   INTRATHECAL OR INTRAVENTRICULAR

1. Since available antineoplastic agents are unable to enter the **cerebrospinal fluid (CSF)** in sufficient concentrations to kill cancer cells resulting from leukemia, breast cancer, lymphoma, and rhabdomyosarcoma, chemotherapy is injected directly into the intrathecal or intraventricular space as prophylaxis or to manage existing disease.
2. The **intrathecal** route of drug instillation is achieved by performing a lumbar puncture and injecting 10–12 ml of drug. This is done on a daily or weekly basis, depending on the treatment protocol.
   a. The drug may reach only epidural or subdural spaces, and **therapeutic levels are usually not reached in the ventricles.**
3. An **Ommaya reservoir** allows central instillation of drugs into the ventricle. The Ommaya reservoir is placed underneath the skin, with the catheter extending from the reservoir to the ventricle. See **Figure 15-7, text page 311.**
   a. The Ommaya reservoir is accessed using sterile technique with a small-gauge needle and then removed once the drug is administered.
4. Drugs are capable of entering the bloodstream and having systemic side effects. These include nausea, stomatitis, and mild myelosuppression.

III.   VASCULAR ACCESS DEVICES

1. An overview of the major venous access devices (VADs) can be found in **Table 15-8, text page 313.**

A.   GENERAL MANAGEMENT

1. **Nontunneled central venous catheters**
   a. The standard **subclavian line** is often used in urgent situations and is an example of a nontunneled central venous catheter.
   b. **Multilumen subclavian catheters** may be placed to augment long-term devices during a hospitalization.
   c. The **peripherally inserted central catheter (PICC)** bridges the gap between subclavian lines and long-term tunneled catheters or ports.
      (1) PICC lines are the **easiest long-term central venous catheter to insert,** but they often require a caregiver since they are located at the antecubital fossa.
      (2) See **Figure 15-8, text page 314,** for visualization of the PICC placement.
      (3) See **Table 15-9, text page 315,** for a PICC overview.
2. **Tunneled central venous catheters**
   a. The **tunneled central venous catheter (TCVC)** provides an option for almost all hematology/oncology patients who need reliable long-term access (months to years) with a low incidence of infection.
   b. A **Dacron cuff** located near the exit site in the subcutaneous tissue facilitates granulation tissue formation to help hold the catheter in place, and it helps stop bacteria from traveling along the subcutaneous portion of the catheter.
   c. See **Figure 15-10, text page 315,** for placement of a TCVC and **Figures 15-11 and 15-12, text page 316,** for pictures of various catheters.
   d. See **Table 15-10, text page 317,** for an overview of TCVC features.
   e. Risks of catheter insertion include pneumothorax and arterial puncture.
   f. Although standardization of care techniques has not occurred, possible options for policies and procedures can be found on **text page 317,** column 1.
   g. **Repairs** of broken, punctured, or torn TCVC catheters can occur as long as two inches of undamaged catheter exits the skin.
3. **Implantable ports**
   a. A **port** is a hollow housing containing a compressed latex septum over a portal chamber that is connected via a small tube to a silicone or polyurethane catheter that is inserted into a major blood vessel. See **Figures 15-13 and 15-14, text pages 318–319.**

    b.   The port is placed subcutaneously and accessed percutaneously using a special noncoring needle. Ports require very little care and maintenance when not in use.

    c.   See **Figures 15-15 and 15-16, text page 319,** for pictures of different types.

    d.   The five major routes for ports are **venous, arterial, peritoneal, intrapleural, and epidural.**

    e.   The arterial and epidural ports have specially designed catheters with small lumens since the flow rates tend to be low.

    f.   The peritoneal catheter has a very large lumen and multiple exit sites in order to allow rapid fluid infusion.

    g.   The venous ports have varying-sized lumens and flow rates. See **Figure 15-17, text page 321,** for illustration of placement.

    h.   See **Table 15-11, text page 318,** for an overview of port features.

    i.   See **Table 15-12, text page 322,** for nursing issues related to arterial, peritoneal, epidural, and intrapleural ports.

    j.   The major **advantage of implantable ports** over other vascular access devices is that they are implanted and do not require routine care other than flushing every 4 weeks.

    k.   The major **disadvantage is that accessing the port requires a needle to pass through the skin** and into the port.

    l.   **Nursing management** involves assessing the site, accessing the device, infusing or withdrawing fluids, and flushing.

    m.   Portal site choice should be made prior to surgery, so that information regarding fat around the site, who the caretaker will be, what the lifestyle involves, and physical activities allowed can be considered.

    n.   Port **access requires a sterile procedure.** See **text page 321,** columns 1 and 2, for assessment and monitoring parameters to be used when accessing the port.

    o.   There is a venous access device which is a **combination of the PICC and the port.** It allows the peripheral insertion of a port near the antecubital fossa. The insertion and proper placement can be achieved in the physician's office or at the bedside, with the assistance of an electronic device.

B.   **COMPLICATION MANAGEMENT**

    1.   Complications such as occlusions and infections can occur with any of the venous access devices. The incidence and type of complication depend on the device, insertion technique, care regimen, and certain physiologic factors.

    2.   **Intraluminal catheter occlusion**

        a.   Inability to withdraw blood or infuse fluid in a venous access device is most commonly a result of a **blood clot** in the catheter. Other causes include crystallization of drugs or lipids, which then obstructs the catheter.

        b.   Blood clots can build up over time, making the catheter appear sluggish, but occlusion can also occur suddenly.

        c.   See **text page 323** for suggestions to prevent catheter occlusions.

        d.   **Urokinase** is commonly utilized to dissolve blood clots that might be causing a catheter occlusion.

    3.   **Extraluminal catheter occlusion**

        a.   **Fibrin sheath formation and thrombosis** are two extraluminal causes of catheter occlusion, in addition to catheter position. If a catheter flushes easily but withdrawal is difficult, then a fibrin sheath is suspected.

        b.   **Thrombosis** may be as high as 10% and can be caused by **endothelial injury, hypercoagulability, multiple catheters, catheter stiffness, catheter size, and catheter placement.**

        c.   Signs and symptoms of catheter thrombosis are related to impaired blood flow and include **edema of the neck, face, shoulder, or arm; prominent superficial veins; neck pain; tingling of the neck, shoulder, or arm; and changes in skin color or temperature.**

        d.   Management of venous thrombosis involves **anticoagulants or thrombolytic agents.**

    4.   **Infection**

        a.   Infection incidence varies with **insertion technique, care for the device, and the physical condition** of the patient.

        b.   Infections can occur **locally or systemically.**

        c.   Infections are more common in patients with neutropenia.

      d.   *S. aureaus* and *S. epidermis* are common organisms of the skin leading to catheter infections.

      e.   Signs and symptoms include **fever, redness, erythema, tenderness,** and **discomfort.**

      f.   Management of infections usually consists of **intravenous antibiotics and meticulous site care.**

   5. **Other complications**

      a.   Occlusions and device malfunctions can occur for a variety of other reasons and require careful assessment.

      b.   It is important to consider **malpositioning or breakage** when occlusion happens, in addition to considering a blood clot.

PRACTICE QUESTIONS

1.   The initial step in patient and family education regarding chemotherapy administration is
   (A)   clarifying information and dispelling misconceptions.
   (B)   obtaining informed consent.
   (C)   choosing an appropriate venous access device.
   (D)   demonstrating safe gloving and gowning.

2.   Which of the following provides evidence that a nurse is qualified to administer chemotherapy?
   (A)   certification in critical care
   (B)   certification in oncology nursing
   (C)   over 5 years of experience as an oncology nurse
   (D)   certification by an approved chemotherapy administration program

3.   When working with a venous access device, the nurse notices that she is able to flush the catheter with ease but is unable to aspirate. Which of the following is a possible cause?
   (A)   a fibrin sheath at the catheter tip
   (B)   an intraluminal clot
   (C)   drug crystallization and precipitation
   (D)   a kink in the catheter subcutaneously

4.   Examining a patient who has neck and face edema, superficial neck veins, tingling of the neck, and skin discoloration on the arm on the side of the catheter, the nurse recognizes these as signs and symptoms of
   (A)   catheter infection.
   (B)   a hole in the catheter.
   (C)   extraluminal thrombosis.
   (D)   intraluminal clot.

5.   Which of the following practices would **not** be found in the guidelines established by the Occupational Safety and Health Administration for preventing cytotoxic drug exposure to personnel and the environment?
   (A)   Do not use intravenous bottles with venting tubes.
   (B)   Do not expel air from the syringes.
   (C)   Prime IV tubing after adding the cytotoxic drug.
   (D)   Double-glove when cleaning up large spills.

6.   During an intravenous push administration of doxorubicin into a patient's left forearm, the nurse becomes unable to obtain a blood return. The patient has no complaints of discomfort at the site, and there is no swelling noted. What is the appropriate nursing action?
   (A)   Take out the intravenous and restart it at another site.
   (B)   Flush the intravenous with saline to ensure that an extravasation has not occurred.
   (C)   Reposition the needle in hopes of obtaining a blood return.
   (D)   Since the patient has no complaints of pain, continue the injection slowly.

7.   In the event that the nurse notes swelling at the site described in Question 6, the nurse's first action should be to
   (A)   continue working on obtaining a blood return.
   (B)   stop drug administration and attempt to aspirate.
   (C)   flush the line with saline.
   (D)   obtain a new site for drug administration.

ANSWER EXPLANATIONS

1.   **The answer is (A).**   Clarifying information and dispelling misconceptions, especially the "old wives' tales" that exist about cancer and cancer treatment, is the initial step in patient and family education. Nurses are usually responsible for imparting specific information about treatment side effects and ways to recognize them and minimize their consequences. (296)

2.   **The answer is (D).**   The Oncology Nursing Society recommends that all nurses who administer chemotherapy attend an approved chemotherapy administration program. Certification in oncology nursing does not imply skill or knowledge of chemotherapy administration procedures. (294)

3.   **The answer is (A).**   A fibrin sheath at the tip of the catheter is usually characterized by easy flushing and infusing of fluids but an inability to aspirate blood (or difficulty doing so). Choices (B) and (D) would most likely be characterized by complete inability to aspirate or flush the catheter. A kink in the catheter subcutaneously is a rare occurrence. Kinks usually occur at the entrance of the catheter into the subclavian vein if the catheter enters at a ninety degree angle, or it can be compressed by tumor. (323–324, 326)

4.   **The answer is (C).**   An extraluminal thrombosis is characterized by edema of the neck, face, shoulder, or arm; prominent superficial veins; neck pain; tingling of the neck, shoulder, or arm; and changes in skin color or temperature. The characteristic sign of a catheter infection is fever, with or without localized redness at the catheter exit site. Intraluminal clot characterized by an inability to flush the catheter or aspirate blood. Depending on the site, a hole in the catheter might lead to extravasation of infusing fluids into the subcutaneous tissue. (323–324)

5.   **The answer is (C).**   IV tubing should be primed with saline or dextrose prior to adding the cytotoxic drug in the event any fluid spills out in the effort to purge the line of air. (295)

6.   **The answer is (B).**   It is not uncommon to lose a blood return when administering chemotherapy. The key is to stop the drug and assess further. With no evidence of swelling or pain, it is safe to flush with saline (20–30 cc) to ensure that an extravasation has not occurred. Injection of the vesicant can then proceed. Taking out the IV and restarting it elsewhere is no insurance that the blood return will not be lost again. Trying to reposition the IV will only ensure infiltration due to manipulation. Patients can experience doxorubicin extravasations without pain, but not without some evidence of swelling.

7.   **The answer is (B).**   Prompt nursing action will, in general, minimize tissue damage, so choice (D) is inappropriate since nursing actions should be directed toward the suspicious IV site. The drug administration should be stopped and drug delivery to the site prevented, since failure to do so further disperses the infiltrated drug into the tissues. This includes flushing the line with saline or dextrose since there might be vesicant drug remaining in the tubing.

16   Chemotherapy: Toxicity Management

VI. **CHEMOTHERAPY TOXICITIES**

A. **GRADING OF TOXICITIES**

1. Specific therapies can be assessed by comparing their benefits with the occurrence of toxicity.
2. Toxicity is assessed by reviewing **which toxicities occurred, toxicity severity, time of onset, duration of effect, and interventions incorporated to minimize the effect.**
3. **Toxicity grading scales** have been developed by the World Health Organization and various cooperative study groups to provide consistency in reporting toxicities. See **Table 16-1, text page 339,** for a chart on grading toxicity.

B. **SYSTEMIC TOXICITIES**

1. **Bone marrow suppression**
   a. **Myelosuppression** is the most common and the most lethal side effect of chemotherapy.
   b. Proliferating **progenitor cells** that produce mature granulocytes, erythrocytes, and thrombocytes in the peripheral blood are destroyed.
   c. The **nadir** usually occurs 7–14 days after chemotherapy, as immature cells in the bone marrow are destroyed and are unable to mature and move into the peripheral blood.
   d. Antineoplastic agents are most effective against cells that are cycling or are in a specific phase of the cell cycle.
   e. Risk factors that can intensify or prolong the cytopenia include **tumor cells in the bone marrow, prior treatment with chemotherapy or radiation, and a high negative nitrogen balance.**
   f. Differences in the lengths and kinetics of the life cycles of particular blood cells also account for the frequency of neutropenia, thrombocytopenia, and anemia. See **Figure 16-3, text page 340,** for a thrombocytopenia flow sheet.
   g. **Neutropenia** can occur when the total white blood count (WBC) is within the normal range but the actual neutrophil count is less than 1500 cells/mm^3.
   h. It is estimated that 80% of infections arise from **endogenous organisms** (GI or respiratory tract).
   i. Chemotherapy-induced damage to the alimentary canal and respiratory tract mucosa facilitates the entry of infecting organisms.
   j. **Prevention, early detection, good hand-washing technique, and prompt medical management of infections** in patients with neutropenia are vital in order to decrease the risk of sepsis.
   k. **Antibiotics** are used to treat chemotherapy-induced infections once cultures are obtained.
   l. Since infection is the most serious complication of chemotherapy-induced myelosuppression, the use of **hematopoietic colony-stimulating factors to augment neutrophil counts** is increasing.

2. **Fatigue**
   a. Although the specific causative mechanisms are unclear, fatigue is a common, often serious side effect of chemotherapy administration.
   b. Fatigue manifests itself as **weariness, weakness, and lack of energy,** and when unrelieved by a "good night's sleep," it is known as chronic fatigue. Chronic fatigue can be an overwhelming experience requiring **energy conservation, rest, setting priorities for activities, and delegating tasks and responsibilities.**

3. **Gastrointestinal**
   a. **Anorexia,** a declining food intake, contributes to weight loss and implies alterations in food perception, taste, and smell that result from chemotherapy side effects.
   b. **Nutritional assessment,** the first step toward meeting nutritional needs, includes a physical assessment, health history, and the obtaining of specific nutritional parameters.
   c. **Diarrhea,** an increase in stool volume and liquidity leading to three or more bowel movements per day, occurs because of destruction of GI epithelial cells and subsequent atrophy of the intestinal mucosa.
   d. The degree and duration of diarrhea depend upon the agent, dose, nadir, and frequency of chemotherapy administration.
   e. Prolonged diarrhea without adequate management will cause **dehydration, nutritional malabsorption, and circulatory collapse.**
   f. **5-fluorouracil** is the chemotherapy that most commonly causes diarrhea, but other agents may also do so, such as methotrexate, actinomycin-D, doxorubicin, and daunorubicin.

    g. **Clostridium difficile,** an infectious process found in patients who have had prior antibiotic therapy, needs to be ruled out through stool cultures.

    h. Chemotherapy is usually administered despite diarrhea, but diarrhea can be severe enough to be the dose-limiting toxicity of 5-fluorouracil and leucovorin.

    i. **Constipation** (infrequent, excessively hard and dry bowel movements) results from a decrease in rectal filling or emptying.

    j. Risk factors contributing to constipation include **narcotic use, a decrease in physical activity, a low-fiber diet, a decrease in fluid intake, and bed rest.**

    k. **Vincristine and vinblastine,** the most common chemotherapy agents to cause constipation, cause autonomic nerve dysfunction resulting in colicky abdominal pain and ileus.

    l. **Laxative therapy or stool softeners** are recommended prior to administration of vincristine or vinblastine in combination with an increase in high-fiber foods and fluids.

    m. Nausea and vomiting is coordinated by the **vomiting center (VC),** which lies in the medulla. The VC receives impulses from the cerebellum, the vestibular apparatus, the chemoreceptor trigger zone, visceral and vagal afferent pathways from the GI tract, and the cerebrum. These impulses lead to nausea, retching, and vomiting.

    n. **Nausea** is a subjective, conscious recognition of the desire to vomit, manifested by an unpleasant wavelike sensation in the epigastric area.

    o. **Retching** is a rhythmic and spasmodic movement involving the diaphragm and abdominal muscles.

    p. **Vomiting** is a somatic process performed by the respiratory muscles causing the forceful oral expulsion of gastric, duodenal, or jejunal contents through the mouth.

    q. **Acute nausea and vomiting** occur within the first 24 hours of drug administration.

    r. **Delayed nausea and vomiting** persist or develop 24 hours after chemotherapy administration.

    s. **Anticipatory nausea and vomiting** result from previous experiences with chemotherapy in which efforts to control emesis were unsuccessful.

    t. **Management** of nausea and vomiting includes an in-depth emetic history and an antiemetic plan. See **Table 16-2, text page 346,** for the emetogenic potential of chemotherapeutic agents and **Table 16-3, text pages 347–348,** for antiemetic therapy regimens.

C. ORGAN TOXICITIES

  1. Certain chemotherapeutic drugs may cause **direct damage** to **specific cells of an organ** or **indirect damage** by the effects of cellular breakdown by-products.

  2. Organ toxicities are predictable on the basis of **cumulative dose, presence of concomitant organ dysfunction, age of the patient, and the manner in which the drug is given.**

  3. **Cardiotoxicity**

    a. **Acute** forms of cardiotoxicity occur immediately and resolve quickly without serious complications. They consist of transient electrocardiogram (ECG) changes and are not an indication to stop the drug.

    b. **Chronic** effects occur weeks or months after drug administration. They involve cardiomyopathy that is nonreversible and presents as biventricular congestive heart failure.

    c. Signs and symptoms include **nonproductive cough, dyspnea, and pedal edema.**

    d. The **cardiomyopathy** becomes progressively worse, with a 60% mortality, and is poorly responsive to diuretics or digitalis.

    e. Direct damage to the cardiac myocyte cells is caused by **anthracyclines,** with an incidence of 2%–3% after cumulative doses.

    f. **Total cumulative doses** have been established at **550 mg/m^2 for doxorubicin and 600 mg/m^2 for daunomycin,** with a decrease in dose to 450 mg/m^2 if mediastinal radiation has been administered.

    g. Chemoprotectants are being studied to protect the cardiac tissue by blocking the anthracycline's damage to the myocytes.

    h. Analogs that have greater antitumor activity and may have reduced cardiotoxicity have been developed in an attempt to further reduce the cardiotoxicity from the anthracyclines.

    i. **Acute pericarditis** has been reported with high-dose cytoxan therapy used in the bone marrow transplant population. It can then progress to pericardial effusions and cardiac tamponade.

    j. **Cytoxan damage** to the myocytes is similar to anthracycline damage, where swelling and decreased contractility lead to less effective pumping of the heart.

   k. **Myocardial ischemia** has been reported with 5-fluorouracil infusion in some patients.
   l. **Asymptomatic bradycardia** has been reported in about 30% of patients with ovarian cancer who are receiving **taxol.** Atrioventricular conduction blocks, left bundle branch blocks, ventricular tachycardia, and cardiac ischemia symptoms have also been reported in 5% of patients receiving taxol.
   m. Cardiac function is evaluated in patients receiving high dosages of anthracyclines or are at high risk for cardiotoxicity. Methods include ECG, echocardiography, and radionuclide cardiography.
   n. Accurate **documentation and monitoring** of total cumulative dosages are important, in addition to cardiac assessment and monitoring.
   o. Upon development of chronic cardiotoxicity, nursing interventions include teaching the patient about conservation of energy, managing fluid retention, and minimizing the sodium in the diet.
   p. See **Table 16-5, text page 351,** for cardiotoxicity effects of chemotherapy agents.
4. **Neurotoxicity**
   a. Chemotherapy-induced neurotoxicity can arise as direct or indirect damage to the **central nervous system (CNS), peripheral nervous system, cranial nerves,** or any of the three combined.
   b. Neurotoxicity that is significant requires holding the drug until the symptoms subside, and reinstituting the drug at 50% the dose.
   c. **Neurotoxicity severity is dose related,** with symptoms varying.
   d. CNS damage is primarily to the **cerebellum** with resulting **altered gait, altered reflexes, ataxia, and confusion.**
   e. Peripheral nervous system damage produces **paralysis or loss of movement and sensation** to those areas affected by the particular nerve.
   f. Autonomic nervous system damage results in **impotence, urinary retention, or ileus.**
   g. Vincristine causes **peripheral neuropathies** characterized by myalgias, loss of deep tendon reflex at the ankle, areflexia, distal symmetric sensory loss, motor weakness, foot drop, and muscle atrophy.
   h. Cisplatin-related neuropathy is reversible, although there are cases of persistent progression despite drug discontinuation.
   i. Cisplatin, affecting the larger-diameter neural tissue fibers, results in sensory changes. Early signs of peripheral neuropathies are **decreased vibratory sensations** in a classic stocking glove distribution.
   j. **Ifosfamide-related neurotoxicities** characterized by blurred vision, subclinical electroencephalographic changes, urinary incontinence, motor system dysfunction, cranial nerve dysfunction, seizures, or irreversible coma have been reported in 5%–30% of patients.
   k. Methotrexate in high doses occasionally causes encephalopathy after several courses, but the condition is usually reversible.
   l. **Neurologic assessment** is critical in patients receiving potentially neurotoxic agents. See **Table 16-6, text page 353,** for neurotoxicity of chemotherapy agents.
5. **Pulmonary toxicity**
   a. Pulmonary toxicity tends to be **irreversible and progressive.**
   b. The **endothelial cells** tend to be the initial site of damage with an inflammatory-type reaction resulting in a pneumonitis.
   c. Another type of injury is the result of an **immunologic mechanism,** with chronic exposure leading to an extensive alteration of the pulmonary parenchyma, changes in the connective tissue, obliteration of alveoli, and dilatation of airspaces.
   d. Continuous injury and repair lead to **restrictive lung disease,** which is characterized by a thickened, still interstitium, increased work to breathe, and a reduced lung volume leading to impaired gas exchange.
   e. **Hypoxemia** is the end result leading to death because oxygen cannot diffuse in the damaged areas while perfusion continues.
   f. Clinical signs of pulmonary toxicity are **dyspnea, unproductive cough, bilateral basilar rales, and tachypnea.** Chest X-ray results may be normal at first with eventual diffuse interstitial markings.
   g. The **carbon monoxide diffusion capacity measurement test** becomes abnormal before clinical signs occur, making this the most sensitive pulmonary function test.
   h. **Bleomycin** causes pulmonary toxicity in 5% of patients with a cumulative dose of 450 units.

    i.   **Cytarabine** exerts a direct effect on the pneumocytes and pulmonary capillary endothelial cells, leading to increased capillary permeability and a capillary leak syndrome. This can occur 2–21 days after the first dose and is related to high doses and continuous infusion administration.

    j.   **Mitomycin C** causes diffuse alveolar damage with a capillary leak and pulmonary edema in 3%–36% of patients.

    k.   **Cytoxan** causes pulmonary toxicity in 1% of patients and is associated with high doses.

    l.   Detection of early lung damage is imperative in an attempt to stop administering the drug and minimize damage, since lung damage is irreversible and progressive.

    m. **High concentrations of oxygen** and chemotherapy agents administered simultaneously may induce lung damage, so oxygen saturations need to be monitored.

    n.   Nursing care in the patient with pulmonary damage focuses on **easing respiratory efforts** and supporting the patient's oxygenation.

    o.   See **Table 16-7, text page 355,** for pulmonary toxicity of chemotherapy agents.

6. **Hepatotoxicity**

    a.   Chemotherapy drugs cause a variety of reactions, with the parenchymal cells as the initial site of insult. Obstruction to **hepatic blood flow** can result in **fatty changes, hepatocellular necrosis, cholestasis, hepatitis, and veno-occlusive disease.**

    b.   Diagnosis is made initially by transient elevations of hepatic enzymes. Later hepatomegaly, jaundice, and abdominal pain appear.

    c.   Hepatotoxicity is **reversible** unless fibrosis or necrosis has occurred.

    d.   **Veno-occlusive disease** occurs in 20% of patients receiving high-dose chemotherapy for bone marrow transplant and has a 50% mortality.

    e.   Clinical signs of veno-occlusive disease are **insidious weight gain, jaundice, abdominal pain, hepatomegaly, ascites, encephalopathy, and elevated bilirubin and SGOT** laboratory values.

    f.   In veno-occlusive disease, fluid and cellular debris become trapped, and eventually fibrosis of the venous wall occurs because of partial or complete occlusion of the hepatic veins by endophlebitis and thrombosis.

    g.   There are few guidelines for the use of chemotherapy drugs when hepatic dysfunction is present, but hepatotoxic drugs must be avoided when liver test results are abnormal.

    h.   Impaired liver function **delays** excretion and results in increased accumulation in the plasma and tissues, especially from drugs such as doxorubicin, vincristine, and vinblastine.

    i.   See **Table 16-8, text page 357,** for hepatotoxicity of chemotherapy agents.

7. **Hemorrhagic cystitis**

    a.   Hemorrhagic cystitis is a **bladder toxicity** that results from **cyclophosphamide and ifosfamide** therapy.

    b.   Hemorrhagic cystitis results from the metabolized by-products (phosphamide mustard and acrolein) of the chemotherapy drugs binding to the bladder mucosa, resulting in inflammation and ulceration.

    c.   Signs and symptoms are **irritative urination, dysuria, suprapubic pain,** and (if severe) life-threatening **hemorrhage.**

    d.   Extensive chronic bleeding and mucosal inflammation can produce long-term cystitis, irreversible bladder fibrosis, bladder contraction, and an increased risk for bladder cancer.

    e.   **Bladder protection** against cytoxan metabolites is being studied with several drugs. Mesna is a uroprotectant administered with ifosfamide, allowing larger doses to be administered.

    f.   Protection against hemorrhagic cystitis from either drug is attempted with **aggressive hydration, frequent voiding, and diuresis.** Occasionally, a three-way Foley catheter is placed for bladder irrigation, especially if there is bleeding, and then it is infused at a rate to clear developing clots.

    g.   **Vasopressins** may be administered to decrease clotting, and cystoscopy may be necessary to cauterize bleeders.

    h.   During drug administration, urine should be tested for blood and **strict intake and output** measured and recorded.

    i.   See **Table 16-9, text page 358.**

8. **Nephrotoxicity**

    a.   Fluid and electrolyte imbalances are a result of the direct and indirect effects of some chemotherapeutic agents.

    b.   Attempts to prevent nephrotoxicity include **aggressive hydration, urinary alkalization, diuresis,** and careful **monitoring of laboratory values.**

    c.   Chemotherapy damage to the kidneys varies from direct renal cell damage to an obstructive nephropathy as a result of precipitate formation.

    d.   **Cisplatin** can cause a mild to severe nephrotoxicity with damage to proximal and distal tubules. Damage can occur within 3–21 hours after administration.

    e.   **Protection** against nephrotoxicity with a variety of drugs is being studied. Some success has been achieved with WR 2721 and diethyldithiocarbamate.

    f.   See **Table 16-10, text page 360,** for chemotherapy agents resulting in nephrotoxicity.

9.   **Gonadal toxicity**

    a.   Gonadal toxicity depends upon the patient's **gender,** the patient's **age, and the specific drugs.**

    b.   Gonadal function is quantified by elevation in the **gonadotropins, in follicle-stimulating hormone, and in luteinizing hormone.**

    c.   The **alkylating agents** are the most detrimental to fertility.

    d.   In males, there is a progressive dose-related depletion of the germinal epithelial lining of the seminiferous tubule, resulting in the disappearance of the spermatocytes and spermatogonia. This results in **azoospermia, oligospermia, and abnormalities of semen volume, motility, and sperm forms** in postpubertal men.

    e.   In women, ova become nonfunctional by direct or indirect injury resulting from loss of supporting follicular cells.

    f.   Drug-induced menopause is reflected in women **developing amenorrhea, hot flashes, and menopausal blood levels of follicle-stimulating hormone, luteinizing hormone, and estradiol.**

    g.   In general, patients are advised to wait at least **2 years** after therapy completion before attempting to conceive.

    h.   **Nursing care** involves providing accurate information regarding chemotherapy and gonadal toxicity, instructing patients to use contraceptives, and teaching them how to manage the side effects of ovarian dysfunction.

VII.   SECONDARY/THERAPY-RELATED CANCERS

1.   A **second malignancy** refers to a new cancer which is related in some way to a treatment that was not only cytotoxic but also carcinogenic.

2.   Therapy-related malignancies generally have a **poor prognosis,** and treatment is usually not successful.

3.   The highest incidence of secondary malignancies occurs in people who have received and survived treatment for **Hodgkin's disease.**

4.   Risk factors also include primary neoplasm, the natural history of the disease, type of chemotherapy, cumulative dose of the drug, the patient's age, the patient's immune status, and the patient's environment.

5.   The **alkylating agents, nitrosureas, and procarbazine** are the chemotherapy drugs most commonly associated with chemotherapy-related cancers.

6.   Patients have a 1.6%–2.3% risk of developing **acute nonlymphocytic leukemia** within 10 years, peaking after 2–3 years.

7.   Patients need to be taught the importance of **follow-up** after therapy completion, even though the risk of a second malignancy is small.

PRACTICE QUESTIONS

1.   Dose limitations of chemotherapy are determined by
    (A)   the patient's physical status and medical history.
    (B)   the patient's history of previous treatments.
    (C)   the amount of cancer cells in the body.
    (D)   the toxicities of the particular drug.

2.   Patient education regarding treatment results in a number of positive outcomes. Which of the following outcomes does **not** result from patient education?
    (A)   improved patient compliance
    (B)   enhanced self-care participation
    (C)   increased self-confidence
    (D)   increases in the doses of prescribed medications

3. The most common and most lethal side effect of chemotherapy is
    (A) respiratory distress.
    (B) electrolyte imbalance from nausea, vomiting, and diarrhea.
    (C) myelosuppression.
    (D) increased liver function tests.

4. Prolonged diarrhea without adequate management can lead to all of the following **except**
    (A) renal failure.
    (B) dehydration.
    (C) circulatory collapse.
    (D) nutritional malabsorption.

5. Which of the following terms is defined as nausea and vomiting occurring 24 hours after drug administration, usually resulting from uncontrolled nausea and vomiting in the immediate 24 hours following drug administration?
    (A) delayed nausea and vomiting
    (B) acute nausea and vomiting
    (C) retching
    (D) anticipatory nausea and vomiting

6. Direct damage to the cardiac myocyte cells is **most** commonly associated with which group of antineoplastic agents?
    (A) vinca alkaloids
    (B) anthracyclines
    (C) antitumor antibiotics
    (D) alkylating agents

7. Signs and symptoms of altered gait, altered reflexes, ataxia, confusion, impotence, or ileus reflect what type of organ damage toxicity?
    (A) hepatic
    (B) neurologic
    (C) renal
    (D) gastrointestinal

8. What is the end result of progressive pulmonary toxicity?
    (A) respiratory alkalosis
    (B) productive, fulminant cough
    (C) dyspnea on exertion
    (D) hypoxia

9. Diagnostic signs and symptoms of veno-occlusive disease include
    (A) jaundice, hepatomegaly, nausea/vomiting.
    (B) hepatomegaly, elevated bilirubin, anxiety.
    (C) anxiety, nausea/vomiting, elevated bilirubin.
    (D) insidious weight gain, abdominal pain, jaundice.

10. Irritative urination, dysuria, suprapubic pain, and blood in the urine are signs and symptoms of
    (A) thrombocytopenia.
    (B) urinary tract infection.
    (C) renal dysfunction.
    (D) hemorrhagic cystitis.

11. What are the major risk factors influencing gonadal toxicity from antineoplastic agents?
    (A) renal function, specific drugs, blood levels of drugs
    (B) gender, age, specific drugs
    (C) renal function, blood levels of drugs, age
    (D) age, blood levels of drugs, gender

12. Which of the following classes of drugs is **most** likely to be associated with second malignancies?
     (A)   antimetabolites
     (B)   taxanes
     (C)   alkylating agents
     (D)   vinca alkyloids

ANSWER EXPLANATIONS

1. **The answer is (D).**   Although a patient's physical well-being and response to previous therapies are important to know, toxicities of the drug commonly determine the maximum amount of drug that can be administered safely. There are expected side effects that can be managed effectively and generally do not warrant reducing or discontinuing the drug. Toxic effects refer to life-threatening, often dose-limiting effects characteristic of high dosages. (332)

2. **The answer is (D).**   Teaching patients about their treatment reduces fear, increases self-confidence, improves compliance, and enhances their participation in their self-care. It has no effect on how much medication they should take. Patient education should begin early in the diagnostic phase and should serve as a guide through treatment and follow-up care. (333)

3. **The answer is (C).**   Myelosuppression is the most common and lethal side effect of chemotherapy. Since hematopoietic cells divide rapidly, they are vulnerable to chemotherapy, potentially resulting in dangerously low levels of red blood cells (anemia), white blood cells (neutropenia), and platelets (thrombocytopenia). When this occurs, patients are at risk for bleeding, infection, and circulatory compromise. (337)

4. **The answer is (A).**   The degree and duration of diarrhea depend on the agent, dose, nadir, and frequency of chemotherapy administration. Patients may experience abdominal cramps and rectal urgency with 5FU-Leucovorin therapy, which can evolve into nocturnal diarrhea or fecal incontinence, leading to lethargy, weakness, orthostatic hypotension, and fluid/electrolyte imbalance. Without adequate management, prolonged diarrhea will cause dehydration, nutritional malabsorption, and circulatory collapse. Renal failure does not result from untreated diarrhea. (341)

5. **The answer is (A).**   Delayed nausea and vomiting persist or develop 24 hours after chemotherapy, perhaps because of the ongoing effect that the metabolites of chemotherapy continue to exert on the CNS or GI tract. If nausea was controlled within the first 24 hours after therapy, delayed patterns are less likely to occur. Despite effective antiemetic regimens, 93% of patients receiving a high dose of cisplatin experience delayed nausea and vomiting. Anticipatory nausea and vomiting occur in 25% of patients as a result of classic operant conditioning from stimuli associated with chemotherapy. Acute nausea and vomiting occur 1–2 hours after treatment, resolving within 24 hours. The pattern of nausea and vomiting is determined by the emetogenicity of the chemotherapy and pretreatment with an antiemetic agent. (343)

6. **The answer is (B).**   Anthracyclines are known to cause cardiotoxicity by directly damaging the cardiac myocyte cells, with an incidence of 2%–3% after cumulative doses are administered. Cardiotoxicity is described as an acute or chronic process. Acute effects are immediate in onset and resolve quickly without serious complications. They are neither dose related nor a reason to stop the drug. Chronic cardiotoxicity occurring in less than 5% of patients develops from a cumulative drug effect and requires immediate discontinuation of the drug. Chronic effects occur weeks or months after administration, involving nonreversible cardiomyopathy presenting as a classic biventricular congestive heart failure. (345)

7. **The answer is (B).**   The clinical picture of chemotherapy-induced neurotoxicity can arise as a direct or an indirect damage to the central nervous system (CNS), peripheral nervous system, cranial nerves, or any combination of the three. Altered reflexes, altered gait, ataxia, confusion, impotence, and ileus are toxicities or symptoms of damage to the neurologic system. (353)

8. **The answer is (D).**   Pulmonary toxicity as a result of chemotherapy administration usually is irreversible and progressive. Chronic exposure to chemotherapy causes an extensive alteration of the pulmonary parenchyma, with changes in the connective tissue, obliteration of alveoli, and dilation of airspaces. Continuous injury and repair result in restrictive lung disease, with a thickened, still interstitium, increased work of breathing, and a functionally reduced lung volume leading to impaired gas exchange. Hypoxemia results because oxygen does not diffuse in the damaged areas while perfusion continues. (352)

9. **The answer is (D).**   Clinical signs of veno-occlusive disease (VOD) include insidious weight gain and jaundice that precede the development of abdominal pain, hepatomegaly, ascites, encephalopathy, and elevated bilirubin and SGOT laboratory values. The incidence of VOD following bone marrow transplantation is 20%, with a 50% mortality rate. (354)

10. **The answer is (D).**   Hemorrhagic cystitis ranges from microscopic hematuria to frank bleeding, necessitating invasive local intervention with instillation of sclerosing agents. Symptoms range from transient irritative urination, dysuria, and suprapubic pain to life-threatening hemorrhage. (356)

11. **The answer is (B).**   The likelihood that chemotherapy will affect a patient's fertility depends in part on the patient's gender, the patient's age, and the specific drugs. The age of female patients is an important predictor of treatment-induced sterility. Women over the age of 30 are less likely to regain ovarian function because they have fewer oocytes. (359)

12. **The answer is (C).**   One of the most serious long-term consequences of cancer is that the treatment intended to cure the patient may contribute to the occurrence of a second malignancy. A second malignancy is a new neoplasm that is related in some way to treatment that was not only cytotoxic but also carcinogenic. The alkylating agents, nitrosoureas, and procarbazine are the agents most commonly implicated in chemotherapy-related malignancies. (361)

17 Biotherapy

STUDY OUTLINE

I. INTRODUCTION

1. The hypothesis that the immune system can be manipulated to **restore, augment, or modulate** its function has stimulated extensive scientific inquiry.
2. Biotherapy, the therapeutic use of biological response modifiers **(BRMs),** has emerged as the fourth modality of cancer therapy as a result of four technologic advances.
   a. **An increased understanding of the complex cellular structure of the immune system**
      (1) This enables scientists to isolate new cellular components and to accurately measure their function.
   b. **Advances in genetic engineering, specifically the discovery of hybridoma techniques**
      (1) This makes it possible to clone genes and to produce large quantities of highly purified biologic agents for analysis and clinical use.
   c. **Advances in molecular biology**
      (1) This allows scientists to construct and alter molecules synthetically so that they can be investigated or their biologic activities changed.
   d. **Technologic advances in laboratory equipment and computer systems**
      (1) This has facilitated researchers in their search for the unknown.
3. The majority of BRMs are agents that modulate the immune system **(immunotherapeutic agents).** Some, however, are responsible for the **growth and maturation of cells.**
   a. A BRM is defined as **any substance that is capable of altering (modifying) the immune system with either a stimulatory or a suppressive effect.** This includes agents that
      (1) Restore, augment, or modulate the host's immunologic mechanisms.
      (2) Have direct antitumor activity.
      (3) Have other biologic effects, including interfering with tumor cells' ability to survive or metastasize or affecting cell differentiation or transformation.
4. See **Figure 17-1, text page 369,** for an illustration of the use of hybridoma technique to make monoclonal antibodies.

II. HISTORICAL PERSPECTIVE

1. Review **text pages 367–368** for historical information.

III. ANTIBODY THERAPY (SEROTHERAPY)

1. The limiting factor in effective cancer therapy is lack of specificity. **Serotherapy** addresses this limitation by promoting specific targeting of tumor cells through an antibody-antigen response. It is based on the knowledge that tumor cells, like most cells, have antigens on their surface that are specific to that cell type.

A. HYBRIDOMA TECHNIQUES

1. A **hybridoma** is the result of a fusion between two cell lines to form a hybrid that shares genetic information. It can be used in cancer therapy to produce a pure antibody to a known antigen found in tumor cells.
2. A hybridoma can be produced from a single cell clone. Thus all antibodies produced by the hybridoma are exactly the same—they are **monoclonal antibodies (MAbs).**

3. Refinement of the hybridoma technique allowed scientists to obtain a pure antibody to a known antigen and facilitated development of new therapeutic and diagnostic applications of antibodies in cancer therapy.
4. See **Figure 17-1, text page 369,** for an illustration of the use of hybridoma techniques to make monoclonal antibodies.

B. ANTIBODY FUNCTION

1. MAbs may be used alone (**unconjugated**) or in combination (**conjugated**) with radioisotopes, toxins, or chemotherapeutic agents to stain, destroy, or identify cells with specific antigens on their cell surface.
2. **Direct tumor cell kill**
   a. Antibodies may kill tumor cells directly through **antibody-dependent** cell-mediated cytotoxicity (ADCC), which results in cell lysis.
   b. Antibodies may kill tumor cells through **opsonization,** in which tumor cells are coated by the antibody to facilitate clearance by the reticuloendothelial system.
3. **Modulation of differentiation/growth**
   a. Although the effect has not yet been demonstrated in vivo, antibodies are capable of blocking tumor cell surface growth receptors for growth factors, thus providing a direct antiproliferative effect.
4. **Regulation of immunity**
   a. Antibodies may also be used to regulate immunity, and work is ongoing to develop an effective immunization to prevent particular types of cancers.
5. **Anti-idiotype as immunogen**
   a. Antibodies complementary to idiotypes (anti-idiotypic antibodies) can be used as surrogate antigen and thus substituted for the original antigen in the preparation of vaccines against infectious micro-organisms. This provides a solution to the supply and immunogenicity problems of a reliable cancer vaccine.

C. UNCONJUGATED MONOCLONAL ANTIBODIES

1. Mouse (murine) MAbs have been used to treat certain cancers, including forms of leukemia and lymphoma, gastrointestinal cancer, and metastatic melanoma. Responses thus far have been transient or limited despite evidence of antitumor effect.

D. IMMUNOCONJUGATES

1. **Immunoconjugates** are formed when a variety of agents are linked with monoclonal antibodies.
2. MAbs have been combined with **toxins, chemotherapeutic agents,** and **radioisotopes** in an effort to use the antibodies to deliver toxic agents directly to tumor cells, i.e., as **magic bullets.**
3. **Toxins**
   a. A variety of extremely lethal toxins (e.g., ricin, diphtheria toxin) are available for conjugation with antitumor antibodies. Some of these toxins are so powerful that a single molecule of toxin can kill a cell.
   b. Trials of immunotoxins in the treatment of melanoma and of colorectal and breast cancer are underway, but major tumor responses have not yet been achieved.
4. **Chemotherapeutic agents**
   a. **Chemoimmunoconjugates** are chemotherapeutic agents (e.g., chlorambucil, the anthracyclines) conjugated to MAbs. Through conjugation, the antibody targets the chemotherapeutic agent to the tumor cell, alleviating the expected toxicity to normal cells and theoretically allowing higher doses of chemotherapy to be given while minimizing system toxicity.
   b. Clinical trials with these agents are in early phases, and efficacy and toxicity are still to be determined.
5. **Isotopes**
   a. Current **diagnostic imaging** is limited by the lack of tumor specificity. Radio-labeled MAbs facilitate specific binding of radioactive agents to tumor cells, thus enhancing the detection of tumor cells.

      b.   Conjugation of an antibody active against a specific tumor antigen with a radioactive isotope (e.g., iodine, yttrium) creates a **therapeutic radioisotope.** The antibody seeks out the tumor and attaches to it, and the radioactive isotope internally irradiates the tumor.

      c.   MAbs may also be linked to various lymphokines, cytokines, and hormones to create **immunobiologic agents** that can increase antigen expression, enhance the action of the body's own cytotoxic cells, and decrease the viability of tumor cells.

E. CHIMERIC ANTIBODIES

1.   A **chimeric antibody** is a mixture of human and murine antibodies. The murine (mouse) part of the antibody recognizes the tumor antigen, while the human part of the antibody consists of the remainder of the immunoglobulin molecule.

2.   The result is an antibody that is both therapeutically effective and less immunogenic than standard murine MAbs.

F. HUMAN ANTIBODIES

1.   It is now possible to produce human antibodies. Human antibodies currently under investigation in the clinical setting include a human monoclonal antibody against endotoxin.

G. PROBLEMS WITH ANTIBODY THERAPY

1.   Problems with the use of MAbs in therapy include
      a.   **Antigenic specificity:** Only tumor-associated antigens, and not tumor-specific antigens, have been isolated. Antigen density must therefore be higher on tumor cells than on the cells of vital organs.
      b.   **Antigenic modulation:** MAbs must be administered intermittently to overcome the shedding or altering of tumor cell surface antigens.
      c.   **Antimouse antibodies:** Significant toxicity can result from the development of human antimouse antibodies.

2.   These problems have prevented monoclonal antibodies from living up to their expected potential.

H. CLINICAL TOXICITIES

1.   Anaphylaxis is not common, but the nurse should be prepared to deal with it immediately.
      a.   **Onset is predicted by a generalized flush and/or urticaria followed by pallor and/or cyanosis.** Patients may also complain of a tickle in the throat or impending doom; complaints of bronchoplasms are also common. If any of these symptoms occur, stop the MAb infusion immediately and alert the physician.
      b.   Anaphylaxis is treated with 0.3 M_1 aqueous 1:1000 epinephrine injected subcutaneously if the patient is conscious, 1:10,000 by intravenous push if the patient cannot be aroused.
      c.   Additional therapeutic measures include the use of oxygen; the administration of antihistamines, corticosteroids, and aminophylline; and possibly cardiopulmonary resuscitation.

2.   The most common side effects seen with MAb administration appear within 2 to 8 hours. They include **fever, rigors, chills,** and **diaphoresis.**

3.   Other common toxicities include weakness, generalized erythema, dyspnea, nausea, vomiting, diarrhea, hypotension, urticaria, pruritis, and malaise.

IV. CYTOKINES

1.   **Cytokines** (which include **lymphokines**) are substances that are released from activated immune system cells that affect the behavior of other cells.

2.   They may alter the growth and metastasis of cancer cells by
      a.   Augmenting the responsiveness of T-cells to tumor-associated antigens.
      b.   Enhancing the effectiveness of B-cell activity.
      c.   Decreasing suppressive functions of the immune system, thereby enhancing immune responsiveness.

3.   Cytokines may be administered directly to patients for control of cancer, or they may be used to manipulate the immune system to generate products that are used to treat individuals with cancer.

A. **INTERFERONS**

1. Recombinant DNA engineering techniques developed in the 1980s made interferons available for the first time in sufficient quantities for large-scale clinical trials. However, early results were modest and disappointing.

2. **Types of interferons**
    a. **Interferons (IFNs)** are a family of naturally occurring cytokines. Three major types of human IFN have been isolated: α-IFN, β-IFN, and γ-IFN. Each type originates from a different cell and has distinct biologic and chemical properties.
    b. See **Table 17-1, text page 373,** for the three types of IFNs, the cells responsible for their natural production, and their major cellular effects.

3. **Cellular effects**
    a. The cellular activities of IFNs are of three types: **antiviral, immunomodulatory,** and **antiproliferative.**
    b. **Antiviral**
        (1) IFNs protect a virally infected cell attack by another virus.
        (2) IFNs inhibit intracellular replication of viral DNA.
    c. **Immunomodulatory**
        (1) IFNs interact with T-lymphocytes that stimulate the cellular immune response.
        (2) In vitro, the killing potential of natural killer (NK) cells is increased in the presence of IFN.
    d. **Antiproliferative**
        (1) IFNs directly inhibit DNA and protein synthesis in tumor cells.
        (2) IFNs also increase tumor cell recognition by stimulating the expression of human lymphocyte antigens (HLAs) and tumor-associated antigens on tumor cell surfaces.
        (3) IFNs increase all cell phases, prolonging the overall generation time and thus inhibiting the rate of cell growth.

4. **Therapeutic uses/clinical trials**
    a. Most research to date has involved the use of **recombinant α-IFN.**
    b. **Hematologic diseases** have responded best to IFN therapy, with measurable responses occurring in the lymphoproliferative malignancies, such as hairy cell leukemia, non-Hodgkin's lymphoma, and multiple myeloma, and in chronic myelogenous and AIDS-associated Kaposi's sarcoma.
    c. Solid tumors in which good responses have been demonstrated include **renal cell carcinoma, malignant melanoma,** and **malignant carcinoid.**

5. **AIDS-associated Kaposi's sarcoma**
    a. Studies suggest that in AIDS-associated Kaposi's sarcoma (KS), α-IFN functions both in an **antiproliferative** and an **immunomodulatory** manner.
    b. Interferon may have a direct effect against HIV proliferation in individuals with AIDS.
    c. Additional studies are now exploring combinations of α–IFN with zidovudine (azidothymidine, AZT, Retrovir).

6. **Administration**
    a. The best dose, route of administration, and frequency of IFN administration are yet to be determined for most applications of α-IFN. It is known, however, that the route of administration of IFN affects significantly the pharmacokinetics of this agent.

7. **Clinical toxicities**
    a. Most toxicities appear to be **dose-related.**
    b. See **Table 17-2, text page 374,** and review **text pages 374–375** for a summary of potential toxicities of interferon.
    c. In addition to those toxicities cited in Table 17-2, other toxicities reported include **dry mouth** and **inflammation at the subcutaneous injection site.**
    d. A limiting factor in IFN therapy may be the development of **neutralizing antibodies.**
        (1) Many factors influence the antibody response, including the type of malignancy. Renal cell carcinoma and KS have the highest incidence of antibody formation.

8. **Future use of IFN therapy**
    a. Uses of IFN either alone or in combination with other therapies (including radiation, hyperthermia, chemotherapy, or surgery) will probably expand.
    b. IFN may also be used in combination with other cytokine agents such as interleukin.

B. **INTERLEUKINS**

1. **Interleukins (ILs)** are among the most important regulatory substances produced by lymphocytes and monocytes.
2. **Interleukin-1 (IL-1)**
    a. **IL-1,** a lymphocyte-activating factor, plays an immunoregulatory role involving a variety of biologic activities, including
        (1) Activation of T-cells to produce IL-2.
        (2) Induction of fibroblast proliferation.
        (3) Induction of fever, promotion of bone resorption, and initiation of acute-phase protein synthesis.
        (4) Enhancement of antibody responsiveness through stimulation of helper T-cells and B-cells.
        (5) Enhancement of cytotoxicity of lymphocytes.
        (6) Induction of tumor cell markers.
        (7) Provision of radioprotective properties.
    b. IL-1 appears to function as a **multilineage** growth factor that allows M-CSF or IL-3 to stimulate proliferation and maturation of cells.
    c. Hematopoiesis is regulated by IL-1's ability to induce proliferation of other CSFs and its **synergistic action with hematopoietic stem cells.**
    d. Two molecular forms of IL-1 (**IL-1α and IL-1β**) have been identified on purification of human IL-1.
    e. **IL-1α** is just entering phase I clinical trials.
        (1) Potential clinical applications of IL-1α include neutropenia, thrombocytopenia, antiproliferative effects, combination therapy with other cytokines, bone marrow transplantation, infectious disease, and dysmyelopoietic states.
        (2) IL-1α is administered subcutaneously.
        (3) Toxicities include fever, chills, headache, nausea/vomiting, tachycardia, asthenia, anorexia, hypotension (which can be a dose-limiting toxicity), myalgia, and diarrhea.
    f. **IL-1β** appears to play a key role in stimulating the production of IL-2 and other cytokines.
        (1) IL-1β is administered intravenous as an intermittent or continuous infusion.
        (2) Toxicities include fever, chills, rigors, tachycardia, tachypnea, hypertension (which may be followed by hypotension), headache, arthralgia, myalgia, and nausea and vomiting.
        (3) Leukocytosis may be seen 4–12 hours after administration, with a return to 20% of baseline within 24 hours.
        (4) An increased platelet count may be seen 5–6 days after administration, persisting for 20–24 days after the cessation of treatment.
3. **Interleukin-2 (IL-2)**
    a. **IL-2** is a glycoprotein produced by helper T-cells after stimulation by mitogens or specific antigens and IL-1.
    b. It binds to specific receptors on T-lymphocytes and on certain malignant lymphocytes, which may account for its specificity in the immune response.
    c. **Cellular effects**
        (1) **Essential factor in the growth of T-cells.**
        (2) Supports proliferation and augmentation of NK cells.
        (3) Is critical for the generation of LAK cells.
        (4) Augments various other T-cell functions.
        (5) Activates cytotoxic effector cells that play a significant role in the systemic toxicity of IL-2.
    d. **Therapeutic/clinical trials**
        (1) IL-2 can be used by itself or in combination with LAK cells (for **adoptive immunotherapy),** tumor-infiltrating lymphocytes (TILs), other cytokine agents, or chemotherapeutic agents.
        (2) IL-2 therapy produces objective tumor response in 20%–50% of patients with renal cell carcinoma and malignant melanoma.
        (3) **Adoptive immunotherapy** is an experimental approach in which the tumor-bearing host passively receives cells that possess antitumor activity.

        (a)   It involves incubating lymphocytes with IL-2 to generate LAK cells, and then infusing the LAK cells in conjunction with additional doses of IL-2.

        (b)   Phase II studies indicate great promise in treatment of both **malignant melanoma** and **renal cell carcinoma.**

    (4)   **TILs** are lymphocytes able to infiltrate into tumors. Combining TILs with IL-2 offers a technique for treatment of metastatic melanoma and renal cell carcinoma that may be superior to IL-2/LAK therapy.

    (5)   Studies are also investigating IL-2 in combination with other cytokines, including interferon and tumor necrosis factor.

  e. **Pharmacokinetics**

    (1)   Serum half-life of IL-2 increases to a range of from 30 to 120 minutes when it is administered by means of intravenous infusion.

  f. **Clinical toxicities**

    (1)   The multisystem toxicities of IL-2 administration, although life-threatening, are reversible. All pretreatment laboratory values and physiological states, with the exception of fatigue, return within 24–96 hours following cessation of therapy.

    (2)   These toxicities are clearly related to **dose** and **schedule** and may be related as well to IL-2-induced production of other cytokines, IFNs, and TNF.

    (3)   Review **text pages 377–378** for specific systemic side effects.

4. **Interleukin-4 (IL-4)**

  a. Produced naturally by activated T-lymphocytes.

  b. Preclinical studies suggest a role in mediating antiproliferative effects.

  c. May also have anti-inflammatory effects.

  d. Clinical toxicities resemble those of IL-2 and are dose-related.

5. **Interleukin-6 (IL-6)**

  a. Produced naturally by monocytes, endothelial cells, and fibroblasts.

  b. Biologic properties include hematologic, antiproliferative, and inflammatory effects.

  c. Toxicities include elevated bilirubin and transaminases, chills, fever, nausea/vomiting, diarrhea, leukopenia, fatigue, somnolence, and anemia.

6. **Interleukin-7 (IL-7)**

  a. Produced by the bone marrow and thymic stromal cells.

  b. Biologic activities include induction of IL-2 production and expansion of immature lymphoid cells.

  c. Not yet used in clinical trials.

7. **Interleukin-10 (IL-10)**

  a. May function either alone or with IL-7 as a lymphopoietin, producing growth of both B- and T-cells.

C. TUMOR NECROSIS FACTOR

1. **Tumor necrosis factor (TNF)** is a naturally occurring agent produced by activated macrophages. In vitro studies on mouse and human cells indicate that TNF has cytotoxic or cytostatic effects on tumor cells with no effect on normal cells.

2. **Cellular effects**

  a. TNF travels through the bloodstream and binds to designated receptors located on tumor cell membranes.

  b. It produces cell arrest in the G_2 phase of the cell cycle, with extensive cell lysis measurable after 7 hours.

  c. Some cells experience lysis, some cytostasis without lysis, and some are basically resistant to TNF.

  d. Other biologic effects of TNF are summarized in **Table 17-3, text page 379.**

3. **Pharmacokinetics**

  a. The serum half-life of intravenous bolus-administered recombinant TNF (rTNF) is approximately 20 minutes.

  b. Factors affecting half-life are dose and route of administration.

4. **Clinical trials**

  a. Phase II clinical trials are underway to determine further tumor response, immune system modulation, dosage, route of administration, and toxicities.

5. **Administration**

  a. Recombinant TNF (rTNF) is currently administered intravenously in a normal saline solution that contains human serum albumin at a concentration of 2 mg/ml.

6. **Clinical toxicities**
   a. The most common toxicities are a **flulike syndrome,** which includes fever, chills, rigors, headaches, and fatigue, and a local reaction at the subcutaneous or intramuscular injection site.
   b. See **Table 17-4, text page 380,** for a complete list of TNF systemic toxicities.
   c. As with INF, most TNF toxicities appear to be **dose-dependent** and are **reversible,** resolving within 48 to 96 hours after the drug is discontinued.

D. **COLONY STIMULATING FACTORS**

1. **Colony stimulating factors (CSFs)** are a group of naturally occurring glycoproteins that regulate blood cell growth. Specifically, they **stimulate the growth of maturing blood cells from their hematopoietic precursors.**
2. Most CSFs are named for the major target cell lineage they affect, e.g., **granulocyte CSF (G-CSF)** targets only granulocytes.
3. The CSFs are **not,** as previously considered, **lineage specific,** and the effects of various factors probably overlap.
4. **Therapeutic applications**
   a. CSFs hold great promise in the treatment of disease states in which myelosuppression, anemia, and thrombocytopenia prevail and limit therapeutic options, e.g., congenital neutropenia and AIDS.
   b. The **use of CSFs** in clinical practice will be either **prophylactic** (i.e., to prevent expected complications) or **therapeutic** (i.e., administered to the patient once complications/needs arise).
5. **Erythropoietin**
   a. **Erythropoietin** is the first CSF approved by the FDA and available for clinical use. It has firmly established its role in the treatment of anemia caused by end-stage renal disease.
   b. When administered after dialysis treatments, it stimulates erythropoiesis and either reduces or eliminates patient transfusion requirements.
   c. Studies have suggested a role for rHuEPO in reducing the anemia associated with AZT therapy in AIDS patients and rheumatoid arthritis.
   d. Several studies investigating the **effects of EPO** levels within the cancer population have found adequate hemoglobin rises, subjective **improvement in anemia-related symptoms,** and **improvement in performance status.**
6. **Granulocyte colony stimulating factor (G-CSF)**
   a. G-CSF functions in the proliferation, maturation, and activation of granulocytes.
   b. It is clinically used to increase production of granulocytes, especially in the bone marrow transplant population, where it has accelerated platelet and neutrophil recovery following high-dose conditioning chemotherapy. It also has a role in stem cell mobilization prior to leukopheresis.
7. **Granulocyte-macrophage colony stimulating factor (GM-CSF)**
   a. GM-CSF exhibits a broad spectrum of biologic activity, affecting all levels of granulocytes and stimulating the production of monocytes and macrophages. It may also produce a **multilineage** effect, decreasing the requirement of platelet and red cell transfusions in some patients.
   b. It is clinically used to permit dose intensification and enhance myeloprotection by administering it both before and after the chemotherapy treatment.
8. **Clinical toxicities**
   a. **One should never administer any CSF that has an immediate effect on the progenitor cells (G-CSF, GM-CSF, or IL-3) within the 24 hours preceding or following cytotoxic therapy.**
   b. Minimal toxicity has been associated with G-CSF therapy.
   c. GM-CSF therapy produces a wider array of systemic toxicities. Commonly reported toxicities that appear to be route- and dose-related include **low-grade fevers with chills and/or rigors** that occur 4 to 6 hours after administration.
   d. See **Table 17-5, text page 383,** for a list of other CSF toxicities.
   e. Review **text pages 382–383** and **Table 17-6, text page 384,** for additional clinical information regarding the administration of G-CSF and GM-CSF and the nursing management of various clinical toxicities.
9. **Interleukin-3 (multi-CSF)**
   a. IL-3 functions primarily as a myeloid growth factor and appears active on the primitive stem cell and also on the mature cells of multiple lineages.

        b.   A **GM-CSF/IL-3 fusion protein (PIXY321)** has been produced recombinantly and may offer a substantial clinical benefit over either of the individual cytokines.

    10. **Macrophage colony stimulating factor (M-CSF)**

        a.   M-CSF demonstrates strong activity on differentiated macrophages and also affects neutrophil production.

  E. **GENE THERAPY**

    1. Gene therapy is an attempt to further modulate cellular function. **Gene therapy is a technique in which a functioning gene is inserted into the cells of a patient either to correct a genetic error or to introduce a new function to the cell.**

    2. Gene therapy can raise **significant scientific, legal, and ethical issues,** and multiple mechanisms have been established at various levels of the system to promote the safe science of gene therapy.

    3. Future studies in **gene therapy** will seek to identify and clone genes responsible for human tumor-associated antigens, thus **enhancing the specificity of cancer therapy.**

V.   NURSING MANAGEMENT

  A. **GENERAL NURSING IMPLICATIONS**

    1. See **text page 300,** column 1, for a list of critical issues the nurse must address in obtaining specific information about the various BRMs being investigated in humans for their immunomodulatory and/or antiproliferative effects.

  B. **NURSING INTERVENTIONS**

    1. The nurse has an obligation to obtain accurate knowledge concerning all phases of therapy so that appropriate patient and family planning and care through the nursing process may be achieved.

    2. The nurse should be involved in discussions with the patient, family, and physician regarding the **patient history, purpose of therapy, course of treatment and necessary procedures,** and **precautions to be taken to prevent adverse reactions.**

    3. The nurse should encourage the patient to share information and observations concerning personal reactions to the treatment. This information may be important to the ultimate evaluation of treatment efficacy and toxicities.

    4. **Nursing interventions should focus on common biologic and chemical properties shared by BRMs, including the nature of the biologic agent as a medication, the diversity of organ-system toxicities, and the presence of an acute or a chronic flulike symptom, as well as other possible side effects.**

        a.   Nursing assessment for organ toxicity involves

           (1) Establishing the patient risk for development of such toxicity.

           (2) Establishing baseline values for future comparisons.

        b.   Toxicities depend on the particular protocol in use for dose, route of administration, and schedule.

    5. Interferon has been viewed as the prototypic BRM because of its **constellation of toxicities,** its **biologic nature,** and the presence of an **acute and a chronic flulike syndrome.** Management of this syndrome includes

        a.   Changing dose or schedule.

        b.   Administering effective medications to block or minimize the effect, e.g., administration of meperidine at the onset of chills or rigors.

        c.   Practicing noninvasive nursing techniques such as imagery and/or relaxation therapy.

    6. The nurse should provide psychosocial support to the patient during any new treatment. The element of patient responsibility and commitment to complete therapy should be emphasized.

VI.   FUTURE PERSPECTIVES

    1. The ultimate success of BRMs as a fourth modality of cancer treatment lies in further understanding the unique complexities of the human immune system. The goal is to develop specific treatments of cancer without the problem of nonspecific toxicities.

2. Nurses will be active in
    a. Providing nursing care to individuals with complex organ toxicities.
    b. Developing and standardizing policies and procedures for monitoring patients receiving BRMs.
    c. Detecting and analyzing the individual's response to the agent being studied.
    d. Investigating current methods of caring for individuals receiving BRM agents and recommending improvements for that care.
    e. Disseminating new concepts in cancer management to other nurses in order to improve patient care through research, presentations, and publications.

PRACTICE QUESTIONS

1. The emergence of biotherapy as the fourth modality of cancer therapy is the result of several technologic advances, including the discovery of hybridoma techniques. Why was this discovery important?
    (A) It made it possible to clone genes and to produce large quantities of highly purified biologic agents.
    (B) It enabled scientists to isolate new cellular components and to accurately measure their function.
    (C) It allowed scientists to construct and alter molecules synthetically so that they could be investigated or their biologic activities changed.
    (D) It facilitated researchers in their development of new laboratory equipment and computer systems.

2. How do most biologic response modifiers (BRMs) work?
    (A) They control the growth of cells.
    (B) They modulate the immune system.
    (C) They control the maturation of cells.
    (D) They target tumor cells through an antibody-antigen response.

3. The monoclonal antibodies (MAbs) used in antibody therapy are produced from a single clone of hybrid cells (a hybridoma). What are these cells a hybrid of?
    (A) mouse lymphocytes and mouse malignant myeloma cells
    (B) human lymphocytes and mouse malignant myeloma cells
    (C) mouse lymphocytes and human malignant myeloma cells
    (D) human lymphocytes and human malignant myeloma cells

4. MAbs can destroy tumor cells through a variety of direct or indirect mechanisms, including all of the following **except**
    (A) through antibody-dependent cell-mediated cytoxicity (ADCC), which results in cell lysis.
    (B) through opsonization, in which tumor cells are coated by the antibody to facilitate clearance by the reticuloendothelial system.
    (C) by blocking cell surface growth receptors for growth factors, thus interfering with proliferation.
    (D) by augmenting the responsiveness of T-cells to tumor-associated antigens, thus modulating the immune system.

5. The term "magic bullets" in antibody therapy refers to the use of
    (A) MAb-radioisotope immunoconjugates in diagnostic imaging.
    (B) antibodies to deliver toxic agents directly to tumor cells while sparing normal cells.
    (C) hybrids of human and murine antibodies to reduce immunogenicity.
    (D) chemotherapeutic or radioisotopic agents to deliver antibodies directly to tumor cells.

6. The most common side effects seen with MAb administration appear within 2 to 8 hours and can **best** be described as
    (A) flulike symptoms, including fever and chills.
    (B) serum sickness, including generalized adenopathies.
    (C) anaphylaxis, including a generalized flush and/or urticaria.
    (D) hematologic distress, including neutropenia and thrombocytopenia.

7. Which of the following substances is **not** a cytokine?
    (A) α-interferon
    (B) interleukin-2
    (C) levamisole
    (D) tumor necrosis factor (TNF)

8. Included among the therapeutic cellular activities of interferons (INFs) are all of the following **except**
   (A) antiviral activity—protecting a virally infected cell attack by another virus.
   (B) immunomodulatory activity—interacting with T-lymphocytes that stimulate the cellular immune response.
   (C) antiproliferative activity—directly inhibiting DNA and protein synthesis in tumor cells.
   (D) immunoregulatory activity—mediating the proliferation and activation of hematopoietic factors.

9. IFN therapy has been **most** effective in the treatment of what kinds of malignancies?
   (A) solid tumors, especially colon and cervical cancers
   (B) basal cell and other skin carcinomas
   (C) hematologic diseases, including hairy cell leukemia
   (D) metastatic foci when a low tumor burden exists

10. Most of the toxicities that occur with the administration of the various types of IFN appear to be related to
    (A) dose.
    (B) route of administration.
    (C) schedule.
    (D) IFN type.

11. Interleukin-2 (IL-2) appears to exert its greatest cellular effects on the
    (A) induction of fibroblast proliferation.
    (B) growth of T-cells.
    (C) stimulation of helper T-cells.
    (D) replication of viral DNA.

12. Adoptive immunotherapy is an experimental approach in which the tumor-bearing host passively receives both IL-2 and cells that possess antitumor activity. What types of cells are administered along with IL-2?
    (A) tumor-infiltrating lymphocytes (TILs)
    (B) NK cells
    (C) LAK cells
    (D) helper T-cells

13. All of the following are common systemic side effects of IL-2 administration **except**
    (A) anemia.
    (B) a diffuse erythematous rash.
    (C) constipation.
    (D) hypotension.

14. Tumor necrosis factor (TNF) acts principally by
    (A) activating macrophages, which destroy tumor cells.
    (B) stimulating the production of T-lymphocytes, which destroy tumor cells.
    (C) killing tumor cells directly.
    (D) regulating hematopoiesis.

15. A major advantage of colony stimulating factors (CSFs) over other BRMs is their
    (A) ability to modulate the immune system without directly affecting either T-cell or B-cell production.
    (B) ability to bind selectively to tumor cell membranes, killing tumor cells without harming normal cells.
    (C) antiproliferative activity against metastatic foci as well as primary tumors.
    (D) applicability to disease states in which myelosuppression, anemia, and thrombocytopenia prevail.

16. An important aspect of the nursing management of biotherapy is the nurse's role in sharing information and observations concerning patients' personal reactions to treatments. This nursing intervention is of greatest relevance because
    (A) patients' reactions are generally more reliable than is information derived from clinical trials.
    (B) such information is important to the ultimate evaluation of efficacy and toxicities.
    (C) this knowledge allows the nurse to predict the severity of potential toxicities.
    (D) such information forms the basis of appropriate patient and family planning care.

ANSWER EXPLANATIONS

1. **The answer is (A).** Previously, isolation and purification were slow, cumbersome, and costly processes that produced small quantities and impure products for analysis and clinical use. Hybridoma, the result of a fusion between two cell lines to form a hybrid that shares genetic information, made it possible to produce large quantities of biologic agents. It can be used in cancer therapy to produce a pure antibody to a known antigen found in tumor cells. (367)

2. **The answer is (B).** A BRM is any soluble substance that is capable of altering (modifying) the immune system with either a stimulatory or a suppressive effect. It may act by restoring, augmenting, or modulating the host's immunologic mechanisms, by having direct antitumor activity, or by having some other biologic effects, including interfering with tumor cells' ability to survive or metastasize. (367)

3. **The answer is (A).** In the production of MAbs, an animal (usually a mouse) is injected with the desired antigen (human tumor cells). The mouse's lymphocytes recognize the antigen as foreign and produce antibodies. The immunized lymphocytes are removed from the mouse and fused with mouse malignant myeloma cells to form a hybrid capable of unlimited cell division. The end result after purification is a monoclonal antibody directed against specific tumor-associated antigens. (368–369)

4. **The answer is (D).** Unconjugated MAbs may directly kill tumor cells through ADCC or opsonization. They may also modulate differentiation and growth by blocking tumor cell surface growth receptors for growth factors, providing a direct antiproliferative effect. Finally, they may be used to regulate immunity. (369–370)

5. **The answer is (B).** Immunoconjugates are formed when a variety of toxic agents, including radioisotopes, toxins, chemotherapeutic agents, and biologic agents are linked to monoclonal antibodies. These agents can then be transmitted directly to tumor cells by the MAbs, where they may have lethal effects on the tumor cells. The efficacy and toxicity of these "bullets" are being determined. (370)

6. **The answer is (A).** Anaphylaxis occurs infrequently and suddenly and is predicted by the presence of generalized flush and/or urticaria followed by pallor and/or cyanosis. Serum sickness, which includes a variety of symptoms, may occur 2 to 4 weeks after MAb therapy. Dillman reports that the most common side effects of MAb administration—fever, chills, rigors, and diaphoresis—occur within 2 to 8 hours. (371)

7. **The answer is (C).** Cytokines (which include lymphokines) are substances that are released from activated immune system cells that affect the behavior of other cells. They may alter the growth and metastasis of cancer cells by augmenting the responsiveness of T-cells to tumor-associated antigens, enhancing the effectiveness of B-cell activity, or decreasing suppressive functions of the immune system, thereby enhancing immune responsiveness. Included among the cytokines are the interferons and interleukins, tumor necrosis factor (TNF), and colony stimulating factors (CSFs). (371)

8. **The answer is (D).** The IFNs are a family of naturally occurring complex proteins that belong to the cytokine family. Each of the three major types in humans—α-IFN, β-IFN, and γ-IFN—originates from a different cell and has distinct biologic and chemical properties. All three types of IFN exhibit the cellular effects listed in choices (A)–(C). (372–373)

9. **The answer is (C).** Hematologic diseases have responded best to IFN therapy, with measurable responses occurring in the lymphoproliferative malignancies (such as hairy cell leukemia, non-Hodgkin's lymphoma, and multiple myeloma) and in chronic myelogenous and AIDS-associated Kaposi's sarcoma. (373)

10. **The answer is (A).** It appears that most IFN toxicities, as well as toxicities from most other BRMs, are dose-related. Low doses of IFN are well tolerated, whereas high doses often require cessation of therapy. A common reaction to any type of IFN is the occurrence of fever, chills, fatigue, and malaise, referred to collectively as flulike syndrome. (374–375)

11. **The answer is (B).** IL-2 is produced by helper T-cells after stimulation by mitogens or specific antigens and IL-1. It binds to specific receptors on T-lymphocytes and on certain malignant lymphocytes, which may account for its specificity in the immune response. It is an essential factor in the growth of T-cells. It also supports proliferation and augmentation of NK cells, is critical for the generation of LAK cells, augments various other T-cell functions, and activates cytotoxic effector cells that play a significant role in the systemic toxicity of IL-2. (376)

12.   **The answer is (C).**   Adoptive immunotherapy involves incubating lymphocytes with IL-2 to generate LAK cells, and then infusing the LAK cells in conjunction with additional doses of IL-2. LAK cells are capable of selectively lysing tumor cells that are resistant to NK cells without affecting normal cells. (376)

13.   **The answer is (C).**   The side effects of IL-2 administration, although life-threatening, are reversible and are related to dose, schedule, and probably IL-2-induced production of other cytokines, IFNs, and TNF. Other common toxicities include confusion, respiratory dysfunction, weight gain, increased heart rate, azotemia and elevated creatine levels, nausea, vomiting, diarrhea, stomatitis, hypoalbuminemia, thrombocytopenia, and flulike syndrome. (377–378)

14.   **The answer is (C).**   Tumor necrosis factor (TNF) is a naturally occurring agent produced by activated macrophages. In vitro studies on mouse and human cells indicate that TNF has cytotoxic or cytostatic effects on tumor cells with no effect on normal cells. TNF travels through the bloodstream and binds to designated receptors located on tumor cell membranes. It produces cell arrest in the G_2 phase of the cell cycle, with extensive cell lysis measurable after 7 hours. (379)

15.   **The answer is (D).**   Colony stimulating factors (CSFs) are a group of naturally occurring glycoproteins that stimulate the growth of maturing blood cells from their hematopoietic precursors. As such, they hold great promise in the treatment of disease states in which myelosuppression, anemia, and thrombocytopenia prevail and limit therapeutic options. They may also allow increased doses of chemotherapy to be given without the risk of long-term myelosuppression and may be used in other hematologic diseases in which abnormalities of blood cell components exist, e.g., congenital neutropenia and AIDS. (381)

16.   **The answer is (B).**   Because of the investigational nature of BRMs, the nurse should encourage patients to share information and observations concerning personal reactions to the treatment. This represents only one of many ways that nurses play an indispensable role in the research process. (386)

18 Bone Marrow Transplantation

STUDY OUTLINE

I. **INTRODUCTION**

1. **Bone marrow transplantation (BMT)** has evolved over the past 30 years from an experimental procedure to an established, effective treatment for selected cancer patients.

II. **HISTORICAL PERSPECTIVES**

1. Following the institution of histocompatible leukocyte antigen (**HLA**) typing to identify suitable sibling donors in the 1960s, successful human **allogeneic** transplants were carried out in increasing numbers.
2. **Autologous** marrow transplantation originally served as a salvage therapy for end-stage patients but has emerged as an important treatment for patients with hematologic and solid-organ malignancies.
   a. Thousands of patients without a matched donor are able to benefit from an autologous BMT.
   b. Supralethal doses of chemotherapy and irradiation can now be administered as a treatment therapy, and the patient can be "rescued" from death with an infusion of his or her own previously harvested marrow.

III. **CONCEPTS OF BONE MARROW TRANSPLANTATION**

1. The basic concepts of the BMT process are as follows:
   a. The **dose** of most chemotherapeutic agents administered to cure a patient's disease is limited by subsequent dose-related marrow toxicity.
   b. The **availability** of donor marrow for transplantation and engraftment makes it possible to administer chemoradiotherapy in supralethal doses in an effort to kill malignant cells (preparative regimens for BMT).
   c. The patient is then **rescued** with donor marrow to prevent iatrogenic death (bone marrow transplantation).
   d. The infused marrow will **reconstitute** the patient's hematopoietic and immunologic system, and the patient (host) will be rescued (engraftment).
   e. **Complications** that follow BMT are the result of the high-dose chemotherapy and conditioning regimens used to prepare the patient to receive the donor marrow (acute and chronic complications).
2. See **Table 18-1, text page 396,** for the sequence and time of events in the process of allogeneic BMT.

IV. **TYPES OF BONE MARROW TRANSPLANTATION**

1. The three sources of donor marrow for transplantation are **syngeneic, autologous,** and **allogeneic.**

A. **SYNGENEIC**

1. A **syngeneic marrow transplant** is one in which the donor is an identical twin, who by definition is a **perfect HLA match.**

154

B. **ALLOGENEIC**

1. **Allogeneic marrow transplantation** depends on the availability of an HLA-matched donor.
2. **Graft-versus-host disease (GVHD)** is a complication unique to allogeneic transplantation and is a major obstacle to successful transplantation.
3. Intensive supportive care and specialized nursing care are integral to the protection of the patient during transplantation.
4. **Diseases treated with allogeneic BMT**
   a. Allogeneic BMT is performed mostly for acute and chronic leukemia, lymphomas, multiple myeloma, severe aplastic anemia, genetic disease, immunologic deficiencies, and inborn errors of metabolism. See **Figure 18-3, text page 397,** for the diseases and frequencies of allogeneic transplants.
   b. **Genetic disease**
      (1) Successful allografts have occurred in children with **aplastic anemia, thalassemia, and Franconis anemia.**
      (2) The use of BMT for sickle cell anemia is still under investigation.
   c. **Immunologic deficiencies**
      (1) Marrow transplantation is a treatment choice only in the presence of an HLA-matched sibling for patients with congenital immunodeficiency diseases, including severe combined immunodeficiency disease syndrome (SCIDS), Wiskott-Aldrich syndrome, and some rare inherited disorders.
   d. **Inborn errors of metabolism**
      (1) Allogeneic BMT has been successful for patients with inborn errors of metabolism, such as Gaucher disease, chronic granulomatosis disease, osteoporosis, mucopolysaccharidosis (Hurler's syndrome), Sanfilipp B disease, and Maroteaux-Lamy syndrome.

C. **DONORS**

1. **Tissue typing**
   a. **Human leukocyte antigen/mixed lymphocyte culture**
      (1) The selection of an appropriate marrow donor is based on the **major histocompatibility complex,** which in humans is comprised of a series of closely linked genetic loci on chromosome 6.
      (2) The five closely linked genes located on chromosome 6 are referred to as a **haplotype** and are individually designated as **HLA-A, HLA-B, HLA-C, HLA-D,** and **HLA-DR.**
         (a) HLA-A and HLA-B loci are defined serologically.
         (b) A locus identical with or closely related to HLA-D, called HLA-DR, can be serologically typed in a **mixed lymphocyte culture** by means of B-lymphocytes.
   b. **ABO typing**
      (1) Techniques that effectively **remove red blood cells from donor marrow** and the **plasma exchange of patient marrow** have reduced the risk of acute hemolytic transfusion reactions when ABO incompatibilities exist.
2. **Marrow collection**
   a. Donor marrow is **harvested** in the operating room under sterile conditions, with the donor anesthetized under general or spinal anesthesia.
   b. Marrow is obtained from the **posterior iliac crests** in 2- to 5-ml aspirates (10 to 15 mg/kg of recipient body weight); the anterior iliac crests and sternum are also used if necessary.
   c. Only **6 to 10 skin punctures** are made, as the aspiration needles are redirected to different sites under the skin.
   d. The heparinized marrow is screened through a series of progressively finer **mesh screens to filter out bone particles and fat** before being placed in blood administration bags for **infusion within 2 to 4 hours.**
   e. See **Figure 18-5, text page 399,** for the steps of marrow collection and harvest.
   f. **Unrelated donors**
      (1) The **National Marrow Donor Program (NMDP)** has approved 53 BMT centers to perform allogeneic BMT for unrelated donors.
      (2) The use of unrelated volunteer donors **increased** from 5% to 8% between 1988 and 1990.

D. **AUTOLOGOUS**

1. An **autologous (self)** marrow graft is a transplant in which a patient with a malignant disease receives his or her own marrow after preparation with conditioning regimens.
2. **Relapse of malignancy** following autologous transplantation may be due to
    a. Failure of the pretransplantation conditioning therapy to successfully eradicate micro-residual disease in the patient.
    b. The presence of malignant cells in the donor marrow.
3. See **Figure 18-6, text page 400,** for the schematic of autologous bone marrow transplantation.
4. **Diseases treated with autologous BMT (ABMT)**
    a. See **Figure 18-7, text page 400,** for a percentage breakdown of the diseases being treated with BMT.
    b. Clinical trials are studying the use of ABMT in breast, ovarian, colon, and small-cell lung cancers, melanoma, multiple myeloma, and malignant glioma.
    c. **Advantages** of ABMT are the absence of graft-versus-host disease and fewer BMT-related toxicities.
5. **Marrow collection**
    a. The procedure for obtaining aspirates for **autologous transplantation** is similar to that for allogeneic transplantation; however, the marrow may then be **incubated with chemotherapeutic drugs** to purge tumor cells, **cryopreserved** for up to 8 years, or immediately **infused** upon completion of the conditioning regimen.
    b. The three methods used to purge marrow of malignant cells are **physical purging, immunologic purging, and pharmacologic purging.**
6. **Autologous peripheral stem cell transplant (PSCT)**
    a. PSCT candidates are patients who are ineligible for ABMT because their marrow is hypoplastic from prior myeloablative therapies and patients with metastatic marrow disease.
    b. **Collection and mobilization** of peripheral stem cells via apheresis is usually done in the outpatient setting.
    c. **Mobilization** is the process of either stimulating circulating hematopoietic stem cells with myelosuppressive chemotherapy or administering growth factors during the collection period. A combination of these two techniques can produce more hematopoietic stem cells than when either technique is used alone.
        (1) See **text page 401,** column 1, for a description of the collection procedure and cryopreservation before storage.
    d. Immediately prior to **PSCI,** the cells are removed from storage and thawed or washed in a warm-water bath.
    e. After thawing, they are quickly infused through a central or peripheral catheter over 2–4 hours.
    f. Complications of the infusion include nephrotoxicity, cardiac toxicity, and dyspnea.

V. **PROCESS OF BONE MARROW TRANSPLANT**

A. **PRETRANSPLANT EVALUATION AND PREPARATION OF THE PATIENT**

1. See **Table 18-2, text page 402,** for the schedule of required evaluations to determine a candidate's and a donor's ability to participate in BMT.
2. An initial meeting with the patient and the patient's family is important in order to **explain the conditioning regimen and risks of BMT** and to **discuss expected outcomes with the patient.**

B. **PREPARATION OF THE DONOR AND NURSING CARE**

1. Bone marrow donors are **comprehensively evaluated** before surgery. This includes evaluation of their tolerance of general or spinal anesthesia during bone marrow harvest.
2. Because the bone marrow donor often needs to provide platelet and granulocyte support for the patient for up to 3 months after marrow transfusion, the donor should receive adequate **counseling and training** prior to marrow donation.
    a. Long-term psychologic effects have been reported for marrow donors of patients who have died following BMT.
    b. Follow-up care for the donor should include **assessment of the harvest site, evaluation of comfort,** and **psychological support.**

VI.   **THE BONE MARROW TRANSPLANT**

    A.   **ADMISSION TO THE HOSPITAL**

        1.   Once patients have been evaluated for BMT, they are admitted to the hospital and placed in a protective isolation room.

    B.   **PRETRANSPLANT CONDITIONING REGIMENS**

        1.   Patients may receive **high-dose chemotherapy alone** as part of the BMT conditioning regimens.
            a.   **Cyclophosphamide** is commonly used for both tumor kill and immune ablation.
            b.   Other drugs used include daunomycin, busulfan, cytarabine, etoposide, and 6-thioguanine.
        2.   **Total body irradiation (TBI)** may precede chemotherapy because its ability to penetrate sanctuary sites for malignant cells offers optimal cell kill.

    C.   **MARROW INFUSION**

        1.   **The day of marrow infusion is referred to as "day zero,"** and subsequent days are numbered from this time.
        2.   The marrow is infused through a **central line** in a manner similar to a blood transfusion, with the potential for complications similar to blood transfusion reactions.
        3.   Within 2 to 4 weeks the marrow graft becomes functional, and peripheral platelets, leukocytes, and red cells increase in number.

VII.   **COMPLICATIONS OF BONE MARROW TRANSPLANTATION**

    A.   **INTERRELATIONSHIPS OF BMT COMPLICATIONS**

        1.   Complications that may arise after transplantation result from
            a.   The high-dose chemotherapy and irradiation for conditioning regimens.
            b.   GVHD during allogeneic transplant.
            c.   Problems associated with the original disease.
        2.   See **Figure 18-9, text page 405,** for the sequence of major complications following BMT.

    B.   **ACUTE COMPLICATIONS**

        1.   See **Figure 18-4, text pages 406–408,** for possible acute complications that occur several days after BMT.
        2.   **Gastrointestinal toxicity**
            a.   **Gastrointestinal toxicity** may be exhibited by severe mucositis throughout the gastrointestinal tract.
            b.   **Nausea and vomiting** are a consistent problem during BMT. They may be caused by **GVHD, CMV esophagitis,** or **gastrointestinal infections.**
            c.   **Diarrhea** may occur as a result of **chemoradiotherapy,** but it seldom persists beyond day 15.
        3.   **Hematologic complications**
            a.   **Hematologic complications** require platelet and red blood cell support until the donor marrow becomes fully engrafted and functional.
               (1)   Blood products must be **irradiated to inactivate T-lymphocytes** that can cause GVHD in the recipient.
               (2)   **Platelet transfusions** from marrow donors yield optimal increments.
               (3)   See **Table 18-5, text page 410,** for clinical manifestations and interventions for hemorrhage management.
            b.   Twenty-four percent of marrow recipients develop hemorrhagic cystitis as a result of cyclophosphamide therapy used in conditioning regimes.
               (1)   Prevention involves aggressive IV therapy and continuous bladder irrigation.
        4.   **Acute graft-versus-host disease**
            a.   **GVHD is an immunologic disease that is a direct consequence of allogeneic marrow transplantation,** occurring in 30%–50% of HLA-identical recipients in either the acute or the chronic form.

    b. **Acute GVHD** targets the skin, liver, and gut when grafted donor T-lymphocytes recognize disparate non-HLA antigens and initiate cytotoxic injury against host tissue.

    c. See **Table 18-6, text page 410,** for the clinical stages of acute GVHD.

5. **Renal complications**

    a. **Renal complications** occur in more than 50% of marrow recipients due to factors that include the **use of nephrotoxic medication, septicemia,** and **volume depletion.**

    b. Nursing assessment is aimed at recognition of the early symptoms of either prerenal or intrarenal failure.

6. **Veno-occlusive disease of the liver**

    a. **Veno-occlusive disease (VOD)** is a serious problem for 40% of adult marrow recipients.

       (1) **Preparative chemotherapy** for BMT is the cause of VOD.

       (2) Risk factors for VOD are a **history of hepatitis before transplant, age greater than 15 years,** and **hematologic malignancy.**

    b. Clinical manifestations of VOD result from **sinusoidal obstruction** and **intrasinusoidal hypertension** and include **fluid retention, sudden weight gain, pain in the right upper quadrant of the abdomen, jaundice, hepatomegaly,** and **encephalopathy.**

    c. Treatment of VOD consists of **fluid management, restriction of sodium,** and keeping the patient with a **hematocrit of greater than 35%** to maintain intravascular volume and renal perfusion.

    d. Nursing assessment includes **close tabulations of fluid balance, twice-a-day weights, abdominal girth measurements,** and **postural blood pressure measurement.**

7. **Pulmonary complications**

    a. **Pulmonary complications** may be early- or late-appearing, occurring as a result of **chemoradiotherapy toxicity** or **bacterial, fungal, or viral infection** in severely immunosuppressed patients.

    b. Clinical manifestations of pneumonia may include **nonproductive cough, dyspnea, hypoxemia, fever, chest radiograph changes,** and **blood gas abnormalities.**

    c. **Interstitial pneumonia** is a nonbacterial, nonfungal process occurring in the interstitial spaces of the lungs in approximately 35% of allogeneic marrow recipients.

    d. **Cytomegalovirus pneumonia** is the leading cause of infectious pneumonia during BMT, occurring in 20% of allogeneic marrow recipients.

    e. **Idiopathic pneumonia,** diagnosed when no causative organism is isolated, is believed to result from high-dose irradiation. It accounts for 30% of all interstitial pneumonia in transplant recipients.

    f. **Bacterial and fungal pneumonias** are not a major cause of death in the marrow recipient, but along with viral pneumonias they account for 15% of pneumonias in BMT patients.

    g. Median time of onset for interstitial pneumonias is **60 to 70 days after BMT;** thus nursing assessment for respiratory compromise during this follow-up period is crucial to initiating prompt treatment.

8. **Neurologic complications**

    a. Neurologic nursing assessments should be incorporated into the evaluation of the BMT patient, as **leukoencephalopathy** has been reported in 7% of all patients who have received prior cranial irradiation and intrathecal methotrexate.

9. **Cardiac complications**

    a. **Cardiomegaly, congestive heart failure,** and **fluid retention** are cardiac complications that may develop within several days after high-dose cyclophosphamide administration.

10. **Infection**

    a. Marrow recipients are at high risk for **bacterial, viral, and fungal complications,** which peak at predicted times after transplantation; days 0–30 preengraftment and days 30–90 postengraftment.

    b. **Preengraftment (days 0–30)**

       (1) The **herpes simplex virus (HSV)** types I and II, **Epstein-Barr** virus, **cytomegalovirus,** and **varicella zoster** virus are major **viruses** occurring in the first 30 days after BMT.

       (2) Neutropenia with concomitant damage to mucosal surfaces contributes to **Gram-negative bacteremia** immediately after transplantation.

       (3) Profound immunosuppression with resulting neutropenia concomitant with denuding of the mucosa in the gastrointestinal tract places marrow recipients at risk for *Candida* infection.

        (4) *Aspergillus* is a major infectious problem during days 0–30. The portal of entry for *Aspergillus* infection is the respiratory tract, and the risk for *Aspergillus* infection increases with the duration and degree of neutropenia.

  c. **Early engraftment (days 30–90)**

        (1) **Cytomegalovirus (CMV)** infection is the most significant infection during this phase, accounting for a 15%–20% mortality rate.

        (2) Risk factors for CMV are presence of **positive serologic titers, GVHD, and the degree of HLA tissue typing** between patient and donor.

        (3) Bacterial infections are less frequent in the early engraftment period.

        (4) **Gram-positive infections** associated with the central lumen catheter present a major risk for systemic infection.

        (5) **Fungal infections** are problematic during this period, and marrow recipients with GVHD have a higher risk than those without GVHD.

  d. **Fever** is the cardinal sign of infection in the pancytopenic marrow recipient, since he or she is unable to mount the classic immune response to infection.

  e. See **Table 18-7, text pages 414–415,** for risk factors associated with life-threatening infections and measures to treat and prevent infections.

  f. Prevention and treatment of infection in the marrow recipient are aimed at **identifying the invasive organism through surveillance cultures** and **treating the accompanying infection with appropriate antibiotics.**

  g. Nurses need to be alert to subtle signs of infection, because there are other factors (such as GVHD, blood products, and drugs) that may also result in a fever response.

VIII. DISCHARGE FROM THE HOSPITAL

  1. See **Table 18-8, text page 416,** for patient guidelines upon discharge.

  2. See **text page 417,** column 1, for common discharge criteria.

IX. CLINICAL MANAGEMENT OF THE BMT OUTPATIENT

  1. Comparative studies of home health care for BMT patients discharged early versus hospital care have been encouraging in terms of patient well-being and reduction of cost.

A. OUTPATIENT HOME CARE

  1. Clinical outpatient staff need to be knowledgeable and able to distinguish signs and symptoms of problems patients are at risk for, including acute and chronic GVHD, herpes, *varicella zoster, cytomegalovirus, Pneumocystis carinii* pneumonia, sexually transmitted diseases, infections and other transplant problems. See **Table 18-9, text page 418.**

  2. See **Table 18-10, text page 419,** for the assessment, procedures, and tests for BMT outpatients.

B. 100-DAY EVALUATION

  1. The 100-day workup evaluates the recipient's stability and risk factors for discharge home. See **Table 18-11, text page 419.**

C. ANNUAL ASSESSMENTS

  1. Patients return to the BMT center for annual evaluations for up to 3 years following BMT.

X. LATE COMPLICATIONS OF BMT

  1. See **Tables 18-12 and 18-13, text pages 420–423,** for the incidence, time period, manifestations, and interventions of late effects of BMT.

A. CHRONIC GRAFT-VERSUS-HOST DISEASE (ALLOGENEIC BMT)

  1. **Chronic GVHD** is a multisystem disorder occurring in 30%–50% of long-term survivors, with clinical and pathological findings resembling those of several naturally occurring autoimmune diseases, such as scleroderma, systemic lupus erythematosus, and rheumatoid arthritis.

2. **Onset and classification**
   a. **Progressive onset of chronic GVHD,** which is a direct extension of acute GVHD, has the poorest prognosis.
   b. **Quiescent onset** develops in patients who have had a resolution of acute GVHD. It has a fair prognosis.
   c. **De novo onset** occurs in patients with no prior acute disease and has the best prognosis.
   d. Chronic GVHD may be **limited to the skin and liver** and have a favorable course, or it may be **extensive,** meaning that **multiple organs are involved** and that treatment is mandatory to achieve improvement.
3. **Clinical manifestations of GVHD**
   a. The **skin** is affected in more than 95% of patients.
   b. **Liver disorders** are observed in about 90% of patients with chronic GVHD.
   c. **Oral mucosa** involvement will develop in approximately 80% of patients.
   d. **Ocular involvement** occurs in 80% of patients.
   e. **Esophageal abnormalities** have been documented in 36% of patients.
   f. Significant **vaginal problems** may occur in many women with chronic GVHD.
4. **Treatment**
   a. Screening studies for GVHD are done at approximately **day 100** in order to implement early treatment if it is detected.
   b. **Combination therapy of immunosuppressive, cytotoxic,** and **supportive antibiotics** given over a period of 1 year to 18 months has improved morbidity and mortality rates.
   c. **Clinical studies**
      (1) **Removal of T-cells** believed to be responsible for GVHD has decreased its incidence but has resulted in **increased graft rejection** and **leukemic relapse.**
      (2) The combination of **methotrexate and cyclosporine,** given prophylactically to prevent GVHD, has led to 80% one-year survival rates in patients with early stage leukemia who are given HLA-identical marrow.
   d. In a curious phenomenon known as the **graft-versus-leukemia effect,** recipients of allogeneic BMT in whom clinically significant GVHD develops have a **lower relapse rate** than those patients without GVHD.

B. **LATE INFECTIOUS COMPLICATIONS**

1. **Late infectious complications** are more prevalent in marrow recipients who develop chronic GVHD.
2. **Varicella zoster virus (VZV)** develops in 30%–50% of long-term survivors within the first year of transplantation.
   a. **All marrow recipients with chronic GVHD are at risk for infection from encapsulated bacteria.**

C. **PULMONARY COMPLICATIONS**

1. Among **pulmonary complications** in BMT survivors are
   a. **Restrictive pulmonary disease,** which is rare and has an incidence peaking 1 year post-BMT.
   b. **Obstructive pulmonary disease,** which occurs in 15% of long-term survivors with chronic GVHD.
   c. **Late interstitial pneumonia,** which develops in 10%–20% of long-term survivors with chronic GVHD and carries a 50% mortality rate.

D. **GONADAL DYSFUNCTION**

1. Most transplant recipients who were preconditioned with TBI will demonstrate **gonadal dysfunction,** although patients who have received chemotherapy alone often recover fertility.
2. Sexual counseling before BMT is important for all candidates for marrow transplantation.
3. **Growth in children**
   a. High-dose cyclophosphamide conditioning for BMT does not interfere with normal growth and development in children, in contrast to TBI, which does result in abnormalities in those processes.
   b. All children have **decreased growth rates after TBI,** and those affected by GVHD have the most marked growth retardation.

      c.   Bone age is not as markedly affected as are **adrenocortical function, growth hormone levels,** and **thyroid function,** particularly in children who have received prior prophylaxis with cranial irradiation.

      d.   **Establishing parental awareness of the late effects of irradiation is a prime nursing function.** Growth patterns should be annually evaluated, and those who demonstrate decreased growth rate should be referred to a pediatric endocrinologist.

E. THYROID DYSFUNCTION

1. **Thyroid dysfunction** occurs in 30%–60% of patients treated with a regimen that includes single-dose total-body irradiation (TBI).

F. OPHTHALMOLOGIC EFFECTS

1. **Cataract development** is primarily related to **TBI administration** and/or long-term **steroid therapy for GVHD.**
2. Lens shielding is not used during TBI because the eye is a potential site of leukemic relapse.
3. Peak time for cataract development is 3 to 6 years after transplantation.

G. GRAFT FAILURE

1. **Graft failure** is more frequent in patients who have had transplantation with HLA-nonidentical or T-cell-depleted marrow compared with unmodified HLA-identical marrow recipients.

H. ASEPTIC NECROSIS

1. **Aseptic necrosis** tends to develop in the humerus or femur head due to softening of the bone from steroid therapy.

I. DENTAL EFFECTS

1. **Dental effects** of the cytoablative regimen or chronic GVHD can lead to oral hygiene effects and dental decay.

J. GENITOURINARY EFFECTS

1. Until recently, genitourinary toxicity had not been reported as a long-term sequela of BMT.
2. Total-body irradiation, drug toxicity related to antimicrobial therapy, and cyclosporine are **causative factors.**
3. The median time of **onset** is 9 months, with a range of 4.5–26 months.
4. **Renal insufficiency** is characterized by increased serum creatinine, decreased glomerular filtration rate, anemia, hypertension, and proteinuria.

K. RADIATION NEPHRITIS

1. **Radiation nephritis** may occur about 5 months after BMT.

L. NEUROLOGIC COMPLICATIONS

1. **Neurologic complications** such as leukoencephalopathy may not appear for months or years after BMT and may be manifested by learning disabilities in children.

M. SECOND MALIGNANCY

1. Secondary malignancies have been observed in a small number of patients who receive BMT. They are considered to be a **late sequela of BMT.**
2. **Relapse** remains a major problem, with most patients experiencing relapse due to **disease in host cells (sanctuary sites).**
3. Patients who relapse after BMT need **intensive supportive care,** because they may feel they have exhausted medical options as well as psychologic and financial resources.

XI.   **PSYCHOSOCIAL ISSUES**

A.   **PATIENTS**

1.   See **Table 18-3, text page 305,** for **stresses** that patients have identified with each phase of the BMT process.

B.   **DONORS**

1.   Donors experience a variety of psychologic reactions before and after their marrow donation.

C.   **FAMILY/CAREGIVERS**

1.   Families incur considerable psychologic, emotional, and social problems before and after marrow transplantation due to
   a.   Transplantation centers often being located far from familiar support systems.
   b.   The long-term issues that confront the family of a recovering BMT patient.
2.   The involvement of a **strong social work team** is beneficial in transplantation settings.

D.   **STAFF**

1.   There is the potential for staff stress related to caring for BMT patients whose conditions may change rapidly.
2.   Nurses are challenged by family interactions as well as patient concerns, and they become part of a psychosocial team caring for acutely ill patients who may die.
3.   **Staff support programs** can be developed that will help maintain emotional health, clinical excellence, and staff retention.

E.   **QUALITY OF LIFE**

1.   BMT recipients surveyed 10 years after BMT report a quality of life similar to that of other cancer survivors.

F.   **ETHICAL ISSUES**

1.   Marrow transplantation may involve complex ethical consideration of issues such as
   a.   **The rights of children.**
   b.   **Effectiveness of informed consent.**
   c.   **Life support in the event of irreversible organ failure.**
   d.   **Allocation of resources.**

XII.   **FUTURE APPLICATIONS**

A.   **STEM CELL TECHNOLOGY**

1.   Research techniques that allow **separation of hematopoietic stem cells** are being developed with the hope that they will allow for infusion of **leukemia-free marrow in autologous transplantation.**

B.   **GENE TRANSFER**

1.   In the future, application of gene technology to BMT may allow replacement of defective genomic material with healthy genes in patients who have genetic diseases and are candidates for marrow transplantation.

PRACTICE QUESTIONS

1.   A bone marrow transplant in which the marrow donor is a perfect HLA-match to the recipient is known as a(n)
   (A)   allogeneic transplant.
   (B)   syngeneic transplant.
   (C)   xenogeneic transplant.
   (D)   autologous transplant.

2.   Which of the following statements about the bone marrow donor for an allogeneic transplant is correct?
   (A)   The donor may need support for potential long-term psychologic effects if the marrow recipient does not have a favorable outcome from BMT.
   (B)   The donor should not be informed of unfavorable results from BMT.
   (C)   The donor typically has no special needs, because marrow donation is relatively risk free.
   (D)   The donor typically receives a local anesthetic prior to bone marrow harvest.

3.   Which of the following statements about idiopathic pneumonia is true?
   (A)   It is identical to interstitial pneumonia.
   (B)   It is diagnosed when no causative organism is isolated.
   (C)   It can be easily treated with antibiotics.
   (D)   It is a manifestation of GVHD.

4.   Among the potential growth abnormalities that TBI can cause in children is
   (A)   early puberty.
   (B)   suppressed bone age, which occurs more frequently than does suppressed adrenocortical function.
   (C)   a decreased growth rate, especially for those affected by GVHD.
   (D)   an exaggeration of secondary sex characteristics.

5.   Nurses are responsible for giving parents of children undergoing BMT all of the following information **except**
   (A)   cataract development is possible for as long as 3 to 6 years after TBI.
   (B)   a decreased growth rate may be an indication for the child to see a pediatric endocrinologist.
   (C)   learning disabilities may represent a late effect of cranial radiation.
   (D)   in all likelihood, their children will never be able to have children.

6.   Monitoring a BMT recipient for signs of infection may be complicated by the
   (A)   patient's lack of signs characteristic of a classic immune response.
   (B)   fact that patients who are neutropenic for prolonged periods generally do not have fevers.
   (C)   limited contact that caregivers have with patients as a result of isolation procedures.
   (D)   fact that BMT patients must be on high-dose steroids during the transplant period.

7.   Ethical considerations related to the complexities of BMT may revolve around
   (A)   allocation of resources.
   (B)   the fact that BMT is palliative and not curative.
   (C)   the ambivalent feelings of nurses caring for BMT patients.
   (D)   the prolonged isolation of the neutropenic BMT patient.

8.   Among the following, the factor that is **least** likely to contribute to family stress when a family member is undergoing BMT is
   (A)   distance from familiar support systems.
   (B)   financial uncertainties.
   (C)   the long-term issues that confront the family of a recovering BMT patient.
   (D)   the active caregiving role families are expected to assume during BMT.

9.   Which of the following is **most** likely to produce staff stress?
   (A)   the responsibility of protecting family members from the distressing changes in the BMT patient
   (B)   the uncertainties of caring for patients whose medical conditions change rapidly
   (C)   a lack of communication with physicians about the care of BMT patients
   (D)   fear of acquiring a malignancy through exposure to high-dose chemotherapy

10.   Which of the following side effects is **most** likely to persist until the donor marrow becomes fully engrafted and functional?
   (A)   acute GVHD
   (B)   diarrhea
   (C)   hematologic complications
   (D)   cardiotoxic manifestations

11. The major dose-limiting factor in administering conventional chemotherapy in high enough doses to achieve a cure is
     (A)   cardiac toxicity.
     (B)   body surface area.
     (C)   bone marrow toxicity.
     (D)   increased risk of veno-occlusive disease.

ANSWER EXPLANATIONS

1.   **The answer is (B).**   A syngeneic marrow transplant is one in which the donor is an identical twin, who by definition is a perfect HLA match. (396)

2.   **The answer is (A).**   Mood changes, lack of self-esteem, altered relationships, and guilt have all been identified as long-term sequelae, which are based on the donor's perception of the success or failure of the BMT. (403)

3.   **The answer is (B).**   Idiopathic pneumonia accounts for 30% of all interstitial pneumonias in marrow recipients and is believed to result from high-dose irradiation. (412)

4.   **The answer is (C).**   All children have decreased growth rates after TBI, and those children who have chronic GVHD are the most significantly affected. (428)

5.   **The answer is (D).**   The adverse effects of high-dose chemotherapy on gonadal function depends on the age of the patient at the time of BMT. (427)

6.   **The answer is (A).**   Fever is the cardinal symptom of infection. The cytopenic condition of marrow recipients masks the classic infection-related symptoms of inflammation, pus formation, and elevated white blood cell counts. (416)

7.   **The answer is (A).**   Marrow transplantation may involve complex moral and ethical considerations relating to informed consent, the rights of children, and allocation of resources. (430)

8.   **The answer is (D).**   The patient's family may be expected to play an emotionally supportive role during BMT, but they would not be expected to have an active caregiving role until the patient has returned home. (430)

9.   **The answer is (B).**   Nurses are challenged by family interactions as well as by patient concerns, and they become part of a psychosocial team caring for acutely ill patients who may die. (430)

10. **The answer is (C).**   Recipients of grafts are at high risk for hemorrhage and must be supported with red blood cells until the marrow becomes fully engrafted and functional. (409)

11. **The answer is (C).**   The theory of replacing diseased marrow with healthy marrow is simple in concept but difficult to implement successfully because of the toxicities related to high-dose chemotherapy and irradiation in preparative regimens. Bone marrow toxicity is the dose-limiting toxicity for giving most chemotherapeutic agents in high enough doses to cure a patient's disease. (395)

19   Overview: Psychosocial Aspects of Cancer

STUDY OUTLINE

I.   INTRODUCTION

1. The **psychosocial** dimension of cancer care focuses on
   a. **The unique needs of the individual at risk for or with cancer.**
   b. **The social groups affected by that individual.**
      (1) Each individual brings to the cancer experience unique personality traits and a personal socialization pattern different from all others.
2. Recent studies have looked at psychosocial variables as a risk factor in carcinogenesis, especially the role of the immune and endocrine systems as mechanisms of causation.
3. Other studies have looked at ways of **maximizing self-actualization** and **minimizing psychosocial distress** in cancer patients.
   a. Such studies offer new understanding about the meaning of the diagnosis of cancer and response patterns of individuals and groups to the actual or perceived threat.
4. Psychosocial responses to the cancer experience are determined by the characteristics of cancer, the person with or at risk for cancer, and the social system and environment of the individual.

II.   CHARACTERISTICS OF CANCER

A.   CANCER POSES A UNIVERSAL THREAT

1. For most people, cancer risks are the product of unmeasurable, cumulative lifestyle and environmental exposure. The particular risk will vary with **age, geographic location,** and **lifestyle,** but no individual or social sector is exempt.
2. For most people, cancer is among the most feared of all diseases. The reasons for this are several:
   a. **Cancer occurs without warning.**
   b. **Cancer often spreads uncontrollably.**
   c. **Cancer is incurable beyond a certain point.**
   d. **Cancer treatments can be mutilating.**
   e. **The cause of cancer is unknown.**
   f. **Cooperation with treatment does not necessarily lead to a successful outcome.**
3. The uncertainty of cancer's diagnosis, spread, and recurrence disrupts normal perceptions of health, such as the ability to adapt or to strive for self-actualization goals.

B.   THE STIGMA OF CANCER PERSISTS

1. The persistent social stigma of cancer is seen in **insurance cancellations, job and military discrimination,** and **problems with reintegration into the school and workplace.**
2. Only in the past 50 years has cancer been met head-on, with the fighting spirit exemplified by the phrase the "war on cancer."

C. **DISEASE AND TREATMENT ARE MARKED BY UNCERTAINTY**

1. The uncertainties associated with cancer may be compounded by delays in diagnosis, unpredictable prognoses, and short illness trajectories resulting in early death in apparently healthy individuals.
    a. Uncertainty can be defined as the inability to determine the meaning of illness-related events.
    b. Uncertainty results from the inability to structure the meaning of illness-related stimuli into a **cognitive schema.**
    c. It is not inherent in the situation but is a perception of the individual. It may be interpreted as a danger or as an opportunity for growth.
    d. Uncertainty may be influenced by
        (1) **Ambiguity concerning the state of the illness.**
        (2) **The complexity of treatment and the system of care.**
        (3) **Lack of information about the diagnosis and seriousness.**
        (4) **Unpredictability of the disease course and prognosis.**
2. Four stages of uncertainty in illness are proposed: **the antecedents** that generate uncertainty; the **cognitive appraisal** of uncertainty as either **danger** or **opportunity; coping efforts** to either reduce uncertainty perceived as danger, or to maintain uncertainty appraised as opportunity; and the **state of adaptation** resulting from effective coping.
    a. Disease- and treatment-related symptoms as well as the emotional responses to illness can alter perception, attention, and cognition and thus can influence the accuracy of stimuli perception.
    b. The more **accurate the cognitive schema** formed of the illness, the less **uncertainty** one experiences.
    c. **Structure providers** are resources that assist the person in interpreting illness-related events. They include credible authority, social support, and education.
    d. **Trust and confidence** in health care professionals lessen uncertainty.
    e. **Social support systems** can both validate perceived meanings of the illness situation and provide feedback used for **social comparisons** with other individuals in similar situations.
    f. **Education of the individual** is one resource that can enhance familiarity with illness events and facilitate interpretation of information received from physicians, nurses, and other sources.
    g. See **Figure 19-1, text page 439,** for a model of perceived uncertainty in illness.

D. **THE CANCER TRAJECTORY IS MANIFEST BY CHRONICITY**

1. Simple crisis resolution models are not sufficient to address the scope of problems encountered with cancer. This is because
    a. Patients must deal with a **continuing series of stressors rather than a single, time-limited crisis.**
    b. Treatment is complex, often extended, and may cause irreparable damage to physical, mental, or social functioning.
    c. Cancer may recur.
2. The concept of a **chronic illness trajectory** can be applied to incorporate the diversity, multiplicity, and complexity of problems that an illness such as cancer brings over time.
    a. Within the trajectory there is interaction between the disease and treatment experience and the person's sense of personal identity, goal attainment, and performance of activities of daily living.
    b. The illness trajectory can be shaped and managed over time.
    c. The eight phases of the chronic illness trajectory are presented in **Table 19-1, text page 441.**
    d. This model may not be applicable to all cancer patients, especially given the longer survival and higher cure rates that are common today.
3. The concept of a **trajectory of cancer recovery** has also been proposed.
    a. This model is oriented toward survival versus dying and emphasizes self-care over professional intervention.
    b. Recovery is multidimensional and has physical, functional, cognitive and affective dimensions.
    c. The **Integrated Cancer Recovery Model** is presented in **Figure 19-2, text page 442.**

III. **INDIVIDUAL RESPONSES TO CANCER**

    A. **HELP-SEEKING RESPONSES**

        1. The search for psychosocial resources to deal with the threat of cancer begins with **self-appraisal,** then extends to **significant others** and ultimately to **health care professionals.**

        2. In contrast, the return to health is manifested by the health care professional giving responsibility back to the individual.

    B. **CULTURALLY DETERMINED RESPONSES**

        1. The **specific culture** of the individual shapes his or her view of life and health. For example, cancer may be less threatening in a culture in which life expectancy is short.

        2. Socioenvironmental factors also shape health behavior. For instance, the socioeconomically disadvantaged must expend most of their material and psychosocial resources on daily survival, so coping and health promotion actions may, of necessity, be compromised.

        3. **Socialization** into culture shapes the attitudes, beliefs, and values that constitute one's personality. Cancer can challenge these values and beliefs and may result in changed responses.

            a. The most common responses are **anxiety** and **depression.**

            b. The "appropriate" response is largely based on

                (1) The individual's psychosocially constructed reality of the situation.

                (2) The adaptability of the social network in acquiring new patterns of response.

    C. **STRESS, EMOTIONS, AND COPING RESPONSES**

        1. Stress is defined as a **relationship between person and environment** in which demands tax or exceed the person's resources.

        2. Stress is not an inherent characteristic of the person or environment but is defined by the constantly changing **individual appraisal** of **threat, harm,** or **challenge** in the situation.

            a. **Appraisal** is influenced by personality, developmental level, values, and perceived resources.

            b. **Primary appraisal** includes perceptions of the meanings and potential outcomes of the situation. Primary appraisal influences the emotional response.

            c. **Secondary appraisal** influences the coping strategies selected to deal with the situation.

            d. **Problem-focused coping strategies** include confrontative and interpersonal strategies such as seeking information and taking problem-solving actions.

            e. **Emotion-focused coping strategies** include distancing, escape-avoidance, and accepting responsibility or blame.

        3. **Stress management theory** is useful in understanding psychosocial responses to cancer.

            a. It makes the health care professional attentive to outmoded adaptive responses used by patients. For instance, denial may be adaptive initially but may later interfere with adaptive health behavior.

            b. It considers the effect of cumulative stressors on the ability to adapt. Individuals most vulnerable to psychosocial distress are likely to be those who

                (1) **Have been unsuccessful in resolving past stress situations.**

                (2) **Are dealing with a number of stressors simultaneously.**

                (3) **Perceive minimal social support in the situation.**

        4. Recent theory integrates stress models into theory about **emotion.**

            a. **Emotion is a complex of psychophysiological reactions** consisting of cognitive appraisals, action impulses, and somatic reactions.

            b. **Theories of emotion** may serve to integrate the various dimensions of the human response to stressful situations. This model also provides a framework for including the effects of positive emotions such as love or happiness, as well as the negative emotions such as anger, and thus **may provide a more inclusive model for understanding the effects of both positive and negative emotions on health.**

IV. **SOCIAL AND FAMILY RESPONSES TO THE STRESS OF CANCER**

        1. **Supportive relationships** at home and in the community may buffer the stressful effects of the cancer diagnosis.

a. **Mechanisms of this buffering effect** are postulated to include
   (1) Diminishing the level of the perceived stress of the situation.
   (2) Facilitating coping effectiveness.
   (3) Lessening the reactions of the individual to stressors.
b. Efforts at school and workplace reintegration are based on the recognition of the role of social networks in facilitating coping with daily stress and the stress of illness.

2. The family of origin or choice generally constitutes the most important social support for the individual throughout the life span.
   a. Increased heterogeneity of lifestyles has **changed the form and definition of the family.**
   b. Each patient will have her or his own definition of what constitutes her or his family and will have personal family values. Health care providers should not impose their values on others or interfere with family interactional processes.
   c. The family can be a source of **information, nurturance, and validation.**
   d. The diagnosis of cancer changes the family system with respect to **daily activities, expectations, roles, boundaries, patterns, and values.**

3. **There are numerous theoretical frameworks** available for studying and working with families. **Table 19-3, text page 444,** provides an overview of the theoretical components of each framework.

V. PROFESSIONAL RESPONSES TO CANCER

A. DISTANCING

1. **Distancing** is an unconscious response of professionals, especially to persons who are dying. Distancing behaviors enhance the loneliness and fear experienced by seriously ill individuals.
   a. Behaviors that manifest distancing include
      (1) Delays in answering call lights.
      (2) Infrequent visitations.
      (3) Failure to communicate.
      (4) Maintaining "professionalism" in emotionally charged situations.
   b. Professionals will be less likely to practice distancing if they learn to deal effectively with the repeated losses that are inevitable in the oncology clinical setting. Ways of coping with losses may include
      (1) Coming to terms with death as a part of humanity.
      (2) Working through the grieving process that accompanies death of a patient.
      (3) Developing personal qualities of flexibility, genuine concern, and listening skills.
2. **Strategic communication** with patient and family can be used to establish and maintain relationships, effect behavioral changes, promote comfort and positive self-image for the patient, and relay information. These communication skills can be enhanced with study, evaluation, and the use of feedback.

B. CARING

1. **Caring** is a process that helps a person attain or maintain health or a peaceful death.
   a. Caring generally refers to the quality of nurse-client interactions and relationships. The caring commitment includes the commitment to protect human dignity and is grounded in human values such as kindness, helpfulness, concern, and love.
   b. For the nurse, two potentially negative outcomes of caring are overinvolvement and burnout, which may be countered with supportive collegial relationships.

VI. PSYCHOSOCIAL OUTCOMES

A. SELF-CARE

1. **Self-care** includes attempts of the individual to promote optimal health, prevent illness, detect symptoms, and manage chronic illness.
2. Processes for achieving these goals include selecting healthful lifestyles, self-monitoring and assessing symptoms, evaluating the severity of the situation, and determining treatment alternatives.

3. **Nursing strategies for promoting patient self-care** include mutual goal setting, information giving, assisting with decision making and problem solving, providing opportunities and support for the expression of personal preferences and decisions.

B. **SURVIVAL**

1. Most psychosocial intervention research tends to use improvements in mood, psychological adjustment, or level of symptom distress as the outcome measure, rather than the effect of the psychosocial care intervention on overall survival. Studies are beginning to examine prospectively the effects of psychosocial intervention (such as group therapy, hypnosis, and coping skills training) on long-term disease-free survival.

C. **QUALITY OF LIFE**

1. The concept of **quality of life** addresses the effects of the disease and its treatment on the patient, family, and community. Quality of life is subjective (it reflects the concerns of the patient) and involves physical, functional, emotional, and social dimensions.
2. Concern about **quality of life** may be reflected in **care goals** that address the alleviation of disease and treatment-related symptoms, the reduction of negative emotional responses, the promoting of well-being, and the maximizing/normalizing of physical, psychological, and social functioning.

PRACTICE QUESTIONS

1. The psychosocial dimension of cancer care focuses on both the unique needs of the individual at risk for or with cancer and the
   (A) unique needs of other individuals in society.
   (B) clinical training of health care professionals.
   (C) social groups affected by that individual.
   (D) role of specific therapies in cancer treatment.

2. The treatment or diagnosis of cancer can be characterized in terms of all of the following **except**
   (A) the psychosocial origins of its incidence.
   (B) the uniqueness of its meaning to the individual.
   (C) the uncertainty of the disease and its treatment.
   (D) the disease's effect on the individual's sense of identity and on his or her entire social system.

3. The text points out that in Western societies, health is a value and illness is experienced as a barrier to the achievement of valued goals. One reason why cancer disrupts our perception of health is that
   (A) cancer alone among common diseases carries the threat of recurrence.
   (B) individuals are never certain that they are free of the disease.
   (C) cancer is so frequently diagnosed and so rarely cured.
   (D) self-actualization goals often supersede safety and survival needs.

4. Cancer patients who are **most** likely to exhibit psychosocial distress include all of the following **except**
   (A) those who have been unsuccessful in resolving past stress situations.
   (B) those who are dealing with a number of stressors simultaneously.
   (C) those who perceive minimal social support in the situation.
   (D) those who cope principally through adaptive and defense mechanisms.

5. Which of the following statements about psychosocial aspects of cancer care is true?
   (A) Denial or minimization may be an effective coping strategy, allowing individuals to assimilate the impact of the illness in manageable increments.
   (B) Psychosocial responses to cancer can be clearly identified as either adaptive or maladaptive.
   (C) A perception of uncertainty in a situation results in an appraisal of danger.
   (D) Distancing behaviors of health professionals are helpful in preventing overinvolvement.

ANSWER EXPLANATIONS

1.   **The answer is (C).**   Each individual brings to the cancer experience unique personality traits and a personal socialization pattern different from all others. Understanding the uniqueness of the individual is achieved only through study of the commonalities of the personality and social psychological (psychosocial) aspects of illness. (438)

2.   **The answer is (A).**   Other aspects of cancer's actual or potential threat are that the disease is a chronic illness and that it can result in a changed identity and social stigma. (438)

3.   **The answer is (B).**   According to Smith's study of the impact of cancer on health in general, perceptions of health range from the most prohibitive level of absence of pathology (not being ill), to disruption of role functioning, to ability to adapt, to the highest level, self-actualization. Because of the problems associated with diagnosing cancer and determining its spread and recurrence, the disease is capable of disrupting each of these dimensions of health, beginning with the perception of being free of the disease. With cancer, this can never be certain. (438)

4.   **The answer is (D).**   According to stress theory, individuals come to the cancer experience with a history of stress responses. Those who have been unsuccessful in resolving past stress situations, who are dealing with a number of stressors simultaneously, and who perceive minimal social support in the situation are at higher risk for psychosocial distress. (443)

5.   **The answer is (A).**   Denial or minimization may be an effective coping strategy, particularly in early stages of the disease and at particularly stressful points in the illness trajectory (such as recurrence). Psychosocial responses cannot be clearly identified as either adaptive or maladaptive; this depends largely on the situation and on the adaptive potential of the particular response in that situation. A perception of uncertainty can result in an appraisal of danger or opportunity, depending on the individual's definition of the situation. Distancing behaviors by health professionals enhance patients' sense of loneliness and fear. Overinvolvement with patients can be countered through supportive collegial relationships. (443)

20   Psychosocial Responses:
        The Patient

STUDY OUTLINE

I.   INTRODUCTION

1. Efforts of health care professionals to understand the unique psychosocial responses of persons with cancer have been assisted by several research approaches and methodologies, including
   a. **Clinical case studies** of individuals and groups experiencing cancer.
   b. **Qualitative studies** of the relationship of selected psychosocial variables to
      (1) Physiological factors, such as site of cancer.
      (2) Care settings, including hospitals, outpatient clinics, and the home.
      (3) Temporal elements of the disease trajectory, from screening through long-term survival.
      (4) Developmental stage of the individual, with emphasis on the responses of children and older adults.
   c. **Qualitative research methods.**
   d. **Advanced statistical modeling procedures** to study the interaction of psychosocial responses.

II.   ANXIETY

1. **Anxiety,** along with **depression,** has been described as the most common psychosocial reaction experienced by people with cancer. It is a recurring response that
   a. Is often associated with transitions in the course of the disease.
   b. Varies in level of intensity throughout the cancer experience.

A.   OPERATIONAL DEFINITION

1. An operational definition of anxiety includes the following:
   a. An individual exists with the ability to respond affectively to changes in the environment.
   b. The individual perceives certain beliefs, values, and conditions essential to a secure existence.
   c. The individual experiences a nonspecific internal or external stimulus that is perceived as a threat to the secure existence.
   d. **The individual responds to the perceived threat affectively with an increased level of arousal associated with vague, unpleasant, and uneasy feelings defined as anxiety.**

B.   MEASUREMENT INSTRUMENT: STATE-TRAIT ANXIETY

1. The instrument most commonly used to measure anxiety in cancer patients is the **State-Trait Anxiety Inventory (STAI),** which consists of two scales, the **A-trait** and the **A-state.**
   a. The **A-state** is designed to measure the **level of transitory anxiety** characterized by feelings of apprehension, tension, nervousness, and worry. Responses are summed to measure how the subject feels at a particular moment.
   b. The **A-trait** is designed to measure **general levels of arousal** and to **predict anxiety proneness.** Responses are summed to measure disposition to respond to a stressful situation with varying levels of intensity and the degree to which presenting stimuli are perceived as dangerous or threatening.

C. **PATTERNS OF OCCURRENCE**

    1. Various studies indicate an association between a diagnosis of cancer and increased levels of anxiety.

    2. Patients treated with surgery, radiation therapy, and chemotherapy also report mild or moderate levels of anxiety, which may actually be motivating for the patient.

D. **IMPACT OF ANXIETY ON PATIENT OUTCOMES**

    1. Initial empirical data indicate that **anxiety is associated with selected patient outcomes,** including critical thinking ability and behavior therapy outcomes.

    2. The strength and direction of the relationships between anxiety and selected psychosocial intervening and outcome variables remain to be defined.

E. **ASSESSMENT CRITERIA**

    1. Anxiety has been recognized as an accepted nursing diagnosis category by the North American Nursing Diagnosis Association (NANDA). However, additional clinical research is needed to test the NANDA recommendations for definition and diagnostic criteria of anxiety.

    2. Patient validation of a diagnosis of anxiety is therefore mandatory.

    3. See **Table 20-1, text page 453,** for various nursing diagnoses that address anxiety.

F. **NURSING INTERVENTIONS**

    1. Interventions are based on helping the patient to
        a. **Recognize various manifestations of anxiety.**
        b. **Determine if the patient desires to do anything about the response (exploration and evaluation).**
        c. **Activate coping strategies to control anxiety levels.**

    2. Patients may or may not acknowledge their anxiety, and they may regard the anxiety they acknowledge in either a positive or negative light. If the patient desires to reduce the anxiety, the nurse can help the patient
        a. Identify the threat.
        b. Learn to modify responses to stimuli.
        c. Channel the responses constructively.

    3. Often the intervention of exploration and evaluation will help the patient focus on the threat and appraise the stimuli in a different way, thus reducing anxiety.

    4. Interventions may also focus on treating the symptoms by **activating previously effective coping strategies** or on **teaching new strategies** to control the anxiety.
        a. The nurse has the opportunity to help the patient identify these strategies and to evaluate their effectiveness in reducing anxiety.
        b. The nurse may also help the patient learn new strategies through
            (1) Formal and informal education programs.
            (2) Assistance on problem solving through counseling.
            (3) Role modeling with anxiety-reducing techniques such as relaxation training or music therapy.
            (4) Referral to support groups within the care institution and the community.
        c. These various behavioral interventions have been used successfully to alleviate anxiety associated with cancer diagnosis and treatment. Each represents an independent nursing action to modify the anxiety response.

G. **FUTURE DIRECTIONS FOR NURSING RESEARCH**

    1. Further research using more controlled study designs is needed to evaluate the effectiveness of a variety of independent nursing interventions on the anxiety level of individuals with cancer.

III. **DEPRESSION**

    1. A diagnosis of **depression** in cancer patients is complicated by
        a. The coexistence of signs and symptoms of disease and treatment that are **similar to those of depression.**

    b. Some patients' normal **predisposition toward depression,** which must be differentiated from depression associated with cancer.

2. Studies indicate that depression among cancer patients is probably underdiagnosed and undertreated.

A. OPERATIONAL DEFINITION

1. An operational definition of depression includes the following:
    a. An individual exists with the ability to respond cognitively, behaviorally, and affectively to stimuli in the environment.
    b. The individual perceives certain goals for the future and attributes the possibilities for success to the self.
    c. The attempts of the individual to attain goals are blocked.
    d. The individual attributes the failure to attain goals to personal inadequacies.
    e. **The perceived loss of self-esteem results in a cluster of**
        (1) **affective (worthlessness, hopelessness, guilt, sadness),**
        (2) **behavioral (change in appetite, sleep disturbances, lack of energy, withdrawal, dependency), and**
        (3) **cognitive (decreased ability to concentrate, indecisiveness, or suicidal ideation) responses defined as depression.**

B. MEASUREMENT INSTRUMENTS

1. The majority of instruments used to assess depression were developed to assess depression in psychiatrically ill patients. Limited reliability and validity data with respect to use with cancer patients have been reported.
2. Instruments include the **Hamilton Rating Scale for Depression, Beck Depression Inventory, Minnesota Multiphasic Personality Inventory (MMPI), Psychosocial Adjustment to Illness Scale (PAIS),** and **Profile of Mood States (POMS).**

C. PATTERNS OF OCCURRENCE

1. The focus of research on depression among cancer patients has been largely descriptive rather than involving intervention studies.
2. Research has been limited by the
    a. Lack of assessment of **preexisting depressive symptoms** before the diagnosis of cancer.
    b. Presence of **confounding physical and psychosocial responses** related to the disease and treatment.
    c. **Minimal reliability and validity estimates for instruments** used among cancer populations.
3. Empirical studies that focus on independent nursing interventions to modify depressive symptoms are needed.

D. ASSESSMENT CRITERIA

1. **Reactive (situational) depression** is defined as "an acute decrease in self-esteem or worth related to a threat to self-competency." The characteristics of situational depression are outlined in **Table 20-3, text page 456.**
2. The psychosocial characteristics described for cancer patients may be the result of the disease, its treatment, or its side effects.
3. The primary criteria for assessment of depression include characteristics that
    a. **Are a change from previous functioning.**
    b. **Are persistent.**
    c. **Occur for most of the day.**
    d. **Occur more days than not.**
    e. **Are present for at least 2 weeks.**

E. NURSING INTERVENTIONS

1. The selection of nursing interventions for the treatment of patients with depression is based on
    a. **Identification of stimuli that have resulted in a loss of self-esteem.**
    b. **The defining characteristics present for the particular patient.**

2. Concentration on the psychosocial and behavioral responses associated with depression offers initial cues for selecting nursing interventions.
3. The nurse should then encourage the patient to
   a. **Acknowledge feelings** associated with depression, including hopelessness, despair, anger, and guilt. The nurse can do this by
      (1) Giving permission to the patient to discuss those feelings.
      (2) Demonstrating acceptance of feelings by attentive listening.
      (3) Exploring methods to deal positively with the feelings.
      (4) Consulting with other health care professionals as needed.
   b. **Appraise the situation cognitively** with respect to aspects of the cancer experience and perceptions of self-esteem and self-competency. The nurse can do this by
      (1) Providing accurate information about the plan of care and personal responses to treatment.
      (2) Helping the patient focus on immediate goals of care.
      (3) Focusing on positive abilities of the patient.
      (4) Contracting short-term goals of care that the patient can achieve.
      (5) Reinforcing patient attempts to meet established goals.
      (6) Enhancing self-esteem and self-competency by
         (a) Providing information about and role modeling self-care behaviors.
         (b) Negotiating goals for increasing independence in self-care and decision making.
         (c) Facilitating social interaction with others.
         (d) Encouraging physical mobility.

F. **FUTURE DIRECTIONS FOR NURSING RESEARCH**

1. Research is needed to establish the criteria for diagnosing depression in the psychiatrically ill versus the medically ill patient.

IV. **HOPELESSNESS**

1. **Hopelessness** appears not to pervade the experience of the cancer patient but rather to wax and wane with changes in perceived health, relationships, and spirituality.

A. **OPERATIONAL DEFINITION**

1. Hopelessness is defined as the **interaction of thoughts, feelings, and behaviors resulting from the inability to mobilize internal and external resources sufficient to**
   a. **Achieve a probability of success greater than zero or to**
   b. **Create an understandable, meaningful, or constructive outcome in the future.**
2. See **text page 457,** column 2, for other aspects of this definition.

B. **MEASUREMENT INSTRUMENTS**

1. Instruments used to measure hopelessness in psychiatrically ill patients are also used with cancer patients. These include the **Beck Hopelessness Scale, Nowotny Hope Scale,** and **Herth Hope Scale.**

C. **PATTERNS OF OCCURRENCE**

1. The study of the relationship of hope and hopelessness to the cancer experience consists of numerous anecdotal articles, a few descriptive studies, and a limited number of intervention studies.
2. Hope and hopelessness have been implicated in the development of cancer and in the quantity and quality of life after diagnosis of cancer. However, the empirical studies done to date have yet to produce a consistent conceptualization of their role.

D. **ASSESSMENT CRITERIA**

1. Hopelessness has been characterized by cognitive, affective, and behavioral responses (see **Table 20-5, text page 458**).

2. Assessment is limited, however, by
    a. An absence of studies that establish the reliability and validity of defining characteristics among clinical populations.
    b. The difficulty faced by clinicians in differentiating hopelessness from depression, powerlessness, and other similar concepts using the accepted defining characteristics.

E. NURSING INTERVENTIONS

1. Among the nursing interventions used to decrease hopelessness and foster hope among cancer patients are **enhancing reality surveillance, fostering supportive relationships, enhancing power and abilities, and creating a future perspective.**

F. FUTURE DIRECTIONS FOR NURSING RESEARCH

1. Further nursing research is required to define the characteristics of hope and hopelessness, describe the relationships between hope and hopelessness and other psychosocial variables, and evaluate the effectiveness of nursing interventions designed to foster hope.

V. ALTERED SEXUAL HEALTH

1. **The diagnosis of cancer poses potential threats to sexuality, how one perceives the self, how one perceives how others see the self, and how one behaves as a sexual being.**

A. OPERATIONAL DEFINITION

1. The inability to express one's sexuality consistent with personal needs and preferences is defined as **altered sexual health.** See **text page 461,** column 1, for other aspects of the definition.

B. MEASUREMENT INSTRUMENTS

1. Two commonly used instruments for measuring sexuality are the **Derogatis Sexual Functioning Inventory** and the **Sexual Adjustment Questionnaire.**

C. PATTERNS OF OCCURRENCE

1. The sequelae associated with radical surgery, radiation, chemotherapy, and biotherapy may threaten the sexual health of persons with cancer.
2. Anecdotal reports and descriptive studies have provided the basis for identifying the potential risks to sexual health for site-specific and treatment-specific patient populations. Emphasis has been on the effects of cancer and treatment on the **frequency of sexual behaviors,** particularly intercourse and orgasm.
3. Recent studies have expanded the concept of sexual health to include issues of **self-concept** and **perceptions and behaviors of significant others.**
4. **Sexual behaviors**
    a. With women, data indicate that
       (1) Women with **gynecologic cancer** in general and **those treated with radiation therapy** are at risk for changes in sexual activity.
       (2) The diagnosis of breast cancer and treatment with surgery do **not** appear to place the patient at increased risk for changes in the frequency of sexual intercourse but, rather, for **changes in self-concept.**
    b. With men, researchers have identified the potential assaults to sexual health among males with genitourinary cancers.
5. **Self-concept**
    a. **Self-concept** is defined as the total self-appraisal of appearance, background and origins, abilities, resources, attitudes, and feelings.
    b. The majority of empirical studies dealing with the relationship of cancer to self-concept have focused on women with **gynecologic and breast cancer** or on males with **testicular and prostate cancer.**

    c. Additional empirical data are needed on the issues of
      (1) Perception of significant others' responses to the physical and psychological sequelae of cancer.
      (2) Interaction of other variables, such as age, depression, and activity status, on the physical as well as psychosocial aspects of sexual health.

D. **ASSESSMENT CRITERIA**

    1. Two nursing diagnoses related to sexual health have been approved by NANDA: **sexual dysfunction** and **altered sexual patterns.** Defining characteristics for each diagnosis are presented in **Table 20-7, text page 463.**
      a. These defining characteristics emphasize both subjective and objective criteria for evaluating sexual health.
      b. The subjective responses and perceptions of the individual and significant others must be considered when identifying a problem and planning care.

E. **NURSING INTERVENTIONS**

    1. The **PLISSIT model (Table 20-8, text page 464)** implies that
      a. For many problems, the simple acknowledgment and discussion of the perception of change in sexual health may be sufficient to solve the problem.
      b. For other problems, especially those that existed prior to the diagnosis of cancer, referral to a professional for intensive individual or couple therapy may be indicated.
    2. **Education** and **counseling** are two basic approaches to treatment of changes in sexual health. A few studies have demonstrated their effectiveness, but more need to be done.
    3. Two problems with respect to counseling interventions are that
      a. Effectiveness is often measured in terms of resumption of sexual intercourse rather than the effect of the intervention on self-concept or on relationships with others.
      b. Patients are generally not screened for participation.
        (1) Screening would increase the probability of identifying those patients and partners with preexisting problems that may require more intensive therapy.

F. **FUTURE DIRECTIONS FOR NURSING RESEARCH**

    1. Nursing research is needed to develop **psychometrically robust instruments for the assessment of sexual health** dimensions among people with cancer. **Multimethods of assessing sexual health** not only in the patient, but also from the perspective of significant others, are required if the interrelationships among the complex factors that contribute to sexual health are to be understood.

PRACTICE QUESTIONS

1. Anxiety is defined operationally as an increased level of arousal associated with vague, unpleasant, and uneasy feelings that occurs in response to a perceived threat. What is the source of this perceived threat?
    (A) a nonspecific external stimulus
    (B) a specific external stimulus, often a physical threat
    (C) a nonspecific internal or external stimulus
    (D) a specific internal stimulus, usually pain or inflammation

2. Empirical data suggest that anxiety is associated with selected patient outcomes. In one study, for example, women with high anxiety related to breast biopsy were found to have
    (A) a higher than average mortality rate.
    (B) elevated diastolic blood pressure.
    (C) recurrent nausea.
    (D) positively correlated critical thinking ability.

3. Among the nursing interventions that have been shown to be effective with cancer patients experiencing anxiety are all of the following **except**
    (A) helping the patient learn new coping strategies through anxiety-reducing role playing.
    (B) helping the patient focus on the perceived threat and appraise the stimuli in a different way, thus reducing anxiety.
    (C) helping the patient identify stimuli that have resulted in a loss of self-esteem.
    (D) exploring perceived patient concerns and helping patients evaluate these concerns.

4. One major reason a diagnosis of depression among cancer patients is often complicated is because
    (A) some cancer patients had preexisting depressive symptoms before the diagnosis of cancer.
    (B) instruments have yet to be developed to measure depression among cancer patients.
    (C) symptoms of depression are often identical to symptoms of anxiety.
    (D) the signs and symptoms of cancer are markedly different from those of depression.

5. With depression, responses to a perceived loss of self-esteem may be affective, behavioral, or cognitive. Which of the following is an example of a **behavioral** response associated with depression?
    (A) lack of energy
    (B) guilt
    (C) indecisiveness
    (D) suicidal ideation

6. The primary criteria for assessment of depression include all of the following characteristics **except**
    (A) characteristics that are a change from previous functioning.
    (B) characteristics that are persistent.
    (C) characteristics that were preexistent.
    (D) characteristics that occur more days than not.

7. A nursing intervention for the treatment of patients with depression that deals with the patient's **affective** responses would be
    (A) negotiating goals for increasing independence in self-care and decision making.
    (B) giving permission for expression of feelings.
    (C) contracting short-term goals of care that the patient can achieve.
    (D) encouraging physical mobility.

8. Unlike anxiety and depression, which of the following is true of hopelessness as a response of patients to the cancer experience?
    (A) It involves a combination of affective, behavioral, and cognitive responses.
    (B) It has not been implicated in the development of cancer or in the quantity and quality of life after diagnosis of cancer.
    (C) It can be clearly distinguished from other similar concepts using the accepted defining characteristics.
    (D) It appears to wax and wane with perceived changes in the patient's life.

9. Research on the effects of cancer and cancer treatment on sexual health has tended to focus on
    (A) the perception of significant others' responses to the physical and psychological sequelae of cancer.
    (B) the frequency of sexual behaviors, particularly intercourse and orgasm.
    (C) issues of self-concept.
    (D) the total self-appraisal of appearance, background and origins, abilities, resources, attitudes, and feelings.

10. The majority of empirical studies dealing with the relationship of cancer to self-concept have focused on
    (A) the total self-appraisal of cancer patients, both men and women.
    (B) the effects of various treatments on relationships of cancer patients with significant others.
    (C) women with gynecologic or breast cancer or males with testicular or prostate cancer.
    (D) the interaction of variables such as age, depression, and activity status on the psychosocial aspects of sexual health.

11. Two basic approaches to nursing intervention for alterations in sexual health of cancer patients are
    (A) education and counseling.
    (B) screening and role playing.
    (C) affective therapy and role modeling.
    (D) enhancing reality surveillance and reinforcing personal power.

ANSWER EXPLANATIONS

1. **The answer is (C).** Anxiety is most likely to occur when an individual experiences a nonspecific internal or external stimulus that is perceived as a threat to certain beliefs, values, and conditions essential to a secure existence. (450)

2. **The answer is (D).** In this study by Scott, anxiety levels (STAI scores) among the 85 patients studied were above the norms for acutely ill psychiatric patients. In addition to the above finding, critical thinking was substantially reduced at hospitalization when compared with 6 to 8 weeks after discharge. (452)

3. **The answer is (C).** Loss of self-esteem is more commonly a symptom of depression. In general, nursing interventions that focus on anxiety are based on helping the patient to recognize various manifestations of anxiety, determining if the patient desires to do anything about the response, and activating coping strategies to control anxiety levels. (452)

4. **The answer is (A).** In addition, the coexistence of signs and symptoms of disease and treatment that are similar to those of depression make the diagnosis of depression difficult. (454)

5. **The answer is (A).** Choice (B) is an affective response; other affective responses include worthlessness, hopelessness, and sadness. Choices (C) and (D) are cognitive responses; another cognitive response is a decreased ability to concentrate. Other behavioral responses include change in appetite, sleep disturbances, withdrawal, and dependency. (454)

6. **The answer is (C).** Critical to establishing a diagnosis of reactive (situational) depression in cancer patients is the evaluation of selected defining characteristics commonly attributed to depression among the psychiatrically ill. Some common characteristics of depression, however, may also occur in the cancer patient as a result of the disease, its treatment, or its side effects, or they may have existed in the patient prior to diagnosis. Therefore, the primary criteria for assessment of depression are that the characteristics are a change from previous functioning, are persistent, occur for most of the day and on more days than not, and are present for at least 2 weeks. (456)

7. **The answer is (B).** The other interventions listed are cognitive or behavioral in approach. Before these interventions are attempted, it is important for the nurse to acknowledge the patient's feelings associated with depression, including hopelessness, despair, anger, and guilt. The nurse can do this in many ways, starting with giving permission to the patient to discuss those feelings, then demonstrating acceptance of them by attentive listening and by exploring methods for the patient to deal positively with them. (456–457)

8. **The answer is (D).** Hopelessness appears not to pervade the experience of the cancer patient, unlike anxiety and depression. Rather, it waxes and wanes with changes in perceived health, relationships, and spirituality. (457)

9. **The answer is (B).** Most reports and studies that have been done on altered sexual behavior as a consequence of the cancer experience have dealt with the effects of cancer and treatment on the frequency of sexual behaviors, particularly intercourse and orgasm. Recent studies, however, have expanded the concept of sexual health to include issues of self-concept and perceptions and behaviors of significant others. (461)

10. **The answer is (C).** Self-concept is defined as the total self-appraisal of appearance, background and origins, abilities, resources, attitudes, and feelings. The majority of empirical studies dealing with the relationship of cancer to self-concept have focused on women with gynecologic or breast cancer or on males with testicular or prostate cancer. Additional empirical data are needed on the issues of perception of

significant others' responses to the physical and psychological sequelae of cancer and on the interaction of other variables, such as age, depression, and activity status, on the physical as well as psychosocial aspects of sexual health. (462–463)

11.   **The answer is (A).**   Recent studies have indicated the effectiveness of education and counseling as approaches to treatment of changes in sexual health. One problem with respect to such interventions is that effectiveness is often measured in terms of resumption of sexual intercourse rather than effect of the intervention on self-concept or on relationships with others. Another problem is that patients are generally not screened for participation. Screening would increase the probability of identifying those patients and partners with preexisting problems that may require more intensive therapy. (464)

21 Psychosocial Responses: The Family

STUDY OUTLINE

I. **INTRODUCTION**

   1. The diagnosis of cancer can precipitate significant changes in the lives of the individual, members of the family unit, and the community.
      a. Responses experienced vary among family members depending upon the developmental stages of the family, illness demands, and available economic and psychosocial resources.
      b. Predictability with respect to family routines, relationships, and communication patterns is threatened.
      c. Family members are challenged to learn new roles, self-care skills, and ways of relating to each other and to others outside the family.
      d. Life becomes more complex as demands on the family increase.
   2. Most of the research on the family cancer experience has focused on the responses of individual family members, especially the spouse's experience and the experiences of the young, adolescent, and adult children of women with breast cancer. Research should be done examining the responses, functioning, and development of nontraditional, multigenerational, or culturally diverse family units experiencing cancer.

II. **INSTRUMENTS FOR EVALUATING THE FAMILY**

   1. **Family APGAR**
      a. The **Family APGAR** is a screening questionnaire designed to assess family **A**daptability, **P**artnership, **G**rowth, **A**ffection, and **R**esolve.
      b. It defines the family as a "psychosocial group consisting of the patient and one or more persons, children or adults, in which there is a **commitment for the members to nurture each other.**"
      c. A strength of the Family APGAR is that it does not assume the structural, institutional, or cultural boundaries of the traditional family.
      d. Reliability and validity data are not reported by the author.
   2. **Family Functioning Index**
      a. The **Family Functioning Index (FFI)** is designed to assess the dynamics of family interaction. Questions assess areas of marital satisfaction, frequency of disagreement, communication, problem solving, and feelings of happiness or closeness.
      b. Validity and reliability estimates appear to be high.
   3. **Feetham Family Functioning Survey**
      a. The Feetham Family Functioning Survey is designed to assess the family's ability to function as a unit within the community and within their own internal system. Items assess family interactions with the community, the family relationship to various subsystems, and reciprocal relationships within the family structure.
      b. Validity and reliability estimates appear to be high.
   4. **Family Inventory of Resources for Management**
      a. This instrument is designed to assess the ability of the family to deal with stressors. Factors evaluated include family strengths (esteem, communication, mastery, and health), extended family support, and financial well-being.
      b. Reliability estimates are satisfactory.

5. **Family Adaptability and Cohesion Evaluation Scales**
   a. This instrument is designed to classify families into three general and 16 specific types on adaptability and cohesion dimensions. The instrument can be administered to individuals, couples, or families.
   b. Reliability estimates are modest, but the instrument appears to be sensitive to differences among individual family members.

III. NEEDS OF THE FAMILY

1. Each family member may have **different needs** at different points in time across the cancer trajectory, depending on the **developmental stage** of the individual and the family, **organization** of the family, **roles** within the family, and **patterns of interaction.**

A. INFORMATION

1. Increased use of ambulatory cancer services has resulted in the family assuming a more active role in the care of the person with cancer across the disease trajectory.
2. Despite the fact that obtaining information is one of the primary tasks facing family members of persons with cancer, few studies have identified either the nature of the information needs of families or the strategies used to obtain the needed information.
3. A review of 20 primary studies suggests that family members need information, in understandable language, about the **status of the patient, treatment plans, side effects, prognosis, emotional responses of the patient, caregiving skills, and available support services.**
4. Needs of family members change as the setting for care changes, and across three phases of illness. Review **text pages 470–471** for a description of the kinds of information and support needs experienced by families coping with a cancer diagnosis.
5. Information needs of families facing cancer can be addressed through a variety of strategies, including **individual instruction, audiovisual or written materials, group sessions, and resources to meet daily demands of family life.**

B. COMMUNICATION

1. **Communication patterns** can become strained between the patient and the spouse facing cancer.
   a. Spouses became **more protective of the patient** with respect to discussing distressful information and reported not sharing their feelings with patients.
   b. However, the majority of subjects reported **increased closeness in patient-spouse and parent-child relationships.**
2. The potential impact of communication issues on the care of the patient and the well-being of family members is far-reaching.
3. Communication becomes a primary issue among family members as caregiving demands increase.
   a. Family members express concern over the difficulty in obtaining necessary information.
   b. **Mood disturbances** among family members become more prominent.
   c. Professional care for family members has been limited, and family members are reluctant to communicate their concerns and responses to health care professionals.
4. The nurse can assume an important role in assessing communication styles and can strengthen communication patterns through **one-on-one counseling, group sessions, role modeling, and role playing.**

C. COPING SKILLS

1. Family responses of **anxiety, depression, hopelessness,** and **altered sexual health** in response to a diagnosis of cancer have been shown to be similar to those of the patients themselves.
2. Concerns of spouses of newly diagnosed patients center on managing their feelings and the feelings of others, relationships, and the demands imposed by cancer.
3. Studies have examined the magnitude and pattern of **crisis development** among spouses of cancer patients, the effectiveness of **crisis counseling,** and factors that predict crisis development.

4. The acute hospitalization period precipitates significant psychological responses among spouses of patients with cancer that continue through the postdischarge home care period and even into the terminal phase of illness (Cassileth, Oberst, and James).

5. Depression has been noted as a primary response of family members experiencing cancer. Spouses of patients with lung cancer experienced shock, fear, and depression at diagnosis; they reported more symptoms of stress than did patients; and they reported feelings of aloneness and helplessness in response to the cancer experience.

6. Home care places additional demands on the physical, social, and emotional resources of the family. **Table 21-1, text page 473,** lists the psychosocial problems experienced by family members of the home-bound cancer patient. **Table 21-2, text page 473,** lists the caregiving demands experienced by spouses when the patient has advanced cancer.

7. **Age** has a significant impact on the family cancer experience. Research suggests that
   a. Families of **patients 70 years or older** were more likely to be overwhelmed by home care demands.
   b. Role disturbances were more likely to occur in families of **patients age 50 years or younger.**
   c. Mood disturbances were more likely to occur in families of **patients 50 years or older.**

8. The **specific cancer disease** type can also affect the needs and experiences of families coping with cancer. Research suggests that
   a. Families of **patients with lung cancer** were more likely to exhibit mood disturbances and to be overwhelmed by the demands of home care.
   b. Families of **patients with cervical cancer** were more likely to experience disturbances in family relationships.
   c. Spouses of **patients with lung cancer** had a high incidence of depression.

9. **Gender differences** have also been noted in several studies of caregiver burden.
   a. Families of **male patients** were more likely to feel overwhelmed by the demands of home care and were more likely to experience a severe mood disturbance than were families of female patients.
   b. Female caregivers had more difficulty with observing the **physical deterioration of the spouse** while male caregivers had more difficulty with **home management.**

10. Strategies used by family members coping with the stressors and demands of the cancer experience include seeking support from and talking with family, friends, and coworkers, seeking information, maintaining a positive attitude, worrying, preparing for the worst, prayer and religious faith, distraction, and taking positive action.

11. The nurse has an important role in evaluating the effectiveness of coping skills and behaviors of the family throughout the cancer experience.

12. Group programs on stress reduction techniques, referrals to self-help groups, or individual counseling may be used to address coping needs. For families with preexisting problems, referral to a mental health professional may be warranted.

D. SUPPORT SERVICES

1. Historically, we have focused on support services designed to meet the physical care needs of the patient at home.

2. Family members and caregivers may have needs for a variety of additional services, including home management, financial counseling, anticipatory guidance, transportation, and child care. However, few programs designed to meet these needs have been described in the literature.

3. Families and caregivers may experience a decreasing amount of support as their needs become protracted, and they may feel reluctant to ask for support and assistance from family members, friends, and the community.

4. Important nursing roles include helping family members recognize the importance of giving friends and family an opportunity to help and assisting family members to clearly communicate about and contract for meeting their specific support needs. Role playing the asking for help may help families to reduce the anxiety associated with making the actual request.

IV. EFFECT OF FAMILY AND CAREGIVER RESPONSES ON PATTERNS OF CARE AND ADAPTATION

1. Limited data exist to determine the **impact of family responses** on **patterns of care,** and on individual-member or family-level **adaptation.**

A.   **PATTERNS OF CARE**

   1.   **Treatment choice**
      a.   Little is known of the effect of treatment choices on adjustment in spouses, particularly spouses from various cultures.
   2.   **Use of hospice**
      a.   Research suggests that patients who experience more physical symptoms or whose symptoms were uncontrolled were more likely to use inpatient hospice services.
      b.   Increased demand for hospice service has also been associated with increased anxiety and fatigue of family members.

B.   **INDIVIDUAL OR FAMILY-LEVEL ADAPTATION**

   1.   Longitudinal study of the family adaptation to the cancer experience suggests that poorly functioning family members had a **lower sense of personal control,** perceived **inadequate emotional support,** and were experiencing **greater stress from noncancer-related sources.**
   2.   **Caregiver health**
      a.   Studies have demonstrated that the experience of caring for an individual with cancer can affect family caregivers' health status.
      b.   Lower income, minimal insurance coverage, and limited education negatively affect caregiver health status.
      c.   Nurses have a responsibility to evaluate the effects of the physical and psychosocial caregiving demands on family members and to decrease the negative effects of cancer on the family by facilitating coping, providing information, and ensuring access to resources.
   3.   **Marital relationships**
      a.   Research suggests that the cancer experience can both negatively and positively impact the marital relationship. A study of long-term survivors of testicular cancer indicates that most couples were experiencing increased **sense of cohesion, intimacy, communication, and sensitivity to feelings as outcomes of their cancer experience.**
      b.   On the other hand, in a study of men who reported divorcing after their cancer experience, **nearly 40% indicated that cancer had interfered with their marriage.**
   4.   **Relationships with and adaptation of children**
      a.   Communication patterns also change between parents and children within the family. Approximately **half** of patients reported changes in the relationships with children. The changes were characterized as **improved** (73%) and **permanent** (76%). Deteriorated relationships were correlated with a **poor prognosis for the patient.**
      b.   Patients with poor adjustment scores reported **more changes and negative changes in relationships with children.** The frequency and magnitude of problems with fears related to prognosis, rejection, and refusal to discuss cancer were greatest in **mother-daughter relationships.**
      c.   **Loss of a parent** during adolescence has been documented as a critical event in the life of a child.
      d.   Adolescents described open information sharing among the family during the illness.
      e.   After the death, adolescents assumed the **protector role** in shielding the remaining parent from discussing distressful feelings. These adolescents found the protector role extremely stressful and indicated that they lacked sufficient support during this period.
      f.   Children tend to cope with the experience by focusing on how they can help the ill parent, rather than how the parents and family could help them, and by maintaining a "business as usual" attitude and minimizing the effects of the illness.
      g.   Adult children reported several major issues in dealing with the cancer experience, including involvement in the parent's illness, disruption of current family relationships, unresolved relationship problems, and illness demands.
      h.   The relationship with adult children can become more complex when the **adult child is a health care professional.** Nurse/daughter perceptions of roles changed positively with the diagnosis of cancer.
      i.   Roles expanded from that of information source to decision maker, intermediary, and caregiver. Patient and family members were perceived to be more open, closer, and dependent after the diagnosis of cancer.
      j.   The effects of cancer in the family on the behaviors of adult children with respect to cancer surveillance have also been evaluated. While one study found no differences between

groups on frequency of breast self-examination, findings of poor adherence to recommended breast cancer screening practices have been noted among high-risk relatives of women with a breast cancer diagnosis.

k. The nurse should assess for the presence of children in the family and for the quality of communications and relationship that existed prior to the diagnosis of cancer. For families with relationships that were less than satisfactory prior to the diagnosis, referral for counseling or family therapy may be helpful.

l. Open discussions with children about the illness, treatment, and ongoing plans for childcare should occur. Children should be encouraged to maintain contact with the ill parent, even during lengthy hospitalizations, and should be encouraged to talk about concerns related to changes in family life.

5. **Family-level adaptation**

a. Family-level adaptation to the cancer experience has also been examined. Findings suggest that individuals who report high levels of family cohesion also report more positive adjustment to cancer.

b. Studies also suggest that "well-adjusted families" tended to have higher levels of spousal communication, included older children who could assume some of the role function, used coping behaviors such as family discussion, feedback, and reflecting, had strong well-parent-child relationships, and were able to find some positive meaning in their cancer experience.

V. ASSESSMENT CRITERIA FOR FAMILY PROBLEMS

1. There are four nursing diagnoses identified by the North American Nursing Diagnosis Association (NANDA) that address the family:
   a. **Alteration in family processes**
   b. **Ineffective family coping: compromised**
   c. **Ineffective family coping: disabling**
   d. **Family coping: potential growth**
2. See **Table 21-3, text page 479,** for a comparison of the definitions and characteristics of these nursing diagnoses.

VI. FAMILY-LEVEL NURSING INTERVENTIONS

1. Nursing interventions may be directed toward the individual members or the family unit.
2. Strategies for family care include
   a. Family-level **teaching** with respect to the disease, treatment, rehabilitation, or prognosis.
   b. **Anticipatory guidance** of family members throughout the cancer experience.
   c. Single and multiple family **group counseling.**
   d. Mobilization of **health care or community resources**.
   e. **Referrals** for intensive family therapy.

A. CANCER INFORMATION SERVICE

1. A Cancer Information Service (CIS) can be helpful in meeting the information needs of family members. CIS callers ask most often for information about site-specific cancers, treatment, and referral sources for second opinions.

B. FORMAL INFORMATION SERVICES

1. Research suggests that a formal, deliberative informational intervention including individual formal information, counseling, referral, and cancer-related literature can produce a positive impact on information needs, satisfaction, and coping.

C. SPOUSAL SUPPORT GROUPS

1. One study looked at the responses of **husbands of 24 patients who had undergone a mastectomy.**
   a. The husbands had strong reactions of disbelief, alarm, isolation, and anxiety related to the role of support-giver for the wife.

b. After the wife's surgery, the husbands assumed the role of **protector** to shield the wife from both his and her emotional reactions to the cancer experience, which resulted in **strained communication patterns, distrust,** and **resentment.**

c. The six husbands who elected to attend a support group **communicated significantly more with their wives** about mastectomy issues than did husbands who did not attend the group sessions.

D. **RISK COUNSELING**

1. Kelly has described a program of risk counseling designed specifically for relatives of persons with cancer. Outcome data have not yet been reported.

E. **PSYCHOTHERAPY**

1. While the majority of cancer patients and significant others are well adjusted without the need for psychotherapy, selected patients and families may benefit from psychotherapy designed to encourage **communication, promote the expression of feelings, and maintain the integrity of the patient support system.**

F. **FORMALIZED SUPPORT SERVICES**

1. The effect of formalized cancer care services on home caregiving has not been extensively investigated. However, one study found no specific differences in psychological functioning between users and nonusers of formalized home caregiving services.

G. **SOCIAL SUPPORT**

1. Examination of the effects of social support on grief resolution following death of a family member from cancer suggest that perceived social support decreases from 1 to 6 months after the death, while mood improves. Spouse subjects were found to be significantly more distressed than child subjects throughout the study period.

VII. **FUTURE DIRECTIONS FOR NURSING RESEARCH AND PRACTICE**

1. Several issues relating to family responses to a diagnosis of cancer require further study or development, including
   a. The effects of the interaction of individual responses within the context of the family unit.
   b. The need for reliable and valid screening instruments for use with families facing cancer.
   c. The delineation of critical defining characteristics that predispose the family to dysfunctional responses.
   d. Studies are needed to evaluate the responses to the experience of cancer of nontraditional, multigenerational, and culturally diverse families.
2. In addition, multiple services and programs designed to meet a spectrum of family needs are needed, and the effectiveness of these services and programs must be evaluated.
3. Methodologic issues to be considered include the need to address consistent definition of the family and to optimize sample size. In addition, data should be collected from more than one or two members of the family, and the limitations associated with aggregation of data from multiple family members in evaluating family-unit-level responses must be addressed.

PRACTICE QUESTIONS

1. Which of the following statements most accurately describes the relationship between family responses to a diagnosis of cancer and the responses of patients themselves?
   (A) Family responses are similar to patient responses.
   (B) Responses of anxiety and depression are less common among family members than among patients.
   (C) Responses of hopelessness and altered sexual health are less common among family members than among patients.
   (D) Family responses generally are not similar to patient responses.

2. In a study by Cassileth, psychological responses of cancer patients were compared with those of their next-of-kin. Which of the following was observed?
    (A) Patient and next-of-kin scores showed weak correlation.
    (B) Psychological status was better for patients than for next-of-kin during follow-up care but not during active treatment.
    (C) Psychological status was better for next-of-kin than for patients during follow-up care but not during active treatment.
    (D) Scores for both groups indicated a decrease in psychological status related to the phase of the cancer experience.

3. Which of the following families is **most** likely to feel overwhelmed by the home care demands of cancer patients?
    (A) families of male patients over the age of 70 with lung cancer
    (B) families of male patients under the age of 70 with prostate cancer
    (C) families of female patients over the age of 70 with breast cancer
    (D) families of female patients under the age of 70 with cervical cancer

4. In Cooper's study of psychological responses of spouses of patients with lung cancer, which of the following was observed?
    (A) Most subjects reported decreased closeness in the patient-spouse relationship.
    (B) Spouses reported more symptoms of stress than did patients.
    (C) Spouses had a relatively low incidence of depression.
    (D) Spouses reported a high level of sharing of feelings with patients.

5. A deterioration in the relationship between patient and child is most likely to occur when the
    (A) relationship is father-son rather than mother-daughter.
    (B) patient is well adjusted.
    (C) relationship is father-daughter rather than mother-daughter.
    (D) prognosis for the patient is poor.

6. According to Berman, a typical reaction of an adolescent following the death of a parent is to
    (A) blame the remaining parent and/or other family members for the parent's death.
    (B) shield the remaining parent from discussing distressing feelings.
    (C) withdraw from family relationships during a protracted period of grieving.
    (D) openly share information and feelings with the remaining parent and other family members.

7. Which of the following is one of the key issues for adult children of cancer patients?
    (A) disruption of current family relationships
    (B) behavior problems
    (C) lack of involvement in decision making regarding the parent's illness
    (D) assuming the protector role and shielding parents from discussing feelings

8. According to a study by Hays, which of the following cancer patients is **most** likely to require inpatient hospice services?
    (A) a patient who experiences more physical symptoms but fewer symptoms that are uncontrolled
    (B) a patient who assumes the role of protector in an attempt to shield family members from emotional reaction
    (C) a patient who experiences fewer physical symptoms but more symptoms that are uncontrolled
    (D) a patient whose family experiences increased anxiety and fatigue in response to uncontrolled symptoms

9. According to NANDA'S family-related nursing diagnoses, family coping that is ineffective and compromised involves
    (A) the neglectful care of the patient in regard to basic human needs.
    (B) family members who take on illness signs of the patient.
    (C) a usually supportive primary person providing insufficient comfort to the patient.
    (D) actions by family members that are detrimental to the health of the patient.

10. Which of the following is **not** a strategy for family care?
    (A) family-level teaching with respect to the disease, treatment, rehabilitation, and/or prognosis
    (B) anticipatory guidance
    (C) mobilization of health care and/or community resources
    (D) the provision of intensive family therapy to all families of cancer patients

ANSWER EXPLANATIONS

1. **The answer is (A).** Family responses of anxiety, depression, hopelessness, and altered sexual health in response to a diagnosis of cancer have been shown to be similar to those of the patients themselves, as indicated by studies by Cassileth, Oberst and James, and others. (472)

2. **The answer is (D).** In Cassileth's study, patient and next-of-kin scores on three outcome measures were correlated significantly. Scores for both patients and next-of-kin indicated a decrease in psychological status related to phase of the cancer experience; that is, their status was better during follow-up versus active treatment versus palliative care. (472)

3. **The answer is (A).** Gender, age, and type of cancer all appear to affect family responses to home care demands. According to studies by Wellisch et al. and others, those families or spouses most likely to feel overwhelmed by home care demands are those caring for an elderly male with lung cancer. In contrast, families of patients with cervical cancer and those of patients under the age of 50 were more likely to experience disturbances in family relationships. (473)

4. **The answer is (B).** Spouses of patients with lung cancer experienced shock, fear, and depression. In addition, they reported more symptoms of stress that did patients, and they reported feelings of aloneness and helplessness in response to the cancer experience. (472)

5. **The answer is (D).** In Lichtman's study of communication patterns between breast cancer patients and children within the family, deteriorated relationships were correlated with a poor prognosis for the patient and with poor adjustment scores on the measurement instruments used. The frequency and magnitude of problems with fears related to prognosis, rejection, and refusal to discuss cancer were greatest in mother-daughter relationships. (476)

6. **The answer is (B).** Loss of a parent during adolescence has been documented as a critical event in the life of a child. Berman found that during the illness adolescents described open information sharing among the family. After the death of the parent, however, adolescents assumed the protector role in shielding the remaining parent from discussing distressful feelings. These adolescents frequently found the protector role extremely stressful. (476)

7. **The answer is (A).** Behavior problems may become a key issue in the younger child, and assuming the protector role is a documented response of many adolescents to the death of their parent. Other major issues for adult children include involvement in the parent's illness, unresolved relationship problems, and coping with illness demands. (476–477)

8. **The answer is (D).** In Hays's study of 100 patients during the last 10 days of their lives, patients who experienced more physical symptoms and more symptoms that were uncontrolled were more likely to require inpatient hospice services. In addition, patients whose families experienced increased anxiety and fatigue in response to the patient's uncontrolled symptoms also showed an increased use of inpatient hospice services. (475)

9. **The answer is (C).** All of the other choices indicate a diagnosis of **Ineffective family coping: disabled.** A diagnosis of **Ineffective family coping: compromised** is made when a usually supportive primary caretaker provides insufficient, ineffective, or compromised support, comfort, assistance, or encouragement

that may be needed by the patient to manage or master adaptive tasks related to health challenges. (478 and Table 21-3, 479)

10.   **The answer is (D).**   Intensive family therapy may be helpful in selected situations. However, research indicates that the majority of cancer patients and significant others facing cancer are well adjusted without the need for intensive intervention. (480)

22 Psychosocial Issues of Long-Term Survival from Adult Cancer

STUDY OUTLINE

I. **INTRODUCTION**

1. Early detection and effective multimodal therapies have greatly increased the numbers of cancer survivors to the extent that cancer is now considered a chronic, life-threatening rather than a terminal disease. **Table 22-1, text page 485,** lists the cancers with high 5-year survival rates.
2. The number of cancer survivors has been increasing dramatically.
   a. This burgeoning population of survivors makes evident the need to address issues of **survival** and the **psychosocial consequences of cancer and its therapies.**
   b. Long-term survivors may experience problems ranging from minor short-term difficulties to major psychosocial crises.
   c. Determining which individuals are at greatest risk for psychosocial morbidity is critical for clinicians.

II. **DEFINITIONS OF SURVIVORSHIP**

1. Historically, cancer survivors have been defined as "cured" if there is no evidence of disease with minimal or nonexistent chance for recurrence, with the "cured" state commencing 5 years after diagnosis.
2. Cancer survivorship can be described as the experience of living through or beyond the illness; as such it is a process, not a stage or a component of survival.
3. Survivorship is more accurately based on **control** rather than **cure.** This is because
   a. Cancer consists of many different diseases, each with it own distinct stages and behaviors and treated with a wide range of modalities.
   b. Some cancers are "cured" once the cancer is physically removed, e.g., melanoma or early breast cancer.
   c. Others may be considered cured following several courses of intensive multimodal therapy, e.g., stage I and II Hodgkin's disease, acute lymphocytic leukemias, and osteogenic sarcoma.
      (1) They may be, by definition, "cured" before the fifth year following diagnosis, but they are still not "medically" cured until the 5-year mark.
   d. Still others may not be "curable" but, with continued treatment, can be controlled, enabling patients to live several years, e.g., multiple myeloma or chronic leukemia.
   e. Finally, some cancers are "incurable," with expectations of inevitable death.
4. A **cancer survival paradigm** allows health care providers to rank the importance of the issues a survivor might identify. In descending order of importance, it focuses on
   a. **Basic survival** (food, shelter, medical care).
   b. **Physical self-concept** (attractiveness, fitness, physical function).
   c. **Psychologic self-concept** (self-respect, integrity, autonomy).
   d. **Proximal affiliation** (intimate relationships).
   e. **Distal affiliation** (social relationships).
   f. **Avocation** (recreation, play).

5. The critical elements and cancer-related barriers in this paradigm are summarized in **Table 22-2, text page 486.** Although physical self-concept has a higher importance rating, psychosocial components comprise the bulk of the model.

III. SURVIVORSHIP AS A CONTINUUM

1. Using the control definition enables cancer survivorship to be viewed as a **continual, ongoing process** rather than as an explicit event occurring at a predetermined time period.
2. A continuum of survival stages, or **seasons,** can be used in lieu of the word *cure.*
   a. The **acute survival stage** begins at diagnosis, when patients must deal with immediate effects of therapy in addition to their mortality.
   b. Social support is critical in the acute survival stage.
   c. The **extended survival stage** begins when the disease has gone into remission or the patient has finished the primary treatment course and starts consolidation or adjuvant therapy.
   d. During the extended survival stage, patients begin to deal with issues such as altered body image and vocational changes.
   e. The **permanent survival stage** is most frequently associated with "cure" and evolves from the time when cancer activity or the chance of its return decreases and the disease can be arrested permanently.
   f. During the permanent survival stage, economic problems and concern for long-term and late effects of cancer treatment often surface.
3. Psychosocial issues of long-term survivorship can arise at any stage or phase of the **survival continuum.**
4. Survivorship interventions should therefore begin at diagnosis, rather than when the patient is considered medically "cured."

IV. PSYCHOSOCIAL THEMES

1. Studies confirm a relative lack of psychopathology in long-term survivors of cancer. The major psychosocial themes that can be anticipated in significant cohorts of adults surviving cancer are
   a. **Psychosocial effects of long-term physiologic alterations.**
   b. **Fears of relapse and death.**
   c. **Dependence on health care providers.**
   d. **Survivor guilt.**
   e. **Uncertain sense of longevity.**
   f. **Social adaptation dilemmas.**
   g. **Contagion effect—the family as survivor.**

A. PSYCHOSOCIAL EFFECTS OF LONG-TERM PHYSIOLOGIC ALTERATIONS

1. Physiologic effects, including symptom distress, depression, and altered sexual behavior, can affect a cancer patient's ability to cope within the trajectory of extended or permanent survival.
2. Heightened anxiety may prompt frequent self-monitoring of even vague physical symptoms.
3. Survivors may benefit from information to help manage physical changes and access to health maintenance programs.

B. FEAR OF RELAPSE AND DEATH

1. Not knowing when and if cancer will reappear often negatively affects the survivor's sense of control over his or her life. This is often referred to as the "Damocles syndrome" (after the courtier of ancient Syracuse held to have been seated at a banquet beneath a sword hung by a single hair).
2. Survivors may continue to feel a heightened sense of vulnerability to illness and may benefit from continued support, reassurance, and access to information.

C. DEPENDENCE ON HEALTH CARE PROVIDERS

1. Near the end of treatment, patients are often elated over the prospect of discontinuing therapy yet fearful of distancing themselves from the health care team.
2. Routine checkups and yearly comprehensive examinations can engender pronounced anxiety and may lead to avoidance.

D. **SURVIVOR GUILT**

1. As comparisons are made among patients, some may wonder, "Why am I doing well and others aren't?"

E. **UNCERTAIN FUTURE**

1. Many survivors change their lifestyle as a reaction to the possibility of dying younger than expected. In addition, a significant value reassessment may lead to heightened awareness of things taken for granted and lessened concern for the trivial: "life re-kindled."

F. **SOCIAL ADAPTATION DILEMMAS**

1. Confusing reactions to available social support may deter a patient's social adaptation. The patient does not want to be treated like a patient, yet may react negatively to the withdrawal of the social support that characterized the initial diagnosis phase.
2. The continuing social stigma of cancer remains as a pervasive potential barrier to successful social reorientation after recovery from cancer.
3. With increasing numbers of cancer survivors, we are witnessing the development and expansion of cancer support and of mutual aid networks to provide support and reduce the isolation of individuals who are recovering from cancer.

G. **FAMILY EFFECTS**

1. Even the most supportive family may experience long-term psychologic stress throughout the cancer continuum. "Conversational isolationism," in which families are hesitant to discuss mutual concerns about the recurrence of cancer, may occur.

V. **EMPLOYMENT AND INSURANCE DISCRIMINATION**

1. Many cancer survivors encounter ongoing socioeconomic impediments to full recovery. Concerns include **regaining financial and work-related stability** and **maintaining insurance coverage.**

A. **EMPLOYMENT DISCRIMINATION**

1. Studies indicate that
    a. Up to 80% of cancer patients return to work after being diagnosed.
    b. The work performance of cancer survivors differs little, if any, from others hired at the same age for similar assignments.
2. Yet cancer patients may face various employment-related problems, including
    a. **Dismissal, demotion, and reduction or elimination of work-related benefits.**
    b. Situations arising from **coworkers' attitudes** about cancer.
    c. Problems related to **survivors' attitudes** about how they should be perceived by others in the workplace.
    d. **"Job-lock,"** or fear of leaving an undesirable position because of the potential loss of medical insurance and other benefits.
3. Certain federal and state laws prohibit employment discrimination against qualified people with a history of cancer.
    a. There can be a problem, however, when the legal system attempts to label all cancer survivors as "handicapped or disabled" when there is often no visible evidence of their being either.
    b. More explicit legislation may be needed.

B. **INSURANCE PROBLEMS**

1. Studies suggest that 25%–30% of cancer survivors experience some form of insurance discrimination.
2. Barriers to insurability can be financially and emotionally devastating to cancer survivors.
3. Several local, state, and national resources are available to cancer survivors experiencing employment and insurance problems, including

a. **COBRA,** a federal law passed in 1986, which offers a continuance of group medical coverage to those whose circumstances warrant reducing or changing work hours or leaving the job.
   (1) The employee is eligible for extended coverage up to 18 months, while spouse and dependents receive these benefits for 36 months.
b. **State insurance commissions,** which provide assistance for insurance problems.
c. **"High-risk pools"** offered by many states for those considered medically uninsurable.
d. **Table 22-3, text page 489,** summarizes other resources.

VI.   REHABILITATION PARALLELS

1. Cancer rehabilitation addresses the quality of survival—not how long a person lives, but how well that individual lives within the constraints of the disease.
2. Early efforts to address cancer rehabilitation focused on hospitalized patients with physically disabling impairments such as amputations and colostomies. Less emphasis was given to other areas of human functioning.
3. Many survivors do not return to prior levels of functioning. These survivors must develop strategies to cope with new situations and alterations in health status and functional abilities.
4. The nurse's role in cancer rehabilitation is to **help the patient reduce the extent to which the cancer-related disability becomes a handicap or interferes with the ability to function in everyday life.**
5. **Table 22-4, text page 490,** offers a list of the foci and objectives of a comprehensive and aggressive **assessment and intervention program** for adult long-term cancer survivors.
   a. This program is based on the notion that rehabilitation is a dynamic process that involves **ongoing reassessment** and **redefinition of goals.**
   b. Preventive and restorative goal setting are seen as critical to the enhancement of a long-term survival trajectory characterized by **minimal debilitation** and a **wellness orientation.**
   c. Particular attention must be paid to the financial burden imposed by cancer.
6. Significant policy statements have been made that encourage future investigation into the development of rehabilitation models of cancer care.
   a. See **text page 492** for a list of ONS recommendations and **Figure 22-1, text page 491,** for the American Cancer Society's **Cancer Survivors' Bill of Rights.**

VII.   RESOURCES AND INTERVENTIONS

1. The availability of **education, counseling,** and **supportive services** becomes crucial in caring for those diagnosed with cancer.
2. Areas for consideration in planning interventions for long-term survivors include **undertaking individualized needs assessments, addressing educational needs, engaging in research,** and **developing model programs.**

A.   ASSESSING INDIVIDUAL NEEDS

1. Included are strategies that **help resolve crisis intensity** and **enhance self-care.**
2. Examples of nursing diagnoses related to individual needs assessment include
   a. Ineffective patient or family coping related to ongoing surveillance for long-term effects from disease or treatment.
   b. Grieving related to loss of job after successful treatment for cancer.
   c. Alterations in sexuality related to difficulties in establishing intimate relationships.
   d. Knowledge deficit related to the recognition of cancer recurrence symptomatology.

B.   ADDRESSING EDUCATIONAL NEEDS RELATED TO SURVIVORSHIP

1. Nurses can help reduce the stress associated with the unknown by **anticipating crisis points** and **sharing this information with survivors.**
   a. **Time-related crises** include anniversaries of diagnosis and treatment cessation, yearly examinations, etc.
   b. **Situation-specific crises** include diagnosis disclosure to friends or coworkers, hearing stories about cancer, establishing intimate relationships, etc.

2. If a crisis becomes unmanageable or persistent, **nursing referrals** can be made for appropriate intervention.
3. Survivors and their families may also want to know about **potential secondary benefits** of the cancer experience, e.g., newfound zest for life.

C. **ENGAGING IN RESEARCH**

1. A comprehensive assessment format is currently needed to study the long-term needs of adult survivors. Several areas need further research.

D. **DEVELOPING MODEL PROGRAMS**

1. Once survivor-specific assessments identify areas of individual need, a more general assessment of community resources already available for cancer survivors can be performed.
2. These two steps lead to the development of formal survival programs.
3. The success of any cancer survival program depends on
   a. The commitment of the health care team to provide **ongoing evaluation and planning for change** in the lives of survivors.
   b. The identification of **key individuals to coordinate activities** within and among team members.
   c. The **involvement of the patient and family** in the program from initial diagnosis.
   d. The effectiveness of **communication** among team members.
4. Most programs are non-hospital based and include **national and local cancer hotlines, regional chapters of national organizations,** and **community networks that focus on peer support.**
5. Hospital- or community-based survivor programs can include a variety of components, including **follow-up clinics, survivor reunions,** and programs that provide **information about cancer survival to coworkers and employers.**

PRACTICE QUESTIONS

1. Why is a definition of cancer survivorship more accurately based on the concept of **control** rather than on the concept of **cure**?
   (A) because, according to a medical definition, most types of cancers cannot be cured
   (B) because different cancers have different stages, behaviors, treatments, and definitions of "cure"
   (C) because only cancers that can be physically removed, such as early forms of breast cancer, can be considered technically "cured"
   (D) because a definition of "cure" carries with it a social stigma that may interfere with cancer treatment

2. According to Vought et al.'s survival paradigm, which of the following issues is a cancer survivor likely to regard as **most** important?
   (A) distal affiliation (social relationships)
   (B) physical self-concept (fitness)
   (C) psychological self-concept (autonomy)
   (D) proximal affiliation (intimate relationships)

3. Which of the following statements about cancer survivorship is correct?
   (A) Using the cure definition enables cancer survivorship to be viewed as a continual, ongoing process.
   (B) The permanent survival stage begins when the disease has gone into remission or the patient has finished the primary treatment course.
   (C) Psychosocial issues of long-term survivorship can arise at any stage of the survival continuum.
   (D) The extended survival stage is most frequently associated with "cure" and evolves from the time when cancer activity decreases.

4. Which of the following psychosocial responses is **least** likely to be observed in a cancer survivor?
   (A) a fear of relapse and death
   (B) survivor guilt
   (C) confusing reactions to available social support
   (D) growing dependence on health care providers

5. Which of the following statements about employment problems among cancer survivors is correct?
    (A) Approximately 40% of cancer patients return to work after being diagnosed.
    (B) The work performance of cancer survivors differs little from others hired at the same age for similar assignments.
    (C) "Job-lock" refers to the situation in which cancer survivors are reluctant to accept new jobs that might involve increased responsibilities.
    (D) Most federal and state laws specifically include cancer survivors among the "handicapped or disabled."

6. Which of the following does COBRA, a federal law passed in 1986, do?
    (A) It offers continued medical coverage to those who leave jobs.
    (B) It provides low-cost insurance to cancer survivors and other high-risk individuals.
    (C) It provides free group health insurance to individuals not otherwise covered by medical plans.
    (D) It prohibits employment discrimination against cancer survivors.

7. A program that regards rehabilitation in cancer care as a dynamic rather than a passive process is **most** likely to emphasize both ongoing reassessment and
    (A) customary convalescence.
    (B) a hospital or community base.
    (C) redefinition of goals.
    (D) frequent nursing referrals.

8. An example of a situation-specific crisis that might be experienced by a cancer survivor would be
    (A) an anniversary of diagnosis cessation.
    (B) a yearly examination.
    (C) waiting for the 5-year survival mark.
    (D) waiting for results of a follow-up examination.

9. All of the following are typical components of a hospital- or community-based survivor program **except**
    (A) a follow-up clinic that provides surveillance for physical and psychological long-term effects.
    (B) a program that provides information about cancer survival to coworkers and employers.
    (C) a national or local hotline that offers various information to cancer survivors.
    (D) survivor reunions for those who live with cancer, their family and friends, and their health care providers.

ANSWER EXPLANATIONS

1. **The answer is (B).**   Cancer consists of many different diseases, each with its own distinct stages and behaviors and treated with a wide range of modalities. Some cancers are "cured" once the cancer is physically removed; others may be considered "cured" following several courses of intensive multimodal therapy; still others may not be "curable" but, with continued treatment, can be controlled, enabling patients to live several years; finally, some cancers are "incurable," with expectations of inevitable death. Using the control definition enables cancer survivorship to be viewed as a continual, ongoing process rather than as an explicit event occurring at a predetermined time period. (485)

2. **The answer is (B).**   After basic survival (food, shelter, medical care), cancer survivors are likely to regard physical self-concept, including attractiveness, fitness, and physical function, as most important, followed by psychological self-concept, proximal and distal affiliation, and avocation. (485)

3. **The answer is (C).**   Viewing cancer survivorship as an evolving process allows recognition of the fact that psychosocial issues of long-term survivorship can arise in any stage—acute, extended, or permanent—of the survival continuum. Survivorship interventions should therefore begin at diagnosis, rather than when the patient is considered medically "cured." The definitions in choices (B) and (D) are reversed. (486)

4. **The answer is (D).**   Near the end of treatment many patients experience significant ambivalence toward the health care team: they are often elated over the prospect of discontinuing therapy yet fearful of distancing themselves from the individuals who have helped them get to this extended survival stage. Also, the fear of recurrence along with the fear of the physician's finding disease can lead to such behaviors as hypochondriasis or avoidance of physicians. (487)

5. **The answer is (B).**   Up to 80% of cancer patients return to work after being diagnosed, and their performance differs little, if any, from others hired for similar assignments. "Job-lock" refers to survivors' fear of losing medical coverage were they to change jobs. Only a few states explicitly protect those with a history of cancer. (488)

6. **The answer is (A).**   Under COBRA, group medical coverage is assured to those whose circumstances warrant reducing or changing work hours or leaving the job. The employee is eligible for extended benefits up to 18 months, while spouse and dependents receive these benefits for 36 months. (489)

7. **The answer is (C).**   The success of any cancer survival program depends on the commitment of the health care team to provide **ongoing evaluation** and **planning for change** in the lives of survivors. Under such a dynamic program, preventive and restorative goal setting become critical to a long-term survivorship trajectory that is characterized by minimal debilitation and a wellness orientation. Particular attention is also paid to the ongoing and long-range implications of financial burden imposed by cancer. (490)

8. **The answer is (D).**   All of the other examples are time-specific crises that may be experienced by survivors. Other situation-specific crises include diagnosis disclosure to friends, hearing stories about cancer, revealing past medical history, and establishing intimate relationships. Since fear of recurrence and worries about health are common among survivors, nurses can help reduce the stress associated with the unknown by anticipating these crisis points—both time- and situation-specific—and sharing information with survivors about cancer recurrence or anticipated problems relative to their diagnosis. (492)

9. **The answer is (C).**   Choice (C) is an example of a non-hospital-based program. (493)

23 Pain

STUDY OUTLINE

I. **INTRODUCTION AND BACKGROUND**

   A. **DEFINITION OF PAIN**

      1. In 1979, the International Association for the Study of Pain (IASP) developed the following definition of pain, which has become commonly accepted and used by most pain specialists: **Pain is an unpleasant sensory and emotional experience associated with actual or potential tissue damage, or described in terms of such damage.**

   B. **THEORIES AND MECHANISMS OF PAIN**

      1. Prior to the mid-twentieth century, there were several traditional or "classical" pain theories, including the **specificity theory, pattern theory, summation theory,** and **sensory interaction theory.**

      2. Most notable of the current theories of pain is the **gate control theory** proposed by Melzack and Wall in 1965. **Table 23-1, text page 501,** provides an overview of the major tenets of both classical and current theories of pain.

      3. The perception and response to pain are due to four distinct processes that operate simultaneously and are all required for pain to occur: **transduction, transmission, modulation,** and **perception.** See **Table 23-2, text page 502,** for a description of these four processes.

      4. See **Figure 23-1, text page 503,** for a diagram of the pain transmission and modulation pathways.

   C. **CANCER PAIN AS A MULTIDIMENSIONAL PHENOMENON**

      1. A multidimensional model of cancer-related pain has been hypothesized that suggests that at least six complex and interrelated dimensions contribute to an individual's perception of, and response to, pain.

      2. The **physiologic dimension** of cancer pain refers to the organic origin or etiology of pain.

         a. Foley described three different types of pain in the person with cancer, each with a different cause. These three types of pain are pain associated with direct tumor involvement, pain associated with cancer treatment, and pain unrelated to either the tumor or its treatment (for example, osteoarthritis).

         b. **Table 23-3, text page 503,** lists examples of tumor-related and treatment-related pain.

         c. Three specific **pain syndromes** that occur in cancer patients have been identified: somatic, visceral, and neuropathic pain. Each of these syndromes is characterized by pain of different qualities, located in different anatomic locations, and caused by different mechanisms. See **Figure 23-2, text page 504,** for elaboration.

         d. The physiologic dimension includes two other characteristics: duration and pattern. **Duration** refers to whether pain is acute or chronic. The **pattern** the pain displays can be transient, rhythmic/intermittent, or continuous.

      3. The **sensory dimension** of cancer pain is related to where the pain is located and to what it feels like. There are three specific components to the sensory dimension:

         a. The **location** of pain is a critical component.

   b. **Intensity** of pain, or how strong it feels, is a perceived and therefore subjective phenomenon, subject to the individual pain threshold and affected by factors like mood and environment.
   c. **Quality** of pain refers to how it actually feels.
4. The **affective dimension** of cancer pain consists of psychological or personality factors associated with pain.
   a. Psychological variables important to a particular patient's pain experience must be identified and dealt with if pain is to be effectively managed.
5. The **cognitive dimension** of cancer pain encompasses the manner in which the pain influences a person's thought processes **or the manner in which he or she views himself or herself.** It may also include the meaning that the pain has for the person.
   a. Studies have examined the effects of opioid analgesics on the cognitive function of patients with pain. Results indicated that cognitive deficits occurred as opioids were first prescribed and with upward dose adjustments. However the deficits were transient, and functioning returned to baseline when drug doses were stabilized for approximately 2 weeks.
   b. Cognitive changes may influence the ability of the individual to report pain.
   c. Knowledge about pain and its management is another aspect of the cognitive dimension of pain. Such knowledge can affect responses both to pain and to interventions.
   d. Cognitive strategies used to cope with pain include various forms of distraction, use of coping self-statements, reinterpretation of painful sensations, selective inattention, withdrawal, and acceptance of the pain.
6. The **behavioral dimension** of pain includes a variety of observable behaviors related to pain, such as verbal and nonverbal communication of pain and strategies or activities engaged in to control pain.
7. The **sociocultural dimension** consists of a variety of demographic (e.g., age, sex, race), ethnic, cultural, spiritual, and related factors that influence a person's perception of and response to pain.
8. Each of the dimensions of the model outlined above (physiological, sensory, affective, cognitive, behavioral, and sociocultural) contributes to nursing assessment and management of pain and facilitates an understanding of cancer pain that is complete, interrelated, interactive, and dynamic.

II. SCOPE OF THE CANCER PAIN PROBLEM

A. PREVALENCE

1. Patients in hospice and specialty units report a higher prevalence of pain than patients in other settings.
2. Pain is more prevalent with certain malignancies and in those patients with advanced stages of disease.
3. Review **text page 508** for additional information regarding the **prevalence of pain** for different types of cancers, levels of disease progression, and in pediatric cancer care.

B. SIGNIFICANCE

1. While health professionals in general are hampered by a lack of research-based knowledge about the prevalence of cancer pain and its impact on patients and others, there is a great deal of evidence to suggest that cancer pain is poorly managed worldwide.
2. Activities in the areas of clinical research, health policy, and sociocultural, political, and professional arenas have increased knowledge about pain and have influenced in both positive and negative ways how it is managed.
3. Current issues in the area of cancer pain include quality of life, family and home care issues, suicide risk, ethical concerns related to use of advanced technologies, financial costs associated with cancer pain, regulatory influences on the use of controlled substances, legal impediments to adequate management of pain, health policy initiatives in pain, increased federal and private research funding opportunities, and increased emphasis on cancer pain by national and international agencies.
4. Review **text pages 508–510** for a discussion of these issues.

C. **PROFESSIONAL ISSUES**

1. Organizational efforts
   a. Organizations and agencies involved with cancer treatment and pain management are directing their efforts toward improving pain management. **Table 23-4, text page 511,** lists the major agencies and organizations involved with cancer pain initiatives.
   b. A variety of **position papers, guidelines, and recommendations** have developed, in part, because of the compelling evidence that unrelieved cancer pain continues to be a significant clinical problem.
   c. Key organizational initiatives include the **Oncology Nursing Society** *Position Paper on Pain,* **the National Institutes of Health consensus statement, the American Pain Society (APS) quality assurance standards on pain management, the American Society of Clinical Oncology (ASCO) formal statement on the rights of patients to receive adequate pain management, an ASCO educational curriculum for oncologists and oncologists-in-training, and the Agency for Health Care Policy and Research (AHCPR) clinical guidelines for management of cancer-related pain.**

2. **Obstacles to successful management**
   a. **Table 23-5, text page 511,** identifies several of the major obstacles to successful pain management.
   b. Review **text pages 511–512** for a discussion of these obstacles.

3. **Improvements in management**
   a. There are several approaches that may be helpful in bringing about a change in practice related to pain management.
   b. Structured and systematic educational content in formal education programs (basic, graduate, and continuing education programs). Research suggests that change in knowledge and attitudes with regard to pain management can occur following even brief educational programs.
   c. Additional **approaches to improving analgesia for patients in pain** include making pain visible, providing practitioners with useful tools, communicating effectively with patients, increasing clinicians' accountability for pain management, facilitating innovation and idea exchange, and increasing the availability of opioids.
   d. Implementation of a **quality assurance program** for the relief of cancer pain sends a clear message regarding the value of pain management in a clinical setting.
   e. **Through their budgetary control, nursing and other administrators are in a position to make the assessment and management of cancer pain an important clinical and organizational priority.**
   f. Major **multidisciplinary program initiatives** such as the World Health Organization Cancer Control Program are helpful in overcoming sociopolitical obstacles to pain management.

4. **Delivery of pain management services**
   a. Practitioners who take care of oncology patients should **possess basic skills in assessment and management of pain.**
   b. Referral to a **pain specialist** or to a **multidisciplinary pain team** for pain management may be helpful in augmenting the services of the primary care team.
   c. Keys issues to be resolved when **referring to a specialist or pain team** include the roles and responsibilities of primary providers and specialists, costs, and clinical decision making among the options suggested during the consultation.

III. **PRINCIPLES OF ASSESSMENT AND MANAGEMENT**

1. **Nursing and medicine have different yet complementary** responsibilities in the assessment and management of cancer pain.
2. According to the **ONS position paper on pain,** the nursing role in pain assessment and management includes describing pain, identifying aggravating and relieving factors, determining the meaning of pain, determining its cause, determining individuals' definitions of optimal pain relief, deriving nursing diagnoses, assisting in the selection of interventions, and evaluating the efficacy of interventions.
3. Other principles of assessment and management that are implicit in the successful nursing management of cancer pain are explored in the following sections.

A. **MULTIDISCIPLINARY APPROACH**

    1.   There is no one best way to treat cancer pain, and no one best person to do it; a multidimensional conceptualization of cancer pain involves multiple health care disciplines.

    2.   Each of the dimensions of cancer pain requires different approaches, different actions, and the input from various health care providers.

B. **NURSING'S SCOPE OF PRACTICE AND RESPONSIBILITIES**

    1.   Oncology nurses, by virtue of their prolonged contact with cancer patients in a variety of settings and their relationships with these persons and their families, are best prepared to assume a leadership role in the assessment and management of cancer pain.

    2.   Scopes of practice have been delineated for nurses with different levels of expertise, including **nurse generalists** and **oncology clinical nurse specialists.**

    3.   **Nurses are responsible for identifying pain as a problem, assessing it, developing a plan of care, implementing this plan, and evaluating and revising the plan as needed.**

    4.   Pain relief is one of several **moral and ethical professional responsibilities with regard to cancer pain** management contained within the Oncology Nursing Society (ONS) position paper on pain. Review the ONS position paper on pain contained in **Table 23-6, text page 515.**

C. **ASSESSMENT AND DIAGNOSIS**

    1.   **Rationale and basic principles**
       a.   The focus of nursing assessment is on the individual as a whole person and on the person's response to pain.
       b.   Collection of pain assessment data should be **systematic, organized,** and **ongoing.**
       c.   Nurses must be aware of and avoid the following **"pitfalls"** in the assessment of pain:
          (1)   The belief that patients with pain display overt behavioral manifestations of pain.
          (2)   The belief that all pain should have a documented organic cause.
          (3)   The belief that pain in cancer patients may be of psychogenic origin.
          (4)   Ascribing all pain in cancer patients to the tumor.
          (5)   Becoming insensitive to patients' pain.

    2.   **Assessment parameters**
       a.   Key assessment parameters using the multidimensional conceptualization of cancer pain are listed and described in **Table 23-7, text page 516.**

    3.   **Assessment tools**
       a.   **Table 23-8, text page 516–517,** presents clinical, psychometric, and practical information about useful tools for assessing cancer pain in adult populations.
       b.   **Unidimensional tools** for pain assessment focus on one dimension of the pain experience, such as sensory, and within that dimension focus on a specific parameter, such as pain intensity (e.g., visual analog scales).
       c.   **Multidimensional tools** for pain assessment, the best known example of which is the McGill Pain Questionnaire, focus on two or more dimensions of the pain experience.
       d.   The choice of which tool or tools to use for assessment of pain in both adults and children depends on several factors, including the **purpose** of the assessment, **the information required,** the **patient characteristics** (such as age, cognitive abilities, and type of pain), **environmental variables,** and the **available time and skills** of the nursing staff.
       e.   Less important than the actual tool used for assessment is the performance of a thorough baseline assessment followed by regular, systematic ongoing assessments.

    4.   **Nursing diagnoses and documentation**
       a.   The outcome of a thorough baseline assessment of the cancer patient with pain should include a number of nursing diagnoses (e.g., anxiety, constipation, ineffective individual coping) that serve to structure the design and implementation of the management plan.
       b.   Assessments and nursing diagnoses related to the problem of pain should be documented in a manner appropriate to the clinical setting. It is suggested that pain assessment (particularly pain intensity and pain relief) be incorporated into routine institutional records such as patient flow sheets.
       c.   The use of **standardized pain assessment and documentation** appears to have a positive impact on pain intensity and to facilitate management of pain.

D. **INCORPORATION INTO PRACTICE**

1. Successful management of cancer pain will ultimately depend on the extent to which systematic processes, tools, documentation procedures, and lines of formal accountability and responsibility for pain management are incorporated into institutional settings.
2. According to the ONS position paper on pain, responsibility for coordination of pain management **lies with the oncology nurse.** The challenge is **how** to meet this responsibility.
3. Application of the APS **quality assurance standards** and the AHCPR guidelines for the management of acute pain and the management of cancer pain may be helpful in developing, implementing, and evaluating better ways of managing cancer pain in any clinical setting.

E. **SPECIAL POPULATIONS**

1. **Children**
    a. Assessment and management of pain in children with cancer have received little attention in the research arena.
    b. The **developmental level** of children is directly related to how they perceive, interpret, and respond to pain, regardless of etiology.
    c. Important facts related to children's pain:
        (1) Neonates, including premature neonates, do feel pain.
        (2) Children who are verbally fluent may deny they have pain when in fact they have pain. This may occur when they have certain fears about pain or when they have adapted to it and do not realize it is worsening.
        (3) Children's lack of willingness or ability to express pain or request treatment for it does not mean they do not have pain.
        (4) The child who sleeps, plays, or is otherwise distracted may still have a good deal of pain.
        (5) Children **do not** tolerate pain better than do adults.
        (6) **Opioids may be used safely in children of all age groups, provided there is an understanding of the pharmacokinetics and the children are properly observed.**
        (7) **Pain is not a harmless entity** in children. Stress reactions to prolonged pain may include prolonged crying leading to hypoxemia and increased heart rate and blood pressure. There is also the possibility of long-term psychological consequences from repeated episodes of acute pain or prolonged periods of unrelieved pain.
    d. **There is evidence that undertreatment of pain is a problem in the care of pediatric patients.** Research suggests that one explanation for this undertreatment is that professionals have **concerns about the risks of addiction** when using opioids with children.
    e. The report of the **consensus conference on the management of pain in childhood cancer** in 1990 provides information regarding assessment and methodologic issues in managing pain, disease-related pain, management of pain associated with procedures, and research priorities.
    f. Interventions for pain in children with cancer should be tailored to the type of pain they are experiencing. Use of an **algorithm** in managing pediatric cancer pain is **recommended.**
        (1) Acute, postoperative pain may be treated in the same manner as adult postoperative pain. The AHCPR guidelines for acute pain management explicitly address the management of pain in children.
        (2) Acute, procedure-related pain (e.g., bone marrow aspiration) is usually accompanied by anxiety and fear. A number of authors recommend the **combined use of premedications and cognitive/behavioral techniques** for procedures such as bone marrow aspiration.
    g. The management of pain due to terminal disease is a challenge. Oral analgesics administered around the clock are often very helpful. **Since children metabolize opioids more quickly than adults,** drugs with a longer duration of action (such as methadone) are advisable, and have been shown to provide adequate pain relief.
2. **The elderly**
    a. A misconception that lay persons have about pain and the elderly is that pain is a normal sequela of aging.

b. Chronic problems, such as arthritis or degenerative disk disease, may confuse the pain problem for individuals who also have cancer-related pain.

c. The elderly may experience significant **sensory and cognitive impairments** requiring the health care professional to be especially astute in obtaining a careful, detailed pain history.

d. **A very important piece of assessment data is any change from baseline behaviors, usual routines, and social interactions that may result from pain.**

e. Another major problem is the sensitivity of elderly patients both to the perception of pain and to pharmacologic interventions.

f. **The risk of toxic effects of narcotics may be higher in the elderly due to decreased drug clearance and to the interactions of multiple drug therapies.**

g. **Text page 523** lists twelve guidelines for the management of medications in the elderly.

3. **Substance abuse history**

a. There are unique and different management challenges for health care professionals when pain and substance abuse coexist. Three patient groups in this special population are
   (1) Patients currently in a methadone maintenance program.
   (2) Patients actively using illicit drugs.
   (3) Patients who previously used illicit drugs.

b. With all patients who have any previous or current substance abuse history, it is important that an adversarial relationship not begin or escalate between patient and staff.

c. Communication among all members of the health team, including the patient, about how pain will be managed should be instituted early in the course of the working relationship with the patient.

d. Individuals with a substance abuse history may require much higher doses of opioids for pain because of **tolerance.**

e. The **assistance of professionals experienced in substance abuse,** analgesic management, and cognitive-behavioral approaches to pain may be helpful in developing an effective plan of care.

4. **Critical care**

a. Management of pain in oncology patients who require **intensive critical care monitoring** (for problems such as sepsis, acute respiratory distress, cerebral edema, and severe graft-versus-host disease) is a challenge. Many of these individuals are unable to speak because of endotracheal intubation or CNS dysfunction and therefore must **rely on other means of communicating about their pain experience.**

5. **Culturally diverse populations**

a. It is important to realize that different **ethnic groups express pain and suffering differently.** The nurse should have knowledge of how the patient's culture views responses to pain.

b. In **providing care to people who are culturally diverse,** it is important to
   (1) Learn as much as possible about the individual's ethnocultural background and its influences on health and illness beliefs and behaviors.
   (2) Identify and achieve mutual goals.
   (3) Compromise and integrate different health care practices into the health care plan.
   (4) Use negotiation to achieve feasible treatment plans and to enlist the patient's and family's participation in reaching goals.
   (5) Identify teaching materials oriented to the needs of particular cultural groups.
   (6) Seek additional information and assistance from cultural organizations as needed.

6. **Palliative and terminal care**

a. **The focus of terminal care is on relief of pain and other symptoms, as well as psychological support of both the patient and the family.**

b. Interventions may include **narcotic analgesics, palliative treatments such as radiotherapy, the use of adjuvant drugs,** and **nonpharmacologic, noninvasive interventions.**

7. **Summary**

a. A multidisciplinary approach is the key to **providing care to special populations with cancer pain.**

b. The approach should also be based on a thorough understanding of the scope of nursing practice, accurate assessment and diagnosis, appropriate attention to developmental, clinical, and ethnocultural issues, and knowledge about palliative care.

IV.   **INTERVENTIONS**

1. Methods for managing cancer pain can be categorized into three main approaches:
    a. Treat the underlying pathology.
    b. Change the patient's perception or sensation of pain.
    c. Diminish the emotional or reactive component of the patient's pain.
2. See also **Figure 23-3, text page 528.**

A.   **TREATMENT OF UNDERLYING PATHOLOGY**

1. **Chemotherapy and hormonal therapy**
    a. **Chemotherapeutic agents** may provide some relief of pain in some types of tumors. For gastrointestinal tumors, lung cancer, esophageal and prostate tumors, where chemotherapy is unlikely to significantly increase survival time, it might palliate symptoms.
    b. **Hormonal therapy** provides significant pain relief with few side effects for prolonged periods of time in such tumors as breast and prostate cancers.
2. **Radiotherapy**
    a. **Radiation therapy** may be helpful in relieving pain due to bone metastases, epidural cord or nerve root compression, and hepatic metastases.
    b. There appears to be little correlation between dose of radiation and extent of relief; relief of pain can begin to occur within 24 to 48 hours after initiation of treatment.
3. **Surgery**
    a. Surgery as a modality for treating cancer pain can take many forms, but the primary goal is palliative.
    b. **Table 23-9, text page 528,** lists clinical conditions and tumors that may benefit from various types of palliative surgeries.

B.   **CHANGE IN THE PERCEPTION/SENSATION OF PAIN**

1. **Pharmacologic therapy**
    a. The pharmacologic management of cancer pain accounts for the major source of pain treatment.
    b. Familiarity with the terminology used to describe analgesics and their effects is important to understanding the actions of opioid drugs (see **Table 23-10, text page 529).**
    c. **Nonopioids** may be used as the first step of pain management or in combination with narcotics.
    d. **Table 23-11, text page 530,** provides a comprehensive list of nonopioids used in cancer pain.
    e. The indication for using nonopioid drugs in patients with cancer is pain that is mild to moderate in intensity.
    f. **Nonsteroidal anti-inflammatory drugs (NSAIDs)** are useful for
        (1) Metastatic bone pain.
        (2) Pain from mechanical compression of tendons, muscles, pleura, and peritoneum.
        (3) Nonobstructive visceral pain.
    g. The combination of nonopioids and opioids administered simultaneously is designed to enhance analgesia and decrease toxicity.
    h. **Table 23-12, text page 530,** outlines several clinical considerations in the use of nonopioid analgesics.
    i. **Opioid analgesics,** which interfere with the perception of pain in the central nervous system, are classified into three groups:
        (1) **Morphine-like opioid agonists** bind with mu and kappa receptors.
        (2) **Opioid antagonists** have no agonist receptor activity.
        (3) **Opioid agonists-antagonists and partial agonists** have very limited usefulness in the management of cancer pain due to the propensity of these drugs to induce narcotic withdrawal.
    j. **Table 23-13, text page 531,** contains information about the relative potencies of analgesics commonly used for mild to moderate pain and for severe pain.
    k. All opioid analgesics share common side effects as a result of their action.
        (1) **Table 23-14, text page 532,** lists central nervous system, respiratory, cardiovascular, gastrointestinal, genitourinary, and dermatologic effects.

      (2)   If **respiratory depression** occurs, it can be easily treated with **naloxone,** which should be titrated to changes in respiratory rate.

      (3)   **Nausea and vomiting** can be controlled through the administration of any of a number of antiemetic agents.

      (4)   Patients should be placed on a bowel regimen to avoid **constipation,** which can become a significant problem if preventive measures are not taken. **Table 23-15, text page 533,** lists several laxatives suitable for the management of opiate-induced constipation.

      (5)   Three concepts of importance are defined on **text page 532: tolerance, physical dependence,** and **addiction.**

l.   Analgesic research and initiatives to create a systematic approach to pain management can be used in **specific analgesic drug selection.** The analgesic ladder developed by the World Health Organization is one such example.

m.   **Morphine** is probably the most frequently used opioid analgesic for moderate to severe pain.

      (1)   The availability of **long-acting morphine** has contributed to improvements in patients' quality of life.

      (2)   The oral absorption rate of morphine is variable; one study has shown oral bioavailability ranging from 15% to 64%.

n.   Both **methadone** and **levorphanol** have prolonged plasma half-lives, which do not correspond to the average duration of action. Patients on these medications are at risk for the development of significant sedation and respiratory depression as their plasma level rises.

o.   **Adjuvant analgesics** are defined as those medications that enhance the action of pain-modulating systems.

      (1)   **Antidepressants** have been used in cancer pain for the treatment of neuropathic pain, which is often due to tumor infiltration of nerves. **Table 23-16, text page 534,** lists antidepressants used for cancer-related pain with the usual starting doses and daily doses.

      (2)   **Anticonvulsants** may be beneficial for patients who have neurogenic or neuropathic pain that is described as lancinating or stabbing. **Table 23-14, text page 535,** lists common doses and toxicities of four anticonvulsants.

      (3)   **Psychostimulants** such as amphetamines are useful in countering the sedation that accompanies narcotic analgesics if pain occurs when the narcotic dose is lowered.

      (4)   While **phenothiazines/antihistamines** have long been thought to potentiate the effects of analgesics, most of the drugs in this class have not been found to potentiate analgesia. Rather, they may serve to intensify the sedative effects of narcotics. Methotrimeprazine is the only phenothiazine with demonstrated analgesic properties.

      (5)   **Steroids** are essential for managing the pain caused by epidural cord compressions but the use of these agents as adjuvant analgesics early in the course of a patient's pain problem is not recommended.

      (6)   **Diphosphonates** are power inhibitors of bone resorption and are often used in the treatment of Paget's disease and hypercalcemia of malignancy. Preliminary evidence suggests that these drugs may also be useful for treating bone pain from metastatic disease.

p.   **Routes of opioid administration**

      (1)   There are several available **routes for opioid administration,** thus allowing the clinician to individualize a patient's analgesic regimen based on changing needs.

      (2)   The **oral route** is an effective, comparatively inexpensive, and safe way for patients to receive opioids.

          (a)   Changing a patient to another route should be considered if high doses of oral opioids are ineffective or if toxicities occur that cannot be successfully treated.

          (b)   The scheduling of oral medications should be on a fixed-interval basis.

      (3)   Patients with acute pain often receive **intermittent intramuscular or subcutaneous injections.**

      (4)   **Continuous intravenous narcotic infusions** provide the patient with steady blood levels of the opioid and can avoid the potential side effects and the return of pain associated with intermittent dosing. Guidelines for initiating and managing continuous intravenous infusions are provided in **Table 23-18, text page 537.**

(5) With the availability of new infusion devices, **continuous subcutaneous infusions** have become a common means of analgesic delivery especially for patients in whom there is no venous access.

(6) One of the newest opioid delivery systems is **transdermal** administration. It has been used in postoperative and cancer patients, and while well-controlled clinical trials are lacking, open-label studies suggest that this delivery system provides effective pain relief.

    (a) Review **text page 537** for discussion of some of the unique features of this delivery system that have important clinical implications.

    (b) **Table 23-19, text page 538,** compares the advantages and disadvantages of transdermal fentanyl.

(7) With the advent of transdermal medications and ambulatory infusion pump technology, the use of the rectal route may not be as common an alternative to orally administered analgesics. **Rectal opioid** administration has several advantages and disadvantages, which are reviewed in **Table 23-20, text page 538.**

(8) The identification of opiate receptors in the brain and spinal cord provided the basis for the use of **intraspinal opioid administration. Text pages 538–539** contain a summary of considerations in the initiation and management of intraspinal opioids, including criteria for determining the appropriateness of this approach to analgesia for a particular patient.

(9) **Patient-controlled analgesia (PCA)** is designed to allow the patient to self-administer analgesics within preset guidelines from special infusion pumps, thereby avoiding the peaks and troughs of conventional prn parenteral administration.

2. **Anesthetic and neurosurgical modalities**

  a. Anesthetic and nerve-block procedures help modulate a patient's neural responses to noxious stimuli.

  b. **Nondestructive nerve blocks** serve two functions.

    (1) They are used for intractable pain such as neuropathic pain caused by invasion of intraspinal nerve roots.

    (2) They are used for prognostic/diagnostic purposes in which they help differentiate between visceral and somatic pain and help predict the efficacy of more permanent neuroablative procedures.

  c. **Neurolytic (destructive) nerve blocks** can lead to more prolonged pain relief.

    (1) Destructive neurosurgical procedures are most often used when standard pharmacologic and nonpharmacologic strategies are no longer effective.

    (2) Patients are carefully selected for these procedures because of the potential for motor and sensory losses associated with them.

  d. **Text page 541** describes the neurosurgical procedures most often used when standard pharmacologic and nonpharmacologic strategies are no longer effective.

C. DIMINISHING THE EMOTIONAL AND REACTIVE COMPONENTS OF PAIN

1. Interventions in this category include strategies that help patients cope with their pain in a positive and proactive way and may be considered as an adjuvant to pharmacologic therapy.

2. These methods are aimed at treating the affective, cognitive, behavioral, and sociocultural effects of pain by

  a. **Increasing the sense of personal control.**

  b. **Reducing feelings of helplessness.**

  c. **Allowing active involvement in care.**

  d. **Reducing stress and anxiety.**

  e. **Elevating mood.**

  f. **Raising the pain threshold.**

3. Most of these interventions are simple and can be initiated when ongoing assessment of pain suggests a need for them.

4. **Counterirritant cutaneous stimulation** is thought to relieve pain by somehow physiologically altering the transmission of painful stimuli. Examples are **massage, application of heat/cold,** and the use of **transcutaneous electrical nerve stimulation (TENS).**

5. **Complete or partial immobilization of parts of the body, positioning,** and in other circumstances **mild exercise or stretching** may be helpful.

6. **Distraction** is directing one's attention away from the sensations and emotional reactions

produced by pain. Examples include conversation, reading, watching television, breathing exercises, visualization, and imagery.

7. **Relaxation training** helps produce physiologic and mental relaxation. The two most common methods are **progressive muscle relaxation** and **autogenic relaxation. Guided imagery,** in which an individual visualizes pleasant places or things, is often used in conjunction with relaxation.

8. **Biofeedback** is a process in which a person learns to reliably influence physiologic responses in order to decrease muscle tension and/or sympathetically mediated responses, such as vasoconstriction, which may produce or worsen pain.

9. **Hypnosis** is a state of aroused, attentive focal concentration with a relative suspension of peripheral awareness. It may block the pain from awareness, substitute another sensation, change the meaning of pain, or increase pain tolerance.

10. Comprehensive treatment packages for cancer pain utilize **cognitive and behavioral methods** with the goal of helping individuals to **modify thoughts, beliefs, or actions/behaviors** that may exacerbate pain, depression, and anxiety and providing them with **specific skills to cope** with pain. There are few data on the efficacy of this type of treatment approach. However, there is some indication that cognitive approaches may help patients **better understand and adhere to pharmacologic treatment regimens.**

11. Preliminary research suggests that **music therapy** and **laughter therapy** may serve to diminish the emotional and reactive components of pain.

12. **Table 23-21, text page 544,** presents the most commonly used **nursing interventions** for decreasing the emotional and reactive components of pain. It also outlines examples, as well as the advantages and disadvantages, of each technique.

V. CONCLUSIONS AND FUTURE DIRECTIONS

1. The nurse has a pivotal role in the multidisciplinary management of cancer pain.
2. There is considerable information available for application to the care of individuals experiencing cancer pain. The challenge is to **utilize this knowledge** to its fullest, to **continue experimenting** with new ways to treat pain, and to **share information with colleagues.**

PRACTICE QUESTIONS

1. Which of the following processes associated with the occurrence of pain is considered vague and subjective in that it encompasses complex behavioral, psychologic, and emotional factors?
   (A) transduction
   (B) transmission
   (C) modulation
   (D) perception

2. The dimension of pain that encompasses the meaning that the pain experience has for a person is the
   (A) behavioral dimension.
   (B) affective dimension.
   (C) sensory dimension.
   (D) cognitive dimension.

3. Assessment of **behavioral** parameters in cancer pain would include an evaluation of
   (A) the quality of the pain.
   (B) associated psychologic problems.
   (C) the effect of pain on activities of daily living.
   (D) the duration of the pain.

4. Which statement regarding the treatment of cancer pain in children is true?
   (A) When children do not physically or verbally indicate that they are having pain, it means that pain is not present.
   (B) It is unsafe to use narcotics in children less than five years of age.
   (C) Children metabolize narcotics more rapidly than adults do, so they may need to be medicated more frequently.
   (D) Whereas adults often require several different medications at once to control their cancer pain, children generally require only one.

5. One misconception about pain in the elderly person is that
    (A) age effects the absorption, distribution, metabolism, and excretion of analgesic drugs.
    (B) an elderly person is better qualified to describe their pain than is an informed son or daughter.
    (C) the risk of toxic effects of narcotics is higher in the elderly due to interactions of multiple medications.
    (D) pain is a common aspect of normal aging.

6. Which of the following nonnarcotic analgesics will **not** significantly decrease inflammation?
    (A) naproxen
    (B) acetylsalicylate
    (C) ibuprofen
    (D) acetaminophen

7. Nonsteroidal anti-inflammatory drugs (NSAIDs) are **most** useful for which of the following?
    (A) phantom limb pain
    (B) nonobstructive visceral pain
    (C) postoperative pain
    (D) pain due to leukemic infiltrates

8. Antidepressants such as amitriptyline may be used to treat pain that is due to
    (A) tumor infiltration of nerves.
    (B) narcotic withdrawal.
    (C) brain metastases.
    (D) surgery.

9. Anticonvulsants may be used to treat
    (A) neurogenic pain.
    (B) acute procedural pain.
    (C) pain secondary to spinal compression.
    (D) the pain of bone metastases.

10. Steroids are sometimes used in the management of pain related to
    (A) bowel obstruction.
    (B) spinal cord compression.
    (C) trigeminal neuralgia.
    (D) tumor pressing on a vital organ.

11. A type of therapy that has few side effects and that has been effective in treating the pain related to bone metastasis in breast cancer is
    (A) surgery.
    (B) hormonal therapy.
    (C) chemotherapy.
    (D) radiation therapy.

12. A nonopioid analgesic that may be helpful for severe pain is
    (A) acetaminophen.
    (B) codeine.
    (C) hydromorphone.
    (D) phenytoin.

13. The drug used to treat respiratory depression related to narcotics is
    (A) naproxen.
    (B) methadone.
    (C) meperidine.
    (D) naloxone.

14. Which of the following statements is true of the nausea and vomiting that sometimes accompany narcotics use?
    (A) It cannot effectively be controlled with antiemetics.
    (B) Most patients find it a "tolerable" side effect.
    (C) Its presence may be an adequate reason to change analgesic agent(s).
    (D) It frequently is a consequence of too much narcotic.

15. Scheduling of oral analgesics generally should be
     (A)   at fixed intervals.
     (B)   every two hours.
     (C)   as needed (prn).
     (D)   related to a patient's activity level.

16. The transdermal route of narcotic administration was first used with which opioid?
     (A)   methadone
     (B)   fentanyl
     (C)   morphine
     (D)   levorphanol

17. An example of counterirritant cutaneous stimulation is
     (A)   subcutaneous administration of morphine.
     (B)   minor surgery.
     (C)   massage.
     (D)   imagery.

18. Directing one's attention away from the sensations and emotional reactions produced by pain is known as
     (A)   distraction.
     (B)   biofeedback.
     (C)   autogenic relaxation.
     (D)   hypnosis.

ANSWER EXPLANATIONS

1. **The answer is (D).**   The neural activities that occur in transmission and modulation culminate in the mechanism of pain known as perception. Because perception varies considerably from one individual to the next, it is the mechanism that contributes to the great diversity in response to noxious stimuli/events. This process is the least understood of all those related to pain. (501)

2. **The answer is (D).**   Of the five dimensions of the cancer pain experience described by Ahles et al., the cognitive dimension relates to the manner in which pain influences a person's thought processes, view of self, and the meaning of the pain. (505)

3. **The answer is (C).**   An assessment of behavioral parameters of pain should include the effect of the pain on activities of daily living (ADLs), such as eating, mobility, and social interactions, as well as activities/ behaviors that increase or decrease the intensity of pain. A behavioral assessment would also consider pain behaviors used, including grimacing or other nonverbal communication and the use of medications or other pain control interventions. (506)

4. **The answer is (C).**   A child's lack of willingness or ability to express pain or request treatment does not mean that he/she is not experiencing it. Children may deny pain because they have certain fears about it, or because they have developed adaptation or coping mechanisms to deal with the pain. Narcotics are used safely in children less than five years old. Children as a group do not tolerate pain better than adults, and their pain/response to pain must be addressed according to the same multidimensional approach as one would utilize for an adult. (520)

5. **The answer is (D).**   Pain is not a normal sequela of aging. Although it may be true that people develop more chronic conditions as they age, it does not necessarily follow that pain accompanies the aging process and that complaints of pain by an elderly person should be dismissed. Because of this common misconception, elderly patients may not report pain as a problem and interventions to control their pain may not be implemented. (521)

6. **The answer is (D).**   Naproxen, acetylsalicylate, and ibuprofen are all nonsteroidal anti-inflammatory drugs. Acetaminophen is not significantly anti-inflammatory and therefore often is considered a separate type of nonnarcotic. (529)

7. **The answer is (B).**   Nonsteroidal anti-inflammatory drugs (NSAIDs) act on the peripheral nervous system by preventing the conversion of arachidonic acid to prostaglandin. These medications have a maxi-

mum ceiling effect for analgesic potential, and their indication for use in cancer patients should be pain that is mild to moderate in intensity. (529)

8. **The answer is (A).** Antidepressants (e.g., amitriptyline, desipramine, imipramine) control pain by inhibiting the uptake of neurotransmitters into nerve terminals. They are used in the treatment of many types of nonmalignant pain such as migraine headaches but are also felt to be useful in neuropathic pain that is due to tumor infiltration of nerves, often described as having a continuous, burning quality. (534)

9. **The answer is (C).** Although their mechanism of action in treating cancer-related pain is not well understood, anticonvulsants (e.g., phenytoin, clonazepam) have been found to be effective in neurogenic or neuropathic pain that is described as stabbing or lancinating. Side effects of the anticonvulsants include sedation/drowsiness, dizziness, ataxia, and behavioral disturbances. (534)

10. **The answer is (B).** Steroids are extremely efficacious for managing the pain caused by epidural cord compression. Some side effects of steroid use such as mood elevation and increased appetite may also be desirable in some patients. However, the use of these drugs as adjuvant analgesics early in the course of a patient's pain problem is not recommended. (535)

11. **The answer is (B).** Hormonal therapy (e.g., estrogen, androgen, progestin, aminoglutethimide, and corticosteroids) has been used effectively to control painful bone metastases in breast and prostate cancers. Hormonal therapy can provide palliation and relief of pain, sometimes for long periods of time, with relatively few side effects. (535)

12. **The answer is (C).** Acetaminophen is a nonopioid analgesic. Phenytoin is an anticonvulsant. Codeine is an opioid analgesic and is commonly used for moderate pain. Large doses of codeine would need to be administered in order for it to be effective against severe pain. According to **Table 20-15, text page 418,** 200 mg of oral codeine would be equivalent to approximately 7.5 mg of oral hydromorphone, another narcotic analgesic. (531)

13. **The answer is (D).** Naloxone is the drug of choice in the treatment of respiratory depression related to opioid overdosing. The amount of naloxone a patient receives should be titrated to changes in respiratory rate. Rapid injections of naloxone should be avoided in opioid-tolerant patients, so as not to precipitate an abstinence syndrome that may include intense pain. (532)

14. **The answer is (C).** Nausea is a common side effect of opioid usage that is not necessarily indicative of toxicity. This side effect can often be controlled with antiemetics, but if after a reasonable trial of antiemetic agents the patient continues to experience nausea, a different analgesic should be tried. (532)

15. **The answer is (A).** Except in a few circumstances, oral pain medication should be on a fixed-interval basis. While the evidence is not conclusive, most caregivers agree that round-the-clock scheduling is most effective in treating pain. (536)

16. **The answer is (B).** Fentanyl, 75 times more potent than morphine, is currently being administered via transdermal patches that are changed at prescribed intervals. This delivery system is an exciting new option for cancer patients who are experiencing pain, but it is not without its side effects, among them a prolonged effect after patch removal secondary to the long half-life of fentanyl. (537)

17. **The answer is (C).** Counterirritant cutaneous stimulation (e.g., massage, heat or cold therapy, transcutaneous electrical nerve stimulation) is thought to help relieve pain by somehow physiologically altering the transmission of nociceptive stimuli referred to in Melzack and Wall's gate control theory of pain. It is also felt that the relief achieved may outlast the actual application of the counterirritant. (542)

18. **The answer is (A).** Distraction (e.g., conversation, imagery, breathing exercises, watching television) directs one's attention away from the sensations and emotional reactions produced by pain and blocks one's awareness of the pain stimulus and its effects. It can be very helpful in reducing pain, but caregivers must remember that the mere fact that a patient is effectively distracted from the pain does not mean that he or she is pain-free. (542)

24 Infection

STUDY OUTLINE

I. **SCOPE OF THE PROBLEM**

   A. **INCIDENCE**

   1. Infections are implicated as the cause of death in 50% of persons with solid tumors and in 80% of those with leukemia. They are a major cause of morbidity and mortality.

II. **ANATOMY AND PHYSIOLOGY**

   A. **INTEGUMENTARY, MUCOSAL, AND CHEMICAL BARRIERS**

   1. **Intact skin** is the most important physical barrier against bacteria. Breaks in the skin can lead to microbes entering the body and causing infection.
   2. The mucociliary activity of **mucous membranes** is another major defense against infection.
       a. **Microorganisms** constitute up to 60% of the weight of the stool; therefore, an intact mucous membrane is essential to prevention of infection.
   3. **Acid pH and microbicidal elements** of fluids and tears inhibit bacterial growth and provide a protective effect.

   B. **LEUKOCYTES**

   1. **Leukocytes, particularly PMNs, are a significant defense against infection. Polymorphonuclear neutrophils (PMNs),** often referred to as polys or segs, constitute 50%–70% of the circulating white blood count (WBCs). PMNs respond quickly to bacterial invasion.
   2. The primary function of PMNs is the destruction and elimination of microorganisms through **phagocytosis,** the process of engulfing and ingesting foreign matter.
   3. PMNs secrete **chemotactants,** chemical substances that alert the body to the presence of an invader and stimulate increased production of PMNs and macrophages.
   4. Without sufficient numbers of PMNs, the body's ability to mount an inflammatory response is compromised.

   C. **MONOCYTES AND MACROPHAGES**

   1. Monocytes and macrophages constitute what was previously referred to as the **reticuloendothelial system.**
       a. Monocytes are released from the bone marrow before they complete the maturation process and are capable of only limited phagocytosis.
       b. After monocytes migrate into the tissues, full maturation occurs; the cells are then referred to as **macrophages.**
   2. Macrophages are **highly phagocytic,** playing roles in inflammation and in cellular and immune responses.

   D. **LYMPHOCYTES**

   1. Lymphocytes are responsible for cellular and humoral immunity. They constitute 25%–30% of the total WBC count.
   2. **B-lymphocytes** produce antibodies and are responsible for **humoral immunity.**

3. **T-lymphocytes** provide **cellular immunity** and result in the elimination of microorganisms.
4. **T-helper cells** comprise 75% of the total T-lymphocyte population, serving as a regulator of immune function by secreting **protein mediators known as cytokines.**

E. **CYTOKINES**

1. Cytokines are protein hormones synthesized by leukocytes.
2. The cytokines produced by mononuclear phagocytes are referred to as **monokines.**
3. The cytokines produced by B- and T-lymphocytes are referred to as **lymphokines.**
4. Cytokines initiate or regulate a number of inflammatory responses.

III. **PATHOPHYSIOLOGY**

A. **ALTERATIONS IN NONSPECIFIC DEFENSES**

1. **Disruptions in protective barriers**
   a. Skin integrity can be altered by invasive metastatic tumor growth, chemotherapy, and radiation therapy.
   b. Procedures associated with diagnosis and surgery also alter skin and mucous membrane integrity. These procedures include biopsy, aspiration, venipuncture, venous catheter, etc.
   c. Neurologic impairments due to cancer can compromise host defenses (such as the gag reflex).
2. **Changes in normal flora**
   a. **Endogenous** microbial flora that normally exist can lead to over 80% of infections in cancer patients.
   b. Poor hand washing by medical personnel is the most significant factor leading to infections in hospital patients.
   c. Antibiotics alter the normal flora, allowing the overgrowth of pathogens.
3. **Obstruction**
   a. Normal **clearing and drainage mechanisms** can be altered by obstruction usually associated with solid tumors or lymphoma. This can contribute to the risk of infection.

B. **GRANULOCYTOPENIA**

1. There is a direct relationship between number of circulating PMNs and incidence of infection.
2. Individuals show granulocyte count is less than **1000/mm^3** are considered **granulocytopenic** and at risk of infection. If the granulocyte count is less than **500/mm^3,** the risk is significant.
3. As length of therapy and duration of granulocytopenia increase, so does incidence of infection.
4. For granulocytopenic patients, PMN count is determined daily because their life span is so short. See **text page 558** for directions as to how to determine an absolute granulocyte count.

C. **IMMUNOSUPPRESSION**

1. **Infection**
   a. Certain **infections** actually contribute to the impairment of immune function. They include cytomegalovirus (CMV), herpes simplex virus (HSV), and Epstein-Barr virus.
   b. Lymphocyte and macrophage function may be abnormally suppressed by infections, thereby extending susceptibility.
2. **Acquired immune deficiency syndrome (AIDS)**
   a. Acquired immune deficiency syndrome is characterized by loss of T-helper cells, resulting in progressive loss of immunocompetence, development of opportunistic infections and chronic wasting, impairment of the central nervous system, and emergence of unusual malignancies.
   b. The virus that causes AIDS, human immunodeficiency virus (HIV), has been isolated in blood, saliva, tears, urine, cerebrospinal fluid, semen, vaginal secretions, and breast milk.
   c. Common **opportunistic infections** associated with AIDS include CMV, HSV, herpes zoster, *Candida albicans, Cryptococcus, Pneumocystis carinii, Toxoplasma gondii, Cryptosporidium, Mycobacterium avium,* and tuberculosis.
   d. AIDS is part of a **continuum** of illnesses related to infection with human immunodeficiency virus. Infections may not be present early in the disease course.

  e. **AIDS-related complex (ARC)** is a vague term first applied to those persons with symptoms of immune deficiency but without opportunistic infections or AIDS-related malignancy.

 3. **Tumor-associated abnormalities**

  a. The types of infections that affect patients with cancer are somewhat predictable and occur often.

  b. Patients with **abnormal cell-mediated immunity** (as in Hodgkin's disease and acute leukemia) usually experience infection and intracellular pathogens, including herpes zoster.

  c. Advanced lung cancer and intracranial tumors are associated with decreased sensitivity and ability to respond to a challenging antigen.

  d. Patients who are **without a spleen** are at a 50 times greater risk of sepsis and death than the normal population.

  e. Fifty-five to seventy percent of **fevers** in individuals with cancer occur from infection, and not from the underlying cancer, especially during periods of granulocytopenia.

 4. **Nutrition**

  a. Cancer can affect an individual's nutritional status by interfering with the functional capacity of gastrointestinal structure, causing inlet or outlet obstruction or vascular impairment.

  b. **Cachexia** is a state of malnutrition and wasting.

  c. There is a relationship between malnutrition and a variety of immune deficiencies.

 5. **Cancer therapy**

  a. The incidence of infectious complications can increase in the cancer patient undergoing a **surgical procedure.** Predisposing factors include duration of preoperative hospitalization, extent of surgery, length of the procedure, presence and degree of hemorrhage and tissue ischemia, nutritional status, prior chemotherapy or corticosteroid therapy, and presence of infection or wound contamination during surgery.

  b. In the postoperative period, the surgical wound is the most common site of infection.

  c. Radiation therapy and chemotherapy interfere with essential metabolic functions of the cell and can cause **inflammation** and **ulceration** of normal tissues, predisposing to infection.

  d. **Blood counts** should be monitored during radiation, especially if a large area is treated or if significant areas of bone marrow are included in the radiation field.

IV. TYPES OF INFECTIONS

A. BACTERIA

 1. **Changing patterns** in bacterial infections are primarily the result of improvements in antibiotic therapy.

 2. **Empiric use of combination antibiotic** therapy, incorporating third-generation cephalosporins, has greatly reduced the number of documented Gram-negative infections.

 3. **Gram-negative organisms**

  a. Gram-negative organisms are the primary cause of infection in the granulocytopenic patient. *E. coli, K. pneumonia, and P. aeruginosa* are the most common organisms cultured.

  b. **Endotoxic or systemic shock** is the most significant consequence of Gram-negative infection, which can quickly lead to death.

  c. Without **early detection** and **prompt** initiation of treatment, endotoxic shock leads to hypotension, tissue ischemia, multisystem failure, and death.

 4. **Gram-positive organisms**

  a. *S. aureus* and *S. epidermidis* are the Gram-positive organisms most commonly responsible for infections in granulocytopenic patients.

  b. The most well-known endotoxin, produced by *S. aureus*, is associated with **toxic shock syndrome.**

 5. **Treatment**

  a. **Empiric antibiotic therapy** is initiated before the organism is identified.

  b. **Selection** of antibiotic agents must be individualized to consider the probable cause of infection and the likely site of origin, as well as institutional patterns of infection and antibiotic resistance.

  c. In general, the empiric antibiotic regimen selected should cover a **broad spectrum of pathogens** without significant risk for the emergence of resistant organisms or drug-related toxicity.

B. **MYCOBACTERIA**

1. Mycobacterial infections are uncommon in cancer patients and are associated more with cellular immunity defects.
2. **Treatment**
   a. Combination therapy has been more successful in treating MAI, including amikacin, rifampin, ciprofloxacin, ethambutol, and clarithromycin.

C. **FUNGI**

1. **Fungal infections** are a major cause of fatal infections with risk factors of prolonged granulocytopenia, venous access catheters, administration of parenteral nutrition or corticosteroids, prolonged use of broad-spectrum antibiotics, and damaged GI mucosa from disease or treatment.
2. *Candida*
   a. *Candida* is the most common cause of invasive fungal infection.
   b. The presence of *Candida* in the sputum, mouth, or throat cannot be definitively correlated with infection because *Candida* can reside harmlessly in the healthy host.
      (1) The immunosuppressed person is at risk when granulocytopenia occurs and/or when **cellular immunity** is impaired.
   c. **Dermatologic** infections with *Candida* occur most frequently in skin folds, such as the groin, perineum, and perianal areas and under the breasts.
   d. **Oral candidiasis (thrush)** is a common yeast infection that can disseminate throughout the GI tract.
3. *Aspergillus*
   a. *Aspergillus* is another common fungus that causes serious infections in persons with cancer, particularly in those who are granulocytopenic and/or receiving immunosuppressive therapy.
   b. The fungus enters the host through the upper airway and typically causes pneumonia or sinus infection.
   c. Aspergillosis is characterized by blood vessel invasion, which can lead to thrombosis and infarction of pulmonary arteries and veins.
4. *Cryptococcus*
   a. ***Cryptococcus neoformans*** is a yeast found in soil and pigeon excreta and generally is acquired by inhalation.
   b. It appears most often in people with Hodgkin's disease and other lymphomas.
   c. It commonly occurs as an insidious meningoencephalitis.
      (1) Headache, vomiting, and diplopia without fever are typical symptoms.
   d. Cryptococcal infection can also occur in the lungs and disseminate to visceral organs.
5. *Histoplasma*
   a. Histoplasmosis generally occurs as a pulmonary infection, usually in individuals with lymphoreticular neoplasms.
   b. The infection commonly disseminates, causing adenopathy and hepatosplenomegaly, which may be confused with the underlying neoplasm.
   c. **Histologic examination** of biopsy material for *Histoplasma* is necessary if this organism is suspected as a cause of infection.
6. **Phycomycetes**
   a. The Phycomycetes (***Mucor, Rhizopus,*** and ***Absidia***) are opportunistic fungi widespread in dust and air.
   b. The lungs, nasal sinuses, and GI tract are the three major sites of infection, although the disease may disseminate to other body sites after the fungi are inhaled into the lungs.
7. *Coccidioides*
   a. *Coccidioides* is found in the soil of the southwestern United States and typically enters the body by inhalation.
   b. Immunocompromised persons are susceptible to the development of serious pulmonary infections.
8. **Treatment**
   a. Two major problems in treatment of fungal infections are the difficulty associated with culturing organisms from infected tissues and the limited number of effective agents available to manage severe fungal infections.

b. **Amphotericin B** is the drug of choice for treatment of systemic fungal infections.
   (1) It is associated with significant side effects and toxicities, including fever, chills, rigors, nausea, hypotension, bronchospasm, vomiting, and occasionally seizures.
   (2) The major toxicity of amphotericin B is **nephrotoxicity.**
   (3) **With continued administration, elevated levels of creatinine and blood urea nitrogen can occur.**
   (4) **Electrolyte imbalances,** particularly hypokalemia, are common and warrant careful monitoring and treatment.
c. **Flucytosine** (5-FC) is an antifungal agent used to treat *Candida* and *Cryptococcus*.
   (1) The major limitation to its use is the rapid onset of drug resistance.
   (2) 5-FC is commonly used in **combination** with amphotericin.
d. **Fluconazole** is an oral antifungal agent that is well absorbed and is able to penetrate cerebral spinal fluid, the eye, and peritoneal fluid.
   (1) It most often is used to treat cryptococcal meningitis and oropharyngeal, esophageal, and systemic *Candida* infections.
   (2) Side effects include exfoliative skin disorders (blistering, peeling, etc.), hepatotoxicity, and (less frequently) GI disturbances and headaches.
e. **Ketaconazole,** another oral antifungal agent, is used to treat disseminated and pulmonary coccidioidomycosis, candidiasis, and histoplasmosis.
   (1) The most frequent side effects are nausea, vomiting, and diarrhea.
f. **Miconazole** is a parenteral antifungal agent considered to be primarily a second-line therapy.
   (1) It may be prescribed for treatment of candidiasis, coccidioidomycosis, and cryptococcus.
   (2) Side effects include hypersensitivity reactions, phlebitis, GI disturbances, and (less frequently) anemia and thrombocytopenia.

D. VIRUSES

1. Common viruses cause measles, mumps, rubella, respiratory infections, colds, and bronchitis.
2. Most viral infections in granulocytopenic patients are caused by herpes viruses (HSV), varicella zoster (VZV), and CMV.
3. **Herpes simplex (HSV)**
   a. HSV can cause serious infection in persons with cancer, either from primary exposure or from reactivation of a latent virus.
   b. Major sites of infection are the oropharynx, esophagus, urogenital tract, perianal area, skin, and eyes.
      (1) In rare cases of HSV dissemination, pulmonary, CNS, and hepatic involvement may be seen.
   c. Patients with impaired cell-mediated immunity are at increased risk for recurrent HSV infections resulting in extensive mucocutaneous ulceration.
4. **Varicella zoster**
   a. **Varicella zoster virus (VZV)** can cause serious vesicular eruption in individuals with cancer, especially children, and results in a mortality rate of about 7%.
   b. Following primary VZV infection, **reactivation ("shingles")** can occur, because the virus remains dormant in the spinal ganglia.
      (1) **Incidence** of reactivation ranges from 5%–10% in patients with solid tumors to 35%–50% in those with Hodgkin's disease or who have had a bone marrow transplant.
   c. **Diagnosis** is based on a history of chickenpox, characteristic dermatomal distribution of vesicular lesions, and positive culture results.
   d. The major complication of VZV infection is **visceral dissemination** resulting in pneumonitis, hepatitis, and meningoencephalitis.
   e. Varicella is highly contagious, and the risk of spread to other seronegative immunocompromised persons is substantial, especially in adults with Hodgkin's disease and children with leukemia.
   f. Because of the severity of VZV infection in persons with cancer, infected patients have been treated with varicella zoster immune globulin (VZIG).
5. **Cytomegalovirus**
   a. **Cytomegalovirus (CMV)** infection is usually a result of viral reactivation, particularly in association with immunosuppression.

    b. **CMV is a common cause of interstitial pneumonitis** in persons with impaired cellular immunity or following bone marrow transplant.

    c. CMV retinitis is the most common opportunistic **ocular** infection noted in immunocompromised persons, especially those with AIDS.

6. **Hepatitis virus**

    a. Hepatitis virus can occur as a primary infection with one of the hepatitis viruses [A, B (HBV), or non-A non-B (NANBV)] or as a secondary infection.

    b. Viral hepatitis occurs as an acute or chronic infection.

    c. Although transfusions of blood products constitute the primary route of transmission, nonparenteral transmission occurs through sexual intercourse and contact with contaminated saliva, urine, and feces.

    d. See **Table 24-1, text page 565,** for the Centers for Disease Control **(CDC) guidelines** on universal precautions.

7. **Treatment**

    a. **Acyclovir** is an antiviral agent preferentially taken up by cells infected with HSV and VZV.

       (1) Treatment with acyclovir decreases viral shedding from infected cells, accelerates healing of lesions, and decreases pain and itching.

       (2) Acyclovir offers significant **prophylaxis** against recurrent infection for immunocompromised individuals, especially those who have had allogeneic bone marrow transplant.

       (3) **Side effects** are minimal, consisting primarily of nausea, vomiting, diarrhea, and anorexia.

       (4) **Phlebitis** is common with IV administration.

    b. **Vidarabine** is an antiviral agent used primarily for VZV and HSV infections.

       (1) Best used **early** in the course of infection, vidarabine is not particularly effective with disseminated infection.

       (2) **Toxicities** include bone marrow suppression, GI disturbances, and neurologic effects such as tremor, confusion, and ataxia.

    c. **Ganciclovir** is used in treatment of CMV infection.

       (1) It is a virostatic agent and therefore does not eliminate existing CMV but rather suppresses viral replication.

       (2) **Foscarnet** is another virostatic agent that suppresses CMV replication and may be prescribed for CMV infection that is resistant to ganciclovir.

       (3) Primary **side effects** include anemia, nephrotoxicity, and hypocalcemia; with less common effects of mild CNS disturbances, including irritability, tremor, and headache.

E. **PROTOZOA AND PARASITES**

1. Infections caused by protozoa and parasites are associated with defects in **cell-mediated immunity.**

2. *Pneumocystis carinii*

    a. *Pneumocystis carinii* (*P. carinii*) is a protozoan that causes infection in malnourished infants, children with primary immunodeficiency disorders, persons with AIDS, and those with cancer who are undergoing immunosuppressive therapy.

    b. **Clinical manifestations** of infection include fever, nonproductive cough, tachypnea with intercostal retraction, and potentially life-threatening respiratory compromise.

3. *Toxoplasma*

    a. *Toxoplasma gondii* (*T. gondii*) is an obligate intracellular parasite found in soil, cat excreta, and improperly cooked meats.

    b. Persons at greatest risk include those with AIDS and those receiving immunosuppressive therapy for hematologic malignancies or prevention of organ transplant rejection.

4. *Cryptosporidium*

    a. Although it is a common cause of enteritis in persons with AIDS, cryptosporidiosis has only occasionally been observed in other immunocompromised patients.

    b. When severe deficiencies in cell-mediated immunity are present, cryptosporidiosis results in voluminous watery **diarrhea** and secondary malnutrition, dehydration, and electrolyte imbalance.

5. **Treatment**

    a. Untreated *P. carinii* is fatal.

    b. The treatment of choice for *P. carinii* is **trimethoprim-sulfamethoxazole.**

    c. Side effects, however, are troublesome and include azotemia, hypocalcemia, and hepato-toxicity.

    d. Prophylactic treatment of high-risk patients most often is accomplished with trimethoprim-sulfamethoxazole.

V. NURSING CARE OF THE PATIENT AT RISK FOR INFECTION

A. PREVENTION

1. **Reducing environmental pathogens**
   a. Since most cancer care is delivered in the ambulatory setting, nursing care focuses on prevention of infection, measures to optimize the person's health, and aggressive interventions when needed.
   b. See **Table 24-2, text pages 566–567,** for nursing measures to prevent life-threatening complications in a patient at risk for infection.
   c. The single most important measure to prevent infection is meticulous **hand washing by every person who enters the room or comes in contact with the individual at risk for infection.**
   d. When the ACG is **less than 1000,** live plants, cut flowers, and fresh fruit should not be brought into the patient's room.
   e. During granulocytopenic episodes, **invasive procedures** are kept to a minimum, with adherence to strict aseptic technique when they are performed.

2. **Optimizing health status**
   a. **Adequate nutritional intake during periods of increased risk requires a high-calorie, high-protein diet.**
      (1) If severe neutropenia is present, a low-bacteria diet may be prescribed, eliminating fresh fruit, raw vegetables, fresh eggs, cold cuts, and skim or chocolate milk.
   b. Fluid intake is monitored to ensure adequate hydration, especially during periods of nausea, vomiting, and diarrhea and when therapy includes agents with bladder and renal toxicity.
   c. Activities are organized to allow for periods of **rest.**
   d. Strategies to maintain skin and mucous membrane integrity are implemented.
   e. The optimal plan for **oral hygiene** includes use of a soft to medium toothbrush, toothpaste, and dental floss.
   f. Enemas, rectal temperatures, and suppositories are likely to traumatize fragile rectal mucosa and are avoided as much as possible in the high-risk patient.
   g. **Activity** consistent with current health status is encouraged, to maintain optimal circulatory and pulmonary function.
   h. Persons with cancer, especially those with acute leukemia, should receive pneumococcal and other vaccines only while in remission, since antibody response is limited during chemotherapy.
   i. Education about infection risk begins at the time of diagnosis.

B. EARLY DETECTION

1. **Physical assessment**
   a. In spite of strict adherence to protective measures, prolonged or severe neutropenia will allow rapid progression of a localized infection to potentially life-threatening sepsis.
   b. During neutropenic periods, patients need nurses with diligent **physical assessment** skills, including the ability to listen carefully to information provided by the patient and significant others and to identify subtle clues indicative of infection.
   c. Classic signs and symptoms of infection may not be present when the inflammatory response is diminished.
   d. The most reliable indicator of infection is a low-grade **fever.**
   e. **Respiratory system**
      (1) The high incidence of **pneumonia** in immunocompromised patients mandates thorough assessment of the respiratory system.
      (2) During hospitalization, **chest auscultation** is performed every 2–4 hours, depending on the extent of risk, and with each nursing visit when at home.
      (3) Assessment findings for upper respiratory infection range from pain, swelling,

erythema, and discharge in nonneutropenic patients to vague discomfort and possibly mild erythema in neutropenic patients.

f. **Oropharynx**
   (1) The oral mucosa is often traumatized by chemotherapeutic agents, especially the **antimetabolites** and **antibiotics.**
   (2) Local infections can occur if inflamed or injured mucosal surfaces become colonized with bacteria, predisposing to systemic infection.
   (3) The oral cavity is inspected regularly for white plaques, gingival edema, erythema, bleeding, and ulceration.
   (4) Oral pain and dysphagia should be followed up with bacterial, fungal, and viral **cultures.**

g. **Gastrointestinal system**
   (1) If a granulocytopenic patient receiving broad-spectrum antibiotics complains of dysphagia and/or retrosternal burning, Candida or HSV esophagitis must be considered.
   (2) **Disruptions** of intestinal mucosa by anticancer therapy facilitate bacterial invasion and increase the potential for sepsis.
   (3) The perirectal area should be inspected routinely for signs of inflammation, infection, hemorrhoids, and fissures. Complaints of perianal itching, perianal tenderness, constipation, or pain with defecation can indicate early stages of perirectal cellulitis.

h. **Central nervous system**
   (1) Subtle changes in neurologic function can signify either the onset of an infection or the progression of malignancy.
   (2) Typical CNS complaints include headache, fever, meningismus, personality changes, focal neurologic signs, nuchal rigidity, altered mental status, and seizures.

i. **Urinary tract**
   (1) Classic signs of a urinary tract infection are typically absent in neutropenic patients.
   (2) Observation of urine characteristics—specifically, cloudy and foul-smelling—is usually more helpful.
   (3) *Candida* infection can result in erythema and pruritus in the perineal area.

j. **Skin**
   (1) Skin **integrity** should be assessed regularly, with special attention given to known areas of disruption or at increased risk of breakdown.

k. **Cardiovascular system**
   (1) Symptoms of cardiovascular infection generally are **nonspecific:** fever, chills, malaise, night sweats.

C. **NURSING CARE DURING EPISODES OF INFECTION**

1. Infection in the neutropenic patient is always considered a potentially life-threatening emergency.
   a. **Fatality** rates during the first 48 hours range from 18% to 40%.
2. **Cultures** are obtained from all potential sites of infection, including urine, sputum, wound, stool, and blood.
3. **Empiric** broad-spectrum antibiotic therapy is initiated promptly, and the patient's response is observed closely.
4. Monitoring for efficacy of antimicrobial treatment includes
   a. Assessing vital signs every 2–4 hours.
   b. Reviewing reports of chest X rays and laboratory data, including arterial blood gases, blood counts, chemistry profiles, culture results, and peak and trough antibiotic levels.
   c. Observing for signs of septic shock.
5. Other supportive nursing care strategies include
   a. Restoring circulatory fluid volume by administering IV fluids, blood or blood products, and vasopressors.
   b. Maintaining adequate oxygenation through the use of supplemental oxygen and, when necessary, mechanical ventilation.
   c. Promoting optimal nutritional status by monitoring dietary intake, consulting with the dietician, and conferring with the physician when enteral or parenteral nutrition is indicated.

VI.   **TREATMENT OF INFECTION**

     A.   **APPROACH TO THE PATIENT WITHOUT GRANULOCYTOPENIA**

         1.   Patients without granulocytopenia can be treated with appropriate antibiotic therapy for the specific infectious agent identified.

         2.   Cultures are performed before the initiation of therapy, and if necessary, antibiotics are changed when the results of sensitivity testing are known.

     B.   **APPROACH TO THE PATIENT WITH GRANULOCYTOPENIA AND FEVER**

         1.   Persons with cancer who have fever during periods of granulocytopenia will have a thorough physical examination, chest radiograph, and appropriate laboratory studies.

         2.   **Empiric antibiotics**

             a.   Empiric antibiotic therapy in the patient with fever and granulocytopenia reduces the number of infections that could become severe enough to be demonstrated by microbiologic culture or clinical documentation.

             b.   The particular empiric antibiotic regimen selected should meet the following criteria:

                 (1)   Provide broad-spectrum coverage for major pathogenic organisms.

                 (2)   Be synergistic and contain one bactericidal agent.

                 (3)   Have minimal organ toxicity.

                 (4)   Satisfactory absorption by the route administered.

                 (5)   Consistent distribution to infected tissues.

                 (6)   Adequate excretion.

         3.   **Isolation precautions and protected environments**

             a.   Persons with cancer who are receiving intensive therapeutic regimens with total body irradiation, steroids, and chemotherapy are significantly more susceptible to infection than those receiving less intensive therapy.

                 (1)   These severely immunocompromised persons often are placed on "protective" regimens intended to reduce the risk of infection.

                     (a)   Efforts to exclude all microorganisms through use of patient isolator rooms, nonabsorbable prophylactic antibiotics, and sterilization of the patients' food and water may prevent or delay the onset of some infection.

         4.   **Granulocyte replacement**

             a.   Limited efficacy, high cost, and serious complications (including development of lymphotoxic antibodies) made granulocyte transfusion impractical.

             b.   Studies have shown that the duration of granulocytopenia following chemotherapy is markedly decreased when G-CSF or GM-CSF is used.

     C.   **APPROACH TO THE PATIENT WITH GRAM-NEGATIVE SEPSIS**

         1.   **Shock** develops in 27%–46% of patients with Gram-negative bacteremia, resulting in inadequate tissue perfusion and circulatory collapse.

             a.   Mortality rate approaches 80% unless vigorous treatment is begun promptly.

         2.   The clinical syndrome is a result of a number of interrelated factors that include the direct effect of bacterial endotoxin on the cardiovascular system, activation of the protein cascade system, nutritional and hydration status of the patient, and the nature of the underlying disease.

         3.   The **first sign** of impending shock in the immunocompromised patient may be limited to low-grade fever, shaking chills, and/or mild hypotension.

         4.   **Early (warm) shock**

             a.   The early phase consists of vasodilation, decreased peripheral vascular resistance, normal to increased cardiac output, and mild hypotension; duration may vary from 30 minutes to 16 hours.

             b.   The patient may appear flushed, with warm extremities and adequate urinary output; central venous pressures are low, as are left ventricular and diastolic pressures, and respiratory alkalosis is present.

             c.   Peripheral vasodilation results in loss of fluid to the interstitial spaces.

         5.   **Late (cold) shock**

             a.   The late phase of septic shock is characterized by a profound reduction in cardiac output, increased peripheral vascular resistance, oliguria, and metabolic acidosis.

6. **Treatment of septic shock**
   a. The treatment of septic shock is based on two objectives: reversing the shock and treating the underlying sepsis.
   b. Individuals in shock require adequate oxygenation, effective circulation and tissue perfusion, nutritional support, and immediate, appropriate broad-spectrum antibiotic therapy.
   c. In low to moderate doses, **dopamine,** the vasoactive agent of choice, increases arterial pressure without causing significant vasoconstriction and selectively increases renal, coronary, cerebral, and mesenteric flow.
   d. Any change in blood pressure, mental status, or urinary output in high-risk patients alerts the nurse to the probability of early shock.
   e. Once treatment has been initiated, nurses monitor closely for complications of shock, including disseminated intravascular coagulation (DIC), renal failure, gastrointestinal bleeding, and hepatic abnormalities **(Table 24-5, text page 572).**
7. Care is taken to meet the psychosocial needs of patients with septic shock and their significant others.
8. See **Table 24-4, text page 571,** for assessment of patients with early and late septic shock.

D. **APPROACH TO THE PATIENT WITH HIV INFECTION**

1. Patients with HIV are at increased risk of opportunistic infection because of HIV-related **impairment of cellular immunity** and because of **granulocytopenia secondary to cancer treatment and/or antimicrobial therapy.**
2. Most opportunistic infections are the consequence of **T-helper cell depletion** and are caused by mycobacterial, viral, fungal, or protozoal organisms.
3. Antimicrobial therapy usually is continued indefinitely, since discontinuing treatment commonly results in recurrent symptoms of infection.
   a. The side effects of long-term antibiotic therapy and the progress of AIDS typically result in anorexia, nausea, vomiting, diarrhea, and malabsorption, which further compromise the person's immune function.

PRACTICE QUESTIONS

1. The body's first line of defense against bacteria, which is commonly altered by cancer or the cancer process, is
   (A) granulocytes.
   (B) the skin.
   (C) macrophages.
   (D) the acid pH of fluid.

2. The type of white blood cell that constitutes 50%–70% of circulating white blood cells and that responds quickly to bacterial invasion is the
   (A) polymorphonuclear neutrophil.
   (B) monocyte.
   (C) macrophage.
   (D) lymphocyte.

3. What is the name given to the microbes that normally live in the body and lead to over 80% of infections in cancer patients?
   (A) exogenous organisms
   (B) intracellular organisms
   (C) extracellular organisms
   (D) endogenous organisms

4. Which of the following variables do **not** influence the incidence of sepsis?
   (A) type of radiotherapy and chemotherapy
   (B) length of myelosuppressive therapy
   (C) absolute granulocyte count less than 500/mm^3
   (D) duration of granulocytopenia

5. The complication of infection with Gram-negative organisms that can quickly lead to death is
    (A) dehydration.
    (B) gastrointestinal bleeding.
    (C) endotoxic shock.
    (D) anaphylaxis.

6. Since fungal infections are a major cause of fatal infections in patients with cancer, a risk factor that should be avoided is
    (A) use of corticosteroids.
    (B) fresh flowers and plants.
    (C) contact with numerous visitors.
    (D) enteral nutrition.

7. Since amphotericin B is the major antifungal agent used, what is the common major electrolyte that the nurse needs to monitor frequently for?
    (A) sodium
    (B) calcium
    (C) potassium
    (D) bicarbonate

8. Meticulous skin care is required when caring for the patient with reactivated varicella zoster virus, in order to
    (A) minimize spread to other areas of the body.
    (B) prevent a secondary bacterial infection.
    (C) promote drainage of the vesicles.
    (D) provide the primary source of pain relief.

9. *Pneumocystis carinii* is potentially fatal and requires treatment with
    (A) foscarnet.
    (B) ganciclovir.
    (C) trimethoprim-sulfamethoxazole.
    (D) an aminoglycoside.

10. The single **most** important measure to prevent infection when caring for the patient with granulocytopenia is
    (A) promptly instituting empiric antibiotics.
    (B) washing the hands meticulously.
    (C) providing optimal nutrition.
    (D) restricting the giving of live flowers and plants.

ANSWER EXPLANATIONS

1. **The answer is (B).** The skin is the first line of defense against invading bacteria and subsequent infection. When a break in the skin occurs, environmental microbes and those that normally inhabit hair follicles and sebaceous glands can enter the body and cause infection. (558)

2. **The answer is (A).** Polymorphonuclear neutrophils comprise 50%–70% of white blood cells and are the first to respond to invading bacteria. The primary function of PMNs is the destruction and elimination of microorganisms through phagocytosis, the process of engulfing and ingesting foreign matter. (558)

3. **The answer is (D).** Undisturbed, endogenous microbial flora exist as a carefully balanced synergistic microenvironment within the host. Alterations in normal flora predispose persons with cancer to serious opportunistic or nosocomial infection. Over 80% of infections developing in cancer patients arise from endogenous organisms, nearly half of which are acquired during hospitalization. (559)

4. **The answer is (A).** There is a direct relationship between the number of circulating PMNs and the incidence of infection. When the granulocyte count is less than 500/mm³, risk of infection is significant. As the length of therapy and the duration of granulocytopenia increase, so does the incidence of sepsis. Although concurrent radiotherapy and chemotherapy might increase the degree of myelosuppression, the incidence of sepsis is not increased. (559)

5.   **The answer is (C).**   The most significant consequence of Gram-negative infection is the potential for endotoxic or systemic shock. The release of endotoxins initiates a cascade of events that, unless interrupted, will rapidly lead to death for the neutropenic patient. (562)

6.   **The answer is (A).**   Factors predisposing to fungal infection include severe, prolonged granulocytopenia, implanted vascular access catheters, administration of parenteral nutrition or corticosteroids, prolonged use of broad-spectrum antibiotics, and damage to oropharyngeal or GI mucosa due to disease or treatment. (562)

7.   **The answer is (C).**   The major toxicity of amphotericin is nephrotoxicity. With continued administration, elevated levels of creatinine and blood urea nitrogen can occur. Electrolyte imbalances, particularly hypokalemia, are common and warrant careful monitoring and treatment. (563)

8.   **The answer is (B).**   Diagnosis of VZV infection is based on a history of chickenpox, characteristic dermatomal distribution of vesicular lesions, and positive culture results. Since skin lesions (vesicles) can become confluent, meticulous skin care is required to prevent secondary bacterial infection. (564)

9.   **The answer is (C).**   *P. carinii* is a protozoan that causes infection in malnourished infants, children with primary immunodeficiency disorders, persons with AIDS, and those with cancer who are undergoing immunosuppressive therapy. Untreated, *P. carinii* is fatal, and even with therapy, mortality is high. The treatment of choice is trimethoprim-sulfamethoxazole. (565)

10.   **The answer is (B).**   Meticulous hand washing, by every person who enters the room or comes in contact with the individual at risk, is the single most important preventive measure against infection in the patient with granulocytopenia. Neutropenic individuals are advised of their risk and are encouraged to remind family, visitors, and staff about hand washing precautions. (568–569)

25   Bleeding Disorders

STUDY OUTLINE

I. **INTRODUCTION**

    1. Multiple hemostatic abnormalities may be involved in bleeding associated with cancer.
        a. Minor bleeding may be the initial symptom that leads to the diagnosis of cancer.
        b. Severe bleeding may indicate the onset of a progressive or terminal disease.
    2. The numerous and unique complications of each type of cancer create a difficult problem in the diagnosis and management of a bleeding disorder. This may be further complicated by the often toxic effects of various cancer treatments.
    3. Rapid recognition, assessment, and treatment of the hemorrhagic complications of cancer may significantly improve quality of life and possibly survival for the person with cancer.

II. **NORMAL HEMATOPOIESIS**

    1. **Blood cells** are formed primarily in the bone marrow through the process of **hematopoiesis.**
    2. The major sites of **blood cell development** in adulthood include the vertebrae, ribs, sternum, skull, proximal epiphyses of long bones, pelvis, and spleen.
    3. The **pluripotent stem cell,** or common progenitor cell, is **the cell from which all blood cells arise.**
    4. The **process** of **proliferation, differentiation,** and **maturation** of the stem cell into the various blood cell lines is mediated by various humoral factors called **colony stimulating factors (CSFs)** or hematopoietic growth factors.
    5. Stem cells in their earliest form are uncommitted to one cell line, but upon division and differentiation they become committed. See **Figure 25-1, text page 577,** for a **diagram of hematopoiesis,** with identification of colony forming units of blood cells early in their development.

A. **COLONY STIMULATING FACTORS (CSFs)**

    1. **CSFs** are hormone-like glycoproteins that act within the microenvironment of the bone marrow to **mediate hematopoiesis for all** of the blood cell lines. Some CSFs affect more than one blood cell line. See **text page 578,** column 1, for a list of common CSFs and the cell lines they mediate.

B. **ERYTHROCYTE PHYSIOLOGY AND FUNCTION**

    1. The **erythrocyte** or red blood cell (RBC) shape allows for **oxygen transport** and easy movement throughout the body.
    2. RBCs are produced in the bone marrow, and the early stage of their development is influenced by the following CSFs: BPA (burst promoting activity, GM-CSF, and IL-3. Once committed to the erythroid line, **red blood cell** development is induced by **erythropoietin (EPO).**
    3. The **kidneys** produce **EPO** in response to hypoxia or anemia.
    4. The major function of the **RBC** is the **transport of hemoglobin, carrying oxygen** to all tissues.

C. **PLATELET PHYSIOLOGY AND FUNCTION**

    1. **Platelets (thrombocytes) are anucleated, disk-shaped fragments of large marrow cells or megakaryocytes.**

    a.   Megakaryocytes mature in the bone marrow and fragment to form platelets.

    b.   Platelets are released in the marrow and then into the bloodstream.

    c.   **Normal platelet counts** for men and women are approximately **150,000–400,000.**

    d.   The platelet nuclei are removed by the reticuloendothelial system.

    e.   The process of maturing and budding takes approximately **10 days.**

    f.   Platelet formation is controlled by a regulatory hormone called **thrombopoietin.**

    g.   Under normal circumstances any reduction in the platelet count causes an increased production of megakaryocytes and platelets in the bone marrow.

2.   **Platelets remain in the vascular system and are not found in extravascular fluid.**

    a.   Normally about **two-thirds** of the total platelet mass circulates in the bloodstream, and the rest are concentrated in the spleen.

    b.   Platelets move freely between bloodstream and spleen.

    c.   Removal of the spleen (splenectomy) will cause a sharp but transient rise in the platelet count.

    d.   In a patient with an enlarged spleen, the platelet count is reduced greatly as the platelets become trapped in the spleen.

    e.   Platelets survive on the average about 10 days and then die.

3.   **Circulating platelets perform several functions.**

    a.   They are vital to **hemostasis,** the formation of a mechanical hemostatic plug (or clot).

    b.   They furnish a **phospholipid surface necessary for the interaction of the clotting factors** of the intrinsic (blood) system.

    c.   They are responsible for **fibrinolysis,** or lysis of the fibrin clot and vessel repair.

4.   **Hemostasis**

    a.   **Hemostasis** is the process by which the fluid nature of blood becomes altered so that a solid clot develops.

    b.   The process is initiated by **vascular or tissue injury** and culminates in the formation of a firm mechanical barrier, a **platelet plug,** which prevents free escape of blood from the damaged vessels.

    c.   Hemostasis is the end result of two dynamic processes, both of which are necessary to arrest bleeding.

    d.   When blood vessel injury occurs, vessels constrict and platelets are immediately attracted to and adhere to collagen fibers of the exposed subendothelial tissue.

    e.   Platelets release various components, including nucleotide adenosine diphosphate **(ADP),** which causes platelets to swell and platelet membranes to become sticky.

    f.   As platelets stick together, large platelet aggregates, or a **hemostatic plug,** form.

    g.   This initial phase of hemostasis depends on **platelet number and function** and the **ability of blood vessels to constrict.**

    h.   It produces only temporary cessation of bleeding.

5.   **Coagulation**

    a.   Blood **coagulation** may be considered a mechanism for rapid **replacement of an unstable platelet plug** with a **stable fibrin clot.**

    b.   When enzymes or coagulation factors are stimulated to interact, it is referred to as the **coagulation cascade.** See **Table 25-1, text page 579,** for a list of normal coagulation factors and **Figure 25-2, text page 579,** for a diagram of the **coagulation cascade.**

    c.   Two separate pathways: the **intrinsic** and **extrinsic,** cause the formation of a **fibrin clot.**

    d.   The **intrinsic** pathway is initiated by **activation** of **factor XII;** components of whole blood are necessary, as are calcium ions.

    e.   The **extrinsic pathway** begins with **trauma to tissues** that lie outside vessels and requires the activating substance of tissue factor or **"thromboplastin"** in addition to whole blood components.

    f.   **Both pathways** lead to stimulation of **factor X,** which is necessary for **conversion of prothrombin to thrombin.** At this point thromboplastin formation is complete.

    g.   **Thrombin** acts on **fibrinogen to form fibrin,** which is the essential portion of a clot.

    h.   **Hemostasis** becomes complete when the **clot becomes a stable insoluble clot** by conversion from **factor XIII** and is able to resist the hydrostatic pressure in the vessel.

    i.   **Fibrin formation** is an essential component of **hemostasis, inflammation,** and **tissue repair.** After fibrin has done its job, it must be removed to restore normal tissue structure and function and normal blood flow, which is done by the **fibrinolytic system.**

6.   **Fibrinolysis**

    a.   **Fibrinolysis,** or clot dissolution, is initiated by enzymes that are present in most body fluids and tissues.

    b.   These enzymes, called **plasminogen activators,** activate the substance **plasminogen,** which converts to **plasmin** in the presence of thrombin. **Plasmin** is responsible for the lysis of fibrin clots.

    c.   The breakdown of fibrin and fibrinogen produces **fibrin degradation products (FDPs)**, which neutralize thrombin, inhibit fibrin polymerization, and interfere with normal platelet formation. This process is summarized in **Figure 25-3, text page 580.**

    d.   A delicate balance between fibrin clot formation (coagulation) and clot dissolution (fibrinolysis) is necessary for effective hemostasis.

III. CAUSES OF BLEEDING IN CANCER

A. TUMOR EFFECTS

1. **Bleeding** is a **common presenting symptom** of cancer. It generally occurs as a result of tumor extension and local tissue invasion.
2. Bleeding can present as subtle pinkish sputum or as frank blood.
3. **Tumors** in close proximity to major **blood vessels** or involved with **vascular tissue** are at risk for causing bleeding because of **invasion or erosion.**
4. Other **structural** causes of bleeding include **cavitational and ulcerative** effects of local infections at vessel sites, destructive effects of radiotherapy, or denuded remains of vessels at radical cancer surgery sites.
5. Minor vascular bleeding may also occur in individuals whose **neoplasms produce abnormal proteins** of very high viscosity (paraprotein), e.g., multiple myeloma, Waldenstrom's macroglobulinemia, and acute leukemia.
6. **Bone marrow infiltration by tumor** can result in **replacement of normal blood cell components,** affecting hematopoiesis. This process is called myelophthisis and can result in anemia, thrombocytopenia, granulocytopenia, and impaired natural killer cell activity.
7. **Manifestations**
   a. Specific bleeding symptoms depend on the **site** and **extent of damage.**
   b. Internal bleeding may result from massive hemoptysis, severe hematemesis, vaginal hemorrhage, loss of consciousness, or hypovolemic shock.
   c. Gradual bleeding is more difficult to diagnose. **Melena** caused by colorectal carcinoma or macroglobulinemia may be manifested by **iron deficiency anemia.**
   d. Anemia may be serious before symptoms appear. Therefore the onset of symptoms, including fatigue, weakness, irritability, dyspnea, and tachycardia, may better reflect the **rate of progression** of the anemia rather than its **severity.**
8. **Management**
   a. **Acute bleeding is best managed by prevention.**
      (1) Tumors lying near or on major vasculature are generally **shrunk** by radiotherapy and/or chemotherapy, or if possible are removed by surgery.
      (2) If vascular integrity is threatened by infection, **antibiotic therapy** generally is initiated.
      (3) If acute bleeding does occur, **direct and steady pressure** at the site of bleeding is applied (if the site is exposed) or **mechanical pressure** may be used (if the site is not directly exposed), e.g., insertion of an occlusion balloon catheter into the bronchus or nasal packing during epistaxis.
      (4) Hypovolemic shock must be avoided. **Whole blood** is typically used to restore or maintain blood volume in acute hemorrhage.
   b. **Minor bleeding** as a result of capillary destruction is controlled by treating the underlying malignancy.
      (1) **Iron therapy** or, in severe cases, **blood replacement,** is used to treat anemia.
      (2) **Packed cells** usually are the therapy of choice in blood replacement. They provide more than 70% of the hematocrit of whole blood with only one-third of the plasma.
      (3) Clinical trials are under way to investigate the treatment of anemia of cancer with **recombinant human erythropoietin (rHuEPO). rHuEPO is a colony stimulating factor** found to be effective in **stimulating erythropoiesis** and in reducing or eliminating the need for transfusion.

B. PLATELET ABNORMALITIES

1. Abnormalities of platelet production, function, survival, and metabolism frequently occur in persons with cancer. Generally, they result from mechanical or humoral effects of the tumor itself or from tumor-induced abnormalities in the host.

2. Quantitative abnormalities
    a. **Thrombocytosis** is a disorder in which there is an increased number of circulating platelets. Individuals usually have no symptoms and do not require treatment.
        (1) It is particularly common in the myeloproliferative disorders such as chronic granulocytic leukemia.
        (2) It is seen frequently in many other cancers (e.g., lung, ovarian, pancreatic) and in persons whose spleens have been removed.
        (3) In only rare cases does it lead to **thrombosis.**
        (4) Symptomatic thrombocytosis may be treated by **thrombocytopheresis,** which rapidly removes large numbers of circulating platelets.
        (5) Alkylating agents and radiation are frequently used to suppress the marrow.
        (6) A drug called **anagrelide** has a hyperproliferative antiaggregating effect on platelets and lowers the platelet count without altering the leukocyte count or the hemoglobin level.
    b. **Thrombocytopenia,** a **reduction** in the number of circulating **platelets,** is the platelet abnormality most frequently associated with cancer.
        (1) It may be due to a **decrease in platelet production, a change in platelet distribution, platelet destruction, or vascular dilution.**
        (2) **One cause of thrombocytopenia is the decreased production of platelets in the bone marrow due either to tumor involvement or to the consequences of cancer therapy on the marrow.**
            (a) The low platelet count is directly proportional to the degree of bone marrow infiltration by tumor cells.
            (b) Marrow infiltration may represent metastatic disease or an intrinsic neoplastic proliferation of marrow elements, e.g., leukemia.
            (c) **Chemotherapy-induced platelet toxicity** usually is caused by the **destruction of the proliferating cells** of the platelet line CFU-MG (colony forming unit megakaryocyte).
                i. The **degree and duration of platelet toxicity** related to various antineoplastic agents are the result of a number of factors, including the **natural nadir** of the drug, its **potential for suppression,** and **cellular recovery time** after the nadir.
                ii. See **Table 25-2, text page 583,** for a list of chemotherapeutic **agents** associated with **moderate to severe thrombocytopenia.**
                iii. The **risk of bone marrow depression** related to radiation therapy is most significantly related to the **volume of productive bone marrow in the radiation field.**
        (3) **Platelet distribution** can be abnormal, causing thrombocytopenia in patients with hypersplenism. An **enlarged spleen may sequester up to 90% of the platelet population,** making them unavailable in the circulation.
            (a) A **palpable spleen** upon physical exam is required for diagnosis.
            (b) If the **primary cause of thrombocytopenia is platelet sequestration,** the bone **marrow will contain normal to increased numbers of megakaryocytes.**
        (4) Platelet **destruction can also cause thrombocytopenia.** It is characterized by a dramatically **shortened platelet life span** and an abundance of precursors in the bone marrow.
            (a) This occurs in **immune thrombocytopenia,** or idiopathic thrombocytopenic purpura, often associated with chronic lymphocytic leukemia and lymphoma and the use of alpha-interferon therapy.
            (b) The rapid destruction of platelets is due to an autoimmune process in which antibodies are formed against the person's own platelets.
            (c) Rapid platelet destruction is also seen in conditions of increased platelet consumption, e.g., disseminated intravascular coagulation.
        (5) **A fourth cause of thrombocytopenia is platelet dilution,** which may occur from the use of platelet-poor blood in blood transfusions.
        (6) **Manifestations**
            (a) **Thrombocytopenia** is the most frequent platelet abnormality associated with cancer and can lead to life-threatening bleeding.
            (b) **Platelet count** is the single most significant factor for predicting bleeding in the cancer patient. In acute leukemia, for example, patients with platelet counts below 20,000 cells/mm^3 have a greater than 50% chance of bleeding.

(c) **Infections** and the **rapidity with which the platelet count is falling** also increase the risk of bleeding in individuals with thrombocytopenia.

(7) **Management**

  (a) The target of therapy for patients with thrombocytopenia is the **underlying cause of the decreased platelet level,** rather than thrombocytopenia itself.

  (b) When thrombocytopenia is due to marrow infiltration with tumor, the best therapy involves **treatment of the tumor itself by chemotherapy and/or radiotherapy.**

  (c) The use of the **CSF-GM** is presently under investigation for **stimulating platelet recovery** after chemotherapy. Some studies are suggesting fewer platelet transfusions in patients receiving GM-CSF.

  (d) GM-CSF can be administered **subcutaneously** as well as **intravenously,** thereby allowing patients to be discharged earlier and to live in the outpatient setting. **Side effects** tend to be **mild** and range from a temporary generalized rash to mild to **moderate bone pain, fever, chills, headaches, nausea, and flushing.**

  (e) Other treatments include **platelet transfusions,** the administration of **epinephrine** (to release platelets from the spleen), and the administration of corticosteroids (to help minimize the bleeding potential of thrombocytopenia).

  (f) In the case of active bleeding, the use of high-dose **immunoglobulins** has been advocated.

  (g) In the absence of bleeding, high-dose **methylprednisone** is equally effective.

  (h) **Splenectomy** is indicated if these methods fail to control sequestration of platelets.

3. **Qualitative abnormalities**

  a. **Alterations in platelet function may also cause bleeding.** This can be caused by

    (1) A decrease in the **procoagulant activity** of platelets.

    (2) Decreased **platelet adhesiveness** and decreased **aggregation in response to adenosine diphosphate (ADP).**

    (3) **Thrombocytosis** associated with myeloproliferative disorders.

    (4) Increased activation of **coagulation factors** in individuals with cancer, causing a buildup of fibrin degradation products, which coat platelets.

    (5) **Pharmacologic agents,** including aspirin and other nonsteroidal anti-inflammatory agents.

    (6) **Beta-lactam antibiotics** commonly used with cancer patients can cause a **prolonged bleeding time** and abnormal platelet aggregation. These effects are seen after several days of high-dose intravenous therapy.

    (7) See **Table 25-3, text page 587,** for a list of **commonly used cancer care drugs that inhibit platelet function.**

  b. Management is aimed at the underlying cause of platelet malfunction, often starting with aggressive therapy directed at the tumor itself.

4. **Hypocoagulation**

  a. **Etiology and pathogenesis**

    (1) Malignancy or the metabolic alterations that accompany malignancy may precipitate an **imbalance in coagulation factors,** leading to decreased hemostasis. These imbalances are related directly to **tumor burden.**

    (2) **Liver disease** is the most significant factor that leads to a state of hypocoagulability. Liver disease may result from tumor invasion, chemotherapy, infection, or surgical resection.

    (3) Other factors include

      (a) A **deficiency of vitamin K.**

      (b) The use of large amounts of **frozen plasma.**

      (c) A **nonspecific plasma antagonist** of several coagulation proteins that has been described in acute leukemias and other disease states in which white cell turnover is rapid.

      (d) Isolated **coagulation factor deficiencies** that have been reported in some malignancies. Some of these are inhibitors of coagulation proteins.

  b. **Manifestations**

    (1) Decreased coagulability less frequently causes serious bleeding when it occurs.

(2) Hemorrhages tend to develop in the **joints** and in the deeper areas of the body such as the **subcutaneous or intramuscular tissue.**

(3) Mucosal bleeding occurs in acquired von Willebrand's syndrome.

  c. **Management**

(1) **Successful tumor therapy combined with infection control generally is the best means of controlling hypocoagulability disorders.**

(2) **Replacement therapy** with fresh or frozen plasma, prothrombin complex, cryoprecipitate, and other substances is sometimes effective in augmenting the production of coagulation factors by the liver.

(3) Vitamin K deficiency can be corrected with dietary sources of vitamin K or with parenteral phytonadione.

5. **Hypercoagulability**

  a. **Disseminated intravascular coagulation (DIC) is the most common serious hypercoagulable state that occurs in persons with cancer.**

  b. It represents an overstimulation of normal coagulation in which **thrombosis and hemorrhage may occur simultaneously.**

(1) Small clots are formed in the microcirculation of many organs at the same time clots and clotting factors are being consumed.

(2) The result is hemorrhage as the body is unable to respond to vascular or tissue injury.

  c. DIC is always secondary to an underlying disease process such as malignancy.

  d. The syndrome often remains undetected until severe hemorrhage occurs.

  e. DIC contributes strongly to morbidity and mortality in patients with cancer, particularly in those with thrombosis or bleeding in the **lung, central nervous system,** or the **gastrointestinal tract.**

  f. **Etiology**

(1) **The most common cause of DIC is infection.** Bacterial endotoxins activate factor XII (Hageman factor), which initiates coagulation by means of the intrinsic pathway of hemostasis and stimulates fibrinolysis.

(2) **Tumors themselves** may stimulate intravascular coagulability. Tumors associated with DIC include acute promyelocytic leukemia and the adenocarcinomas.

(3) Cytotoxic agents used to treat adenocarcinomas may contribute to DIC.

(4) See **Table 25-4, text page 589,** for a complete list of common causes of DIC.

  g. **Pathogenesis**

(1) **DIC always results from an underlying disease process that triggers abnormal thrombin formation.**

(2) Excess circulating thrombin may then abnormally activate both coagulation and fibrinolysis.

(3) Thrombin converts fibrinogen to fibrin. Fibrin thrombi are deposited in various organs, trap platelets, impede blood flow, and cause tissue damage.

(4) Thrombin also converts plasminogen to plasmin, which breaks down fibrinogen and fibrin. The FDPs that are formed interfere with fibrin clot formation and aid in the consumption of clotting factors and platelets.

(5) Bleeding is caused by many factors, including the consumption of platelets and certain clotting factors, plasmin's fibrinolytic properties, and the anticoagulant properties of the FDPs.

  h. **Manifestations**

(1) In chronic DIC the patient is not critically ill, and few if any clinical manifestations may be present.

(2) Acute DIC occurs rapidly over hours to days. Symptoms may include

    (a) **Widespread purpura and significant gastrointestinal and genitourinary hemorrhage.**

    (b) **Signs of shock and associated organ hypoxia.**

    (c) **Hemoptysis, intraperitoneal hemorrhage, and intracranial bleeding that may be life threatening.**

(3) See **Table 25-5, text page 590,** for a list of tests generally done to support the diagnosis of DIC. No specific laboratory finding is absolutely diagnostic.

  i. **Management**

(1) Treatment of the underlying malignancy is vital in treating the patient with a hypercoagulability disorder. All other therapy provides only an interval of symptomatic relief.

(2) **Heparin therapy** often is the primary treatment for DIC in malignancy.
  (a) It is controversial in that it carries the potential for unnecessarily exposing the patient to the risk of bleeding.
  (b) Heparin inhibits the formation of new clots and may decrease the consumption of clotting factors.
  (c) Therapy is maintained until symptoms disappear and laboratory values return to normal.
(3) **Epsilon-amino caproic acid (EACA; Amicar)** may be used when the fibrinolysis of DIC has been resolved but uncontrolled bleeding persists.
  (a) It prevents the binding of plasminogen or plasmin to fibrin or fibrinogen.
  (b) Administration is intravenous or oral.
(4) **Blood component therapy** often is necessary in DIC. This may include packed cells, fresh frozen plasma, antithrombin III, and cryoprecipitate.
(5) Prevention of further complications is another important goal in managing DIC.
  (a) Thrombophlebitis and edema should be closely monitored.
  (b) Loose clothing and elastic support stockings may help.
  (c) Assisting patients in exercising the legs is also useful.
  (d) Patients should avoid compressing the knee vessels, e.g., crossing the knees or legs.
(6) Patient education is a necessary component of care for the patient at risk for DIC.

IV. PATIENT ASSESSMENT

1. Patient assessment begins with a thorough history and physical examination.

A. PATIENT/FAMILY HISTORY

1. See **text page 592,** column 1, for a list of key aspects of a comprehensive history for patients at risk for bleeding.
2. Questions should focus on activities of daily living, for example, excessive bleeding while shaving or prolonged bleeding after minor cuts and scrapes.

B. PHYSICAL EXAMINATION

1. **Observation** is the most important measure in early detection of bleeding. Diagnostic signals may be subtle, e.g., traces of blood during tooth brushing, skin petechiae, or oozing from venipuncture sites.
2. **Hemorrhage** is the major problem associated with active bleeding. Common sites of hemorrhage include the gums, nose, bladder, gastrointestinal tract, and brain.
3. Occult blood in urine and stools should be routinely monitored.
4. See **Table 25-6, text page 592,** for physical signs and symptoms of bleeding.

C. SCREENING TESTS

1. The most common screening tests are
    a. **Bleeding time,** which measures the time it takes for a small skin incision to stop bleeding.
    b. **Platelet count,** which measures the actual number of circulating platelets per cubic millimeter of blood.
    c. **Whole blood clot retraction test,** which measures the speed and extent of blood clot retraction in a test tube.
    d. **Prothrombin time,** which measures the time it takes for a mixture of tissue thromboplastin, ionized calcium, and citrated plasma to clot compared with the time needed for a normal sample of blood to clot.
    e. **Partial thromboplastin time (activated),** which measures the intrinsic and common pathways of the clotting mechanism.
    f. **The fibrin degradation products (FDP) test,** which measures the activity of the fibrinolytic system.
2. See **Table 25-6, text page 593,** for a comprehensive list of the screening tests of hemostatic function, what each test measures, and what the normal value of each test is.

V.   **GENERAL NURSING CONSIDERATIONS FOR THE PERSON EXPERIENCING BLEEDING**

1. **The physical safety of the patient is always ensured to prevent trauma in those with diminished thrombocytic activity.** This means taking all precautions to help the patient avoid bumps, bruises, cuts, punctures, scrapes, irritations, or any activity that might break the skin or damage underlying tissue.
2. All **unnecessary procedures should be avoided,** including intramuscular or subcutaneous injections, rectal temperatures or suppositories, and indwelling catheters.
    a. If the patient requires parenteral administration of medication, the **intravenous route** should be used whenever possible.
    b. Injections, if unavoidable, are given with a needle of the **smallest possible gauge.** Pressure to the injection site is administered for several minutes, followed by application of a **pressure bandage** to avoid hematomas.
3. Severe **uterine hemorrhage** may be avoided by suppressing menses with pharmacologic agents. If menses is not suppressed, careful napkin counts are done during menses to help determine the volume of blood loss.
4. **Epistaxis** may be life threatening. The patient with epistaxis is placed in high Flower's position. Ice packs, nasal packing, or topical epinephrine may be used to decrease bleeding caused by a small vessel rupture within the nasal mucosa.
5. **Constipation** and associated strained bowel movements can be reduced by stool softeners and proper diet.
6. **Physical and emotional rest** is essential to the patient when active bleeding occurs. A calm approach and reassurance by the nurse are essential. Sedation may be used as needed to decrease anxiety levels.

VI.   **BLOOD COMPONENT THERAPY**

1. **Transfusion therapy** is provided to correct deficiencies in a specific **component of whole blood.** Aggressive transfusion support for patients with cancer who receive highly toxic treatment regimens has led to a decrease in the morbidity and mortality of cancer and its treatment.

A.   **RED BLOOD CELL THERAPY**

1. The decision to transfuse red blood cell replacement is usually based on the adverse physiologic effects of anemia the patient is experiencing.
2. **Physiologic signs of anemia** include **hyperventilation, rapid pulse, shortness of breath on exertion, rapid pulse, pallor, and fatigue.** These can often be relieved when the patient is transfused to keep the hemoglobin above 10 or 11 g/100 ml.

B.   **PLATELET THERAPY**

1. **The use of platelet transfusions has proved to have tremendous therapeutic value in controlling and preventing hemorrhage in individuals with cancer.**
2. Generally, the patient is transfused when
    a. There is **actual bleeding** associated with thrombocytopenia, or in the presence of infection or a rapid decrease in circulating platelets.
    b. The platelet count is greater than 20,000 cells/mm^3 yet bleeding is present.
    c. Patients with abnormally functioning platelets have bleeding.
3. Prophylactic platelet transmission may be given to maintain a platelet count greater than 20,000 cells/mm^3 or during periods of intense chemotherapy.
4. **Platelet survival**
    a. Several factors have been identified as important in determining failure of posttransfusion platelet survival in a patient, including
        (1) Infection and associated increased hemorrhage, fever, DIC, and splenomegaly.
        (2) Refractoriness to the platelet transfusion due to repeated exposure of patient/recipient platelets to the HLA antigens on donor platelets.
        (3) Leukoagglutinin reactions directed at non-HLA leukocyte antigens, causing an antibody reaction.
5. See **Table 25-8, text page 596,** for a description of **platelet transfusion therapy.**

C. **PLASMA THERAPY**

    1. **Plasma is removed from whole blood** and spun down to an average yield of 50 cc and frozen, in which form it is called **fresh-frozen plasma.** It contains all the clotting factors and the plasma proteins of albumin and cryoprecipitate.

    2. Plasma is used for **replacing clotting factors** in patients with coagulation disorders.

D. **TRANSFUSION COMPLICATIONS**

    1. Complications of platelet transfusions are similar to those of any blood product and may be **immediate** or **delayed.**

    2. The major hazards include **hemolytic and nonhemolytic transfusion reactions, transmission of diseases, and complications associated with intravenous therapy and transfusions.**

    3. Platelets generally can be transfused across incompatibilities of major **red blood cell antigen (ABO)** unless there is gross red blood cell contamination. If there is spillage and if donor and recipient A, B, and O antigens are not matched, hemolytic reactions are likely.

    4. Serious transfusion complications in patients who are significantly immunosuppressed include the risk of developing graft-versus-host (GVH) disease and the rare transfusion-related acute lung injury (TRALI).

    5. It is generally recommended that all blood products given to the severely immunocompromised host be **exposed to irradiation** before transfusion.

       a. Irradiation inhibits proliferation of lymphocytes without impairment of platelets, red cells, or granulocytes.

       b. Leukocyte-poor-blood filters can serve as an alternative approach to preventing GVH disease.

E. **LEUKOCYTE-DEPLETED BLOOD PRODUCTS**

    1. Since **leukocytes** remaining in donor blood collected for transfusion are **responsible for many of the complications** related to transfusion therapy, their removal from stored blood products is done extensively to prevent febrile nonhemolytic reactions as well as other complications.

    2. See **Table 25-10, text page 599, for complications** of transfusions.

    3. See **Table 25-11, text page 599,** for the nursing management of transfusion reactions.

    4. **Leukocyte depletion methods** include the traditional methods as well as **laboratory filtration and bedside filtration** of blood components.

F. **HOME TRANSFUSION THERAPY FOR THE CANCER PATIENT**

    1. There are a number of benefits to **home transfusion therapy** for the cancer patient. They include **decreased cost, convenience for the family and patient, psychological benefits, and the ability to be treated in a familiar environment** with family available.

    2. One drawback is that the patient is at **greater risk for complications** in the absence of sophisticated emergency equipment.

    3. See **text page 600** for seven basic selection criteria for a home transfusion therapy program.

    4. See **Figure 25-4, text page 601,** for a **home transfusion flow sheet** and **Table 25-13, text pages 602 and 603,** for a home transfusion protocol.

PRACTICE QUESTIONS

1. The typical response of the body to a reduction in the platelet count, such as that caused by bleeding, is a(n)

    (A) increase in the fibrinolytic activity of remaining platelets.

    (B) release of ADP into the bloodstream, which increases the oxygen-carrying capacity of available platelets.

    (C) sequestering of red blood cells in the spleen.

    (D) increased production of megakaryocytes in the bone marrow.

2. Circulating platelets perform several vital functions, including all of the following **except**

    (A) fibrinolysis, or the lysis of fibrin clots and vessel repair.

    (B) the release of plasminogen activators required for clot formation.

(C) furnishing a phospholipid surface for the biochemical phase of hemostasis.
(D) the formation of a mechanical hemostatic plug at the site of vessel injury.

3. Which of the following pairings of substances and functions in hemostasis is **incorrect?**
(A) fibrin: the actual substance of a clot
(B) thrombin: acts on fibrinogen to form fibrin
(C) plasmin: breaks up clots
(D) thromboplastin: acts on plasminogen to form plasmin

4. Bleeding as a symptom of cancer is most often due either to the mechanical pressure of tumors on organs or to
(A) interference with vasculature.
(B) damage to the spleen.
(C) hypocoagulability of the blood.
(D) infection.

5. Acute bleeding that occurs as a result of tumor-induced structural damage to vasculature is best managed by prevention. If acute bleeding does occur, however, and the site is not directly exposed, the best management approach is often
(A) radiotherapy combined with chemotherapy.
(B) oral or parenteral iron supplements to reduce anemia.
(C) mechanical pressure, e.g., nasal packing during epistaxis.
(D) direct and steady pressure at the site of bleeding.

6. The single most significant factor for predicting bleeding in the individual with cancer is
(A) tumor site.
(B) platelet count.
(C) abnormal platelet function.
(D) an imbalance in coagulation factors.

7. Thrombocytopenia in cancer patients may be caused by any of the following factors **except**
(A) an abnormal distribution of platelets that results in increased platelet sequestration.
(B) rapid platelet destruction characterized by a shortened platelet life span.
(C) overstimulation of normal coagulation causing rapid platelet thrombosis.
(D) decreased production of platelets in the bone marrow due to tumor involvement.

8. Patients with cancers may at times have bleeding despite normal platelet counts and coagulation factors. An example is bleeding caused by
(A) platelet sequestration.
(B) disseminated intravascular coagulation (DIC).
(C) decreased platelet adhesiveness.
(D) hypocoagulability.

9. Malignancy or the metabolic alterations that accompany malignancy may lead to an imbalance in coagulation factors, leading to decreased hemostasis (hypocoagulability). The most significant factor that leads to a state of hypocoagulability is
(A) liver disease.
(B) a deficiency of vitamin K.
(C) thrombocytosis.
(D) DIC.

10. The symptoms of disseminated intravascular coagulation (DIC) seem paradoxical because
(A) both platelet function and platelet numbers are implicated in DIC.
(B) patients may experience fever at the same time their bodies are hypothermic.
(C) DIC may be both the cause and effect of malignancy.
(D) thrombosis and hemorrhage may occur simultaneously.

11. Therapy for disseminated intravascular coagulation (DIC) often involves the administration of several substances. Which of the following is **not** a common treatment for DIC?
(A) heparin
(B) epsilon-amino caproic acid (EACA or Amicar)

(C)   vitamin K
(D)   platelet replacement

12.   The **most** important measure in the early detection of bleeding is
      (A)   accurate screening, beginning with a platelet count.
      (B)   observation for subtle diagnostic signals such as skin petechiae.
      (C)   a family history, focusing on possible congenital bleeding disorders.
      (D)   diagnostic testing of the complete cardiovascular system.

13.   The prothrombin time is a screening test of hemostatic function that is performed when tissue thrombo-
      plastin and ionized calcium are added to citrated plasma. Clotting time is then recorded and compared
      with the clotting time of a normal blood sample. This test is a measure of
      (A)   the ability of platelets to aggregate.
      (B)   the concentration of functional factor in plasma.
      (C)   platelet plug formation.
      (D)   extrinsic and common pathways in the clotting mechanism.

14.   Nursing care of the cancer patient at risk for bleeding should incorporate all of the following measures
      except
      (A)   avoidance of trauma.
      (B)   use of intramuscular rather than intravenous injections.
      (C)   avoidance of unnecessary procedures, including rectal temperatures or suppositories.
      (D)   suppression or monitoring of menses.

15.   Under which of the following circumstances would administration of a single donor platelet concentrate
      be preferable to that of a random donor platelet concentrate?
      (A)   when the patient is severely immunosuppressed
      (B)   when cost is a major factor
      (C)   when a patient's red blood cell antigens (ABO) are not known
      (D)   when time is a major factor

16.   Mrs. Ryan has metastatic cancer and presents with severe shortness of breath. The body's physiologic re-
      sponse to shortness of breath includes which of the following?
      (A)   Erythropoietin stimulates the stem cells of the bone marrow to produce red blood cells.
      (B)   Red blood cell production occurs in response to erythropoietin, which is produced by the bone
            marrow.
      (C)   Erythropoietin stimulates red blood cell production from the liver.
      (D)   Erythropoietin, which is produced by the kidney, stimulates red blood cell production.

17.   Colony stimulating factors (CSFs) act on the stem cells to mediate which of the following steps in hemato-
      poiesis?
      (A)   cellular proliferation only
      (B)   cellular differentiation only
      (C)   stem cell maturation only
      (D)   all of the above

18.   There are numerous steps in the cascade of events leading to blood clot production. Which of the follow-
      ing substances results from both the intrinsic and the extrinsic pathway and is necessary for conversion of
      prothrombin to thrombin?
      (A)   factor XII
      (B)   factor VII
      (C)   thromboplastin
      (D)   fibrinogen

19.   The occurrence of bleeding is common in the patient with cancer. It can occur for a number of reasons.
      Which of the following are two direct causes of such bleeding?
      (A)   chemotherapy administration and radiation therapy
      (B)   vascular tissue erosion from tumor and neutropenia
      (C)   the cavitational effects of infection and chemotherapy administration
      (D)   vascular tissue erosion from tumor and the cavitational effects of infection

20. The person with cancer who presents with dyspnea on exertion, rapid pulse, pallor, and fatigue following many months of cancer therapy should be evaluated for
     (A) myelophthisis.
     (B) dehydration.
     (C) hypercalcemia.
     (D) anemia.

ANSWER EXPLANATIONS

1. **The answer is (D).**   Megakaryocytes mature in the bone marrow and fragment to form platelets, which are then released into the bloodstream. Under normal circumstances any reduction in platelet count—from bleeding, malignancy, chemotherapy or radiotherapy, or other causes—will cause an increase in the production of megakaryocytes and platelets in the bone marrow. This activity is controlled by a regulatory hormone called thrombopoietin. (576)

2. **The answer is (B).**   Plasminogen activators are enzymes that are present in most body fluids and tissues. They are responsible for the conversion of plasminogen to plasmin in the presence of thrombin. It is plasmin that is responsible for the lysis (and not the formation) of fibrin clots. (580)

3. **The answer is (D).**   Thromboplastins are enzymes released from damaged tissue walls that catalyze the conversion of prothrombin to thrombin, the most powerful of the coagulation enzymes. It is thrombin that catalyzes the conversion of plasminogen to plasmin during fibrinolysis. (580)

4. **The answer is (A).**   All of the other choices can be factors in bleeding, but erosion and rupture of vessels precipitated by tumor invasion or pressure is the other major cause of bleeding in persons with cancer. Any tumor involvement of vasculature tissue or any tumor lying in close proximity to major vessels is seen as a threat of bleeding. Bleeding may also be the result of radiotherapy or radial cancer surgery and various platelet and coagulation abnormalities. (580)

5. **The answer is (C).**   If acute bleeding does occur, direct methods to halt the hemorrhage should be instituted immediately. Choices (A) and (B) are preventive methods; choice (D), while immediate and direct, applies to an exposed bleeding site. Another example of the use of mechanical pressure to stop acute bleeding is the insertion of an occlusion balloon catheter into the bronchus. (581–582)

6. **The answer is (B).**   Although all of the other choices are factors in bleeding as well, platelet count is the single most important factor in predicting bleeding in the individual with cancer. In acute leukemia, for example, patients with platelet counts below 20,000 cells/mm^3 have a greater than 50% chance of bleeding. Low platelet count (thrombocytopenia) is also the most frequent platelet abnormality associated with cancer. (582)

7. **The answer is (C).**   The other choices all result in lowered platelet count. (A) is often associated with splenomegaly, an enlarged spleen; (B) is frequently due to an autoimmune response in which antibodies are formed against the person's own platelets; (D) may also be the consequences of cancer therapy on bone marrow. A fourth cause of thrombocytopenia is platelet dilution caused often by the use of stored platelet-poor blood. (582–583)

8. **The answer is (C).**   Choices (B) and (D) are coagulation abnormalities; choice (A) is a quantitative abnormality. Qualitative abnormalities such as choice (C) refer principally to alterations in platelet function, which may include a decreased procoagulant activity of platelets, decreased platelet adhesiveness and decreased aggregation in response to ADP, thrombocytosis associated with myeloproliferative disorders, and the coating of platelets by fibrin degradation products as a result of the increased activation of coagulation factors. (585–586)

9. **The answer is (A).**   Liver disease may result from a variety of causes, including tumor invasion, chemotherapy, infection, or surgical resection. Regardless, it may either interfere with the synthesis of plasma coagulation factors or interfere with their functioning, decreasing hemostasis. Other causes of hypocoagulability include vitamin K deficiency, the use of large amounts of frozen plasma, the presence of coagulation protein antagonists, and coagulation factor deficiencies. (588)

10. **The answer is (D).** DIC always results from an underlying disease process that triggers abnormal activation of thrombin formation. Thrombin is both a powerful coagulant and an agent of fibrinolysis. Thus small clots may be formed in the microcirculation of many organs at the same time clots and clotting factors are being consumed. The result is hemorrhage as the body is unable to respond to vascular or tissue injury. (589–590)

11. **The answer is (C).** Vitamin K might be administered to a patient experiencing **hypo**coagulability, but not the **hyper**coagulability caused by DIC. All of the other therapies may provide short-term relief of DIC symptoms. Treatment of the underlying malignancy is vital in treating the patient with DIC, inasmuch as the tumor is the ultimate stimulus. (591)

12. **The answer is (B).** Because diagnostic signals may be subtle, including skin petechiae that may be noticed while bathing the person, traces of blood during tooth brushing, etc., it is important for the nurse to be keenly observant. A family history and various screening tests may be valuable in assessment, but they do not substitute for observation. (591–592)

13. **The answer is (D).** This screening test is called **prothrombin time (PT).** Choice (A) is the platelet aggregation test; (B) is the specific factor assays test; (C) is the bleeding time test. (593)

14. **The answer is (B).** If the patient requires parenteral administration of medication, the intravenous route is used whenever possible. Intramuscular and subcutaneous injections place the patient at risk for the development of hematomas. Injections, if unavoidable, are administered with a needle of the smallest possible gauge. (594)

15. **The answer is (A).** Because a random donor platelet concentrate consists of four units of platelets from four different donors, it may expose the recipient to multiple tissue antigens leading to platelet refractoriness. A single donor platelet concentrate is taken from one donor; patients are therefore not exposed to multiple antigens. This may be important with patients who are severely immunosuppressed, such as those who have undergone bone marrow transplantation. (596)

16. **The answer is (D).** Choice (A) is wrong because erythropoietin acts on the erythroid cell line, not on stem cells. Choice (B) is wrong because erythropoietin is produced only by the kidneys. Choice (C) is wrong because RBCs are produced by the bone marrow. (578)

17. **The answer is (D).** CSFs mediate all of these steps. (576–578)

18. **The answer is (C).** Thromboplastin is needed for conversion of prothrombin to thrombin, and its formation results from both pathways of the clotting cascade—the intrinsic and extrinsic pathways. (580)

19. **The answer is (D).** Tumor effects on the body can lead to bleeding for numerous reasons, which include invasion into nearby vascular tissue, cavitational or ulcerative effects from infection, and such destructive effects of radiotherapy as tissue fibrosis. Chemotherapy does not have a direct effect on bleeding other than to cause myelosuppression and thrombocytopenia. (580–581)

20. **The answer is (D).** The patient presents with typical symptoms of anemia of chronic illness associated with long-term therapy. Myelophthisis can also cause these symptoms, but not before fever neutropenia, etc. (581)

26   Fatigue

STUDY OUTLINE

I.   INTRODUCTION

1. **Acute fatigue** is a relatively temporary state that is relieved by rest. When fatigue persists over time, it is known as **chronic fatigue** or **chronic fatigue syndrome.**
   a. Chronic fatigue may not respond to rest, persists over time, and often interferes with performance of daily activities.
2. Individuals with cancer may experience both acute and chronic fatigue as a result of the **disease,** as a **side effect of treatment,** and as a result of the **psychological distress** produced by the diagnosis.
3. The incidence of fatigue in cancer patients treated with surgery, radiation therapy, chemotherapy, or biologic response modifiers (BRMs) is **90%.**
4. Despite evidence of the incidence and importance of fatigue among individuals with cancer, research has been limited.

II.   DEFINITION OF FATIGUE

1. Fatigue has been defined in terms of both **objective performance** and **subjective experience.**
2. Research into the **objective performance** view of fatigue focused initially on job or athletic performance. The aim was to identify the causes of fatigue and find ways to improve performance.
   a. Fatigue is defined in terms of some **objective indicator** of the point at which performance declines, e.g., accuracy of completion of some mental task.
   b. Physical weakness represents a muscular performance deficit demonstrated on objective testing.
3. In the **subjective experience** approach, fatigue is considered both a **feeling state** and the **impact of that state on the individual's perception of his or her ability to engage in usual activities.**
   a. Subjectively defined fatigue has a **voluntary** component, since individuals may push themselves to engage in a valued activity.
4. The subjective view of fatigue is more relevant to the nursing care of cancer patients.
   a. Patients' actions will most often be based on their **perceptions** rather than on some objective indicator.
   b. Some will define their fatigue in terms of **sensations,** others in terms of their **perception of their ability to engage in usual activities.**
   c. Nursing care focuses on helping those who are at risk for fatigue or experiencing fatigue to plan for and deal with the experience.

III.   PATHOPHYSIOLOGY OF FATIGUE

A.   THEORIES OF CAUSATION

1. Although no clear support for any of the major hypotheses for fatigue has emerged, all of the different hypotheses are potentially relevant to explaining at least some aspects of the fatigue experienced by individuals with cancer.
2. These major hypotheses include
   a. The **accumulation hypothesis,** which proposes that a buildup of waste products in the body produces fatigue.
   b. The **depletion hypothesis,** which proposes that muscular activity is impaired when certain substances (e.g., carbohydrates) are not readily available.

    c.   Hypotheses based on **biochemical and physiochemical phenomena,** which focus on changes in the production or balance of substances such as muscle proteins, glucose, electrolytes, and hormones.

    d.   Hypotheses based on **central nervous system control,** including Grandjean's neurophysiologic model, which focuses on the balance between the reticular activating system and inhibitory system.

    e.   Selye's hypothesis based on **adaptation and energy reserves,** which suggests that every individual has a certain amount of superficial energy available for adaptation and that fatigue occurs when the energy supply is depleted.

        (1) It incorporates elements from other hypotheses and focuses on the individual's response to stressors.

    f.   The **psychobiologic-entropy hypothesis** seeks to associate activity, fatigue, symptoms, and functional status based on clinical observations that individuals who become less active due to disease and or treatment-related symptoms lose energizing metabolic resources.

        (1) This hypothesis is summarized in four propositions.

            (a)   Too much as well as too little rest contributes to feelings of fatigue.

            (b)   Too little as well as too much activity contributes to feelings of fatigue.

            (c)   A balance between activity and rest promotes restoration; an imbalance promotes fatigue and deterioration.

            (d)   Any symptom that contributes to decreased activity will lead to increased fatigue and decreased functional status.

        (2) Fatigue can be a **primary symptom,** a direct consequence of preexisting conditions or a **secondary symptom** in which it is a result of the person's physiologic or psychosocial response.

        (3) Three strategies for nursing interventions are aimed at mitigating fatigue:

            (a)   symptom alleviation

            (b)   individualized activity/exercise program

            (c)   combination of (a) and (b).

  3. Individuals with cancer require energy to deal with symptoms and side effects. They may also experience disruption in their usual restorative activities when nausea, pain, or urinary frequency interferes with sleep and rest.

IV.   CANCER AND FATIGUE: PATHOPHYSIOLOGY AND PATHOPSYCHOLOGY

A.   TREATMENT EFFECTS

  1. Fatigue is a consistent finding in patients who are recovering from **surgery** and is generally assumed to have multiple causes.

  2. Fatigue is the only systemic side effect of local **radiation treatment** and has been reported to be the most severe side effect of radiation during the last week of treatment.

    a.   In most forms of cancer, fatigue appears to **increase throughout treatment** and decline gradually following treatment.

    b.   In lung cancer, fatigue is highest at the **beginning of treatment** and declines before the end of treatment.

        (1) This may have to do with the increased energy expenditure required for breathing through partially obstructed airways.

        (2) Radiation therapy may decrease tumor size, reopen airways, and thereby reduce fatigue.

  3. Despite the variation among treatment regimens, fatigue is the most prevalent side effect experienced by patients receiving **chemotherapy** for cancer.

  4. **Biotherapy** appears to produce fatigue that is more severe than that associated with surgery, radiation treatment, and the most commonly used chemotherapy regimens.

    a.   The severity may exceed the individual's level of tolerance, causing the person to terminate treatment.

    b.   Since fatigue is a dose-limiting side effect of biologic response modifiers (BRMs), including interferons, a high priority of nursing care of individuals receiving BRM therapy is preventing and ameliorating fatigue.

B. **OTHER ETIOLOGIC FACTORS**

    1. In addition to direct effects of treatment, cancer patients experience a variety of problems that may produce fatigue, including both **physical** and **psychosocial factors.**

        a. **Physical factors**

            (1) **Physical problems** such as pain, pruritis, urinary frequency, nausea, and vomiting may interfere with patients' ability to sleep.

            (2) A number of other factors, including anorexia, hepatic and renal damage, side effects of medications, diabetes, bone marrow depression, amputation, and alcohol and drugs may contribute to these and other symptoms and therefore to fatigue.

        b. **Psychosocial factors**

            (1) **Anxiety** and **depression** can result from the disruption in lifestyle produced by fatigue. This may occur when fatigue experienced as a side effect of cancer treatment forces the individual to give up usual social roles or makes it impossible to reach desired goals.

                (a) Fatigue affects different people different ways. Some find its impact on normal activity acceptable while others do not.

            (2) Some individuals may try to combine cancer treatment with their usual daily activities. Fatigue may be the result of expending too much energy.

V. **NURSING CARE OF THE CANCER PATIENT WITH FATIGUE**

    1. **In helping the cancer patient maintain the highest quality of life, the nurse must understand the possible causes of the fatigue as well as the patient's values, coping resources, usual activities, and perception of fatigue.**

A. **ASSESSMENT**

    1. **Level of fatigue**

        a. Patient **self-reporting** of fatigue is generally more accurate than nurses' judgments or observations. Various self-report measures may be used.

        b. Level of fatigue can be assessed by the nurse using observations of the individual's **appearance, level of consciousness, activity level,** or **patient reports of activity level.** However, such measures may represent a response to a variety of problems, such as nausea or pain, and they generally are not very sensitive.

        c. Level of fatigue should be assessed at multiple points in time. The nurse must obtain information about both the daily pattern of fatigue and variations in fatigue in relation to the treatment cycle.

    2. **Usual activities**

        a. **Figure 23-2, text page 491,** contains a list of questions that can be used to assess the cancer patient's level of fatigue and patterns of usual activities.

        b. Patients should be asked to **describe a typical day.** Those who report fatigue should be asked to describe **what they do about it** and to indicate **the extent to which their self-care activities are effective in relieving their fatigue.**

        c. The nurse should also

            (1) Determine who might be available to assume some of the individual's usual responsibilities.

            (2) Learn the meaning and value of each of the individual's activities.

    3. **Additional assessment data**

        a. The assessment includes **potential causes of fatigue,** including other chronic diseases as well as infection, pain, acute CNS changes, sleep disruption, overexertion, dehydration, electrolyte imbalances, malnutrition, anxiety, and depression.

        b. A careful **review of the patient's medical and social history,** including previous and current cancer treatment, laboratory data, and a thorough physical assessment, are essential in obtaining information about potential causes of fatigue.

B. **INTERVENTIONS**

    1. The types of interventions that are suggested for dealing with fatigue include

        a. **Providing preparatory information** to structure the person's expectations about receiving chemotherapy or radiation therapy.

b. **Decreasing activities** and **increasing sleep or rest,** which may mean controlling the side effects that interfere with sleep and rest.
(1) Medication may be used with some individuals to induce sleep or reduce anxiety.
c. **Rearranging activities** to allow for rest periods or to shorten the time that high-energy output is required.
(1) Subjects can learn to limit energy expenditure through careful planning and scheduling, decreasing activities, and depending on others.
d. **Planning activities to coincide with the time the individual feels most energetic,** e.g., doing errands when energy levels are highest.
e. **Encouraging exercise,** including short walks or the patient's usual exercise.
f. **Manipulating the environment** to allow undisturbed sleep and rest as well as providing adequate stimulation to prevent boredom-related fatigue.
(1) The nurse or family member may at times have to perform the daily activities for the person so that he or she can conserve energy.
g. **Extending interventions** after treatment ends and until normal activities can resume.
(1) Individuals with advanced cancer may require the use of assistive devices such as wheelchairs and grab rails and other measures that conserve energy and maintain the best possible quality of life.
h. See **Figure 26-2, text page 616,** for a teaching guide for fatigue.

PRACTICE QUESTIONS

1. Individuals with cancer may experience acute or chronic fatigue as a result of a number of factors. Which of the following is **least** likely to be a cause of cancer-related fatigue?
(A) the side effects of cancer treatment
(B) the psychological distress of cancer diagnosis
(C) the effects of cancer on objective performance
(D) the disease itself

2. Several hypotheses have been proposed to explain fatigue. Which of the following statements concerning these hypotheses is correct?
(A) The accumulation hypothesis proposes that muscular activity is impaired when certain substances (e.g., carbohydrates) are not readily available.
(B) Selye's hypothesis based on adaptation and energy reserves incorporates elements from other hypotheses.
(C) Grandjean's neurophysiologic model has gained universal acceptance among cancer researchers.
(D) The depletion hypothesis proposes that a buildup of waste products in the body produces fatigue.

3. The form of cancer therapy that appears to produce the **most** severe fatigue is
(A) surgery.
(B) local radiation treatment.
(C) most common forms of chemotherapy.
(D) biologic response modifiers.

4. In most forms of cancer, fatigue appears to increase throughout treatment and decline gradually following treatment. In lung cancer, however, fatigue is highest at the beginning of treatment and declines before the end of treatment. This is probably because
(A) radiation therapy decreases tumor size, thereby facilitating breathing and consequently reducing fatigue.
(B) lung cancer is more likely to be treated with total body irradiation than are other types of cancers.
(C) the effects of radiation therapy are greatest at the cellular level.
(D) lung cancer is more likely to be treated with local irradiation than are other types of cancers.

5. Fatigue may produce anxiety or depression in some individuals with cancer. The **best** explanation for this effect is that
(A) fatigue-induced electrolyte imbalances often trigger feelings of anxiety or depression.
(B) fatigue and anxiety and depression have the same etiology.
(C) treatment-induced fatigue may force the individual to give up usual social roles.
(D) anxiety or depression frequently forces individuals with cancer to expend too much energy.

6. In assessing levels of fatigue in cancer patients, the nurse generally will receive the **most** relevant information from
   (A) the physical examination.
   (B) objective ratings of fatigue.
   (C) patient self-reports of fatigue.
   (D) assessment measures based on levels of activity.

7. Among the following assessment measures, the one **least** likely to be a valuable source of information in assessing fatigue in the individual with cancer is the patient's
   (A) self-report of fatigue.
   (B) description of a typical day.
   (C) medical and social history.
   (D) level of consciousness.

8. The types of interventions that are suggested for dealing with fatigue in cancer patients include all of the following **except**
   (A) providing preparatory information to structure the person's expectations about receiving chemotherapy or radiation therapy.
   (B) manipulating the environment to provide adequate stimulation to prevent boredom-related fatigue.
   (C) discouraging exercise to avoid increasing levels of fatigue.
   (D) rearranging activities to allow for rest periods or to shorten the time that high-energy output is required.

ANSWER EXPLANATIONS

1. **The answer is (C).** The patient's assessment of fatigue is likely to be based on subjective experience, especially on his or her perceptions, rather than on some objective indicator of performance. A subjective experience definition of fatigue considers both a feeling state (how do I feel?) and the impact of that state on the individual's perception of his or her ability to engage in usual activities (what do I feel like doing?). Any of the other factors, often in combination with the others, can produce fatigue. (609)

2. **The answer is (B).** Selye's hypothesis based on adaptation and energy reserves suggests that every individual has a certain amount of superficial energy available for adaptation, and that fatigue occurs when the energy supply is depleted. It incorporates elements from other hypotheses and focuses on the individual's response to stressors. The definitions in choices (A) and (D) are reversed. No clear support for any of the major hypotheses for fatigue, including Grandjean's, has emerged, although all are potentially relevant to explaining aspects of fatigue as it relates to cancer. (609–610)

3. **The answer is (D).** Based on the limited information available on the incidence and characteristics of fatigue associated with the use of biologic response modifiers, it appears that this cancer treatment modality is likely to produce fatigue that is more severe than that associated with surgery, radiation treatment, and the most commonly used chemotherapy regimens. (613)

4. **The answer is (A).** The increased energy expenditure required for breathing through partially obstructed airways may cause extreme fatigue in the individual with lung cancer. If radiation therapy is successful in decreasing tumor size, individuals who enter treatment with some degree of airway obstruction are likely to experience some relief of fatigue as a result of the treatment. This is not true with other forms of cancer. (612)

5. **The answer is (C).** Anxiety and depression can result from the disruption in lifestyle produced by fatigue. This may occur when fatigue experienced as a side effect of cancer treatment forces the individual to give up usual social roles or makes it impossible to reach desired goals. (614)

6. **The answer is (C).** Since the patient's perception of fatigue will influence decisions about activities, participation in treatment, and overall quality of life, so-called objective ratings of fatigue made by health care professionals are less relevant to the patient's situation than assessments made by the patient. Various self-report measures are available for use by the nurse. Any measure of activity level as an indicator of fatigue is problematic in that it may represent a response to a variety of problems, such as nausea and pain, rather than a report of fatigue. (615)

7. **The answer is (D).**   Measures of level of consciousness and appearance are likely to represent multiple causes, including physical and psychosocial side effects of treatment other than fatigue. An assessment of fatigue should also focus on potential causes of fatigue, including other chronic diseases as well as infection, pain, acute CNS changes, sleep disruption, overexertion, dehydration, electrolyte imbalances, malnutrition, anxiety, and depression. (615)

8. **The answer is (C).**   Individuals for whom exercise is not contraindicated can be encouraged to try short walks or their usual exercise to see if it relieves their fatigue. Other interventions include decreasing activities and increasing sleep or rest and planning activities to coincide with periods of highest energy. The environment may also be manipulated to allow undisturbed sleep and rest. (617)

27 Nutritional Disturbances

STUDY OUTLINE

I. PATHOPHYSIOLOGY OF MALNUTRITION IN CANCER

    1. **Protein-calorie malnutrition** occurs when the protein-calorie composition of the diet does not meet the individual's physiologic requirements.

    2. Malnourished individuals are more susceptible to infection and are less likely to tolerate or derive benefit from cancer therapy.

  A. METABOLIC EFFECTS OF THE TUMOR

    1. **Cachexia, the most severe malnutrition syndrome in cancer, is characterized by profound and progressive loss of body weight, fat, and muscle.**
      a. One-half to two-thirds of all individuals with cancer experience cachexia, and it is one of the major causes of mortality.
      b. There is little correlation between cachexia and tumor extent, type, and location.
      c. Cachexia may result in part from **paraneoplastic syndromes** arising from the abnormal production of peptides by cancer cells, which lead to metabolic alterations in the host.
    2. **Altered carbohydrate metabolism**
      a. Tumors predominantly use **anaerobic glycolysis** in glucose metabolism, a process far less efficient in energy production than **oxidative respiration.**
        (1) The tumor uses glucose for its own growth, demanding increasing amounts as it enlarges.
      b. The lactic acid produced by anaerobic glycolysis is recruited back into glucose production in a process called **gluconeogenesis,** which is quite energy-consuming and occurs at an increased rate in persons with cancer.
      c. A third aberration of carbohydrate metabolism present in individuals with cancer is **glucose intolerance.**
    3. **Altered protein metabolism**
      a. Abnormalities of protein metabolism and protein depletion are common in individuals with cancer, especially those with cachexia.
        (1) Loss of 30% of protein content will cause death.
      b. A number of factors may be responsible for the protein depletion in individuals with cancer.
        (1) The tumor takes up **increased amounts of amino acids,** which are converted to lactic acid and returned to glucose through gluconeogenesis.
        (2) **Protein synthesis is decreased** in persons with cancer, even in those with a normal food intake.
        (3) The **breakdown of muscle protein,** particularly skeletal muscle, is accelerated in humans with cancer.
        (4) Loss of protein through **abnormal excretion and leakage,** e.g., via decubitus ulcers or fistulas, can contribute significantly to depletion of protein stores and decreased muscle mass.
        (5) In the healthy adult, during fasting, fat deposits are the first to be used to meet energy needs. In cancer cachexia, protein use **continues independent of the host's nutritional intake.**
    4. Research results are conflicting regarding the degree to which **lipid metabolism** is altered in individuals with cancer. Some argue that lipid mobilization is increased as a result of the tumor's excessive energy needs. Others find this process unchanged by tumor presence.

5. **Fluid and electrolyte imbalances**
   a. There are several common tumor-related fluid and electrolyte abnormalities that occur in persons with cancer.
      (1) In some tumors (e.g., lung, parathyroid), an ectopic parathyroidlike hormone causes **hypercalcemia** and the deposition of calcium in renal tubules and may result in a gradual or sudden onset of **renal failure.**
      (2) **Hyperuricemia,** due either to tumor lysis syndrome or rapid neoplastic growth, involves a sudden increase of uric acid in the plasma. Urate crystals may be deposited in the kidneys, causing **renal damage.**
      (3) **Hyponatremia** may be seen with some tumors, particularly lung cancer, which causes the **syndrome of inappropriate antidiuretic hormone (SIADH),** characterized by persistent urinary loss of sodium.
      (4) Renin-secreting tumors (e.g., hypernephromas) cause increased secretion of aldosterone, resulting in **hypokalemia.**
6. **Increased energy expenditure**
   a. **Protein turnover** and **gluconeogenesis** are energy-requiring metabolic processes that are increased in individuals with cancer, causing a tremendous drain on energy reserves.
   b. In cancer, **increased basal metabolic rate** is a frequent feature of advanced disease, even when food intake is decreased.
7. **Altered taste**
   a. Cancer patients often experience a general reduction in taste perception **(hypogeusesthesia)** and/or a perverted sense of taste **(dysgeusia),** causing, for example, a decreased threshold for bitter tastes and an increased threshold for sugar.
   b. Deficiencies of zinc, copper, nickel, niacin, and vitamin A have been implicated in decreased or altered taste sensations.
   c. **Learned aversions,** which may develop when a food is associated with unpleasant symptoms such as nausea, may be a major factor in taste changes.
8. **Anorexia**
   a. **Anorexia** is often an initial symptom of cancer and is sometimes the first evidence of recurrence or progression of disease.
   b. Various factors contribute to anorexia in persons with cancer.
      (1) **Increased circulating lipids and peptides** may create a false interpretation of satiety by the hypothalamus.
      (2) Researchers speculate that **increased brain levels of certain neurotransmitters,** such as **serotonin or tryptophan,** may cause decreased food intake.
      (3) **Taste changes,** outlined above, may lead to altered dietary habits and a lack of interest in food.
      (4) **Physical discomfort** may depress appetite or may impair the motor functions necessary to eating.
9. **Immunosuppression**
   a. **Malnutrition has a number of deleterious effects on the immune system.**
      (1) Lymphatic structures of the immune systems are decreased in size and weight in malnourished persons.
      (2) Decreased phagocytic activity, due to deficiency of protein for synthesis of phagocytes, is a consequence of malnutrition.
      (3) The greater the degree of malnutrition, the larger the decrease of T-lymphocytes in the peripheral circulation, sometimes leading to **anergy,** a total absence of hypersensitivity response.
      (4) The percentage of B-lymphocytes may decrease as malnutrition progresses.
      (5) Malnutrition compromises the complement system, due to a deficiency of protein to synthesize the complement factors, thereby increasing susceptibility to infection.
   b. **Cancer prognosis appears to be closely related to the degree of immunosuppression, and the degree of immunosuppression is related to the degree of malnutrition.**

B. **MECHANICAL EFFECTS OF THE TUMOR**

   1. The nutritional consequences of tumor destruction depend on factors such as tumor location, type, extent, and invasiveness versus encapsulation. **Table 27-1, text page 625,** shows some of the nutritional consequences of expanding tumors.

C.   **NUTRITIONAL CONSEQUENCES OF CANCER TREATMENT**

1.   **Anorexia** may be caused by many of the treatments for cancer.
2.   **Constipation,** caused by factors such as drugs (e.g., vincristine, narcotics), immobility, and certain surgical procedures, creates a full abdominal feeling and contributes to anorexia.
3.   **Diarrhea** is most commonly the result of chemotherapy or abdominal radiation, both of which cause mucosal toxicity. Malabsorption, dehydration, and electrolyte imbalances may occur.
4.   **Gastrointestinal fistulas** may develop due to tissue necrosis adjacent to an expanding tumor, tissue destruction due to chemotherapy or radiotherapy, or surgery.
5.   **Fluid and electrolyte disturbances** occur frequently as a result of cancer therapy, causing vomiting, diarrhea, and fistulas.
6.   All cancer treatment techniques predispose individuals to **infection;** infection increases metabolic demands on the host and may facilitate malnutrition.
7.   **Intestinal malabsorption** may result from
   a.   Interruption to the structure of the bowel and subsequently the absorptive surface through surgery.
   b.   Damage to the absorptive surface of the bowel due to injury to epithelial cells by cytotoxic drugs or radiation.
   c.   Lack of the substances (e.g., bile, digestive enzymes, gastric secretions) necessary for the absorption of nutrients.
8.   **Mucositis** is a consequence of the rapid turnover of epithelial cells of the mucous membranes, which makes them vulnerable to the toxicities of chemotherapy and radiotherapy.
   a.   Chemotherapy, as a systemic treatment, puts all mucous membranes at risk, but the most common sites of mucositis are the **oral cavity** and the **esophagus.**
   b.   Mucosal tissue included in a radiation field is at risk for damage; the development and severity of mucositis following radiotherapy depends on the **dose of radiation** and the **method of administration.**
9.   **Nausea and vomiting** are most commonly associated with the administration of **antineoplastic drugs** (especially cisplatin, doxorubicin, and dacarbazine), mediated by the chemoreceptor trigger zone.
10. **Taste changes** may occur in individuals undergoing antineoplastic therapy.
   a.   Some chemotherapy drugs (cisplatin, cytoxan) cause a metallic taste during administration, while others (5-fluorouracil) cause decreased sensitivity to salty and sweet tastes.
   b.   **Xerostomia,** decreased secretion of saliva, is caused by the destruction of taste buds and salivary cells during radiation to the head/neck, leading to decreased taste perception and difficult mastication.

II.   **NUTRITIONAL ASSESSMENT**

1.   **Nutritional assessment** is the critical first step in developing a plan to improve/maintain the nutritional status of the person with cancer. Its goals are to
   a.   **Identify individuals at risk.**
   b.   **Provide baseline data to develop a nutritional therapy plan.**
   c.   **Provide ongoing data to evaluate therapy.**

A.   **PHYSICAL SIGNS**

1.   Common manifestations of malnutrition include **sparse, thin hair; pallor; dull, sunken eyes; mouth lesions; muscle and tissue wasting;** and **edema.**
2.   **Mental status** should be evaluated for apathy and the ability to follow a nutrition care plan.

B.   **DIETARY HISTORY**

1.   It is important to elicit information about a person's usual **dietary habits,** including likes and dislikes, times of meals, and changes in diet as a result of illness/treatment.
2.   One common method of assessing a person's nutritional intake is a **dietary recall,** in which a person is asked to recall specific types and quantities of foods eaten over a specific period, usually 24 hours.
3.   If a more accurate dietary history is required, the individual may be asked to weigh and measure food (a **weighed inventory**).

4. These methods help to identify areas for intervention as well as tailor a plan to a patient's preferences and habits.

C. **ANTHROPOMETRIC MEASUREMENTS**

1. **Anthropometric measurements** are physical measurements of the human body that provide important information about nutritional status.
2. **Height and weight**
   a. **Height** should be obtained whenever possible.
   b. **Body weight** is one of the most important measurements of the nutritional assessment.
      (1) Weight loss in the person with cancer is associated with increased morbidity and mortality.
      (2) A sensitive index of nutritional status is **percent weight change,** which indicates the extent of tissue loss as a result of inadequate nutrition. A formula for determining this index is provided on **text page 629.** A means of evaluating weight change is given in **Table 27-2, text page 629.**
      (3) **Fluid composition** of the body (presence of edema or dehydration) can profoundly affect weight fluctuations.
3. The **skinfold thickness measurement** is the best single determinant of subcutaneous fat in the body tissues, reflecting changes in total body fat.
4. **Midarm muscle circumference** is a sensitive index of protein status that correlates significantly with serum albumin levels.

D. **BIOCHEMICAL MEASUREMENTS**

1. **Biochemical data** are the most specific of the assessment parameters, detecting **covert nutritional deficiencies.**
2. Standard measures of the **visceral protein compartment** include **serum albumin, serum transferrin,** and **prealbumin.** These measures assess the person's visceral protein status on a long-term, intermediate, and short-term basis, respectively.
   a. Serum protein measurements can be used to identify an individual's risk of developing complications.
3. **Urinary creatinine** is an excellent index of **lean body mass.** In the individual with cancer, creatinine excretion is decreased as muscle protein is degraded and used to meet energy requirements.

E. **IMMUNOLOGIC MEASUREMENTS**

1. **Immune function is a critical measure of nutritional status. The degree of T-lymphocyte depression correlates in an almost linear fashion with protein-calorie malnutrition.**
2. Two measurements that are commonly used to evaluate immune function in relation to nutritional status are **total lymphocyte count** and **skin sensitivity test to recall antigens.**

F. **SUMMARY**

1. **Table 27-3, text page 631,** summarizes the components of a nutritional assessment.
2. The recommended **protocol** for evaluating the efficacy of nutritional therapy includes
   a. **Daily:** body weight.
   b. **Twice weekly:** nitrogen balance (urinary creatinine, serum albumin).
   c. **Weekly:** total lymphocyte count.
   d. **Every three weeks:** anthropometric, skin tests, serum transferrin.

III. **NUTRITIONAL MANAGEMENT**

1. Aggressive **nutritional therapy** for individuals with cancer has been shown to decrease the morbidity and mortality of cancer and its therapy by
   a. **Preventing weight loss.**
   b. **Maintaining or improving nutritional status.**
   c. **Increasing responsiveness to therapy.**
   d. **Improving the individual's sense of well-being.**
   e. **Improving the quality of life.**

A. **CONTROVERSIES IN NUTRITIONAL SUPPORT**

1. Controversy exists over whether nutritional therapy is contraindicated in some individuals with cancer, because it permits or even encourages tumor growth by improving the supply of nutrients.
2. Research suggests that even if tumor stimulation does occur, the benefits to the individual in terms of outcome and well-being warrant nutritional therapy.
3. These benefits include
   a. **Fewer complications of antineoplastic therapies.**
   b. **Enhanced ability to tolerate larger doses of drugs.**
   c. **Positive nitrogen balance and weight gain.**
   d. **Possible enhanced tumor response to chemotherapy.**

B. **ESTABLISHING THE NUTRITIONAL THERAPY PLAN**

1. **Identifying the goal of nutritional therapy** will help determine the most effective method of
   a. Weight gain or weight maintenance.
   b. Restoration of immune function.
   c. Improved sense of well-being.
   d. Prolongation of life.
2. **Establishing the individual's caloric requirements** is accomplished on the basis of the nutritional assessment.
   a. **Basal metabolic rate (BMR)** is a measure of the amount of energy required to sustain life in a fasting, resting individual. It is determined primarily by body size, age, sex, and stress of illness.
   b. Only about 25% of patients with cancer are hypermetabolic; about 40%–50% are normometabolic.
   c. **Text page 632** provides a formula for determining caloric needs.
   d. **Activity level** is the major variable in the energy requirements of individuals.
   e. Once caloric needs have been established, the composition of the diet and method of feeding may be determined.
3. **Composition of the diet**
   a. **The main aim of nutritional therapy is to protect or restore body protein.**
   b. **Nitrogen balance** is an index of protein balance in the body. A negative nitrogen balance implies that body protein is being depleted.
   c. In the normal individual, 7%–8% of the total calories must be provided by protein to maintain a positive protein balance; this amount is doubled in hypermetabolic states.
   d. **Energy requirements, present nutritional deficits, allergies, preferences, and conditions that affect digestion or absorption must all be considered in determining the composition of the diet.**

C. **ENTERAL NUTRITION**

1. The nutritional benefits of enteral (oral and tube feeding) and parenteral nutrition are comparable; the major factor in choosing between them is **bowel function.** If the gastrointestinal tract is normal and patent, **enteral nutrition** is the treatment of choice.
2. **Oral feeding**
   a. If an individual is unable to eat an adequate amount of regular food, the diet may be supplemented or replaced with liquid nutritional formulas.
   b. Composition of the diet may need to be altered based on the symptoms the individual experiences as a result of the tumor or cancer treatments.
   c. **Figure 27-4, text pages 634–635,** offers an extensive list of suggested approaches to problems that interfere with normal nutrition.
   d. Generally, it is the nurse's responsibility to observe and record the person's tolerance of the diet and the quantities of food consumed.
   e. The nurse should be aware that persons with cancer may be following **unconventional diets** that may be deficient in many essential nutrients and calories.
3. **Enteral feeding**
   a. If oral intake cannot prevent weight loss, or if a person's physical condition prevents oral intake for prolonged periods, **tube feeding** may be required.

      b. Tube feedings may be administered by **nasogastric intubation, esophagostomy, gastrostomy, or jejunostomy.**

      c. **Diarrhea** is the most common side effect of tube feeding.

        (1) It is usually treated by decreasing the volume or rate of delivery.

        (2) It may also be caused by the **high osmolarity** of the tube feeding, which can be adjusted by decreasing the concentration of the liquid.

      d. **Blood glucose levels** and **electrolyte status** should be carefully monitored.

    4. **Liquid formulas for enteral nutrition**

      a. The advantage of liquid feedings is that they **can be ingested and digested easily.**

      b. The major disadvantages are their **monotony, cost,** and **lack of satisfaction** associated with foods of varying textures.

      c. Commercially prepared liquid formulas provide approximately 1 to 2 kcal/ml.

    5. The efficacy of an enteral feeding is evaluated primarily by the person's **ability to gain or maintain weight** and by an **improvement in nitrogen balance.**

D. PARENTERAL NUTRITION

    1. **Total parenteral nutrition (TPN)** is the intravenous infusion of a concentrated mixture of proteins, glucose, fluid, minerals, electrolytes, and trace elements into a central vein.

    2. When used appropriately, TPN improves response to cancer therapy and improves quality of life.

    3. **TPN is indicated when it becomes impractical or impossible to administer food through the GI tract or when other feeding methods fail to provide sufficient calories and nutrients to meet metabolic needs.**

    4. A person is considered to be eligible for TPN if enteral therapy has failed or is inappropriate and two or more of the following criteria are met:

      a. **Weight loss of 10% or more from the usual.**

      b. **Serum albumin level below 3.5 g/dL.**

      c. **Immunoincompetence to recall skin test antigens.**

    5. Three categories of complications are associated with TPN therapy.

      a. **Infection**

        (1) Glucose and protein-rich TPN solutions provide an excellent medium for bacterial/fungal growth.

        (2) Infection results from **contamination of the TPN solution, insertion site, or equipment used,** or through **seeding of the catheter tip by blood-borne infection.**

        (3) Skin organisms are the most frequent cause of sepsis (e.g., *S. aureus, S. epidermidis, Klebsiella,* fungi).

      b. **Mechanical complications**

        (1) **Thromboses** of the catheter lumen or, rarely, of the central vein itself are the most common mechanical problems associated with TPN therapy.

        (2) **Air embolism** is a rare but potentially fatal complication.

        (3) **Precipitation of minerals** may occur, especially with calcium phosphate.

      c. **Metabolic complications**

        (1) The most common metabolic complications of TPN are listed in **Table 27-5, text page 638.**

        (2) **Hyperglycemia,** the most common metabolic complication, occurs in approximately 15% of persons receiving TPN. It is best treated by adding crystalline insulin to each TPN solution.

        (3) In order to prevent hypoglycemia, the TPN infusion should be **tapered** for an hour or two before discontinuation, if time permits.

        (4) **Essential fatty acid deficiency** is prevented by administration of lipid emulsions to individuals who receive TPN longer than 14 days without dietary fat intake. **Text page 639** provides a list of guidelines for lipid emulsion infusion.

E. PHARMACOLOGIC TREATMENT OF CACHEXIA

    1. **Megestrol acetate,** a synthetic derivative of progesterone used in the hormonal treatment of breast cancer and prostate cancer, causes weight gain and increased appetite.

    2. The use of megestrol acetate as a treatment of cachexia due to cancer has been proposed.

F.   NUTRITIONAL THERAPY AT HOME

1.   **Home nutritional support is indicated for persons who would otherwise not need to be hospitalized.**
2.   With sufficient instruction to the patient and family, tube feedings, whether by gravity or electronic infusion pump, can be accomplished at home with little difficulty.
3.   The individual who will be receiving long-term TPN at home will have a **Hickman- or Broviac-type catheter** placed, which entails proper instruction in meticulous catheter care.
4.   The most frequent complication of home TPN is **sepsis,** usually requiring removal of the catheter.

IV.   **FUTURE TRENDS**

1.   The major question in research about cancer and malnutrition is whether nutritional depletion in the individual with cancer is purely a manifestation of cancer that will resolve spontaneously after cancer therapy or whether nutritional intervention will actually improve treatment success.
2.   The goal is for nutritional assessment to be a prognosticator of cancer outcome, which requires the identification of assessment parameters that can measure response to nutritional therapy.

PRACTICE QUESTIONS

1.   Protein depletion is a common manifestation of cancer. Factors that may be responsible for this fact include all of the following **except**
     (A)   Protein synthesis is decreased, even in those with normal food intake.
     (B)   Breakdown of muscle protein is accelerated.
     (C)   Protein is lost through abnormal excretion and leakage.
     (D)   Tumors require only small amounts of protein to survive.

2.   Persons with cancer may experience fluid and electrolyte imbalances related to hyperuricemia. In this condition
     (A)   a sudden decrease in levels of serum uric acid causes renal failure.
     (B)   tumor lysis releases calcium deposits in the renal tubules, which leads to renal failure.
     (C)   tumor lysis causes the syndrome of inappropriate antidiuretic hormone secretion (SIADH).
     (D)   urate crystals may be deposited in the kidneys, causing renal failure.

3.   An example of a chemotherapeutic agent that may cause a metallic taste during administration, leading to taste changes, is
     (A)   etoposide.
     (B)   cyclophosphamide.
     (C)   doxorubicin.
     (D)   dacarbazine.

4.   Cancer patients often experience a general reduction in taste perception (hypogeusesthesia) and/or a perverted sense of taste (dysgeusia). One of the conditions implicated in this is
     (A)   sustained hyperglycemia.
     (B)   permanent damage to the chemoreceptor trigger zone.
     (C)   an increase in circulating lipids and peptides.
     (D)   vitamin and mineral deficiencies.

5.   Malnutrition negatively affects the immune system by causing
     (A)   a decrease in the number of circulating T-lymphocytes.
     (B)   an increase in the size of lymphatic structures.
     (C)   an increase in the frequency of immune hypersensitivity reactions.
     (D)   damage to the bone marrow.

6. All of the following are nutritional consequences of cancer treatment **except**
   (A) infection.
   (B) alopecia.
   (C) constipation.
   (D) diarrhea.

7. Xerostomia, a decrease in saliva secretion, is a side effect of
   (A) oral surgery.
   (B) bone marrow transplant.
   (C) cisplatin administration.
   (D) head and neck irradiation.

8. Dietary recall is a method of nutritional assessment in which a person is asked to recount the types and amounts of foods eaten over a specific period. A method that often is more accurate than a dietary recall is
   (A) a physical examination.
   (B) a dietary history.
   (C) a weighed inventory.
   (D) exercise tolerance testing.

9. Which of the following tests is used to determine protein status?
   (A) midarm muscle circumference
   (B) skinfold thickness measurement
   (C) daily weight
   (D) orthostatic vital signs

10. An analysis of biochemical data will often yield information regarding nutritional status. Decreased levels of urinary creatinine may be an indicator of
    (A) decreased mortality.
    (B) fat depletion.
    (C) increased gastrointestinal absorption.
    (D) decreased lean body mass.

11. Some researchers claim that nutritional therapy is contraindicated in persons with cancer because
    (A) it encourages tumor growth by improving the supply of nutrients.
    (B) improved nutritional status does not, over the long run, influence responsiveness to therapy or quality of life.
    (C) certain nutritional therapies put patients at higher risk for developing fatal infections.
    (D) changes in appetite are to be expected in someone undergoing treatment, and they will usually subside when treatment is completed.

12. Basal metabolic rate (BMR) is a measure of the amount of energy required to sustain life, and is determined by all of the following **except**
    (A) age.
    (B) body size.
    (C) presence of cancer.
    (D) sex.

13. In order to maintain a positive nitrogen/protein balance, how much of a normal individual's total caloric intake should derive from protein?
    (A) no more than 4%
    (B) at least 7%
    (C) at least 13%
    (D) at least 20%

14. The nutritional benefits of enteral and parenteral nutrition are comparable. The major factor in choosing between them is
    (A) cost.

    (B)   duration of the therapy.
    (C)   patient's preference.
    (D)   bowel function.

15.   The most common side effect of tube feedings is _____ and is usually treated by _____ .
    (A)   nausea; administration of antiemetics
    (B)   diarrhea; decreasing volume or rate of infusion
    (C)   constipation; increasing the amount of fluid given with the tube feeding
    (D)   infection; aseptic technique and administration of antibiotics as needed

16.   Criteria for selecting individuals with cancer to receive total parental nutrition (TPN) include all of the following **except**
    (A)   weight loss of 10% or more from the usual.
    (B)   a serum albumin below 3.5 g/dL.
    (C)   immunocompetence to a battery of recall skin antigens.
    (D)   a hypometabolic state.

17.   All of the following are potential metabolic complications of TPN **except**
    (A)   hypoglycemia.
    (B)   hyperglycemia.
    (C)   essential fatty acid deficiency.
    (D)   low platelets.

18.   Megestrol acetate, used in the hormonal treatment of breast and prostate cancers, may be effective in the treatment of cancer-induced cachexia because it causes
    (A)   improved immune function.
    (B)   increased appetite.
    (C)   slower rate of protein degradation.
    (D)   strengthening of the gastrointestinal mucosa.

ANSWER EXPLANATIONS

1.   **The answer is (D).**   Protein synthesis is decreased in individuals with cancer due to decreased intake and malnutrition and possibly due to decreased rate of serum albumin synthesis. Muscle degradation, especially skeletal muscle, is increased in individuals with cancer. Abnormal excretion and leakage (for example, through decubitus ulcers and fistulas) also can cause protein depletion. Tumors require large amounts of amino acids in order to fuel the process of gluconeogenesis, thus depriving the body of protein reserves. (622)

2.   **The answer is (D).**   Hyperuricemia involves a release of uric acid in the plasma during the process of tumor lysis. Urate crystals may be deposited in the kidney, causing damage and perhaps renal failure. (623)

3.   **The answer is (B).**   A common complaint during intravenous administration of drugs such as nitrogen mustard, cisplatin, and cyclophosphamide is that they cause a metallic taste. Some individuals become so sensitized to this taste that they become nauseated in anticipation of their administration. (627)

4.   **The answer is (D).**   Although the exact mechanisms responsible for taste changes in individuals with cancer remains unknown, it appears that nutritional deficiencies, among them deficiencies of vitamin A, zinc, copper, nickel, and niacin, may play a role. (623)

5.   **The answer is (A).**   Malnutrition causes a decrease in the number of circulating T-lymphocytes. With fewer T-lymphocytes, the hypersensitivity response to antigens is delayed, causing an alteration in immune function. Other undesirable effects of malnutrition on immunocompetency is a decrease in size of lymphatic structures, decreased phagocytic activity, and decreased B-lymphocyte function. (624)

6.   **The answer is (B).**   Treatment with chemotherapeutic agents such as vincristine may lead to constipation and ileus. Use of narcotics for pain control can also cause constipation. Diarrhea is associated with

both chemotherapy administration and radiotherapy; both cause mucosal toxicity in rapidly proliferating cells. Individuals receiving chemotherapy or radiotherapy have an increased risk of infection because of damage to hematopoietic tissue, which leads to neutropenia; infection increases an individual's metabolic needs and may precipitate malnutrition. (626)

7. **The answer is (D).** Radiotherapy to the head and neck region destroys taste buds and cells responsible for saliva secretion, resulting in xerostomia. A person who is experiencing this effect produces little saliva, and the saliva that is produced is viscid, acidic, and high in organic content. Affected individuals often complain of decreased taste perception and difficult mastication. (627)

8. **The answer is (C).** In a dietary recall, the quantities of food reported often are only estimates of what a person has consumed. A weighed inventory is much more accurate in that it requires actual weighing and recording of all of the food consumed in a specific period of time. (628)

9. **The answer is (A).** Mid-arm muscle circumference (arm circumference minus triceps skin fold) is felt to be an accurate indicator of protein status that correlates with serum albumin levels when done correctly by a trained individual. It is estimated that the measurement of mid-arm muscle circumference in the same person can vary by as much as 5% when calculated by different individuals. (629)

10. **The answer is (D).** Because all muscle produces creatinine, the proportion of creatinine produced is directly proportional to the amount of muscle in the body. In individuals with cancer and in other malnourished individuals, creatinine excretion is decreased as muscle protein is degraded for use as energy. (629)

11. **The answer is (A).** It is speculated by some that because the energy requirements of a tumor take precedence over the energy requirements of its host, providing more and better nutrition to a patient with cancer is actually permitting or encouraging tumor growth. Although this process is known to occur in rats, it is unclear whether it occurs similarly in humans. Other researchers feel that the benefits of nutrition in individuals with cancer outweigh the risks. (632)

12. **The answer is (C).** Basal metabolic rate (BMR) primarily is determined by a person's body size, but age, sex, and stress of illness are also factors. Although advanced cancer increases an individual's caloric needs, it is felt that the majority of persons with cancer are "normometabolic." (632)

13. **The answer is (B).** A normometabolic individual needs to receive 7%–8% of his or her calories from protein to provide a positive nitrogen balance. A person who is hypermetabolic has double the protein requirements and should receive at least 15%–20% of his or her total calories from protein. (632)

14. **The answer is (D).** Although cost, duration of therapy, and acceptability to the individual are all factors to be considered when selecting the methods of feeding an individual, it is patency of the gastrointestinal tract that ultimately determines whether enteral or parenteral nutrition will be the treatment of choice. (633)

15. **The answer is (B).** Diarrhea is the most common side effect of tube feedings, caused by bacterial contamination of formula, high osmolarity of fluid, lactose intolerance, and/or rapid administration. It is most commonly treated by slowing the rate of delivery of the feeding. If slowing the rate is ineffective, the concentration of the liquid can be adjusted to decrease its osmolarity; and if diarrhea persists, in the absence of *C. difficile* toxin, antidiarrheal medications may be indicated. (635–636)

16. **The answer is (C).** Total parenteral nutrition (TPN) is a mixture of proteins, glucose, fluid, vitamins, minerals, electrolytes, and trace elements usually administered through a large, central vein. When used appropriately, TPN improves response to cancer therapy and improves quality of life. TPN is indicated when it becomes impractical or impossible to administer food through the GI tract or when other feeding methods fail to provide sufficient calories and nutrients to meet metabolic needs. A person is considered to be eligible for TPN if enteral therapy has failed or is inappropriate and two or more of the following criteria are met: weight loss of 10% or more from the usual; serum albumin level below 3.5 g/dL; and immunoincompetence to recall skin test antigens. (636)

17. **The answer is (D).** Hyperglycemia caused by excessive total dose or rate of infusion of glucose, or inadequate endogenous insulin production, is a common metabolic complication of TPN therapy. Hypoglycemia, caused by persistence of insulin production secondary to prolonged stimulation of islet

cells by high glucose infusion, also is a possible complication. Essential fatty acid deficiency is possible if individuals are receiving prolonged (>14 days) TPN therapy without associated lipid administration. (637–638)

18.   **The answer is (B).**   Weight gain of 10 to 20 pounds or more, along with increased appetite, are common side effects of megestrol acetate, although the exact mechanism of action that brings about these side effects has not yet been determined. This, and its possible use in the treatment of cachexia in individuals with cancer and HIV infection, is currently being investigated. (639)

28   Hypercalcemia

STUDY OUTLINE

I.   **INTRODUCTION**

    A.   **INCIDENCE**

1. About 10%–20% of cancer patients will develop **hypercalcemia** at some point during the course of their disease. However, not all cancer patients are at the same risk of developing hypercalcemia.
2. **Tumor type** is one factor in the development of hypercalcemia in cancer patients.
    a. Patients with **lung cancer** account for 25%–35% of reported cases, while 20%–40% of cases occur in patients with **breast cancer.** This high frequency is related to high overall incidence of these two types of cancers.
    b. One-third of patients with **multiple myeloma,** a relatively rare cancer, develop hypercalcemia.
    c. Cancers of the stomach, duodenum, colon, rectum, biliary tract, and prostate are rare causes of hypercalcemia.
    d. See **Table 28-2, text page 646,** for a list of the reported frequencies of malignancy-associated hypercalcemia by tumor type.
3. **Tumor histology** is a second factor in the development of the condition.
    a. **Squamous histology** is the predominant histology for lung, esophageal, head and neck, and many female reproductive tumors.
    b. Although rare in patients with small-cell lung cancer, 23% of patients with squamous epidermoid carcinoma of the lung and 13% of those with large-cell anaplastic carcinoma of the lung will develop hypercalcemia.
4. **Hypercalcemia of malignancy is usually progressive, causes unpleasant symptoms, can cause the patient to deteriorate rapidly, and may be the cause of death in patients refractory to treatment.**
    a. Early stages have vague and nonspecific symptoms that can be confused with symptoms resulting from treatments.
5. The pathophysiology is complex and heterogeneous and usually involves a combination of both **bone resorption** and **decreased renal calcium clearance.**
6. Treatment approaches are numerous and vary with
    a. **The degree of hypercalcemia and associated symptomatology.**
    b. **The underlying malignancy.**
    c. **The patient's overall physical status and prognosis.**
7. Nurses play an important role in several aspects of treatment and care, including
    a. Recognition of patients at risk.
    b. Patient and family teaching.
    c. Early recognition and monitoring of symptoms and response to treatment.
    d. If necessary, assisting the patient and family in the terminal phases of illness.

    B.   **DEFINITION**

1. Hypercalcemia is considered to exist when the serum calcium level exceeds **11.0 mg/dL,** compared with the normal range of **8.5 to 10.5 mg/dL.**

II.   **PHYSIOLOGY OF CALCIUM HOMEOSTASIS**

1. Less than 1% of the body's calcium is available in an **extracellular, freely ionized,** and **biologically active** form that is available to influence such physiologic functions as clotting or cell membrane permeability. The rest is bound to phosphate in bone.

A. **NORMAL CALCIUM HOMEOSTASIS**

1. Extracellular calcium levels are controlled tightly within a narrow range, primarily through the effects of **parathyroid hormone (PTH)** and **1,25-dihydroxyvitamin D.**
    a. These two hormones exert their effects by controlling movement of calcium across three organs: **bone, kidney,** and **small intestine.**
    b. Renal regulation of calcium is controlled by PTH and 1,25-dihydroxyvitamin D. Only when pathologic states involving **increased bone resorption** (e.g., some malignancies, Paget's disease) occur do other homeostatic mechanisms come into play.
2. **Calcitonin**
    a. Calcitonin is secreted by thyroid parafollicular cells and acts as a **counterregulator** to PTH.
    b. In healthy adults, calcitonin appears to play a minor role in calcium homeostasis. However, it can be an important inhibitor of **bone resorption** in pathologic states, although its effects are transient.
3. **Parathyroid hormone**
    a. A drop in extracellular calcium stimulates release of PTH from the parathyroid glands. PTH then stimulates production of 1,25-dihydroxyvitamin D, which acts to **increase absorption of calcium from the intestine and thus elevate serum calcium levels.**
    b. PTH also acts directly on the kidneys to rapidly **regulate and fine tune calcium balance.**
    c. Sixty-five percent of calcium filtered by the glomerulus is resorbed in the proximal tubules. When patients are dehydrated, renal blood flow is decreased and sodium resorption is enhanced. **Calcium resorption accompanies sodium resorption, so dehydration can potentiate hypercalcemia by this mechanism.**
    d. In the skeleton, **PTH plays a mediating role in bone resorption by stimulating the number and activity of bone osteoclasts,** leading to the release of calcium and phosphate into the circulation.
4. **1,25-Dihydroxyvitamin D**
    a. 25-hydroxyvitamin D is the major circulating and storage form of vitamin D.
    b. 25-hydroxyvitamin D is hydroxylated in the proximal tubules of the kidney, under the influence of PTH, to form 1,25-dihydroxyvitamin D.
    c. 1,25-dihydroxyvitamin D acts on the gastrointestinal tract to **stimulate the absorption of dietary calcium in response to low circulating levels of calcium.**
    d. In disease states such as primary hyperparathyroidism, sarcoidosis, and T- and B-cell lymphomas, extra renal synthesis of 1,25-dihydroxyvitamin D may occur, thus increasing intestinal calcium absorption and producing hypercalcemia.
5. **Homeostatic responses to increased calcium loads**
    a. The more serum calcium, the less PTH secretion. The less PTH, the less calcium that is released from bone and absorbed from the intestine.
    b. This inhibitory effect of serum calcium occurs as a result of **decreased renal synthesis of 1,25-dihydroxyvitamin D** and **increased urinary calcium excretion.**
    c. The kidney is the principal route by which a calcium load can be cleared; it can increase calcium excretion approximately fivefold.
    d. Mild hypercalcemia impairs kidney function. Impaired renal function contributes to the development of hypercalcemia and renal failure.
6. **The role of bone in calcium homeostasis**
    a. **Skeletal bone serves as the body's calcium reservoir.**
    b. **In the healthy adult before middle life, bone resorption and formation are in balance** and occur in response to the need for repair and in response to local mechanical factors such as weight bearing and fluid pressure.
    c. **In disease states, the contribution of skeletal calcium to extracellular calcium levels assumes an important role.**
7. **Bone remodeling**
    a. **Skeletal bone** serves as the body's calcium reservoir. In the healthy adult before middle life, bone resorption and formation are in balance and occur as a renewal process in

response to the **need for repair** and to **local mechanical factors** such as weight bearing and fluid pressure.

b. Normal bone remodeling is **"coupled"**; bone resorption is coupled with bone formation. **"Uncoupling"** refers to the failure of bone formation to follow the resorption process.

c. Bone remodeling activity is influenced by **mechanical factors** such as weight bearing, by the activity of **osteotropic hormones,** and by **local factors** such as prostaglandins, regulatory proteins, and constituents of the organic matrix.

d. See **Table 28-3, text page 648,** for a list of cells responsible for bone remodeling and **Table 28-4, text page 649,** for a list of hormonal mediators of calcium homeostasis and bone remodeling.

e. At physiologic levels of osteotropic hormones, bone remodeling takes place in an orderly and coupled manner, as described in **Figure 28-1, text page 649.**

f. High levels of PTH and 1,25-dihydroxyvitamin D stimulate large volumes of osteocytic and osteoclastic breakdown and resorption of calcified matrix. Hormones that act as **growth factors for osteoclast progenitors** include the **bone-resorbing cytokines interleukin-1, tumor necrosis factor, and transforming growth factor alpha.**

g. An elevated **serum acid phosphatase** can indicate the presence of osteoclastic bone catabolism, as seen in metastatic skeletal involvement.

h. In pathologic states, including some malignancies, local and humoral factors that influence the liberation of calcium from bone assume more significance than skeletal calcium.

B. PATHOPHYSIOLOGY

1. Malignancy-associated hypercalcemia is a complex metabolic complication in which **bone resorption exceeds both bone formation and the kidney's ability to excrete extracellular calcium.**

2. Both **humoral** and **local factors** have been implicated in this process.
   a. Humoral, or tumor-produced, circulating factors include a **PTH-like factor, transforming growth factors,** and **1,25-dihydroxyvitamin D.**
   b. Local factors implicated include a family of **cytokine osteoclast-activating factors.**

3. **Humoral hypercalcemia of malignancy**
   a. **Hypercalcemia that develops in patients with solid tumors without bone metastases** is thought to be due to **tumor-produced systemic mediators of increased bone resorption.** See **Table 28-5, text page 650,** for a description of the source and action of several humoral factors implicated in the development of hypercalcemia and **Table 28-6, text page 651,** for a description of the source and action of local cytokines and growth factors influencing bone resorption.
   b. Several authors have suggested that a **PTH-related protein** contributes to hypercalcemia by stimulating increased renal calcium resorption while another agent works in concern with the PTH-related protein to enhance bone-resorbing activity.

4. **1,25-Dihydroxyvitamin D**
   a. **Increased** levels of **circulating 1,25-dihydroxyvitamin D** have been observed in hypercalcemia **in patients with Hodgkin's disease and non-Hodgkin's lymphoma without bone metastases.**
   b. This hypercalcemia resolved with effective treatment of the tumor. This suggests that tumors produce substances that act to increase levels of 1,25-dihydroxyvitamin D or to increase synthesis of 1,25-dihydroxyvitamin D by tumor-associated cells.

5. **Tumors with skeletal metastases**
   a. **The cause of hypercalcemia** in cancer patients with **skeletal metastases** such as breast cancer, multiple myeloma, and lymphoma is probably **multifactorial, including both humoral and local cell-mediated mechanisms.** Among the implicated factors are prostaglandin E, TGF-alpha, and the cytokines known as osteoclast-activating factor (OAF).
   b. Hypercalcemia occurs in up to 40% of women with **breast cancer.**
   c. Although the majority of breast cancer patients with hypercalcemia have widespread skeletal metastases, not all patients with metastases develop hypercalcemia.
   d. Evidence suggests that direct bone resorption by tumor cells is a minor component of the bone destruction that occurs with metastatic breast cancer.
   e. Hypercalcemia of breast cancer is generally responsive to osteoclast inhibitors, suggesting that osteoclast activation is the major mechanism associated with hypercalcemia. However, other factors have also been implicated. See **Table 28-7, text page 652,** for a comparison

of the implicated factors and clinical features of hypercalcemia in several types of tumors with skeletal metastases.

f. The presence of breast cancer cells at the bone surface may also stimulate a cell-mediated immune response and production of tumor necrosis factor or IL-1, both of which are potent bone-resorbing factors.

g. **Hematologic malignancies,** including multiple myeloma and lymphomas, are also associated with the development of hypercalcemia.

h. Twenty to forty percent of all multiple myeloma patients experience hypercalcemia at some time during the disease. Hypercalcemia can be either a presenting symptom or an indicator of terminal disease. Hypercalcemia in myeloma can be expected whenever patients become bedridden.

i. The **pathophysiology of hypercalcemia in multiple myeloma** is increased bone resorption (extensive bone destruction occurs adjacent to collections of myeloma cells) and decreased glomerular filtration (resulting in an inability to clear calcium through the glomerulus).

j. Causative factors for the hypercalcemia of multiple myeloma include GM-CSF, tumor necrosis factor, and IL-1, but it is not clear whether these factors are produced by the tumor or produced by normal immune cells in response to the presence of myeloma by the tumor cells.

k. In patients with lymphomas, hypercalcemia is usually seen in patients with bone involvement. However, humoral factors such as elevated levels of 1,25-dihydroxyvitamin D and PTH-related protein have also been implicated.

l. Other factors, including **immobilization, dehydration, inappropriate use of diuretics,** and **generalized wasting,** all play an important role in the pathogenesis of malignancy-associated hypercalcemia.

m. Weight bearing is important in preventing hypercalcemia due to immobilization.

III. **CLINICAL MANIFESTATIONS**

1. Hypercalcemia that develops slowly and gradually is associated with few, if any, symptoms.
2. Conversely, a **rapidly expanding tumor burden associated with a progressively increasing rate of bone resorption may suddenly overwhelm the kidney's ability to maintain calcium homeostasis, producing a rapid and symptomatic rise in serum calcium levels.** This is particularly true of **HHM.**

A. **SIGNS AND SYMPTOMS**

1. **Hypercalcemia produces symptoms in almost all organ systems.** Symptoms are numerous, vague, and nonspecific, and may be confused with those of end-stage disease.
2. Recognition of symptoms is important for early identification and treatment of the syndrome to reduce the risk of **coma, irreversible renal failure,** or a **terminal cardiac event.**
3. Common symptoms are **nausea, vomiting, polyurea, polydipsia, anorexia, weakness, fatigue,** and **confusion.** See **Table 28-8, text page 653,** for a complete list of signs and symptoms, affected systems, and mechanisms involved.
4. **Gastrointestinal**
    a. Elevated extracellular calcium levels **depress smooth muscle contractility,** leading to delayed gastric emptying and decreased gastrointestinal motility.
    b. Anorexia, nausea, vomiting, abdominal pain, and constipation are early common symptoms in patients with hypercalcemia.
5. **Neuromuscular**
    a. **Elevated extracellular calcium levels affect both the central nervous system (CNS) and neuromuscular function.**
    b. Initial CNS dysfunction can present as personality changes (such as extreme restlessness, irritability, and deterioration in cognitive function), impaired concentration, mild confusion, drowsiness, and lethargy.
    c. Neuromuscular involvement is primarily neuropathic, involving decreased muscle strength and a decrease in respiratory muscular capacity.
6. **Renal**
    a. **Hypercalcemia interferes with the action of ADH on the kidney's collecting tubules, causing an inability to concentrate urine and polyuria.** Subsequent volume contraction,

which may be exacerbated by nausea and vomiting, decreases the glomerular filtration rate.

    b. Decreased glomerular filtration stimulates sodium and water reabsorption in the proximal tubule. Since sodium and calcium are absorbed in parallel, hypercalcemia is exacerbated.

  7. **Cardiovascular**

    a. **Calcium ions affect cardiac muscle contractility and cell membrane permeability, as well as influencing the conduction of electrical impulses within the heart.**

    b. Hypercalcemia can produce bradycardia, hypertension, dysrhythmias, atrioventricular lock, and asystole.

    c. In patients taking digitalis, the development of significant dysrythmias is common, **and hypercalcemia may also potentiate digitalis toxicity.**

B. LABORATORY ASSESSMENT

1. An elevated serum calcium is diagnostic. When serum proteins are abnormal, however, as sometimes occurs in multiple myeloma, **ionized serum levels** provide a more accurate means of measuring calcium than does total serum calcium, which includes calcium bound to proteins.
2. When ionized calcium levels are not available, serum calcium levels can be corrected to reflect more accurately ionized serum calcium.

IV. TREATMENT

1. Treatment must be directed both at **excessive bone resorption** and **impaired renal calcium excretion.**

    a. Most important initially is improving renal calcium excretion, usually by **correcting dehydration and diminished GFR.**

    b. Next bone resorption must be inhibited either by **eliminating the underlying cause (treating the primary tumor)** or **inhibiting osteoclast function** to prevent recurrence of hypercalcemia.

    c. Unless the primary tumor or skeletal metastases can be controlled, all antihypercalcemia interventions tend to be **palliative.**

    d. Effective treatment of hypercalcemia in the terminally ill patient can produce improvement of symptoms **and facilitate patient discharge from the hospital during the terminal stages of the illness.**

2. There are several pharmacologic approaches to the treatment of patients with hypercalcemia (see **Table 28-9, text page 655**), but specific therapy regimens for different hypercalcemia etiologies have not yet been developed.
3. The degree of urgency with which hypercalcemia is treated depends on the **serum calcium level** and the **patient's symptomatology.**
4. Early dialogue among physician, patient, and family regarding what constitutes a "quality death" for the patient may be helpful in decision making regarding the treatment of hypercalcemia.

A. GENERAL MEASURES

1. Initial measures include **correcting volume contraction** and **removing factors that may exacerbate hypercalcemia,** including thiazide diuretics, vitamins A and D and in some breast cancer patients, hormonal agents.
2. **Mobilization** should be encouraged, and any **calcium supplementation** should be discontinued.

B. HYDRATION AND SALINE DIURESIS

1. Depending on the severity of hypercalcemia, either **oral or intravenous hydration with normal saline** may be required.
2. Central venous pressure and cardiac function should be monitored in patients with compromised cardiac function or renal failure.
3. Measurement of fluid intake and output, body weight, and assessment of signs of fluid overload are important.

C. **LOOP DIURETICS**

1. Loop diuretics such as **furosemide** may be used to enhance calcium secretion.
2. Patients treated with high doses of furosemide must be monitored to ensure that fluid and electrolyte losses are replaced and that extracellular fluid volume is not depleted.

D. **CALCITONIN**

1. **Calcitonin,** a thyroid secretion, produces transient inhibition of bone resorption. Inhibition is short and costs are high, but calcitonin can buy time while antineoplastic therapy is started.
2. It is the preferred treatment **when saline diuresis or Mithracin therapy is contraindicated** (e.g., thrombocytopenia, renal or cardiac failure).
3. Best responses are seen in patients with **multiple myeloma and other hematologic neoplasms.**
4. Administration is **subcutaneous** or as rectal suppositories and is most effective when **combined with glucocorticoids.**

E. **GLUCOCORTICOIDS**

1. **Glucocorticoids (prednisone and hydrocortisone)** are most effective in hypercalcemia associated with multiple myeloma, other hematologic diseases, and sometimes breast carcinoma.
2. They may work because they inhibit bone resorption mediated by osteoclast-activating factors or because they cause a decrease in calcium either by a direct tumor cytolytic effect or by inhibiting tumor production of prostaglandin.
3. Both can be used in patients with renal or cardiac failure who are dehydrated, and they therefore are useful **when saline diuresis is contraindicated.**

F. **PLICAMYCIN**

1. **Plicamycin** (mithramycin) is a cytotoxic drug with antihypercalcemia effects, probably through its toxic effects on osteoclasts and irreversible impairment of osteoclast bone resorption.
2. It has been associated with thrombocytopenia, renal and hepatic toxicity, hypocalcemia, and tetany. Toxicity is more likely in patients with impaired renal function.
3. Nausea, vomiting, and toxic effects are related to **cumulative dosage** and rarely occur with the first or second dose.
4. Plicamycin's **major advantages** include **its ease of administration** and **lower cost.** Its **major disadvantages** are **cumulative myelotoxicity** and **renal toxicity.**
5. Administration is **intravenous** either as a slow bolus injection or as a 4-hour infusion. The dose may be repeated if no detectable lowering of serum calcium is seen within 48 hours.
6. Its duration of action is variable and unpredictable, lasting from 3 days to a week or more.

G. **PHOSPHATES**

1. **Intravenous injection of inorganic phosphates** rapidly decreases extracellular calcium concentration by promoting skeletal calcification.
2. Because **nephrocalcinosis and other extraskeletal calcification** may also occur, use of intravenous phosphates should not be employed except as a last resort.
3. The most common and limiting side effect is diarrhea.

H. **PROSTAGLANDIN INHIBITORS**

1. Aspirin, indomethacin, and nonsteroidal anti-inflammatory drugs have been tried, but only on occasion is there an antihypercalcemia response.

I. **BISPHOSPHONATES**

1. **Bisphosphonates** act as effective inhibitors of osteoclast bone resorption by binding tightly to calcified bone matrix and preventing osteoclast bone resorption.

2. **Etidronate**
   a. **Etidronate** is available in both intravenous and oral form and has been shown to be more effective than either saline hydration alone or calcitonin after saline hydration.
   b. It is administered intravenously in the hydrated patient, followed by oral maintenance therapy. Serum calcium levels usually normalize within 4–5 days, and the median duration of action may be as long as a month.
   c. Toxicities associated with long-term use include impaired mineralization of bone and increases in serum phosphate.
3. **Pamidronate**
   a. **Pamidronate** has been demonstrated to be more effective than Etidronate, and does not have the toxicity of impairing bone mineralization.
   b. Pamidronate has a rapid onset of action and a longer duration of action than that seen with other therapies.
4. **Clodronate**
   a. **Clodronate** is a highly effective bisphosphonate that has been studied extensively in Europe. However, trials in the United States were halted when it was reported that several patients had developed leukemia after being treated with this agent.

J. **GALLIUM NITRATE**

1. **Gallium nitrate,** another osteoclastic inhibitor, appears to be more effective than calcitonin in achieving normal calcium levels over a longer period of time.
2. A major disadvantage to the use of gallium nitrate is the 5-day continuous treatment regimen, which makes outpatient treatment inconvenient.

V. **CONCLUSION**

1. Counseling of patients and families regarding prevention and recognition of early symptoms of hypercalcemia enables early therapy to commence before extreme debilitation develops. **Table 28-10, text page 659,** outlines the teaching points to be covered in providing patient and family education related to hypercalcemia.

PRACTICE QUESTIONS

1. Which of the following types of malignancies is **least** likely to be associated with hypercalcemia?
   (A) lung cancer
   (B) breast cancer
   (C) multiple myeloma
   (D) colon cancer

2. The pathophysiology of hypercalcemia involves a combination of two factors, bone resorption and
   (A) decreased renal calcium clearance.
   (B) increased osteoclast activity.
   (C) increased glomerular function.
   (D) decreased availability of ionized calcium.

3. Control of extracellular calcium levels within a narrow range is achieved through the action of several agents, including all of the following **except**
   (A) parathyroid hormone (PTH), which controls renal regulation of calcium.
   (B) 1,25-dihydroxyvitamin D, which controls intestinal calcium absorption.
   (C) calcitonin.
   (D) glucocorticoids, which control osteoclast activity.

4. How does the body typically respond to elevated levels of extracellular calcium?
   (A) by reducing PTH secretion
   (B) by increasing bone resorption
   (C) by increasing renal synthesis of 1,25-dihydroxyvitamin D
   (D) by decreasing urinary calcium excretion

5. The location and frequency of bone remodeling activity is controlled by several factors, including all of the following **except**
    (A) local factors such as prostaglandins, regulatory proteins, and constituents of the organic matrix.
    (B) mechanical factors such as weight bearing.
    (C) skeletal calcium, which couples bone resorption and bone formation.
    (D) osteotropic hormones, especially PTH and 1,25-dihydroxyvitamin D.

6. Factors that are produced by tumors themselves have been implicated in malignancy-associated hypercalcemia. Probably the most important of these circulating tumor-produced, or humoral, factors is
    (A) prostaglandin.
    (B) PTH-like factor.
    (C) bisphosphonate.
    (D) osteoclast-activating factor.

7. A patient is found to have a large tumor mass associated with high levels of PTH-related protein but normal levels of 1,25-dihydroxyvitamin D and normal intestinal absorption rates. Bone absorption is found to exceed bone formation. The **most** likely diagnosis is
    (A) primary hyperparathyroidism.
    (B) multiple myeloma.
    (C) humoral hypercalcemia of malignancy (HHM).
    (D) Hodgkin's disease.

8. Which of the following statements about the association between breast cancer and hypercalcemia is correct?
    (A) Bone resorption in breast cancer patients is probably due to cancer cells directly rather than to PGE mediation.
    (B) Tumor flare is thought to be the result of PGE inhibition by breast cancer cells.
    (C) Not all patients with metastases develop hypercalcemia, although most breast cancer patients with hypercalcemia have widespread skeletal metastases.
    (D) Hypercalcemia in breast cancer patients is usually responsive to prostaglandin inhibitors.

9. The symptoms of hypercalcemia in cancer patients are **best** described as
    (A) similar to those of acute renal failure.
    (B) easily identified but difficult to treat.
    (C) distinct from those of end-stage disease.
    (D) numerous, vague, and nonspecific.

10. Among the common early symptoms in hypercalcemic patients are all of the following **except**
    (A) nausea and vomiting.
    (B) diarrhea.
    (C) hypertension.
    (D) polyuria.

11. The most important **initial** treatment of hypercalcemia is
    (A) improving renal calcium excretion.
    (B) treating the primary tumor.
    (C) inhibiting osteoclast function.
    (D) inhibiting bone resorption.

12. A loop diuretic such as furosemide would be used in the treatment of hypercalcemia in order to
    (A) rehydrate the patient.
    (B) correct electrolyte imbalance.
    (C) enhance calcium excretion.
    (D) increase bone resorption.

13. A patient with multiple myeloma and compromised cardiac and renal function is diagnosed as hypercalcemic. Of the following treatments, the one **most** likely to be administered is
    (A) saline diuresis.
    (B) intravenous injection of inorganic phosphates.
    (C) plicamycin.
    (D) calcitonin with glucocorticoids.

14. A patient with acute hypercalcemia may need treatment that rapidly decreases extracellular calcium concentration. Of the following agents, the one **most** likely to be administered under these emergency circumstances is
    (A) plicamycin.
    (B) bisphosphonates.
    (C) phosphates.
    (D) prostaglandin inhibitors.

ANSWER EXPLANATIONS

1. **The answer is (D).** Patients with lung and breast cancer account for the highest percentage of malignancy-induced hypercalcemia. This high frequency is related to the high overall incidence of these two types of cancers. However, multiple myeloma, which is relatively rare, is the underlying cause in 10% of malignancy-associated hypercalcemia cases. (645–646)

2. **The answer is (A).** Hypercalcemia is characterized by excess extracellular calcium. This condition results from bone resorption—the release of skeletal calcium into serum—and from the failure of the kidneys to clear extracellular calcium. As calcium levels rise, symptoms of hypercalcemia appear. (646)

3. **The answer is (D).** Glucocorticoids, including prednisone and hydrocortisone, are used to treat hypercalcemia. They are not part of the body's normal homeostatic mechanism that regulates serum calcium. PTH and 1,25-dihydroxyvitamin D exert their effects by controlling movement of calcium across bone, kidney, and small intestine. PTH's action on the kidney occur through the formulation and action of NcAMP, which acts as a second messenger influencing calcium transport. (646)

4. **The answer is (A).** The body's homeostatic response to increased calcium loads involves suppression of PTH, which decreases bone resorption and inhibits intestinal calcium absorption. This inhibitory effect occurs as a result of decreased renal synthesis of 1,25-dihydroxyvitamin D and increased urinary calcium excretion. The calcium load is cleared principally by the kidney. (646–647)

5. **The answer is (C).** Bone remodeling, the process of bone formation and resorption, involves three types of bone cells: osteoblasts, osteocytes, and osteoclasts. Incitement of bone remodeling is thought to be directed at the osteocyte. Bone remodeling is said to be "coupled"; bone resorption is coupled with bone formation. "Uncoupling" refers to the failure of bone formation to follow the resorption process. Bone remodeling activity is influenced by mechanical factors such as weight bearing, by the activity of osteotropic hormones, and by local factors such as prostaglandins, regulatory proteins, and constituents of the organic matrix. (648–649)

6. **The answer is (B).** Malignancy-associated hypercalcemia is a complex metabolic complication in which bone resorption exceeds both bone formation and the kidney's ability to excrete extracellular calcium. Both humoral and local factors have been implicated in this process. Humoral, or tumor-produced, circulating factors include a PTH-like factor, transforming growth factors (TGF-alpha), and 1,25-dihydroxyvitamin D. Hypercalcemia that develops in patients with solid tumors without bone metastases, including HHM, is thought to be due to PTH-like factor. (650)

7. **The answer is (C).** In humoral hypercalcemia of malignancy (HHM), patients secrete high levels of PTH-related protein but have normal levels of 1,25-dihydroxyvitamin D and normal intestinal absorption rates. Osteoblastic and osteoclastic activities are "uncoupled" so that bone resorption exceeds bone formation. Hypercalcemia and hypercalciuria thus occur. Conversely, in primary hyperparathyroidism a parathyroid adenoma secretes excessive PTH, which stimulates intestinal and renal calcium absorption. Bone remodeling is accelerated, with a "coupled" increase in both osteoclastic and osteoblastic activity. Hypercalcemia occurs due to the combined action of PTH and 1,25-dihydroxyvitamin D on the kidney; and 1,25-dihydroxyvitamin D on the gut. (650)

8. **The answer is (C).** Bone resorption in breast cancer patients is probably due to PGE-mediated osteolysis rather than direct bone resorption. Tumor flare is thought to indicate the release of PGE by a hormonally responsive tumor. Hypercalcemia in breast cancer patients is generally unresponsive to prostaglandin inhibitors. (651)

9. **The answer is (D).** Hypercalcemia symptoms are numerous, vague, and nonspecific, and since many cancer patients with hypercalcemia have large tumor burdens and will die in 3 to 6 months, symptoms of hypercalcemia may be confused with those of end-stage disease. (653)

10. **The answer is (B).** Constipation, and not diarrhea, is more likely to be observed during the early stages of hypercalcemia. Elevated extracellular calcium levels depress smooth muscle contractility, leading to delayed gastric emptying and decreased gastrointestinal motility. (653)

11. **The answer is (A).** Before excessive bone resorption can be treated, impaired renal calcium excretion must be improved, usually by correcting dehydration and removing factors that may exacerbate hypercalcemia, including thiazide diuretics. Oral or intravenous hydration with normal saline may be required. (656)

12. **The answer is (C).** Although loop diuretics such as furosemide may be used to enhance calcium excretion, patients treated with high doses of furosemide must be monitored in an intensive care setting to ensure that fluid and electrolyte losses are replaced and that extracellular fluid volume is not depleted. (656)

13. **The answer is (D).** Both calcitonin and glucocorticoids have been shown to be effective in treating hypercalcemic patients with multiple myeloma. Both inhibit bone resorption. Glucocorticoids also increase urinary calcium excretion and decrease intestinal calcium absorption. Unlike saline diuresis or plicamycin, both calcitonin and glucocorticoids can be used in patients with renal or cardiac failure who are dehydrated. Another substance, gallium nitrate, appears to be more effective than calcitonin in achieving a sustained decrease in calcium levels. (655–658)

14. **The answer is (C).** Intravenous injection of inorganic phosphates rapidly decreases extracellular calcium concentration by promoting skeletal calcification. Because nephrocalcinosis and other extraskeletal calcification may also occur, however, use of intravenous phosphates is limited to a last resort. Both plicamycin and bisphosphonates have a slow onset of action. Prostaglandin inhibitors such as aspirin, indomethacin, and nonsteroidal anti-inflammatory drugs have not proved consistently effective in lowering calcium levels. (657–658)

29 Hormonal Disturbances

STUDY OUTLINE

I. **INTRODUCTION**

1. Abnormal hormone secretion can occur as a consequence of malignant neoplastic growth. This hormone release may be **ectopic** (from nonendocrine tissue that has been transformed by malignancy) or **entopic** (from a primary malignancy of an endocrine gland).

2. The release of hormone from nonendocrine tissue is termed **ectopic hormone secretion,** e.g., the release of ACTH from lung tumors.

   a. If the hormone produced by the malignant cells is biologically active, the target organ for the specific hormone will respond.

   b. If the hormone is produced in sufficient quantity, this abnormal secretion will become clinically evident as an **endocrine syndrome,** e.g., Cushing's syndrome that results from an excess glucocorticoid production by the adrenal glands in response to the ectopic production of ACTH from cancer cells.

   c. Malignant nonendocrine cells that produce these hormones are **not sensitive to the regulatory feedback systems that exist for endocrine glands.** Because hormone production is unchecked, excess secretion of the hormone occurs. The resulting endocrine abnormalities may be more life threatening than the cancer itself.

3. Tumors may also produce **non-hormonal tumor markers** such as alpha-fetoprotein and carcinoembryonic antigen (CEA). The systemic effects of these tumor products are referred to as **paraneoplastic phenomena.**

   a. The tumor produces biologically active substances that enter the circulation and cause some physiologic alteration.

   b. Measurement of these products can be used for tumor detection, diagnosis of disease recurrence, and assessment of tumor response to treatment.

II. **ANATOMY, PHYSIOLOGY, AND SCIENTIFIC PRINCIPLES**

A. **NEUROENDOCRINE STRUCTURES**

1. The neuroendocrine structures of major importance include the **hypothalamus,** the **connecting hypophysial-portal system,** the **pituitary gland,** and the **target endocrine glands and tissues.**

2. The hormones produced by the **endocrine cells** and **some hypothalamic neurons** are the chemical signals that are transported by the circulatory system to their specific sites of action, the peripherally located **endocrine glands.**

   a. These target glands respond to centrally released hormones by **producing and releasing another hormone,** e.g., the release of cortisol by the adrenal cortex in response to the pituitary release of ACTH, or by **exhibiting some other biologic response,** e.g., the conservation of water by the renal tubules.

   b. Some peripheral glands have other regulatory mechanisms, e.g., the circulatory levels of glucose influence the secretion of insulin by islet cells of the pancreas. Other examples involve the parathyroid glands, the thymus gland, and the gastrointestinal endocrine cells.

B. **NEUROENDOCRINE REGULATION AND FUNCTION**

1. Many factors are involved in the normal regulation of neuroendocrine function. See **Figure 29-1, text page 665,** and related text discussion for examples.

2. This regulation includes
    a. The capacity to sense minute environmental changes in the internal milieu and in some cases the external world.
    b. The ability of the system, in response to changes, to **increase or decrease synthesis** and **release hormones or other biologic effects.**
3. The regulatory systems involve a chain of events that result in modulation of the system. In the case of **ectopic hormone production by malignant cells,** the regulatory system is not effective.
    a. Undifferentiated malignant cells produce a hormone **autonomously without regard to the normal regulatory feedback mechanisms** to which normal endocrine cells respond.
    b. The result is excess ectopic hormones that are not subject to the usual control mechanisms.

C. **GLANDS**

1. Important target glands for pituitary gland trophic hormones include the **pineal gland,** the **thyroid gland** (thyroxine), the **adrenal gland** (aldosterone, glucocorticoids), the **ovary** (estrogens), and the **testis** (testosterone).
2. Other hormone-secreting tissues include the **pancreatic A** (glucagon) and **B cells** (insulin), the **parathyroid** (PTH), the **adrenal medulla** (epinephrine), the **C cells of the thyroid** (calcitonin), the **gastrointestinal hormone-secreting cells** (gastrin, substance P, cholecystokinin), and the **placenta** (HCG).
3. The **hypothalamus,** although not considered a gland, synthesizes and secretes hormones (TRH, GnRH or LHRH, somatostatin, ADH, oxytocin) that stimulate the synthesis and secretion of the **pituitary gland** trophic hormones (growth hormone, ACTH, TSH, luteinizing hormone, prolactin, melanocyte-stimulating hormone). It is these hormones that work on the target glands.

D. **HORMONES**

1. **Hormones are produced by glands, carried in the bloodstream, and serve as the highly specialized messengers for their respective target tissue sites.**
2. Hormones are classified by their chemical composition. The four major classifications are
    a. The **amine group,** which includes catecholamines, norepinephrine, and epinephrine. Their time frame of action is milliseconds.
    b. The **iodothyronines** thyronine and triiodothyronine. Their time frame of action is days.
    c. The **peptide, protein,** and **glycoprotein group** that includes a large number of hormones, including insulin, ACTH, vasopressin, oxytocin, and luteinizing hormone (LH). Their time frame of action is minutes to hours.
    d. The **steroids,** including estrogens, glucosteroids, and aldosterone. Their time frame of action is hours.
3. **All ectopically produced hormones observed to occur with malignant tumors have been of the peptide/protein class in which the synthesis occurs via DNA-RNA direction.** The end result of their activity, however, may be an excess secretion of some **nonprotein** such as cortisol.
4. Some hormones, such as ACTH and insulin, are produced as larger molecules **(prohormones)** that must be cleaved or separated to yield the biologically active hormone.
5. Most hormones are transported in the circulatory system attached to carrier proteins specific for the hormone, or to albumin. However, **only the free, or unbound, hormone** is available as the biologically active molecule that is able to interact with its cell-specific receptors.

E. **TARGET TISSUES/RECEPTORS**

1. **Protein receptors in target tissue recognize the hormone specific for the particular target tissue.** These receptors may be **on the surface** (peptide/protein hormones) or **intracellular** (steroid hormones).
2. Some hormones have receptors in many types of tissues (e.g., growth hormone) whereas others have specific receptors in only one or a few types of tissues (e.g., antidiuretic hormone in renal tubule cells).
3. The number of receptors and amount of hormone binding to the receptors influence the magnitude of the hormone response and are probably regulated.

III. **PATHOPHYSIOLOGY**

1. **It is believed that in the malignant transformation of cells, some of the genes that are not normally expressed are, in fact, expressed or become activated in the malignant cells.**
   a. This can account for the expression of genes that code for the synthesis of the peptide/protein hormones in the nonendocrine malignant cells.
2. Only when the tumor product has sufficient biologic activity will a clinical syndrome become evident.
   a. Only some of the peptides synthesized by the malignant cells are exactly like the normally secreted hormone from endocrine cells. Others are fragments or deviate in other ways.
3. For both ectopic hormone secretion and paraneoplastic agents (i.e., tumor markers), the effects may precede the diagnosis of malignancy or may occur at any time after the diagnosis.

IV. **CLINICAL MANIFESTATIONS**

1. The clinical manifestations of the paraneoplastic syndromes vary, depending on the type of ectopic product(s) produced by the malignant tumor.
2. More than one hormone or product may be produced by a tumor. Only those products that are **biologically active** and that are **secreted in sufficient excess** result in a clinical syndrome.

A. **GLANDS**

1. Malignancies arising in endocrine glands may or may not result in hormonal disturbances, and, if they occur, hormonal secretions may be increased or decreased. Secretions are **entopic.**
2. Endocrine glands may also be affected by the ectopic secretions of other malignant cells.

B. **HORMONES AND TARGET TISSUES**

1. Ectopic hormones, which are themselves peptides or polypeptides, may nevertheless be trophic to an endocrine gland that secretes a **steroid hormone,** e.g., ACTH stimulating production of cortisol by the adrenal cortex (Cushing's disease).
2. **Ectopic adrenocorticotropic hormone (ACTH) production**
   a. Ectopic production of ACTH occurs most often in association with **small-cell lung cancer** and in **carcinomas of the pancreas and thymus.** It has also been observed in other lung cancer types and in a variety of other tumors.
   b. Clinical evidence of ectopic ACTH results from the stimulatory effect of ACTH on the adrenal cortex and the subsequent glucocorticoid production. High serum and cortisol levels are diagnostic.
   c. Symptoms include **muscle weakness and atrophy, edema, hypertension,** and **psychosis.**
      (1) Classic features of Cushing's disease, including centripetal obesity, moon facies, buffalo hump, and cutaneous striae, are likely to appear only when tumor growth is **slow.**
   d. If tumor therapy is not effective, levels of cortisol can be decreased with agents that **inhibit cortisol** such as aminoglutethimide, metyrapone, and ketoconazole.
3. **Ectopic antidiuretic hormone production**
   a. **Vasopressin (ADH)** is produced ectopically most often in carcinomas of the **lung (small-cell)** and **colon.**
   b. Patients may have **hyponatremia and inappropriately high urine osmolality** and **water retention.**
   c. If there is excessive fluid intake, symptoms of the **syndrome of inappropriate antidiuretic hormone (SIADH)** may occur and include lethargy; agitation; altered mental status, including confusion and psychotic behavior; seizures and coma; and in some cases, death.
   d. Treatment is directed at the tumor. In addition, several steps may be taken to **increase serum sodium** and **decrease retention of water** to **raise plasma osmolality.**
      (1) Fluid restriction may be needed to control hyponatremia.
      (2) Chemotherapy may be postponed if it requires hydration.
      (3) **Three percent hypertonic saline and furosemide** may be used if the patient has severe symptoms or is comatose.
      (4) Demeclocycline may be used if cancer treatment fails and SIADH recurs.

e. **Neurophysin,** a carrier protein of vasopressin, may be an effective tumor marker in patients with small-cell lung cancer.

4. **Ectopic gonadotropin production**
   a. **Human chorionic gonadotropin (HCG)** is normally produced by the placenta.
   b. The biologically active HCG that has been produced ectopically by tumors has resulted in **gynecomastia** in men, **oligomenorrhea** in women, and **precocious puberty** in children.
   c. HCG secretion has been reported for several tumors, including those in the pituitary gland, ovary and testis, and cancers of the lung, breast, pancreas, GI tract, and prostate. Incidence is low.
   d. Treatment is directed at the tumor.

5. **Ectopic calcitonin production**
   a. Increased calcitonin levels have occurred in patients with lung (especially small-cell) cancer, with breast, gastric and colon cancer, and with carcinoid tumors.
   b. There is to date no recognized clinical syndrome that results from ectopic production.

6. **Ectopic parathyroid hormone production and hypercalcemia**
   a. Hypercalcemia may result from the ectopic production of tumor-produced factors that have parathyroid-like hormone activity. Rarely does PTH itself appear to be involved.
      (1) **PTH-like factor, osteoclast activating factor (OAF),** and **prostaglandins** have been produced by tumors and can cause hypercalcemia.
   b. The resulting effect is **stimulation of osteoclastic bone resorption** and, for some of the factors, **inhibition of renal excretion of calcium.**
   c. Review **Chapter 28, text and guide,** for symptoms and treatments.

7. **Ectopic growth-hormone releasing hormone (GHRH) production**
   a. A number of tumors have produced **growth-hormone releasing hormone (GHRH),** including carcinoid tumors, pancreatic islet cells, small-cell lung cancer, thyroid medullary carcinoma, and endometrial cancer.
   b. **Acromegaly** appears rarely, particularly in slow-growing bronchial carcinoid tumors.

8. **Ectopic production**
   a. Some hormones, including chorionic gonadotropin, growth hormone, and insulin, appear to be found normally in small amounts in **nonendocrine** tissue. This would call into question whether the hormones produced by nonendocrine tumors really are ectopic.
   b. One characteristic of hormone synthesis in malignant nonendocrine tissue, however, is that it appears to be **autonomous**—it does not respond to regulatory feedback mechanisms such as occurs for hormones produced entopically.

V.   **ASSESSMENT**

1. In assessing paraneoplastic syndrome, the nurse should
   a. **Be alert to signs and symptoms that are associated with specific ectopic hormone production.**
   b. **Be knowledgeable about the tumors that are more frequently associated with ectopic hormone production (e.g., small-cell lung cancer) and the more commonly observed syndromes (e.g., SIADH).**

A.   **HISTORY**

1. The history should attempt to identify or to rule out malignancy as the source of any symptoms associated with both cancer and an endocrine syndrome, including any evidence of **weight loss, changes in the diet, fatigue, weakness,** and **other changes in usual patterns.**
2. For the person with a known malignancy, the history includes information about the type, stage, treatment used, and evidence of any paraneoplastic syndromes.

B.   **PHYSICAL EXAMINATION**

1. **Hypertrophy** or other structural changes in the endocrine gland, such as a nodule, may be found during the physical examination.
   a. **Hypertrophy** or **hyperplasia** may result from excess trophic hormone stimulation of the gland.
   b. **Tumor growth** within the gland can also change its structure.
2. The **location** of the gland influences both recognition of these changes during the examination and whether the individual will notice sensations associated with glandular hypertrophy.

3. Changes to be alert to include
   a. **A tightness in the neck or a pressure on the trachea that might be caused by thyroid enlargement.**
   b. **A bilateral loss of the temporal visual field and headache that might be caused by pituitary gland enlargement.**
4. The examination also identifies changes that may be associated with ectopic hormone syndromes such as **hyperpigmentation** (possible evidence of ectopic ACTH) or **gynecomastia** (possible evidence of ectopic HCG).

C. **DIAGNOSTIC STUDIES**

1. Highly sensitive **radioimmunoassay techniques** are used to determine if there are alterations in secretion of the suspected hormone(s). Both blood and urine are used.
2. If alterations exist, **serial monitoring of hormone levels over time** may be used to determine if the alterations are due to a paraneoplastic syndrome, a malignancy of an endocrine gland, or the result of a benign change in endocrine tissue.
3. Responses to the **administration of stimulatory and/or inhibitory hormones** are useful in determining if the hormone production is ectopic. They should **not** effect hormone levels if the secretion is ectopically produced, because ectopic hormones are produced autonomously.
4. The effects of **tumor removal** or **tumor therapy** are also important in determining if the secretion is ectopically produced.
   a. Hormone levels should decrease as the source of hormone is eliminated or reduced.
   b. High concentrations of hormone in the tumor or a difference in hormone concentration across the arteriovenous gradient of the tumor tissue also provide evidence of hormone production by the tumor.
5. In all cases, diagnostic procedures are used that **allow differentiation between an ectopic paraneoplastic syndrome and some other plausible diagnosis.** For example, the presence of a known tumor marker suggests malignancy.
6. The nurse's role includes
   a. **Explaining the specific diagnostic procedures to the patient and family.**
   b. **Ensuring accurate collection of specimens such as urine.**
   c. **Assisting the patient and family to cope with all the attendant circumstances associated with diagnostic procedures.**
   d. **Assisting in the administration of stimulatory or suppressive test agents.**

VI. **INTERVENTIONS**

1. **The most effective therapy for paraneoplastic syndromes is the ablation of the tumor.** This alleviates the excess ectopic hormone secretion and usually results in regression of the syndrome.
2. If tumor therapy is not effective, other symptom-reducing strategies may be used. This may involve, for example, **fluid restriction (for SIADH)** or the use of **drugs that block hormone receptors or hormone synthesis.**

PRACTICE QUESTIONS

1. The feature of all ectopic hormone secretions that distinguishes them from entopic secretions is that they
   (A) enter the circulation and cause remote effects.
   (B) are released by endocrine tissue that has been invaded by malignancy.
   (C) produce symptoms that are indistinguishable from those of malignancy.
   (D) are produced by malignant cells that are of nonendocrine origin.

2. Peripherally located endocrine glands are an essential component of the neuroendocrine system. They typically function by
   (A) controlling the chain of events that results in modulation of the system.
   (B) producing and releasing hormones in response to centrally released hormones.
   (C) stimulating or inhibiting the hormonal activity of the anterior pituitary gland cells.
   (D) synthesizing and secreting hormones that stimulate production of the pituitary gland trophic hormones.

3. Hormones are classified by chemical composition into four groups. All ectopically produced hormones observed to occur with malignant tumors belong to which of these groups?
   (A) the amine group
   (B) the peptide/protein group
   (C) the steroid group
   (D) the iodothyronine group

4. It is now believed that the malignant transformation of nonendocrine cells to ectopic hormone-producing cells is controlled by
   (A) the hypothalamus in conjunction with the anterior pituitary.
   (B) a group of cells with a common embryonic origin in the neural crest.
   (C) genes that become activated in the malignant cells.
   (D) the abnormal secretions of one or more peripheral target glands.

5. For an ectopic product secreted by a malignant tumor to be manifested as a clinical syndrome, it must be biologically active and must
   (A) be a hormone.
   (B) affect a single target gland.
   (C) have receptors in many types of tissues.
   (D) be secreted in sufficient excess.

6. Ectopic production of ACTH is **most** likely to occur in association with which of the following cancers?
   (A) small-cell lung cancer
   (B) Hodgkin's disease
   (C) liver carcinoma
   (D) cancer of the parathyroid

7. Each of the following treatments may be appropriate for the syndrome of inappropriate antidiuretic hormone (SIADH) **except**
   (A) replacement of depleted fluids.
   (B) infusion of 3% hypertonic saline and furosemide.
   (C) administration of demeclocycline.
   (D) postponement of chemotherapy requiring hydration.

8. Some hormones appear to be found normally in small amounts in nonendocrine tissue, which would call into question whether the hormones produced by nonendocrine tumors really are ectopic rather than entopic. One characteristic of hormone synthesis in malignant nonendocrine tissue, however, is that it occurs
   (A) only in cells of common embryonic origin.
   (B) autonomously, without regulatory control.
   (C) without activation of specific genes.
   (D) on the cell surface without direction by DNA and RNA.

9. Physical examination of the individual with a possible ectopic hormone syndrome would be **least** likely to focus on
   (A) hypertrophy or other structural change in an endocrine gland.
   (B) changes such as hyperpigmentation that may be associated with specific ectopic hormone syndromes.
   (C) conditions such as vision loss or tightness in the neck that may be due to pressure from an enlarged gland.
   (D) monitoring hormones over time to determine if any alterations are due to malignancy.

10. Diagnostic studies used to determine if a secretion is ectopically produced include all of the following **except**
   (A) administration of stimulatory and inhibitory hormones.
   (B) monitoring the effects of tumor removal on hormone levels.
   (C) radioimmunoassay to determine the characteristics of specific hormones.
   (D) serial monitoring of hormone levels over time.

ANSWER EXPLANATIONS

1. **The answer is (D).** Ectopic hormone production occurs in malignant cells that are of nonendocrine origin, whereas entopic hormone production occurs in endocrine cells. Tumor markers are also produced by malignant cells but are not hormones. All three types of secretions enter the circulation and cause remote effects. However, malignant nonendocrine cells that produce ectopic hormones are not sensitive to the regulatory feedback systems that exist for endocrine glands. Because hormone production is unchecked, excess secretion of the hormone occurs. (663)

2. **The answer is (B).** Peripheral target glands respond to trophic hormones released by the pituitary gland, under the control of the hypothalamus, by producing and releasing another hormone, e.g., the release of cortisol by the adrenal cortex in response to the pituitary release of ACTH, or by exhibiting some other biologic response, e.g., the conservation of water by the renal tubules. Some peripheral glands have other regulatory mechanisms, e.g., the circulatory levels of glucose influence the secretion of insulin by islets of the pancreas. (665)

3. **The answer is (B).** The only hormones produced ectopically, by nonendocrine cells, are those belonging to the peptide/protein class in which the synthesis occurs via DNA-RNA direction. Included in this group are hormones such as insulin and glucagon, ACTH, vasopressin, and luteinizing hormone. It is important to note, however, that the end result of ectopic hormone production may be an excess secretion of some **nonprotein** such as cortisol (a steroid). (666)

4. **The answer is (C).** It is believed that in the malignant transformation of cells, some genes that are not normally expressed—and that control the synthesis of polypeptide hormones—become activated. This would account for the fact that only polypeptide hormones occur in ectopic production from tumors of nonendocrine origin. (667)

5. **The answer is (D).** The clinical manifestations of the paraneoplastic syndromes vary, depending on the type of ectopic product(s) produced by the malignant tumor. More than one hormone or product may be produced by a tumor. Only those products that are biologically active and that are secreted in sufficient excess result in a clinical syndrome. The ectopic product does not have to be a hormone—it can be a hormone fragment or precursor molecule or some other tumor marker; and it can affect one type of tissue or many. (668)

6. **The answer is (A).** Ectopic production of ACTH occurs most often in association with small-cell lung cancer and in carcinomas of the pancreas and thymus, although it has been observed in other lung cancer types and in a variety of other tumors. Clinical evidence of ectopic ACTH results from the stimulatory effect of ACTH on the adrenal cortex and the subsequent glucocorticoid production. (668)

7. **The answer is (A).** Vasopressin (ADH) may be produced ectopically, most often in carcinomas of the lung (small cell) and colon, with accompanying hyponatremia and inappropriately high urine osmolality and water retention. If there is excessive fluid intake, symptoms of the syndrome of inappropriate antidiuretic hormone (SIADH) may occur. Treatment is directed at the tumor. In addition, several steps may be taken to increase serum sodium and decrease retention of water to raise plasma osmolality, including choices (B)–(D). (669)

8. **The answer is (B).** Chorionic gonadotropin, growth hormone, and insulin have all been found in small amounts in nonendocrine tissue. Thus the question is whether the hormones produced really are ectopic (and whether gene activation can, by itself, explain ectopic hormone production). One general characteristic, however, is that ectopic hormone production appears to be autonomous: it does not respond to the regulatory feedback mechanisms such as occurs for hormones produced entopically. (671)

9. **The answer is (D).** Serial monitoring of hormone levels over time might be included in a diagnostic evaluation in order to determine whether hormone levels are normal or abnormal. It would not be part of a typical physical examination, however, which is more likely to focus on glandular hypertrophy or hyperplasia that might occur from excess trophic hormone stimulation of an endocrine gland, as well as changes that might be associated with specific ectopic hormone syndromes. (671–672)

10.   **The answer is (C).**   Radioimmunoassay techniques are used to measure **levels** (rather than characteristics) of hormones, hormone precursors and fragments, and subunits. Once an excess hormone production is identified by radioimmunoassay, the other diagnostic procedures listed may be used to differentiate between an ectopic paraneoplastic syndrome and some other plausible diagnosis, including a benign change in endocrine tissue. In addition, high concentrations of hormone in the excised tumor or a difference in hormone concentration across the arteriovenous gradient of the tumor tissue provides evidence of hormone production by the tumor. (671–672)

30 Malignant Effusions and Edemas

STUDY OUTLINE

I. INTRODUCTION

1. **Abnormal leakage** from the blood and lymph vessels into tissues (edema) or cavities (effusions) occurs with many kinds of malignancy.
2. Although cancers can metastasize to any of the body's serous cavities, **malignant effusions** occur most commonly in the pleural space of the lung (pleural effusion), the peritoneal cavity in the abdomen (ascites), or the space surrounding the heart (pericardial effusion).
3. The brain and the extremities are frequent sites for **malignant edemas.**

II. NORMAL FLUID REGULATION

1. **First spacing** describes a normal distribution of fluid in both the extracellular and intravascular compartments.
2. **Second spacing** refers to an excess of interstitial fluid accumulation (edema), and **third spacing** is fluid retention in areas that usually have no fluid or a minimum of fluid (effusion).
3. Extracellular fluids are separated into interstitial and intravascular compartments by the semipermeable membranes surrounding capillaries and cells, which serve as the points where exchange takes place between each cell and its respective fluid environment and between the interstitial fluid and the plasma within the circulatory system.
4. See **Figure 30-1, text page 676,** for a diagram of pressures influencing fluid movement.

III. FLUID DISTURBANCES IN CANCER

A. EFFECTS OF CANCER AND CANCER TREATMENT

1. Cancer, either a primary tumor or a metastatic lesion, can negatively affect fluid pressure dynamics in several ways:
   a. Direct extension of tumor.
   b. Seeding of body cavities with malignant cells.
   c. Lymphatic or venous obstruction.
   d. Causing of severe hypoproteinemia.
2. Cancer treatments can affect or be altered by effusions and edemas.
3. See **Table 30-1, text page 677,** for causes of malignant edema.

B. GENERAL CONSIDERATIONS: SIMILARITIES AND DIFFERENCES

1. **Benign versus malignant**
   a. **Lymphedema** is a benign, iatrogenic problem secondary to radical cancer surgery.
2. **Incidence**
   a. The actual incidence of metastases and malignant fluid retention is less clear today, but it is surmised that the incidence of these later complications is on the rise because longer survival after diagnosis is occurring as a result of improved treatments for primary disease.
   b. **Pericardial effusions** tend to be seen in **end-stage** disease, whereas **pleural effusions, ascites, and cerebral edema** may be the first indication of cancer.
3. **Rapid versus slow accumulation**
   a. Cavities and tissues can accommodate surprisingly large volumes of fluids if the abnormal liquid accumulates slowly over time.

b.   A rapid increase in volume, even a small amount, tends to overwhelm compensatory mechanisms, and life-threatening symptoms can occur.

4.   **Assessment**

a.   Many more malignant pleural effusions than pericardial effusions are symptomatic.

b.   The most helpful diagnostic tools for pleural effusions are the **chest X ray** and examination of the pleural fluid, whereas the **echocardiogram** is the most important diagnostic tool in pericardial effusions.

c.   Brain lesions causing cerebral edema are usually diagnosed with CT.

5.   **Transudates versus exudates**

a.   Fluid accumulation at an effusion site can be classified as either a transudate or an exudate.

(1)   A **transudate** is a low-protein fluid that has leaked from blood vessels due to mechanical factors, as in cirrhosis, congestive heart failure, or nephrotic syndrome.

(2)   An **exudate** is high in protein-rich fluid that has leaked from blood vessels with increased permeability.

b.   Most malignant effusions are exudates, caused by irritation of the serous membrane by sloughed cancer cells or solid tumor implants.

6.   **Treatment**

a.   For effusions, systemic treatment is usually employed if the underlying cancer is responsive to chemotherapy.

b.   Otherwise, local therapy for malignant effusions is similar:

(1)   Drain the fluid.

(2)   Attempt to obliterate the third space.

(3)   Prevent reaccumulation.

c.   The main goals of treatment for malignant effusions and edemas are similar (see **Table 30-2, text page 678**).

d.   Specific therapy depends upon the site where the fluid has accumulated and the individual patient and tumor-related factors (see **Table 30-3, text page 678**).

7.   **Nursing care**

a.   Ongoing **assessment** of each cancer patient for signs or symptoms of fluid retention is crucial so interventions can be instituted early.

b.   When fluid accumulation occurs, the patient and family will need **emotional support** to counteract the stress and fears associated with advancing disease, cosmetic appearance changes, and the necessity for further medical intervention.

c.   The nurse will probably assist with potentially painful diagnostic and/or sclerosing **procedures.**

d.   Nursing interventions include **minimizing discomfort, providing reassurance,** and **monitoring** the patient during and after procedures for untoward reactions.

e.   **Prevention** is important, particularly with lymphedema.

f.   **Pain evaluation** and control are often in order since the abnormal fluid accumulation can put pressure on nerve endings in surrounding structures.

g.   If life-threatening cardiac tamponade or brain herniation occurs, **emergency care** is needed.

h.   See **Table 30-4, text page 679,** for a listing of published nursing care plans for patients with malignant effusions or edemas.

IV.   **LUNG: MALIGNANT PLEURAL EFFUSION**

A.   **INCIDENCE**

1.   Although it is usually stated that approximately half of all newly diagnosed pleural effusions in adults are malignant, there have been no recent reports on the incidence of pleural effusion.

a.   See **Table 30-5, text page 679,** for the incidence of pleural effusions with different tumor types.

2.   **Fifty percent** of cancer patients will develop a pleural effusion at some time during the course of the disease.

a.   It may be the first sign of malignancy.

b.   Pleural effusion later in the disease progression is an ominous sign, but it does not necessarily mean the beginning of the terminal stage.

3.   Most patients (90%) will have effusions of more than 500 ml, and approximately one-third will present with bilateral pleural effusions.

B. **PATHOPHYSIOLOGY**

1. Normally, fluid is constantly being filtered across the pleural space from the parietal pleural surface and reabsorbed through the visceral pleura.
    a. Five to 10 liters of fluid moves through the pleural space each 24 hours, and the space between these two pleura contains a small amount of fluid (5–15 ml) that acts as a lubricant allowing the two surfaces to move without friction.
2. In the presence of a massive effusion process, the interpleural space may contain as much as 1500 ml of fluid.
3. There are **five ways** in which fluid equilibrium in the pleural space can be disturbed by cancer, either directly by origination in the pleura or indirectly via metastatic spread.
    a. Most commonly, **implantation** with cancer cells on the pleural surface leads to increased **capillary permeability** and leakage from the intravascular to the interstitial compartment.
    b. **Obstruction** of pleural or pulmonary lymphatic channels by malignant processes can prevent reabsorption of fluid.
    c. The **pulmonary veins** can be obstructed by tumor, leading to increased capillary hydrostatic pressure in the visceral pleura.
    d. The pleural space **colloid osmotic pressure** may be increased by necrotic malignant cells being shed into the pleural space, leading to reduced absorption of fluid by the visceral pleural capillaries.
    e. The thoracic duct may be **perforated,** producing a chylous pleural effusion.
4. Tumor-related pathologies that can cause pleural effusion include superior vena cava syndrome, endobronchial obstruction with atelectasis, postobstructive pneumonitis, and pericardial constriction.

C. **CLINICAL MANIFESTATIONS**

1. The **extent** of alteration of respiratory function depends on the amount and rate of pleural fluid accumulation as well as on the patient's underlying pulmonary status.
2. Fluid accumulation **restricts lung expansion, reduces lung volume, alters the ventilation and perfusion capacity,** and **results in abnormal gas exchange and hypoxia.**
3. When pleural effusion develops in the patient with advanced cancer, it is often difficult to sort out the respiratory effects of the pleural fluid accumulation from shortness of breath due to thoracic muscle weakness and general debilitation.

D. **SIGNS AND SYMPTOMS**

1. Common presenting symptoms and signs are distressing to most patients. See **Table 30-6, text page 681.**
2. Cough is caused by compression of bronchial walls by fluid.
3. Dull, aching, continuous chest pain is the most common symptom and points to parietal pleural metastasis.
4. The degree of subjective symptoms produced by a pleural effusion is not so dependent on the amount of fluid involved as on the rapidity with which it has accumulated.

E. **DIAGNOSIS**

1. **Radiographic examination**
    a. **Chest X rays** are important in visualizing free fluid in the pleural cavity and relating the accumulation to other structures.
    b. The larger the effusion, the more opaque it will appear.
    c. A pleural effusion will not be detected on a posterior-anterior chest film unless it contains at least **200–300 ml** of fluid.
    d. **Clues** to the type of cancer causing the pleural effusion may be seen on X ray.
        (1) Mediastinal shift away from the effusion points to a disseminated nonthoracic tumor.
        (2) If the mediastinum is shifted toward the effusion, carcinoma of the lung, with some degree of bronchial obstruction, is probably involved.
        (3) Mesothelioma or fixed central node metastasis is indicated if no mediastinal shift is seen.

2. **Pleural fluid examination**
   a. Any new pleural effusion must be aspirated to confirm the presence of malignant cells and to rule out nonmalignant causes.
   b. **Pleural fluid cytologic analysis** yields a definitive diagnosis in 70% of patients with malignant pleural effusions.
   c. Thoracoscopy with direct pleural biopsy leads to a diagnosis 100% of the time.
   d. Pleural fluid removal provides immediate relief for the distressing symptoms of large effusions (1000–1500 ml).
      (1) Fluid should be removed slowly to avoid re-expansion pulmonary edema.
   e. The aspirated fluid is sent for cultures, Gram and acid-fast stains, cell counts, and chemistry studies.
   f. A **bloody effusion** is the single strongest indicator of malignancy.

F. **TREATMENT**

   1. Treatment is based upon the tumor type and any previous therapy.
   2. Small, asymptomatic effusions caused by lymphomas, leukemias, breast cancer, small-cell lung cancer, and ovarian cancer are first treated with systemic chemotherapy or hormonal therapy.
   3. Patients with chemotherapy-resistant tumors will require alternative treatment approaches.
   4. **Removal of fluid**
      a. Relief of symptoms is a **short-term goal** achieved with fluid drainage. Long-term goals involve obliteration of the pleural space so that pleural fluid cannot reaccumulate.
      b. **Thoracentesis**
         (1) Pleural fluid is removed by needle aspiration through the chest wall.
         (2) After the thoracentesis is complete and the pleural fluid has been drained, the patient is assessed for complications such as **pneumothorax, pain, hypotension,** or **pulmonary edema.**
         (3) Patient education and support as well as medication and local anesthesia are important measures to prevent anxiety and discomfort during any of these therapeutic procedures.
         (4) Although thoracentesis alone is effective for diagnosis, palliation, or relief of acute respiratory distress, it is of little value for treating recurrent malignant effusions because the fluid usually reaccumulates quickly.
         (5) The risks of **repeated thoracentesis** include hypoalbuminemia, electrolyte imbalance, pneumothorax, fluid loculation, and infection.
         (6) Thoracentesis via an **implanted port** and intrapleural catheter is an alternative approach that can be advantageous for the patient whose cancer is refractory to treatment and who is thus likely to experience repeated pleural fluid reaccumulation. See **Figure 30-4, text page 683,** for a diagram of pleural fluid removal via an implanted port.
      c. **Thoracostomy tube**
         (1) A thoracostomy tube may be inserted to facilitate fluid drainage and then left in place to assess the degree of fluid reaccumulation.
         (2) **Nursing assessments** while a thoracostomy tube is in place include observing for pneumothorax, pain, hypotension, and pulmonary edema, as well as care of the closed-chest drainage system.
         (3) Care is taken to ensure that the chest tube remains **patent** since exudate fluid tends to clot.
   5. **Obliteration of the pleural space**
      a. Obliteration of the pleural space is achieved by instilling a chemical agent that causes the visceral and parietal pleura to become permanently adhered together.
      b. **Chemical agents**
         (1) Chemical sclerosing does not prolong the patient's life but may enhance quality of life by relieving symptoms and reducing the time a patient spends in the hospital.
         (2) Bleomycin and tetracycline, currently the two most commonly used chemical agents, control malignant pleural effusions in 70% or more of patients. Tetracycline has been popular due to its overall efficacy, convenience, low cost, and minimal morbidity.
         (3) The selected sclerosing agent is instilled into the pleural space via the thoracentesis needle or the thoracostomy tube.

(4) **Nursing management** during chest tube insertion and pleural sclerosing includes patient education and reassurance, pain control, positioning, and management of the chest tube drainage, as well as maintainence of the drainage system.

(5) Investigational methods for controlling malignant pleural effusion include antibody-guided radiation and use of a sclerosing agent.

c. **Surgical methods**

(1) If a pleural effusion remains uncontrolled after other approaches have been tried, surgery is another option.

(2) If a patient has a good life expectancy and a good performance status, **pleural stripping** is advocated.

(3) Success rates approach 90%, but there can be serious complications, such as persistent **air leak, bleeding, pneumonia,** and **empyema.**

(4) A **pleuroperitoneal shunt** is inserted into the subcutaneous tissue, and pleural fluid is diverted to the peritoneal cavity via manual compression of the shunt's valve pump. The patients must be motivated, because they are required to conscientiously **pump the valve** intermittently to prevent clogging.

d. **Radiation**

(1) Radiation is limited to treatment of the underlying disease, not the resultant effusion.

V. HEART: MALIGNANT PERICARDIAL EFFUSION

A. INCIDENCE

1. Autopsy series indicate that metastasis to the heart and pericardium occurs in 8%–20% of cases.

2. Pericardial effusion is not easily detected by routine tests and is often not discovered while the patient is alive.

3. See **Table 30-7, text page 684,** for the incidence of pericardial effusion related to tumor type.

B. PATHOPHYSIOLOGY

1. Two layers make up the **pericardial sac:** a tough outer fibrous pericardium called the parietal pericardium and an inner layer of serous pericardium called the visceral pericardium.

a. See **Figure 30-5, text page 684,** for a diagram of the pericardium.

2. The pericardial cavity ordinarily contains less than 50 ml of fluid, which can serve as a lubricant.

3. Pericardial metastasis results from lymphatic or hematogenous spread or from direct invasion by an adjacent primary tumor.

4. The majority of pericardial effusions result from obstruction of **lymphatic and venous drainage** of the heart.

a. This obstruction disturbs the intrapericardial pressure and results in fluid buildup.

5. The effects of pericardial fluid accumulation are largely dependent on the rate of exudation, the physical compliance capacity of the pericardial cavity, ventricular function, myocardial size, and blood volume.

a. Rapid build-up of even 150–200 ml can trigger a cardiac-oncologic emergency.

C. CLINICAL MANIFESTATIONS

1. Pericardial effusion **interferes** with cardiac function as the fluid burden occupies space and reduces the volume of the heart in diastole.

2. Systemic circulatory effects of decreased cardiac output and impaired venous return lead to **generalized congestion.**

a. The body tries to **compensate in several ways.**

(1) A **tachycardia** is created by adrenergic stimulation to offset decreased stroke volume.

(2) Systemic and pulmonary **venous pressure increase** in an attempt to improve ventricular filling.

(3) The **adrenergic stimulation** increases the ejection fraction, leading to increased peripheral resistance that will support arterial blood pressure.

D. **SIGNS AND SYMPTOMS**

1. The patient may have only **nonspecific symptoms** at first: dyspnea, cough, and chest pain.
2. The clinician should have a high index of suspicion for pericardial involvement whenever cancer patients exhibit cardiovascular symptoms.
3. See **Table 30-8, text page 685,** for signs and symptoms of a developing pericardial effusion.
   a. Findings can be subdivided into three clinical stages, from mild effusion to tamponade.
4. Cardiac tamponade is characterized by **impaired hemodynamic function** due to increased intrapericardial pressure that overcomes normal compensatory mechanisms.
5. **Nursing management** of patients in tamponade includes measures to minimize activity and promote adequate respiration, elevation of the head of the bed, and administration of oxygen and medications to relieve anxiety and pain.
6. **Intravascular volume maintenance** with intravenous fluids, vasopressors, and other cardiac medications may be in order while preparation is being made for pericardiocentesis or surgical intervention.

E. **DIAGNOSIS**

1. **Radiography**
   a. **Echocardiography (ECHO)** is the fastest, least invasive, and most precise method of visualization and quantification of malignant pericardial effusion.
2. **Electrocardiography (ECG)**
   a. **ECG changes** with neoplastic pericarditis or effusions include tachycardia, premature contractions, low QRS voltage, and nonspecific ST and T wave changes.
3. **Pericardial fluid examination**
   a. Fluid withdrawn from the pericardial cavity by pericardiocentesis that has a **bloody appearance** is indicative of malignancy, especially with lung cancer.

F. **TREATMENT**

1. See **Figure 30-6, text page 686,** for an algorithm for diagnosis and management of malignant pericardial effusions.
2. **Removal of fluid**
   a. **Pericardiocentesis alone**
      (1) Percutaneous pericardiocentesis guided by ECHO is an important diagnostic tool and is useful for initial drainage of fluid from the pericardium.
      (2) Pericardial drainage alone as treatment for effusion has been equivocal, with most patients relapsing a short time after the tap.
      (3) Nursing care during the pericardiocentesis includes:
         (a) **Explaining** the procedure to the patient and attempting to reduce anxiety and discomfort.
         (b) **Positioning** the patient in a semi-Fowler's position.
         (c) Maintaining **asepsis.**
         (d) Having available a good **light source, defibrillator,** and emergency **medications.**
      (4) The nurse must continuously monitor the patient and the EKG during the pericardiocentesis and must afterwards monitor for complications such as pneumothorax, myocardial laceration, and coronary artery laceration.
   b. **Subxiphoid pericardiotomy**
      (1) Under local anesthesia, subxiphoid pericardiostomy allows for a longer period of drainage and permits examination of the pericardial space as well as obtaining a pericardial biopsy.
3. **Obliteration of the pericardial space**
   a. **Pericardiocentesis with sclerosing agent instillation**
      (1) **Sclerosing agents** such as tetracycline, 5FU, radioactive gold or phosphorus, quinacrine, and thiotepa are instilled into the pericardial cavity via pericardiocentesis, but they are associated with significant toxicity.
      (2) Effusions recur in approximately 50% of the patients thus treated.
   b. **Surgery**
      (1) Surgical intervention, including pleuropericardial window via thoracotomy and pericardiectomy is generally reserved for medically appropriate patients whose

malignant effusion is unresponsive to other therapies or who have required repeated pericardiocentesis.

(2) A **preoperative** nursing care plan for patients with tamponade undergoing pericardial window surgery includes measures to maintain blood pressure and heart rate, maintain urine output and mental status, provide sufficient oxygen, and decrease pain and anxiety.

(3) **Postoperative** nursing measures include prevention of infection, atelectasis, pleural effusion, and pneumothorax. Prevention of anxiety and pain and bleeding due to the catheter and maintaining free-flowing pericardial drainage are important.

c. **Radiation**

(1) The use of external beam radiation is primarily reserved for pericardial effusions due to lymphomas, which are highly radiosensitive.

VI. ABDOMEN: MALIGNANT PERITONEAL EFFUSION

A. INCIDENCE

1. Malignant peritoneal effusion (ascites) is most common in patients with ovarian cancer.
2. Ascites also develops in patients with gastrointestinal malignancies, though it typically develops later in the course of the disease.
3. The appearance of ascites in patients with advanced disease is prognostically grim, and palliation is usually all that can be offered.

B. PATHOPHYSIOLOGY

1. The peritoneal cavity is covered by a serous lining composed of the visceral peritoneum that lines and supports the abdominal organs, and the parietal peritoneum.
2. See **Figure 30-7, text page 687,** for a diagram of the peritoneal cavity.
3. Normally, the volume of peritoneal fluid is regulated by the pressure gradient balances described previously, with **lymphatic channels** draining 80% of all lymphatic peritoneal fluid.
   a. When the production of peritoneal fluid exceeds the ability of the lymphatic channels to drain the cavity, ascites develops.
4. The most common cause of ascitic fluid buildup is **tumor seeding** the peritoneum, resulting in obstruction of the diaphragmatic and/or abdominal lymphatics.

C. CLINICAL MANIFESTATIONS

1. The pressure of ascitic fluid volume on nearby organs is uncomfortable and restrictive for patients. Several liters of ascitic fluid can be accommodated in the abdomen.
2. The massive accumulation of fluid leads to negative body image changes, anorexia, early satiety, and difficulty breathing and walking.
3. See **Table 30-10, text page 689,** for clinical findings on the patient with malignant ascites.
4. Most physical signs appear after one liter or more of fluid is present.

D. DIAGNOSIS

1. Peritoneal effusion is diagnosed primarily by **physical exam,** with malignant characteristics confirmed by **paracentesis.**
2. The following **signs** are characteristic of free fluid: bulging flanks, tympany at the top of the abdominal curve, elicitation of a fluid wave, and shifting dullness.

E. TREATMENT

1. See **Figure 30-8, text page 689,** for an algorithm for diagnosis and management of malignant ascites. Nursing care measures focus on maintaining fluid and electrolyte balance, comfort measures, and early recognition of complications.
2. **Diet and diuresis**
   a. Sodium restriction and diuretics are usually **ineffective** in malignant ascites.
   b. Unless the underlying malignancy causing the ascites **responds to antineoplastic therapy,** the pathophysiology of ascites will remain unaltered, and fluid accumulation will continue despite exogenous fluid restriction measures.

3. **Removal of fluid**
   a. **Paracentesis**
      (1) Because the fluid reaccumulates rapidly, fluid removal is usually reserved until a large volume of fluid has accumulated and the patient is profoundly symptomatic.
      (2) Removal of two to three liters of fluid and repeated paracentesis taps can lead to severe protein depletion and electrolyte abnormalities.
4. **Obliteration of the intraperitoneal space**
   a. Chemotherapy instillation is designed to provoke an inflammatory response leading to **sclerosis of the peritoneal space linings.**
   b. The **Tenchoff catheter** is often used to provide repeated access to the peritoneum. It remains in place indefinitely and allows peritoneal fluid sampling in addition to drug instillation.
5. **Peritoneovenous shunting**
   a. Shunt devices can be used to recirculate ascitic fluid continuously to the intravascular space.
   b. A **pressure differential** between the abdominal cavity and the thoracic vein enables fluid to ascend from the peritoneal cavity into the superior vena cava.
   c. Peritoneovenous shunting is usually reserved until all other treatment options have failed.
   d. Nursing care of the patient with a peritoneovenous shunt includes
      (1) **Teaching** the patient and family the purpose and care of the shunt.
      (2) **Watching for signs** and **symptoms** of problems with the shunt.
      (3) Recognition and prevention of **infection.**
      (4) Alleviating **anxiety.**

VII. BRAIN: MALIGNANT CEREBRAL EDEMA

A. INCIDENCE

1. Cerebral edema results from an **increase in brain volume** caused by an increase in the fluid content of the brain.
2. The three major types of cerebral edema are **vasogenic edema** (extracellular, the most common type); **cytotoxic edema** (intracellular, due to metabolic abnormalities); and **interstitial edema** (due to cerebrospinal fluid blockage).
3. Malignant cerebral edema is the **vasogenic type** caused by increased permeability of the cerebral capillary endothelial cells.
   a. Most cerebral edema accompanies primary or metastatic brain tumors or carcinomatous meningitis.
4. **Brain metastasis** occurs in 25%–35% of all cancer patients, with **lung cancer** accounting for most of the metastatic lesions in the brain (40%–50%), followed by breast cancer (13%), melanoma, renal carcinoma, and others.

B. PATHOPHYSIOLOGY

1. Mechanisms thought to play a role in the formation of malignant cerebral edema are
   a. Injury to the vascular endothelium by expanding tumor.
   b. Dysplastic vascular structures within tumor lesions.
   c. Biochemically mediated alterations of capillary permeability.
   d. A less stable blood-brain barrier integrity.
2. The progression of edema through brain tissue occurs as bulk fluid flow regulated by cerebral perfusion pressure.
3. The tumor continuously produces edema fluid.
4. Cerebral edema probably leads to **neurologic dysfunction** because of its relation to ischemic effects of the mass itself and/or toxic inhibition of local neuron activity induced by metabolic abnormalities in the surrounding extravascular fluid.
5. When the edema exceeds the limits of compensatory mechanism, **brain herniation** can occur.

C. CLINICAL MANIFESTATIONS

1. Malignant cerebral edema produces **diffuse** signs and symptoms reflecting its more global effects on brain functioning, as opposed to the focal signs and symptoms caused by direct destruction of tissue by tumor.

2. Most patients with metastatic brain tumors have regional swelling of tissue, mostly in the cerebrum. In such patients, the clinical deficits manifested are more often caused by peritumoral edema than by the tumor mass itself.
3. Lack of persistence in tasks, undue irritability, emotional lability, inertia, faulty insight, forgetfulness, reduced range of mental activity, indifference to common social practices, and lack of initiative and spontaneity are early symptoms. As time progresses, the symptoms become more pronounced (see **Table 30-11, text page 691**).
4. **Seizure** is the most common acute onset symptom.
5. **Headache,** another common early symptom, is due to distortion and traction of pain-sensitive structures by the edema.
6. Clinical signs may be observed that relate to **specific parts of the brain,** and these can be localized to the affected area by neurological assessment.

D. DIAGNOSIS

1. **Neurologic examination, CT scanning,** and **magnetic resonance imaging (MRI)** are the primary studies used for diagnosing a brain tumor mass.
2. MRI is best for visualizing cerebral edema.

E. TREATMENT

1. Aggressive therapy is warranted to sustain or restore neurologic function.
2. The principal treatment regimen is radiation therapy.
3. Patients receive supportive care and steroids to reduce edema.
4. **Nursing management** focuses on assessment, medication administration, management of side effects associated with these medications, the institution of safety and seizure precautions, and prevention of complications of immobility.
5. Interventions may be targeted to the patient's specific neurologic deficits.
6. With **advanced cerebral edema** and the resultant intercranial hypertension, changes in vital signs (such as bounding radial pulse, elevated temperature, and respiratory impairment) may be seen.
7. Decreased level of consciousness, change in pupil size and reaction to light, and altered motor response, in addition to other vital signs changes, should alert the nurse to impending brain **herniation,** an oncologic emergency.
8. **Steroids and osmotherapy**
   a. **Glucocorticoids** such as dexamethasone and prednisone are the single most important adjunctive treatment to combat the effects of vasogenic cerebral edema since they rapidly reduce the rate of edema fluid formation by the tumor by 30%.
   b. The aim of steroid therapy is to reduce intracranial pressure and increase cerebral blood flow.
   c. **Steroid withdrawal** can result in headache, lethargy, postural dizziness, or nausea, even if there is no laboratory evidence of adrenal insufficiency.
   d. The continued **long-term use of steroids** can lead to serious toxic effects such as cataracts, hyperglycemia, peptic ulcer, and osteoporosis.
9. **Radiation therapy**
   a. Ionizing radiation to the underlying tumor is the most effective way to decrease malignant edema as well as tumor bulk.
   b. Treatment typically lasts 2–3 weeks.
   c. Despite initial response rates of 80%, radiation accomplishes little in terms of survival.
   d. Median survival after treatment is 3–6 months.
10. **Surgery**
    a. **Surgical decompression** may be in order in selected cases of resistant or relapsing cerebral metastasis.
    b. Surgical decompression or debulking can rapidly reduce the effect of the mass and remove the source of edema production.

VIII. ARMS/LEGS: IATROGENIC SECONDARY LYMPHEDEMA

A. INCIDENCE AND PATHOPHYSIOLOGY

1. Lymphedema occurs most commonly in women who have undergone a modified radical mastectomy, with a rate of **5%–10%**.

2. Mechanical interruption (**surgical technique**) and **radiation** often produce lymphatic obstruction, the most common cause of lymphedema.
3. Other **factors** contributing to the development of lymphedema are obesity, insufficient muscle contraction, inflammation, trauma, formation of fibrosclerotic tissue within the lymph vessel, and scarring secondary to radiation therapy or infection.
4. **Chronic lymphedema** is a late postoperative complication that can occur 6 weeks to 20 years after surgery.
5. **Leg lymphedema** may also occur after groin dissection.
   a. Groin dissection is performed for the treatment of metastatic diseases from primary tumors located in the anatomic area drained by the inguinal lymph nodes.
   b. The incidence of leg lymphedema after surgery increases gradually over time, and by the fifth postoperative year is estimated to occur in 80% of patients.
6. Rarely, a malignant lymphedema of the extremities occurs in a patient with an advanced, untreated lymphoma who has ignored earlier symptoms. Cancer cells obstruct lymph vessels or lymph nodes through intraluminal propagation or by external compression.

B. **DIAGNOSIS**

1. **Assessment** for extremity lymphedema includes monitoring the limb circumference, skin condition, mobility of the extremity, signs of infection, nutritional status, circulation impairment, and constriction caused by clothing or other objects.
2. **Measurements** of the arm circumference are taken prior to surgery and at each postoperative visit.
3. Lymphedema is **defined** as present if there is a difference in measurement of 1.0 cm to 1.5 cm compared to the unaffected extremity.

C. **TREATMENT**

1. The **goals of therapy** are primarily aimed at prevention, at increasing the flow of lymph away from the limb, and at minimizing the formation of new lymph fluid.
2. **Elevation, progressive mild exercise,** and **massage** help mobilize fluid out of the limb.
3. **Prophylactic measures** to prevent new fluid from forming include elastic support sleeves or stockings; sodium restriction; and avoidance of infection, excessive limb use, local heat, and trauma to the limb.
4. Nursing care is usually divided into primary, secondary, and tertiary interventions.
   a. **Primary nursing interventions** for lymphedema involve measures to prevent the complication, beginning preoperatively.
   b. The **secondary phase** of nursing management is directed toward the early detection and initial treatment of lymphedema.
      (1) The patient should be alerted to the signs and symptoms of lymphedema.
      (2) The arms/legs should be measured at regular intervals.
      (3) The affected limb should be elevated.
      (4) Massage therapy may be instituted.
      (5) An elastic wrap or sleeve to the affected extremity may be needed.
      (6) Discomfort should be managed.
      (7) Hand and arm care measures and exercises should be continued.
   c. **Tertiary care** is associated with the long-term care of the patient with lymphedema. It includes elevation of the arm; continued hand and arm care measures and exercises; massage therapy, elastic wrap or sleeve to the extremity; pain control; and assessment of the patient for general functioning and ability to perform activities of daily living.
   d. Long-term use of **diuretics** is reserved for cases of generalized low-protein edemas in which the total body sodium content is elevated.

IX. **FEET: MALIGNANT PEDAL EDEMA**

1. Peripheral, or dependent, edema is common in patients with far advanced cancer.
2. Among the multiple causes are the lack of normal muscular activity, which would ordinarily return fluids from the periphery to the central circulation; hypoalbuminemia; venous or lymphatic obstruction; compromised circulation; malnutrition; and hyperaldosteronism.

A. **DIAGNOSIS**

1. **Measurement** of the ankle is useful to record changes in circumference and note the effectiveness of treatment measures.
2. **Pitting** can be assessed by pressing the thumb into the patient's skin over a bony surface.
3. The edema of advanced cancer is **bilateral;** a unilateral edema would lead to a search for a treatable cause such as thrombophlebitis.

B. **TREATMENT**

1. Three approaches to relieving ankle edema are improving nutritional status; elevating the legs while sitting and wearing support stockings, while eliminating constrictive clothing (to improve venous return); and using diuretics on a short-term basis.

PRACTICE QUESTIONS

1. Third spacing is
    (A) the normal fluid distribution in the extracellular and intravascular compartments.
    (B) an excess of interstitial fluid accumulation.
    (C) fluid retention in sites that normally have very little or no fluid.
    (D) lack of normal osmotic pressures.

2. Which of the following conditions is benign and iatrogenic in origin and is usually secondary to radical cancer surgery?
    (A) pericardial effusion
    (B) lymphedema
    (C) pleural effusion
    (D) anasarca

3. Choose the statement that **most** accurately describes the degree of subjective symptoms produced by malignant pericardial and pleural **effusions.**
    (A) Symptoms tend to be related more to the rate of fluid accumulation than to the volume collected.
    (B) Symptoms tend to be related more to the volume of fluid collected than to the rate of collection.
    (C) Symptoms are related more to the underlying disease and length of time the patient has been diagnosed with cancer.
    (D) Symptoms correspond directly to whether the metastatic disease is from microscopic seeding of the cavities or from local extension.

4. Thoracentesis involves fluid removal from
    (A) the pericardial sac.
    (B) the pleural cavity.
    (C) the abdominal cavity.
    (D) the spinal column.

5. The **first** and **most common** means of obliteration of the pleural cavity in a patient with chronic, recurrent malignant pleural effusions is
    (A) pleuroperitoneal shunt.
    (B) pleural stripping.
    (C) sclerosis.
    (D) local radiation.

6. Malignant pericardial effusions
    (A) are extremely rare.
    (B) are easily detected by tachycardia, low blood pressure, and shortness of breath.
    (C) occur in 50% of all patients with cancer, especially the hematologic malignancies.
    (D) are not easily detected by routine tests and are found in 8%–20% of autopsies.

7.   The patient who is experiencing a pericardial effusion shows signs and symptoms that include
     (A)   chest pain, confusion, nausea, and vomiting.
     (B)   confusion, nausea, vomiting, and hypertension.
     (C)   hypertension, bradycardia, and increased cardiac output.
     (D)   decreased cardiac output, dyspnea, cough, and chest pain.

8.   The cancer **most** often associated with malignant ascites is
     (A)   ovarian cancer.
     (B)   pancreatic cancer.
     (C)   breast cancer.
     (D)   esophageal cancer.

9.   The **most** common acute sign of malignant cerebral edema is
     (A)   headache.
     (B)   nausea/vomiting.
     (C)   seizure.
     (D)   disorientation.

10. Prophylactic measures to prevent new fluid from forming in patients with lymphedema of the arm or leg
     include all of the following **except**
     (A)   elastic support sleeves or stockings.
     (B)   pain control.
     (C)   sodium restriction.
     (D)   avoidance of infection.

ANSWER EXPLANATIONS

1.   **The answer is (C).**   The distribution pattern of body water is termed fluid spacing. First spacing describes a normal distribution of fluid in both the extracellular and the intracellular compartments. Second spacing refers to an excess accumulation of interstitial fluid (edema), and third spacing is fluid retention in sites that normally have no fluid or a minimum of fluid (effusion). (676)

2.   **The answer is (B).**   Lymphedema is a benign, iatrogenic problem caused by radical cancer surgery. Arm lymphedema often developed after the most common treatment for all types of breast cancer in the past: radical mastectomy with axillary node dissection followed by radiation. It now occurs much less frequently. Lymphedema of the leg may develop after groin dissection that is performed for the treatment of metastatic disease from primary tumors. Mechanical interruption (surgical technique) and radiation often produce lymphatic obstruction, the most common cause of lymphedema. (677, 692)

3.   **The answer is (A).**   Common presenting signs and symptoms of malignant effusions are distressing to most patients. The degree of subjective symptoms produced by a pleural effusion depends less on the amount of fluid involved than on the rapidity with which it has accumulated. If fluid accumulation is gradual, the heart and lungs can accommodate, but rapid accumulation can trigger an oncologic emergency. (680, 684)

4.   **The answer is (B).**   Relief of pleural effusion symptoms such as dyspnea, cough, and dull, aching chest pain is a short-term treatment goal that is usually achieved when the pleural fluid is mechanically drained. Thoracentesis involves pleural fluid removal by needle aspiration through the chest wall. Fluid tends to reaccumulate when it is not possible to control the underlying cancer. Long-range treatment goals are directed toward the obliteration of the pleural space so that pleural fluid cannot reaccumulate. (681)

5.   **The answer is (C).**   Sclerosis with chemical agents is the most common method used to obliterate the pleural space in patients with malignant pleural effusions. Chemical sclerosing does not prolong the patient's life but may enhance quality of life by relieving symptoms and reducing the time a patient spends in the hospital. Shunts and stripping are surgical methods that become options after other approaches have been tried and the pleural effusion remains uncontrolled. Although external beam radiation may be used as local treatment for mediastinal tumors, hemithoracic radiation is not recommended as a first-line management of malignant pleural effusions because of the hazard of pulmonary fibrosis. (682–684)

6.   **The answer is (D).**   Malignant pericardial effusions are not easily detected by routine tests and are found in 8%–20% of autopsies. Only 30% of affected patients are symptomatic. Since pericardial effusion is not easily detected by routine tests, it is often not discovered while the patient is alive. (684)

7.   **The answer is (D).**   Pericardial effusion interferes with cardiac function because the fluid burden occupies space and reduces the volume of the heart in diastole. Systemic circulatory effects of decreased cardiac output and impaired venous return lead to generalized congestion. The body tries to compensate in several ways: tachycardia, an increase in systemic and pulmonary venous pressure, and increased ejection fraction. (684–685)

8.   **The answer is (A).**   Malignant peritoneal effusion (ascites) is most common in patients with ovarian cancer. Ascites is found at presentation in 33% of these patients, and over 60% will develop ascites at some time before death. (687)

9.   **The answer is (C).**   Malignant cerebral edema produces diffuse signs and symptoms reflecting its more global effects on brain functioning, as opposed to the focal signs and symptoms caused by direct destruction of tissue by tumor. Subtle early changes in the patient's status are vague and usually are observed only by someone who knows the patient well. Seizure is the most common acute onset sign. Headache, another common early symptom, is due to distortion and traction of pain-sensitive structures by the edema. (691)

10.   **The answer is (B).**   Prophylactic measures to prevent new fluid from forming include elastic support sleeves or stockings; sodium restriction; and avoidance of infection, excessive use of the limb, local heat, and trauma to the limb. Preventive nursing measures are categorized as primary nursing interventions. Tertiary care is associated with the long-term care of the patient with lymphedema and includes arm elevation, continued hand and arm care measures and exercises, massage therapy, elastic wrap or sleeve to the extremity, pain control, and assessment of the patient for general functioning and ability to perform activities of daily living. (693)

31

Sexual and Reproductive Dysfunction

STUDY OUTLINE

I.   INTRODUCTION

1. Difficulties with sexual intimacy and childbearing affect all aspects of the patient's and family's lives, sometimes influencing choices for therapy.
2. Alterations in sexual function may be permanent or temporary. Even short-term changes can have long-term effects on the patient and family, affecting lifestyles and life choices.
3. Various factors interact to affect the cancer patient's sexuality, including
   a. **The biologic/physiologic process of cancer,** including infertility and sterility.
   b. **The effects of treatment and the alterations caused by cancer and treatment,** including changes in body appearance and the inability to have intercourse.
   c. **The psychologic issues surrounding the patient and family,** including psychosexual issues of alteration in body image, fears of abandonment, loss of self-esteem, alterations in sexual identity, and concerns about self.

II.   PHYSIOLOGY OF GONADAL FUNCTION

1. See **Figures 31-1 and 31-2, text page 698,** along with accompanying text, for a review of normal testicular and ovarian function, and **Figures 31-3 and 31-4, text page 699,** for a review of ovarian failure and germinal aplasia.
2. The hormones involved in the control of reproduction are
   a. **Luteinizing hormone-releasing hormone (LHRH),** or **gonadotropin-releasing hormone (GnRH),** secreted by the hypothalamus and stimulating the anterior pituitary to produce.
   b. **Luteinizing hormone (LH)** and **follicle-stimulating hormone (FSH),** which stimulate the testis and ovary to produce the appropriate hormones.
3. When blood levels of LH and FSH are adequate, the hormones exert a **negative feedback** on the pituitary, thus decreasing secretion.
4. When blood levels of LH and FSH are inadequate, which may occur as a result of **disease, therapy, psychologic factors,** or any combination of these factors, **ovarian failure** (in women) and **germinal aplasia** (in men) may be the result.

III.   EFFECT OF CANCER THERAPY ON GONADAL FUNCTION

A.   SURGERY

1. Surgery for cancer of the **gastrointestinal** and **genitourinary tracts** may result in removal of or damage to sexual organs, causing sexual dysfunction.
2. In addition, surgery on **head** and **neck** areas and on the **breast** or **amputation** may alter body image and affect sexual identity.
3. **Cancer of the colon and rectum**
   a. The most common surgery for colon cancer is some degree of **colectomy** with or without a **colostomy.** Cancer of the rectum, however, may require **anterior or abdominoperineal resection (APR).**
   b. Sexual dysfunction caused by APR may be related to the **placement of a colostomy** or to **dysfunctions related to removal of or interference with sexual organ function,** or some combination of the two.

    c.   Sexual dysfunction caused by colostomy has been associated with patient's **negative changes in body image and self-esteem,** as well as the **responses by family and friends.**

    d.   **APR** in women may also mean removal of the ovaries or uterus, causing dysfunction from primary **inability to have children** or from **alterations in hormonal patterns.** Vaginal removal or scarring may also interfere with intercourse.

    e.   **APR** in men produces more severe sexual dysfunction associated with **damage to nerves that control erection and ejaculation.** Erectile impotence or problems with ejaculation may result.

    f.   For all patients the **removal of rectal tissue** appears to be the common denominator to organic sexual dysfunction. If the rectum remains intact, there rarely is an associated sexual dysfunction without direct tumor involvement.

  4. **Cancers of the genitourinary tract**

    a. **Bladder cancer**

      (1) **Radical cystectomy** results in sexual dysfunction for both men and women, although **penile replacement** and **revascularization** or **vaginal reconstruction** may reduce dysfunction.

      (2) **Urinary diversion** is also necessary. A **Kock pouch,** or continent reservoir, reduces its effects on body image.

    b. **Penile cancer/cancer of the male urethra**

      (1) **Penile implants** have been used successfully after total penectomy. Cancer of the penis is rare, however.

    c. **Testicular cancer**

      (1) Testicular cancer may be treated by **orchiectomy** (either unilateral or bilateral) and possibly **retroperitoneal lymph node dissection** and/or removal of a pelvic mass.

      (2) Bilateral orchiectomy produces **sterility** and **decreased libido** as a result of the loss of testosterone.

      (3) Retroperitoneal lymph node dissection may result in **temporary or permanent loss of ejaculation,** whereas potency and the ability to have an orgasm remain. New nerve-sparing surgical procedures can spare the loss of ejaculation.

      (4) For those individuals desiring to maintain fertility, sperm banking should be discussed and arranged prior to therapy.

    d. **Prostate cancer**

      (1) Treatments for prostate cancer have a potential to alter sexual function.

      (2) **Prostatectomy** may involve **transurethral, transabdominal,** or **perineal resection.**

        (a) **Retrograde ejaculation** is common with the first two procedures; **erectile dysfunction** also may occur with the second.

        (b) Permanent damage to erectile function with loss of emission and ejaculation may occur with perineal resection, or **radical prostatectomy.**

        (c) The development of **nerve-sparing or potency-sparing** surgery has been a significant development in the surgical treatment of prostate cancer.

      (3) **Bilateral orchiectomy** causes sexual dysfunction through gradual diminution of libido, impotence, gynecomastia, and penile atrophy. **Penile prosthesis** may restore erectile potential, and new surgical techniques reduce retrograde ejaculation and sterility.

      (4) **With new techniques, sterility in individuals with retrograde ejaculation is not as frequent.** Because of the ability to separate sperm from urine, artificial insemination of the mate may be possible.

  5. **Gynecologic malignancies**

    a. Sexual identity, as well as sexual functioning, are often affected permanently by surgery of the vulva, vagina, uterus and uterine cervix, ovary and fallopian tube, or pelvic exenteration.

    b. Reproductive counseling should be provided to patient and family before surgical intervention.

    c. **Vulvar cancer** occurs primarily in postmenopausal women.

      (1) Good cosmetic results occur for all but the **simple vulvectomy,** which removes the labia and subcutaneous tissue, with retention of the clitoris.

      (2) **Radical vulvectomy,** which removes the labia and clitoris and usually includes a groin node dissection, produces a range of side effects, including altered orgasmic potential.

    d. Although **vaginal cancer** is less common, surgery for the majority of gynecologic cancers results in some abnormality and/or need for reconstruction of the vagina.

    e. Invasive **cancer of the uterine corpus and cervix** are the first and second most common gynecologic malignancies, representing 10% of all cancers in women.

        (1) Of the procedures used for cervical intraepithelial neoplasia and carcinoma in situ, only **simple hysterectomy** affects fertility and childbearing. It may also affect sexual identity and/or body image.

        (2) Treatment for invasive disease involves **radical hysterectomy,** consisting of removal of the uterus and cervix, supporting structures, and upper third of the vagina and lymph nodes.

        (3) For **cancer of the endometrium,** the ovaries and fallopian tubes also may be removed, producing **menopausal symptoms.**

            (a) Radical hysterectomy, including oophorectomy, may also decrease sexual desire as a consequence of loss of childbearing potential.

    f. Initial treatment for **ovarian cancer** involves radical hysterectomy with bilateral salpingo-oophorectomy and omentectomy, with associated **loss of fertility** and **occurrence of menopausal symptoms.**

  6. **Pelvic exenteration**

    a. In women, dysfunction related to **removal of all pelvic organs** with resulting ostomies is profound and is associated with changes in body image, sexual identity, and self-esteem.

  7. **Breast cancer**

    a. **Mastectomy** or **lumpectomy** may cause dysfunction as a result of psychologic issues, including regret over the loss of breast-feeding capability, fear of rejection, physical discomfort, anxiety about initiating sexual activities, and feelings of being defective or different.

    b. Although it has been previously reported that lumpectomy caused significantly less alteration in body image and sexual functioning, recent studies showed no difference between women receiving lumpectomy and radiotherapy and women undergoing mastectomy.

    c. What appears to be of significance is the opportunity to select the surgical technique employed. Therefore, choices should be offered whenever possible.

    d. **Breast reconstruction** also bolsters self-esteem and decreases negative reactions to body image alterations.

  8. **Head and neck cancer**

    a. Surgical treatment of head and neck cancer can lead to alterations in self-esteem and body image, resulting in changes in sexuality and intimacy.

    b. Alterations in sensation, breathing, voice, and the ability to use the mouth and tongue may affect sexuality.

    c. Presurgical counseling and long-term follow-up may be helpful in sexual rehabilitation of patients with head and neck cancer.

B. RADIATION THERAPY

  1. Radiation therapy can cause sexual and reproductive dysfunction through

    a. **Primary organ failure,** e.g., ovarian failure and testicular aplasia.

    b. **Alterations in organ function,** e.g., decreased lubrication and impotence.

    c. The **temporary and permanent effects of therapy unassociated with reproduction,** e.g., diarrhea, fatigue, anxiety, low self-esteem.

  2. Permanent effects most commonly are related to **total dose, volume of tissues irradiated, exposure time, age,** and **prior fertility status.**

  3. For woman, movement of the ovaries out of the radiation field (oophoropexy), with appropriate shielding, has helped maintain fertility.

  4. Low-level testicular radiation (caused for example by scatter from a primary field) can cause an alteration in testicular function and reduced/absent spermatogenesis, so patients who do not require primary testicular irradiation should receive additional testicular shielding to alleviate infertility sequelae.

  5. The majority of men treated by external beam for prostate cancer have temporary or permanent impotence. The impotence is thought to be caused by fibrosis of pelvic vasculature or radiation damage of pelvic nerves.

  6. In addition to sterility or transient infertility, radiation therapy can cause decreases in sexual enjoyment, ability to obtain orgasm, libido, and frequency of intercourse and sexual dreams, as well as vaginal stenosis in women.

C. **CHEMOTHERAPY**

1. Chemotherapy-induced reproductive and sexual dysfunction is related to the **type of drug** (e.g., alkylating agents), **dose, length of treatment, age,** and **sex** of the individual receiving treatment and the **length of time after treatment.**
2. Other factors that play a role in infertility or sexual dysfunction include single versus multiple agents and drugs given to combat side effects of chemotherapy.
3. See **Table 31-1, text page 705,** for a list of chemotherapeutic agents that affect sexual or reproductive function.
4. **Men**
   a. Infertility occurs in men primarily through **depletion of the germinal epithelium** that lines the seminiferous tubules.
   b. The chemotherapy regimen **MOPP,** used in the treatment of Hodgkin's disease, produces frequent sexual dysfunction and decreased fertility, as does hormonal manipulation and treatment with **estrogens.**
5. **Women**
   a. Women experience sexual and reproductive dysfunction from chemotherapy as a result of **hormonal alterations** or direct effects that cause ovarian fibrosis and follicle destruction.
   b. **MOPP** combination chemotherapy in women older than 30 years of age has been implicated in amenorrhea and early menopause.
   c. When hormonal manipulation includes **androgens,** both sexual and reproductive functions and body image and feelings of sexual identity are affected.
6. **Children**
   a. Effects of chemotherapy on male children appear to be **age related,** with pubertal males showing greater effects than prepubertal males.
7. **Other issues**
   a. A number of medications used in the treatment of cancer can cause impotence and/or can negatively affect sexual desire, sense of sexual fulfillment, and ability to achieve orgasm. **Table 31-2, text page 706,** lists some cancer-associated drugs that affect sexual and reproductive function.

D. **BIOLOGIC RESPONSE MODIFIERS**

1. Little information presently is available on the sexual and reproductive dysfunctions associated with BRMs, although **interferons** have been associated with decreased libido.
2. The common side effects of BRMs, such as fatigue and flulike symptoms, affect interest in and comfort with sexual activities.

E. **BONE MARROW TRANSPLANTATION**

1. Sexual and reproductive dysfunctions associated with **bone marrow transplantation** may include chronic fatigue, body image alterations, gonadal dysfunction, and infertility. Sexual interest and activity increase as health improves.
2. Following bone marrow transplantation, women experienced decreased sexual desire and satisfaction, vaginal atrophy, decreased vaginal lubrication, and painful intercourse. Men may experience premature ejaculation.
3. Research suggests that most patients receiving BMT with TBI will experience gonadal dysfunction.

F. **SEXUAL COUNSELING**

1. All patients should receive information concerning the possible side effects of disease and treatment on sexuality and reproduction.
2. Potential side effects and possible methods for management should be discussed with the patient (and partner, if available) at diagnosis, throughout treatment, and during follow-up visits.
3. Nurses should include sexuality in their assessments of all patients. The **ALARM** model and the **Auchincloss** model may be helpful in providing a structure for evaluating sexual functioning in the patient and partner experiencing a cancer diagnosis (see **Table 31-3, text page 707**).
4. The **PLISSIT** model (see **Table 31-4, text page 707**) can be used to guide intervention to maintain optimal sexual functioning and to promote adaptation to the sexual and reproductive side effects of disease and treatment.

IV.   **FERTILITY CONSIDERATIONS AND PROCREATIVE ALTERNATIVES**

    A.   **MUTAGENICITY**

        1.   It has been difficult to specifically implicate germ cell mutations from chemotherapy or radiation therapy as the cause of adverse outcomes to pregnancies in humans.

    B.   **TERATOGENICITY**

        1.   Both chemotherapy and radiation therapy are known to have **teratogenetic effects on the fetus,** especially in the first trimester, causing spontaneous abortion, fetal malformation, or fetal death.

        2.   Fetal damage probably does not occur at doses less than 10 cGy of radiation and is only rarely reported at doses less than 50 cGy.

        3.   Chemotherapy (particularly the alkylating agents and antimetabolites) have been most often associated with fetal malformations. **Table 31-5, text page 708,** lists the teratogenic effects of chemotherapy.

    C.   **REPRODUCTIVE COUNSELING**

        1.   Discussions concerning fertility and reproduction issues should be held before the onset of therapy and should continue well into the posttreatment and follow-up stages.

        2.   Issues to be discussed include

            a.   Current fertility status.

            b.   Desire for future childbearing.

            c.   Contraceptive practices.

        3.   **Birth control measures** should be implemented to avoid pregnancy during cancer therapy. However, methods to maintain fertility should be investigated.

        4.   **Shielding of the testes or ovaries** or positioning of the ovaries outside the radiation field is advised.

        5.   For those individuals receiving chemotherapy, **birth control pills for women** and **gonadotropin-releasing hormone analogues for men** may protect the germ cells.

        6.   It has been suggested that after cancer therapy an individual should wait a minimum of 2 years before attempting conception.

            a.   **This suggestion is made both to prevent pregnancy during the time recurrence is most likely and to allow for the recovery of spermatogenesis or ovarian function.**

    D.   **SPERM BANKING**

        1.   **Sperm banking** has been used to preserve procreation abilities in men undergoing cancer therapy, provided they are fertile at diagnosis.

        2.   Even if artificial insemination is never completed, the knowledge that semen has been banked can provide a psychologic boost for the male undergoing therapy.

    E.   **IN VITRO FERTILIZATION AND EMBRYO TRANSFER**

        1.   **In vitro fertilization** may be used for male infertility because of low sperm counts or for female infertility as a result of severe endometriosis.

        2.   Other methods to attain fertility include the use of **cryopreserved oocytes and zygotes,** with pregnancy rates of about 40%.

V.   **PREGNANCY AND CANCER**

    A.   **MEDICAL MANAGEMENT OF COMMONLY ASSOCIATED CANCERS**

        1.   **Breast cancer**

            a.   Breast cancer is the cancer most commonly associated with pregnancy.

            b.   **Breast examination** should be part of the initial prenatal visit. BSE education should be included.

            c.   If a mass is felt, prompt **evaluation, including a mammogram,** is necessary.

    d. Treatment should proceed as in the nonpregnant patient.
      (1) **Biopsy** is safe to the fetus and should be performed without delay.
      (2) Further therapy can be tailored to **time, gestation, physician recommendations,** and **patient wishes.**
      (3) In general, **modified mastectomy with lymph node sampling** is the standard treatment for early disease. Adjuvant chemotherapy can be delayed until after delivery.
      (4) For the woman who desires breast-conserving surgery, **lumpectomy** with lymph node sampling may be done but radiation therapy should be delayed until after delivery.
      (5) For advanced disease, **surgery** and **chemotherapy** should be undertaken without delay.
      (6) **Therapeutic abortion** may be suggested during the first term to prevent chemotherapy exposure to the fetus.
    e. Survival rates are comparable to those of nonpregnant women.
    f. **Further pregnancies following a breast cancer diagnosis have been considered controversial.** Most authors suggest a wait of 1–3 years after treatment for stages I and II and a wait of up to 5 years for stages III and IV. It is also suggested that breast feeding be restricted to the nonirradiated breast.

  2. **Cancer of the cervix**
    a. The second cancer commonly associated with pregnancy is cancer of the cervix. **Carcinoma in situ** is the most common form.
    b. Signs and symptoms are similar to those found in the nonpregnant patient, with the majority of patients experiencing **vaginal bleeding or discharge.**
    c. Diagnosis is typically made by **Pap smear.** If the smear is abnormal, **colposcopy with appropriate biopsies** should be undertaken. **Cone biopsy should be avoided** because it is associated with a 30% complication rate.
    d. For carcinoma in situ the pregnancy should be allowed to continue. Biopsy should be repeated every 6 to 8 weeks and, unless there is progression, **definitive therapy should be delayed until after delivery.**
    e. If frank **invasion** is found, treatment as for nonpregnant women should not be delayed.
      (1) During the first two trimesters, **surgery** or **radiation therapy, without therapeutic abortion,** is usually undertaken.
      (2) Early stage disease (IA and IB) may be treated with **radical hysterectomy** and **pelvic node dissection,** whereas in advanced disease **radiation therapy** is the most common treatment.
      (3) During the third trimester, fetal viability usually can be awaited and the baby delivered by **cesarean section,** after which the appropriate cancer therapy can be given.

  3. **Ovarian cancer**
    a. Ovarian masses are common during therapy. Few are malignant.
    b. **If a malignancy is diagnosed, treatment should proceed as in the nonpregnant patient.**
      (1) **Stage IA** disease of low-grade histologic findings can be managed by **unilateral oophorectomy** and **biopsy of the other ovary.** The pregnancy may be allowed to continue.
      (2) For **all other stages,** standard therapy of **radical hysterectomy, omentectomy, node biopsy,** and **peritoneal washings** should be carried out.
      (3) If the patient is **near term,** a **cesarean section,** followed by appropriate therapy, may be performed.
    c. As many as half of all patients will be diagnosed with stage III or IV disease. A prognosis of long-term survival is poor.
    d. The wishes of the patient should be considered. Women with advanced disease may choose to delay treatment until the fetus is viable.
      (1) **Palliative treatment** should be instituted at the earliest possible time.
  4. **Malignant melanoma**
    a. Malignant melanoma is one of the most rapidly increasing cancers.
      (1) It occurs most often in a **preexisting mole** in fair-haired individuals with blue or green eyes and an inability to tan when exposed to the sun.
      (2) The peak incidence is during the **third and fourth decades.**
    b. Melanoma that occurs during pregnancy is more often found on the **trunk,** a site associated with poor prognosis. In addition, all pigmented areas darken during pregnancy, which makes early diagnosis difficult.
    c. **Biopsy** and **removal of questionable lesions** are indicated.

   d. For patients with advanced disease, **therapeutic abortion** followed by **palliative chemotherapy** is advised.
   e. Because malignant melanoma is **known to metastasize to the placenta and fetus,** the placenta should be carefully evaluated at delivery and the baby monitored for development of melanoma.
   f. Further pregnancies should not be undertaken until at least 2 years after diagnosis and treatment.

5. **Lymphomas**
    a. Both Hodgkin's disease and non-Hodgkin's lymphoma (NHL) are rare in pregnant women.
    b. Hodgkin's disease confined to the neck or axilla can be treated with **radiation therapy used with fetal shielding.**
    c. Because more extensive disease requires combination chemotherapy, a **therapeutic abortion** is suggested during the first half of pregnancy.
    d. During the second half, therapy will be defined by the stage of the pregnancy.
    e. If viability is imminent, therapy may be delayed or single-drug treatment instituted and delivery awaited.
    f. For rapidly progressing disease, **combination chemotherapy** should be instituted immediately.

6. **Leukemia**
    a. **Treatment should be instituted immediately unless the fetus is viable or near viability.**
        (1) If the fetus is viable, delivery should not be delayed.
        (2) If the fetus is near viability, **leukapheresis** may be utilized until delivery is possible.
        (3) **Therapeutic abortion** is suggested during the **first trimester** to avoid fetal exposure to chemotherapy.
    b. Leukemia **may spread to the placenta and fetus;** thus placental and fetal monitoring are important aspects of delivery and postpartum care.

B. **EFFECTS OF TREATMENT AND MALIGNANCY ON THE FETUS**

1. **Surgery**
    a. **Maternal surgery can be safely accomplished with minimal risk to the fetus. Pelvic surgery is more easily accomplished during the second trimester.**
    b. There is little risk to the fetus from short exposure to anesthetic agents after the first trimester, provided ventilation is adequate and hypotension is prevented.
2. **Radiation**
    a. **Low doses of radiation** associated with diagnostic X-ray studies are **not harmful** if adequate fetal shielding is provided.
    b. **Higher doses of radiation** have been associated with fetal damage, including mental retardation, skin changes, and spontaneous abortions.
    c. Radiation to the pelvis should be avoided.
3. **Chemotherapy**
    a. **Chemotherapy during the first trimester** has been associated with fetal wastage, malformations, and low birth weight.
4. **Maternal-fetal spread**
    a. Only a few cancers spread from the mother to the fetus, with **melanoma, NHL,** and **leukemia** the most common.

C. **NURSING MANAGEMENT OF THE PREGNANT PATIENT**

1. Interventions to include **psychosocial, educational,** and **ethical** considerations must be developed. These include
    a. Careful explanations of all aspects of care, with special emphasis on the support of the patient and her family.
        (1) **Issues relating to the diagnosis and treatment of cancer may produce ambivalence toward pregnancy and threaten the establishment of emotional affiliation to the growing child.**
    b. Discussion of **ethical considerations** as plans for pregnancy are contrasted with needs for therapy. In some instances therapeutic abortion may be necessary for optimal treatment; in others, therapy delays may be requested to provide for the safety of the fetus.

PRACTICE QUESTIONS

1. Sexuality in the cancer patient may be affected by several factors, including each of the following **except**
    (A) psychosexual changes associated with mutagenicity.
    (B) physiologic problems of fertility and sterility.
    (C) psychologic issues such as loss of self-esteem and fears of abandonment.
    (D) changes in body appearance resulting from therapy.

2. For patients who undergo surgery for gastrointestinal cancer, possible organic sexual dysfunction is **most** closely associated with
    (A) placement of a colostomy.
    (B) removal of rectal tissue.
    (C) changes in body image.
    (D) responses by family and friends.

3. Treatments for prostate cancer have a potential to alter sexual function, even though prostate cancer occurs mostly in older men. Permanent damage to erectile function with loss of emission and ejaculation is **most** likely to occur with
    (A) radical prostatectomy.
    (B) transurethral resection.
    (C) bilateral orchiectomy.
    (D) transabdominal resection.

4. Which of the following statements about the relationship between gynecologic malignancies and sexual dysfunction is correct?
    (A) Pelvic exenteration results in relatively few problems with sexual dysfunction.
    (B) The procedures commonly used to treat carcinoma in situ are not likely to affect fertility or childbearing.
    (C) Menopausal symptoms are closely associated with radical hysterectomy.
    (D) The majority of gynecologic cancers result in some abnormality of the vagina.

5. A woman wishing to minimize the effects of breast surgery on her sexuality would be **most** likely to elect
    (A) lumpectomy.
    (B) modified mastectomy.
    (C) radical mastectomy.
    (D) any of the above might be selected by an individual woman; it is the opportunity to have input into treatment selection that is significant.

6. Which of the following side effects is **least** likely to occur as a result of radiation therapy?
    (A) alterations in organ function, e.g., decreased vaginal lubrication
    (B) enhanced hormonal activity, e.g., overstimulation of the hypothalamus or pituitary
    (C) general or psychologic side effects of therapy that can alter sexual function, e.g., diarrhea, loss of sexual desire
    (D) primary organ failure, e.g., ovarian failure

7. Which of the following has been implicated in sexual dysfunction in both men and women receiving chemotherapy?
    (A) depletion of the germinal epithelium
    (B) treatment with estrogens
    (C) combination chemotherapy with MOPP
    (D) treatment with androgens

8. It has been suggested that after cancer therapy an individual should wait a minimum of 2 years before attempting conception. One reason for this is to allow for the recovery of spermatogenesis or ovarian function. Another important reason is that
    (A) residues from chemotherapy typically remain in the body for at least 18 months.
    (B) the psychologic effects of cancer therapy may be felt for a prolonged period of time.
    (C) germinal epithelium may have been damaged by chemotherapy and/or radiation therapy.
    (D) recurrence is most likely within the first 2 years after cancer therapy.

9. Which of the following statements about pregnancy and cancer is **false?**
    (A) Most cancers do not adversely affect a pregnancy.
    (B) In general, pregnancy does not adversely affect the outcome of a cancer.
    (C) Therapeutic abortion has been shown to be of benefit in altering disease progression.
    (D) Treatment options should be evaluated as though the patient were not pregnant and therapy should be instituted when appropriate.

10. The standard treatment for early breast cancer diagnosed in a pregnant woman consists of
    (A) immediate surgery and chemotherapy.
    (B) modified mastectomy with lymph node sampling.
    (C) lumpectomy with lymph node sampling if the woman is in the first trimester of pregnancy.
    (D) mammogram followed by biopsy and adjuvant chemotherapy.

11. Invasion of a cervical carcino ma in situ into underlying tissue is found in a woman during the third trimester of her pregnancy. Which of the following treatments is **most** likely to be followed?
    (A) Fetal viability is awaited and appropriate therapy is given after delivery of the baby by cesarean section.
    (B) Surgery or radiation therapy, without therapeutic abortion, is undertaken immediately.
    (C) A radical hysterectomy and pelvic node dissection is performed and combined with radiation therapy.
    (D) Therapeutic abortion is performed immediately and followed by standard treatment for advanced disease.

12. Evaluation of the placenta for evidence of metastasis to the fetus is **most** likely to be carried out under which of the following situations?
    (A) when the mother has received combination chemotherapy during the third trimester of pregnancy
    (B) when the mother has received low doses of radiation during the first trimester of pregnancy
    (C) when the mother has breast cancer or invasive cervical cancer
    (D) when the mother has a melanoma or lymphoma

13. Which of the following is **most** likely to involve risk to the fetus whose mother is being treated for cancer?
    (A) pelvic surgery on the mother during the second trimester of pregnancy
    (B) low doses of radiation associated with diagnostic X rays
    (C) chemotherapy during the first trimester of pregnancy
    (D) the use of anesthetic agents during surgery on the mother during the second trimester of pregnancy

ANSWER EXPLANATIONS

1. **The answer is (A).**   Among the factors that affect the cancer patient's sexuality are those related to the biologic/physiologic process of cancer, the effects of treatment, the alterations caused by cancer and treatment, and the psychologic issues surrounding the patient and family. Physiologic problems of infertility and sterility, changes in body appearance, and the inability to have intercourse are enhanced by psychologic and psychosexual issues of alteration in body image, fears of abandonment, loss of self-esteem, alterations in sexual identity, and concerns about self. Mutagenicity and psychosexual changes are not closely related. (697)

2. **The answer is (B).**   Choices (A), (C), and (D), while all associated with sexual dysfunction resulting from gastrointestinal surgery, primarily are psychosexual and not organic issues. For all patients the removal of rectal tissue appears to be the most common denominator to organic sexual dysfunction. If the rectum remains intact, there rarely is an associated sexual dysfunction without direct tumor invasion. (700)

3. **The answer is (A).**   Permanent damage to erectile function with loss of emission and ejaculation may occur with perineal resection, or radical prostatectomy. Retrograde ejaculation is common with transurethral and transabdominal resection; erectile dysfunction with transabdominal resection. Bilateral orchiectomy causes sexual dysfunction through gradual diminution of libido, impotence, gynecomastia, and penile atrophy. (701)

4. **The answer is (D).**   Sexual identity, as well as sexual functioning, is often affected permanently by surgery of the vulva, vagina, uterus and uterine cervix, ovary and fallopian tube, or pelvic exenteration. Although vaginal cancer is less common than most other gynecologic malignancies, surgery for the majority of gynecologic cancers (except for carcinoma in situ) results in some abnormality and/or reconstruction

of the vagina. In women, dysfunction related to pelvic exenteration (removal of all pelvic organs) with resulting ostomies is profound and is associated with changes in body image, sexual identity, and self-esteem. Simple hysterectomy, used to treat noninvasive cervical cancer, affects fertility and childbearing. Menopausal symptoms are most closely related to removal of the ovaries and fallopian tubes, which is not part of a radical hysterectomy. (702)

5. **The answer is (D).** Although it has been previously reported that the use of breast-preserving surgery (lumpectomy) has been shown to cause significantly less alteration in body image, sexual desire, and frequency of intercourse, recent studies showed no difference between women receiving lumpectomy and radiotherapy, and women undergoing mastectomy. What appears to be of significance is the opportunity or perceived opportunity to **select the surgical technique employed. Thus, choices should be offered whenever possible.** (703)

6. **The answer is (B).** Radiation therapy can cause sexual and reproductive dysfunction through primary organ failure (e.g., ovarian failure and testicular aplasia), through alterations in organ function (e.g., decreased lubrication and impotence), and through the temporary and permanent effects of therapy associated with reproduction (e.g., diarrhea and fatigue). In addition, radiation therapy can cause decreases in sexual enjoyment, ability to obtain orgasm, libido, and frequency of intercourse and sexual dreams, as well as vaginal stenosis in women. (703-704)

7. **The answer is (C).** Chemotherapy-induced reproductive and sexual dysfunction is related to the type of drug, dose, length of treatment, age, and sex of the individual receiving treatment and to the length of time after treatment, as well as to the use of single versus multiple agents and drugs given to combat side effects of chemotherapy. Combination chemotherapy with MOPP (mechlorethamine, vincristine, procarbazine, and prednisone) has been shown to produce sexual dysfunction and to decrease fertility in both men and women. Androgen therapy affects sexual function in women; estrogen therapy affects sexual function in men. Chemotherapy may deplete the germinal epithelium that lines the seminiferous tubules in men. (704-706)

8. **The answer is (D).** Those who do not believe that another pregnancy is contraindicated suggest a waiting period of 2 to 5 years after completion of all therapy inasmuch as recurrence is most likely during this time period. Further pregnancies after a diagnosis of breast cancer have been considered controversial. Some authors suggest that all women refrain from any pregnancies, whereas others suggest that a pregnancy may actually protect against recurrence. Choice (B) is true but should not seriously affect an attempt at conception; choice (C) duplicates the initial reason. (709-712)

9. **The answer is (C).** Therapeutic abortion has not been shown to be of benefit in altering disease progression and should not be considered unless pregnancy will compromise treatment and thus prognosis. Therapeutic abortion is most likely to be called for when the cancer is diagnosed at an advanced stage during the first trimester of pregnancy and the effects of combination chemotherapy are likely to damage the fetus. (710)

10. **The answer is (B).** Treatment of the pregnant women with early breast cancer should be as in the non-pregnant woman, with therapy tailored to time, gestation, physician recommendations, and patient desires. In general, modified mastectomy with lymph node sampling is the standard treatment for early disease. Adjuvant chemotherapy can be delayed until after delivery. For the woman who desires breast-conserving surgery, lumpectomy with lymph node sampling may be done but radiation therapy should be delayed until after delivery. For advance disease, surgery and chemotherapy should be undertaken without delay. Therapeutic abortion may be suggested during the first term to prevent chemotherapy exposure to the fetus. (710)

11. **The answer is (A).** During the first two trimesters, surgery or radiation therapy, without therapeutic abortion, is usually undertaken. Early stage disease may be treated with radical hysterectomy and pelvic node dissection, whereas in advanced disease radiation therapy is the most common treatment. During the third trimester, fetal viability usually can be awaited and the baby delivered by cesarean section, after which appropriate cancer therapy can be given. (710-711)

12. **The answer is (D).** Certain malignancies, notably melanoma, non-Hodgkin's lymphoma (NHL), and leukemia, are known to spread from the mother to the fetus. If the mother has any of these cancers, the placenta should be carefully evaluated at delivery and the baby monitored for development of the disease. (712)

13. **The answer is (C).** Chemotherapy during the first trimester has been associated with fetal wastage, malformations, and low birth weight, although the incidence of fetal malformations is low and may be minimized or avoided with careful selection of agents. Maternal surgery can be safely accomplished with minimal risk to the fetus. Pelvic surgery is more easily accomplished during the second trimester. There is little risk to the fetus from short exposure to anesthetic agents after the first trimester, provided ventilation is adequate and hypotension is prevented. Low doses of radiation associated with diagnostic X-ray studies are not harmful if adequate fetal shielding is provided. (712)

32   Altered Body Image and Sexuality

STUDY OUTLINE

I. INTRODUCTION

1. **Body image** and **sexuality** are integral parts of a person and must be given as much attention in a nursing care plan as other physical, emotional, and spiritual needs.
2. **How changes should be managed depends on the patient's perception of these changes and the reactions of those persons who are important to the patient.**

II. CONCEPT OF BODY IMAGE

1. Body image involves both **self-perception** and **social feedback.** It is a "picture of our body, formed in the mind's eye."
   a. It relates to one's actual appearance and body function as well as to how one perceives the self and what one perceives as an "ideal" body or image.
   b. It is affected by physical factors and sensations (e.g., pain and stress) as well as emotional and social reactions.

III. CANCER AND BODY IMAGE

1. According to one study, a majority of cancer patients perceive the diagnosis and treatment of cancer as changing their physical appearance and that
   a. These changes make them feel worse.
   b. They feel moderately or strongly about these changes.
   c. These changes refer to changed **perceptions of body image or emotional outlook.**
2. The patient must learn to change the image of his or her physical self to make it **consistent with reality.** This is an important part of the adjustment process in cancer.
3. Certain types of cancer are more likely to alter body appearances and functions and affect body image, e.g., breast cancer, head and neck cancer, colorectal or bladder cancer, gynecologic cancer, prostate or testicular cancer.

A. BREAST CANCER

1. Because our society values the breast in terms of **fertility and femininity** and as a **symbol of sexuality,** women who undergo mastectomy may feel rejected, sexually mutilated, and depressed.
   a. These feelings may contribute to poor self-image, a sense of worthlessness, difficulties in interpersonal relationships, a decline in sexual activity, and, in some cases, deterioration of marriage or intimate relationship.
   b. The feelings are **not necessarily related to age.** For example, they may relate to whether the patient is or is not in a strong relationship.
2. The increased use of **lumpectomy** and **radiation therapy** in lieu of modified mastectomy has been oriented to improving the cosmetic outcome of breast therapy.
   a. Nurses cannot assume, however, that lesser surgery or immediate cosmesis will eliminate all distress related to altered body image.
   b. Effects and **side effects of treatment** (e.g., skin discoloration or thickening as a result of radiation therapy) can have an impact on the patient's body image.

3. **Breast reconstruction** is also an option for women who wish to increase their self-esteem, improve their appearance, eliminate their need for prosthesis, and permit them to wear more attractive clothing.

B.   HEAD AND NECK CANCER

1. Procedures viewed as most severe are associated with **major structural alteration in the center of the face,** e.g., orbital exenteration and radical maxillectomy.
2. Unless patients adjust to altered body image, they will not be successfully rehabilitated in spite of the restoration of cosmetic appearance and function.

C.   CANCERS RESULTING IN OSTOMIES

1. Cancer patients with surgically constructed **stomas,** either **colostomies** or **urostomies,** often have disturbances of body image.
2. They often have **poor psychosocial outcomes,** which range from failure to return to occupations, withdrawal from social and intimate contacts, depression, and anxiety.
3. Changes in body image and self-concept may occur as a result of loss of sphincter control, new or accentuated sensory phenomena (e.g., flatus), and the visibility of urine or stools on their bodies.

D.   SIDE EFFECTS OF CHEMOTHERAPY

1. The **symptoms of chemotherapy,** including alopecia, vomiting, diarrhea, weakness, fatigue, muscle atrophy, and neurologic changes can alter body image.
2. The nurse should remember that the impact of changes in body image **may fluctuate during the cancer experience,** and that body image changes **do not mean the same to each person.**
   a.   Loss of hair may seem serious at an early stage, or to some people, but relatively minor later in the disease, or to other people.
3. Side effects of **weakness** and **fatigue** may be especially difficult for individuals who value strength, endurance, and productivity.
   a.   Their expectations may lead them to **attempt too much** and become ill from exhaustion.
   b.   The nurse must be sensitive to patients' disturbed body image caused by failure to live up to past levels of activity and productivity.
   c.   Emphasizing the patent's **remaining abilities** can promote acceptance of altered body image.

IV.   PROMOTING ADJUSTMENT TO AN ALTERED BODY IMAGE

1. The goal of promoting a healthy and realistic attitude requires support for the patient who has to accept a new or changed body image. This support can come from the **nurse,** the **family,** and from **mutual self-help groups.**
2. The nurse can help by
   a.   Providing **emotional support** as patients grieve the loss of a body part or a body function. This means
      (1)   Attentive listening and assurance to the patient that grieving is normal and appropriate.
      (2)   Helping patients express anger and grief and cope with these feelings.
      (3)   Assisting patients to deal with the change and not make it the focus of their lives. This reinforces self-esteem.
      (4)   Encouraging patients to not use cancer as an excuse for unsuccessful relationships but, instead, to resume social relationships.
   b.   Providing **information** and **teaching patients to manage procedures** involved with body changes.
      (1)   Patient self-management can improve perceptions of body image, e.g., irrigation and self-care after head and neck surgery.
   c.   Allowing patients to **accept change at their own pace;** not pushing patients to accept it.
3. The **family** should be prepared for the patient's changes. This involves an ongoing assessment of the family's response to the patient's illness, treatment, and changes.
   a.   **Children** can be particularly helpful in the patient's adaptation to physical change if they have a secure and special relationship with the patient.

4. Orienting patients and their families to **mutual self-help groups** can be very helpful to patients who are adjusting to changes in body image.
   a. Hearing others share their experiences with change may help patients make their own adjustments.
   b. Not all patients benefit from such activities, and nurses should be cautious not to force patients to participate.

V. ALTERATION IN SEXUAL FUNCTIONING

1. Changes in sexuality that occur with cancer or cancer therapy can result from **changes in appearance or function** or from **stress and other psychologic factors** that adversely affect sexual functioning.
2. Sexual disability may be determined less by body-image alteration than by other psychosexual and treatment-related psychologic changes.

VI. BARRIERS TO INTERVENTIONS FOR SEXUALITY

1. **Nurses may be reluctant to discuss sex with patients.**
   a. Sex may seem like a low priority compared with information on treatments or medications.
   b. Nurses may feel uncomfortable discussing sexual matters because
      (1) They feel inadequately informed.
      (2) Their beliefs may be rigid and they do not think such a discussion is appropriate.
      (3) They feel other health professionals can better handle this aspect.
      (4) They feel it would be an invasion of the patient's privacy and the patient may be offended.
2. But avoiding inquiries into sexuality may convey the impression that sex is no longer important to the patient. Nurses need to listen carefully for subtle cues that patients wish to discuss their sexual concerns.

VII. NURSING CARE ISSUES REGARDING SEXUALITY

1. Nurses should recognize their own biases regarding sexuality to be assured they are not
   a. Forcing their own attitudes and biases on the patient.
   b. Failing to inform the patient of options that do not fit into the nurses' own value systems.
2. **It is important for nurses to recognize their own preconceived notions about age, gender, and expectations about sexual behavior.**
   a. **Interviews** can be conducted to discover patients' feelings about sexual aspects of their lives after experiencing cancer, its treatment, and its effect on themselves and their families.
   b. Consideration must be given to the patient's **age, religious and ethnic background, education,** and **specific illness ramifications.**
   c. If there is a conflict of values, the nurse should refer the patient to others who may be more helpful.
   d. The nurse also should not make assumptions about **sexual preference or behavior** or press for information that is not readily given. Heterosexuality should not be assumed, for example.
3. In males, problems of erectile impotence and impairment of sexual function are most likely to occur after **ostomy surgery** or **orchidectomy.**
   a. These problems may have a profound effect on self-image, masculinity, and sexual identity.
   b. Fear of **sexual or social rejection** may result from anxiety about sexual functioning and associated feelings of loss of attractiveness and desirability.
   c. This may lead some cancer patients to isolate themselves and avoid taking the risks necessary to develop intimate relationships.
4. **Antineoplastic drugs** may also affect sexual functioning, e.g., by loss of sensation or muscle control. For these patients there is a need to identify appropriate alternatives for expressing sexuality and receiving sexual pleasure.

VIII.   **INTERVENTIONS TO ENHANCE SEXUAL FUNCTIONING**

1.   **Nurses should work to broaden all aspects of their knowledge about sexuality.**
2.   Qualified **consultants** may be brought in to help nurses cope with the sexual needs of their patients and also to discuss specific issues involving selected patients.
3.   Assessment requires interviewing the patient regarding sexual issues.
   a.   **Table 32-1, text page 728,** provides examples of questions that can be integrated into an interview.
   b.   Interviews should begin with the least sensitive sexual matters, usually starting with general questions.
   c.   Discussion of more intimate aspects of sexuality can begin after an atmosphere of trust has been created.
   d.   Teaching strategies can be used to clarify information, impart facts, and dispel myths.
   e.   A **sexual-adjustment questionnaire (SAQ)** may be used to identify patients at higher risk of postoperative sexual problems.
4.   If fatigue or other symptoms limit sexual activities, couples can be advised that sexual intercourse is not the only expression of sexual experience. Intimacy can be expressed by touching, holding hands, caressing, lying together, etc.
5.   Assessment also should determine any other possible causes of alterations in sexual functioning, including **medications.**
6.   The timing of counseling should be guided by the patient's needs at the specific time.

A.   **SEXUAL COUNSELING**

1.   The **PLISSIT model** (see **Chapter 20, text page 464 and Table 20-8**) consists of four stages of interventions used in sexual counseling: Permission, Limited Intervention, Specific Suggestions, and Intensive Therapy.
2.   **Permission** is first promoted when the nurse asks patients about their sexual concerns or suggests that it is an appropriate topic for discussion.
3.   **Limited information** continues the discussion and provides specific factual information to help clarify concerns the patient may have as well as eliminate myths and clarify misconceptions.
4.   **Specific suggestions** are appropriate when support and limited information alone are not adequate for the particular patient. Follow-up is assured to monitor the effectiveness of the suggestions.
   a.   Suggestions include **strategies for enhancing sexual expression** after the patient and partner express their goals for sexual activity, e.g., fantasy, changing positions, use of lubrication, finding alternative methods to achieve sexual satisfaction.
   b.   Suggestions take into account the patient's and partner's **values** and **attitudes toward sex.**
   c.   Referral for **intensive therapy** is advised if sexual concerns remain unresolved.
5.   **Intensive therapy** is called for when adequate progress is not being made and more depth of counseling is needed for complex needs.
   a.   Referral to a therapist can be one of the nurse's most important functions.
   b.   Intensive therapy may be required to deal with
      (1)   Sexual problems that existed prior to the cancer experience.
      (2)   When reconstructive surgery of genitalia is needed or when the use of prosthetic devices, such as penile implants, may be necessary.
6.   The nurse should be careful not to delve into alternate methods of sexual experiences without gaining permission from the patient. Such discussion can actually increase the sexual concerns of the couple.

PRACTICE QUESTIONS

1.   An individual's body image is affected by several factors, including all of the following **except**
   (A)   feedback from significant others and significant events.
   (B)   what one perceives as an "ideal" body or image.
   (C)   how one's body actually looks and functions.
   (D)   the various elements that refer to psychologic self.

2. According to a study by Frank-Stromborg and Wright, a majority of cancer patients perceive the diagnosis and treatment of cancer as changing their physical appearance. How did patients in this study feel about these changes in appearance?
    (A) They felt positively about these changes and in many cases used them to their advantage in fighting the disease.
    (B) They felt worse about themselves because they also perceived a change in their body image.
    (C) They had no strong feelings about these changes.
    (D) They quickly adapted to these changes because of the psychologic need to match body image with reality.

3. The use of lumpectomy and radiation therapy in lieu of modified mastectomy as a treatment for breast cancer has been oriented to improving the cosmetic outcome of breast therapy. Which of the following statements about these therapies is correct?
    (A) The side effects of radiation therapy can have an impact on the patient's perception of body image.
    (B) Lumpectomy and radiation therapy produce fewer long-term concerns and distress than does modified mastectomy.
    (C) Chronologic age is likely to be the most important factor in making women feel vulnerable to body image disturbances caused by any of these therapies.
    (D) Lesser surgery or immediate cosmesis appears to have little effect on reducing distress related to body image in the immediate postoperative period.

4. Poor psychosocial outcomes associated with perceived changes in body image are **most** likely to develop in which of the following cancer patients?
    (A) patients with surgically constructed stomas
    (B) patients receiving chemotherapy
    (C) patients undergoing breast reconstruction
    (D) patients with even minor disfigurement or dysfunction caused by facial surgery

5. Nurses can help the patient who has to accept a new or changed body image in several ways. Included among the most important nursing interventions are all of the following **except**
    (A) assuring the patient that grieving the loss of a body part or function is normal.
    (B) helping patients deal with the change by making it the major focus of their lives.
    (C) teaching patients to manage procedures involved with body changes, which increases self-esteem.
    (D) orienting patients and their families to mutual self-help groups.

6. Successful nursing interventions for sexuality in the patient with altered body image can be hindered by several factors. Which of the following is **least** likely to interfere with successful intervention?
    (A) the nurse's reluctance to discuss sexuality with the patient
    (B) the nurse's failure to recognize his or her own biases regarding sexuality
    (C) the nurse's reluctance to acknowledge the patient's need for privacy on sexual matters
    (D) the nurse's failure to consider the patient's age, religious and ethnic background, sexual preferences, and education.

7. In interviewing a cancer patient regarding sexual issues, which of the following questions would be **most** appropriate during the early part of the interview?
    (A) "Have you had any difficulties in sexual relationships prior to getting this diagnosis?"
    (B) "Have you experienced a change in sexual desire, excitement, or orgasm?"
    (C) "What place does sexuality have in your relationship with your spouse?"
    (D) "Has treatment affected the way you feel about yourself as a woman (man)?"

8. In counseling an older cancer patient about sexuality, using the PLISSIT model, you find that she and her spouse are reluctant to engage in sexual intercourse because they fear the activity will tire her. Of the following suggestions, the one **most** appropriate for this patient would be:
    (A) "Don't worry. A little bit of fatigue is normal and acceptable."
    (B) "Sexual intercourse actually is not very tiring. That's one of the common myths of sexuality."
    (C) "You needn't have sexual intercourse to be intimate. Try holding or lying next to each other."
    (D) "You two seem to have a conflict on this issue. Perhaps therapy would be good idea."

9. In the PLISSIT model, intensive therapy is called for when adequate progress is not being made and more depth of counseling is required for complex needs. An example is when

(A)   sexual problems existed prior to cancer experience.
(B)   specific suggestions are needed for enhancing sexual expression.
(C)   the nurse is unwilling to delve into the patient's sexual feelings.
(D)   permission to discuss sexuality has not been granted by the patient.

ANSWER EXPLANATIONS

1.   **The answer is (D).**   Body image includes those elements that refer to the **physical** self, including how we perceive our bodies; how our bodies actually look and how they function; the impact of sensory input (e.g., pain); feelings we have about our intelligence, mobility, and physical capacity to endure stress and pain; and what we perceive as an "ideal" body or image. In Schilder's definition, it is the "picture of our body, formed in the mind's eye." (720)

2.   **The answer is (B).**   More than half of the patients in this study perceived the diagnosis and treatment of cancer as changing their physical appearance and that these changes made them feel worse; in addition, the majority felt moderately or strongly negative about these changes. These patients primarily referred to changes in their body image or changes in their emotional outlook as factors affecting their changed feelings about themselves. (721)

3.   **The answer is (A).**   Although in general lesser surgery or immediate cosmesis does reduce distress related to body image in the immediate postoperative period in breast surgery, the concerns and distress of all breast cancer patients are similar at 1 year, regardless of the extent of surgical intervention. In addition, radiation therapy can cause changes in the breast tissue and the contour of the breast, thickening and discoloration of the skin, and other physical effects that can have an impact on the patient's perception of body image. Factors other than chronologic age are more likely to be the issue in making women feel vulnerable to body image disturbances caused by any of these therapies. (728)

4.   **The answer is (A).**   Although the other patients listed may experience changes in perceived body image as a consequence of their therapies, patients with stomas are more likely to have poor psychosocial outcomes, which range from failure to return to occupations, withdrawal from social and intimate contacts, depression, and anxiety. Oberst and Scott found that patients with ostomies were slower to return to preillness functional levels and had greater psychologic distress than nonstomy patients who received surgical treatment for cancer. Changes in body image and self-concept may occur as a result of loss of sphincter control, new or accentuated sensory phenomena (e.g., flatus), and the potential visibility (or detectability) of urine or stools on the patient's body. (723)

5.   **The answer is (B).**   The goal of promoting a healthy and realistic attitude requires nursing support for the patient who has to accept a new or changed body image. Assisting patients to deal with the change and **not** make it the focus of their lives reinforces their self-esteem. Patients need to understand the full situation to avoid placing undue restrictions on themselves because of cancer or its treatment or using cancer as an excuse for unsuccessful relationships. In general, the nurse can help by providing emotional support as patients grieve the loss of a body part or a body function; providing information and teaching patients to manage procedures involved with body changes; allowing patients to accept change at their own pace; participating in an ongoing assessment of the family's response to the patient's illness, treatment, and changes; and orienting patients and their families to mutual self-help groups. (724–725)

6.   **The answer is (C).**   Nurses may be reluctant to discuss sex with patients for a number of reasons. Sex may seem like a low priority compared with information on treatments or medications. In addition, nurses may feel uncomfortable discussing sexual matters because they feel inadequately informed, their beliefs may be rigid and they do not think such a discussion is appropriate, they feel other health professionals can better handle this aspect, or they feel it would be an invasion of the patient's privacy and the patient may be offended. Avoiding inquiries into sexuality, however, may convey the impression that sex is no longer important to the patient. Nurses need to listen carefully for subtle cues that patients wish to discuss their sexual concerns. They also need to recognize diversity in the ages, cultures, and sexual preferences of their patients. (725–726)

7.   **The answer is (D).**   Interviews should begin with the least sensitive sexual matters, usually starting with general questions dealing with the patient's self-concept and feelings of body image. Discussion of more intimate aspects of sexuality can begin after an atmosphere of trust has been established. (727–729)

8.   **The answer is (C).**   In the PLISSIT model, specific suggestions are appropriate when support and limited information alone are not adequate for the particular patient. Suggestions often include strategies for enhancing sexual expression after the patient and partner express their goals for sexual activity, e.g., fantasy, changing positions, finding alternative methods to achieve sexual satisfaction. Suggestions also take into account the patient's and partner's values and attitudes toward sex. In this situation, it may be sufficient to advise the patient that sexual intercourse is not the only expression of sexuality. Intimacy can be expressed in many ways, including close body contact, lying together, showing a caring approach, touching, etc. (729–730)

9.   **The answer is (A).**   Referral to a therapist can be one of the nurse's most important functions, and nurses should learn to recognize when there is a need for more competent and expert sexual therapists to obtain adequate and appropriate support for the patient and partner. Intensive therapy may be required to deal with sexual problems that existed prior to the cancer experience or when reconstructive surgery of genitalia is needed or when the use of prosthetic devices, such as penile implants, may be necessary. The nurse's unwillingness to discuss sexuality should not be a reason for her or him to refer the patient to a therapist. (730–731)

33 Integumentary and Mucous Membrane Alterations

STUDY OUTLINE

I.   **INTRODUCTION**

1. Cancer treatment can affect the skin and mucous membranes, and oncology nurses in all settings can expect to see these common challenges, especially with the now more frequent use of chemotherapy.

II. **ANATOMY AND PHYSIOLOGY**

A. **INTEGUMENT**

1. **Skin**
    a. The skin is the largest organ of the body, making up 15% of the total body weight and receiving one-third of the heart's oxygenated blood.
    b. The skin is composed of three layers (see **Figure 33-1, text page 735**).
        (1) The **epidermis,** the outer layer, renews itself continuously through cell division in its deepest, basal layer.
        (2) The **dermis** provides nutrient support to the avascular epidermal layer.
        (3) **Subcutaneous tissue** is the deepest skin layer.
    c. Intact skin provides **protection from environmental assaults** such as those from bacteria, heat and cold, physical trauma, and radiation. Protection against the environment is accomplished by
        (1) **Eccrine gland sweating.**
        (2) **Insulation by skin and subcutaneous tissues.**
        (3) **Regulation of cutaneous blood flow (vasoconstriction and vasodilation).**
        (4) **Muscle activity (e.g., shivering).**
    d. **Receptors** for heat, cold, pain, and touch in the skin make the skin a sensory organ.
    e. **Excretion** of water and salt by the skin helps regulate the body's water balance.
    f. **Production of Vitamin D** in the skin by the effect of ultraviolet radiation assists with the body's formation of bones and teeth.
    g. **Self-image** and **communication of an individual's feelings** are functions of the skin's visibility.
2. **Hair**
    a. Hair is a product of the epidermis and is distributed widely over the body except for the lips, palms, soles, and nipples.
    b. The growth, loss, and length of hair depends on the length of the various components of the hair growth cycle, as well as on body location. The hair growth phases are the
        (1) **Anagen phase,** during which the hair is growing. Hair grows an average of 1 cm in 28 days.
        (2) **Catagen phase,** a slow or intermittent growth phase.
        (3) **Telogen phase,** during which all growth ceases and hair loss occurs.
    c. Hair has both physical and psychosocial functions in humans. These include
        (1) Protecting the skin and regulating temperature.
        (2) Contributing to body image as a secondary sexual characteristic.

3. **Nails**
   a. Nails are found on the dorsal surfaces of the terminal phalanges of the fingers and toes. They shape the fingers and greatly enhance the coordinated fine motion of the fingers.
   b. Nails rest on the **nail bed,** composed of the germinal layer of the epidermis and the underlying dermis. The visible part of the nail, called the **body,** is highly vascular.
4. **Glands**
   a. **Sweat glands** are of two types.
      (1) **Apocrine glands,** found in limited areas such as axillae and genitalia, are odiferous and increase evaporative heat loss.
      (2) **Eccrine glands** function to cool the body through the secretion of water and its evaporation.
   b. **Sebaceous glands** secrete **sebum,** which lubricates hair and skin to keep them pliable and waterproof.

B. **MUCOUS MEMBRANES**

1. Mucous membranes are continuous with the skin and **line the body cavities and hollow organs** that open to the body's exterior, such as the organs of the respiratory, digestive, and excretory, and reproductive tracts.
2. Formed by **epithelia combined with connective tissue,** the function of the various mucous membranes depend on location, but may include **absorption, transport,** or **secretion of mucus.**
3. **The rapidly proliferating cells of the epithelial layer of the mucous membranes make them very sensitive to the cell-kill effects of radiotherapy and chemotherapy.**

III. **ALTERATIONS TO THE INTEGUMENT**

A. **RADIATION EFFECTS**

1. **Radiation effects** on the skin are related to the rate of cell turnover in the irradiated area. In rapidly proliferating cells and tissues, **acute** radiation damage can be seen during or immediately after radiotherapy; months or years are needed to see **chronic** effects.
   a. **Acute effects** depend more on dose as it relates to time than on total dose alone. Since normal skin is usually included in the radiation therapy field, **skin reactions** are to be expected. The degree of these reactions depends on such factors such as **dose, type of machine, anatomic location,** and **concomitant chemotherapy.** See **Table 33-1, text page 739,** for acute effects on skin.
   b. **Late radiation skin effects** may result from vascular or connective tissue damage, or from parenchymal or stromal cell depletion. These effects limit the total radiation dose that can be administered. Other factors influencing the development of chronic effects include **tissue integrity** and **radiobiologic factors.** See **Table 33-2, text page 740,** for late effects of radiation on skin.
   c. **Care of irradiated skin** involves
      (1) **Assessment** before treatment, every week during treatment, after the completion of treatment, and every few months thereafter.
      (2) **Management of skin reactions,** beginning with patient teaching of anticipated skin reactions and skin care guidelines. See **Tables 33-4 and 33-5, text pages 742–744,** for these guidelines and the rationale for their use.

B. **CHEMOTHERAPY EFFECTS**

1. **Chemotherapy effects** on the skin include
   a. **Hyperpigmentation** or **hypopigmentation,** which can be widespread or occur only over the veins into which certain drugs were given. Its occurrence is related to drug dose, exposure to radiation, and natural complexion.
   b. **Hypersensitivity,** which occurs infrequently.
   c. **Hand-foot syndrome (acral erythema),** which consists of erythema, scaling, and epidermal sloughing from palms and soles followed by desquamation and reepithelialization. This syndrome has been reported with continuous infusions of 5-FU, doxorubicin, and high-dose cytarabine.

2. **Pruritis**
   a. **Etiology** can be related to specific cancer diagnosis, infection, radiation therapy, or a reaction to antibiotics, analgesics, or chemotherapy.
   b. **Assessment** of the patient includes
      (1) Screening for any of the possible etiologies as noted above.
      (2) Eliciting information as to onset, duration, and prior history of pruritis.
      (3) Examining the skin for possible contributing causes.
   c. **Management** of this distressing symptom focuses on skin care, environmental control, and administration of therapeutics.
3. **Photosensitivity**
   a. This **enhanced skin response to ultraviolet light** can be the result of a variety of topical, oral, and parenteral medications.
   b. Photosensitivity reactions can also occur in a **radiation treatment field area,** as the radiation therapy can destroy protective melanocytes in the irradiated epidermis and result in the slower rate of melanin production in new epidermal cells.
   c. Protective measures patients can use include **avoiding sun exposure and tanning booths,** wearing **clothing or a hat** to cover irradiated skin, and using **sunscreen** with a minimum sun protection factor of 15.

C. **VESICANT CHEMOTHERAPY EXTRAVASATION**

1. The most **benign local reaction** to chemotherapy is venous flare, characterized by a localized erythema, venous streaking, and pruritus along the injected vein.
2. **Irritants** are nonvesicant chemotherapy agents that cause a local tissue reaction characterized by pain, venous irritation, and chemical phlebitis.
3. Vesicant infiltration into local tissues that is capable of causing pain, ulceration, necrosis, and sloughing of damaged tissue is known as **extravasation.**
4. In most cases, extravasation is a consequence of **poor venous integrity** more than administration technique.
5. **Prevention and assessment**
   a. **Rapid response** to a suspected extravasation is the first step in ensuring the best possible outcome.
   b. **Bleb formation** may be the first sign of drug infiltration at the injection site.
   c. If **pain** is present, it may be an early or a late symptom.
   d. Vesicant injection is **stopped** at the first sign of discomfort. Once it is determined that an infiltration has occurred, the IV is restarted at another injection site.
   e. A **blood return** should be assessed every 1–2 cc of drug administration.
   f. Occasionally extravasation results from implanted ports and, less commonly, from tunneled catheters.
6. **Management**
   a. See **text pages 754–757** for an outline of what steps to take in the event of an extravasation.

IV. **HAIR**

A. **RADIATION EFFECTS**

1. The damage by radiation on hair follicles occurs in two distinct ways.
   a. Radiation causes the growing hair shafts in the **anagen phase** to shift into the **telogen phase,** when hair growth ceases and hair can fall out.
   b. Radiation **disrupts the mitotic activity** of the epithelial cells in the hair root, halting growth of new hairs and weakening shafts of existing hairs, making breakage likely.
2. The radiosensitivity of hair is, in decreasing order, scalp hair, male beard, eyebrows, axilla, pubis, and fine hairs of the body.
3. **Scalp hair loss can be complete, as in whole brain irradiation, or partial, as when only part of the scalp is irradiated.**
4. Hair thinning occurs at approximately 2500–3000 cGy, and complete loss occurs at radiation doses greater than 4500–5000 cGy.
5. Hair regrowth begins 8–9 weeks after completion of radiation; new hair may have a different texture or color.

B. **CHEMOTHERAPY EFFECTS**

1. **Alopecia**
    a. **Alopecia** due to chemotherapy is temporary and reversible. Hair growth resumes within 1 to 2 months and, as is the case with regrowth following radiation, hair may be of a different texture, thickness, and color.
    b. **Alopecia is not an inevitable side effect of chemotherapy.** It is related to the use of specific drugs (e.g., doxorubicin or cyclophosphamide) or the combination of drugs, doses, and methods of administration.

2. **Prevention of alopecia**
    a. Efforts to decrease or prevent chemotherapy-induced alopecia by use of **scalp tourniquets** or **scalp hypothermia** have met with mixed results in limited, unrandomized studies.
    b. The possibility of **scalp micrometastases** is a risk associated with these hair preservation techniques.

C. **NURSING CARE**

1. Hair contributes greatly to body image and is closely associated with sexuality.
2. Nurses should be sure patients and families know what degree of hair loss to expect.
3. Nurses can also offer emotional support and information on wigs and hair care.

D. **HIRSUTISM**

1. **Hirsutism,** an increase in normal body hair, can be a troublesome side effect for women given **androgens** for the treatment of breast cancer.

V. **NAILS**

1. **Nail loss** can occur with radiation doses of 3000 cGy.
2. **Pigmentation changes of the nail** can occur with chemotherapeutic agents such as doxorubicin, cyclophosphamide, and SFU.
3. **Beau's lines,** a transverse white line or nail depression and separation, can occur with SFU and bleomycin.

VI. **GLANDS**

1. Radiation therapy doses greater that 3000 cGy can **permanently destroy sweat glands,** leaving skin unable to perspire.
2. Sebaceous glands are more sensitive to radiation therapy, and their destruction can cause skin dryness and leave the skin susceptible to fissuring and infection.

VII. **ALTERATIONS OF THE MUCOUS MEMBRANES**

A. **GASTROINTESTINAL MUCOSITIS**

1. **Stomatitis**
    a. Oral complications resulting from treatment may be acute or chronic.
    b. **Acute reactions** include mucosal inflammation and ulceration, infection, and mucosal bleeding.
    c. **Chronic complications** occur as a result of changes in healthy tissue that include xerostomia, taste alterations, trismus, and soft tissue and bone necrosis.
    d. In allogeneic bone marrow transplant patients, acute and chronic graft-versus-host disease is seen.
    e. See **Table 33-13, text page 764,** for factors that contribute to the occurrence and severity of stomatitis.

2. **Chemotherapy-induced stomatitis**
    a. See **Table 33-14, text page 765,** for factors affecting chemotherapy-induced stomatotoxicity.
    b. Patients with **hematologic malignancies** have a two to three times higher rate of oral problems than those with solid tumors.

    c. Preexisting oral disease, poor oral hygiene, and local irritants such as dental prostheses, tobacco, and alcohol predispose chemotherapy patients to an **increased risk** of oral complications.

    d. Stomatitis occurs most commonly with the **antimetabolites and antitumor antibiotics.**

    e. **Direct stomatotoxicity** results from the cytotoxic action of drugs on the cells of the oral basal epithelium, causing a decrease in the rate of cell renewal.

    f. A **dry mucosa, tongue, or lips followed by a burning sensation and increased salivation** can occur in the first 5–7 days. **Ulceration** then occurs 7–14 days after drug exposure. Healing occurs within 2–3 weeks when the granulocyte count returns to normal levels.

    g. **Xerostomia** is a decrease in the quality and quantity of saliva.

    h. Commonly induced **taste alterations** can occur from direct drug injury to taste cells.

    i. **Indirect stomatotoxicity** results from chemotherapy-induced neutropenia and resultant oral infection.

    j. Oral bleeding and hemorrhage are indirect stomatotoxic sequelae from **chemotherapy-induced thrombocytopenia.**

3. **Oral graft-versus-host disease**

    a. Acute and chronic GVHD is a significant complication of patients who undergo allogeneic BMT.

    b. Treatment strategies include systemic immunosuppressive therapy, topical steroids, and fluoride therapy.

4. **Radiation-induced stomatitis and oral complications**

    a. **Radiation treatment** to the oral cavity can result in stomatitis, hypogeusia, and xerostomia.

    b. A baseline examination should be performed by a **dentist** at least 2–3 weeks before therapy begins. **Daily fluoride treatments** and good oral hygiene can significantly reduce oral complications from radiation.

    c. The type of radiation used and the use of multimodality therapy will influence the degree of stomatitis.

    d. Stomatitis resulting from radiation therapy is self-limiting and resolves 2–3 weeks after completion.

    e. **Taste changes** usually occur early in the course of radiation therapy and worsen as the accumulated dose increases. They may take months to resolve.

    f. **Xerostomia** is the most common side effect of radiation to the head and neck. It results from changes in salivary gland function.

    g. Since salivary glands are **highly radiosensitive,** a drastic decrease in secretion occurs after just 10 Gy and is usually permanent after 40 Gy.

    h. Irritants such as tobacco, alcohol, carbonated beverages, and caffeine should be avoided since they are also drying agents.

    i. Lubricating agents such as saliva substitutes are frequently used.

    j. Prompt and early detection of infection helps prevent organisms from spreading systemically.

    k. Although less common, radiation-induced soft tissue and bone necrosis can result from head and neck treatments.

    l. **Trismus** results from fibrosis of the muscles of mastication and/or from fibrotic changes in the capsule of the temporomandibular joint.

5. **Nursing care**

    a. Comprehensive oral and dental assessments assist in early identification and treatment of oral complications secondary to chemotherapy and/or radiation therapy. See **Table 33-17, text page 773,** for an oral assessment guide.

    b. See **text page 772,** column 2, for a grading system depicting degree of severity.

    c. See **Table 33-18, text page 774,** for a protocol for oral care based on assessment and grade of stomatitis.

    d. Lubrication of lips, analgesic topical formulations, and systemic analgesics assist in providing relief of pain and discomfort.

B. INFECTIONS OF THE ORAL CAVITY

1. Infection is the most significant oral complication secondary to treatment and is due to the ideal conditions for microbial growth, particularly in the granulocytopenic patient.
2. *Streptococcus, Candida,* **and herpes simplex** are the major oral infectious pathogens.
3. **Prophylactic drugs** for each pathogen may be indicated.

4. **Esophagitis**
   a. **Esophagitis** is the destruction and inadequate replacement of the mucosal squamous epithelial cells by radiotherapy or chemotherapeutic agents resulting in an inflammatory response.
   b. **Radiation-induced esophagitis**
   c. The onset of esophagitis is dose-related and may be enhanced or hastened by concomitant chemotherapy or alcohol.
   d. **Symptoms** often begin with difficulty swallowing liquids followed by a burning sensation and dysphagia.
   e. **Late complications** include epithelial thickening, microvascular changes, and fibrosis of muscle and connective tissue.
   f. **Nursing considerations** include identifying the risk factors of alcohol, tobacco, ulcer disease, and esophageal exposure to radiation.
   g. See **Table 33-21, text page 782,** for self-care guidelines to assist patients who are experiencing esophagitis or dysphagia.
   h. Local anesthetics are often used, and if pain and discomfort are not relieved, narcotic analgesics are often added.
   i. *Candida* infections of the esophagus may or not be symptomatic and require prompt treatment.
   j. Any patient who experiences oral mucositis from chemotherapy is at risk for chemotherapy-induced esophagitis.

5. **Enteritis**
   a. Radiation-induced enteritis results from radiation treatment for **pelvic and abdominal malignancies.**
   b. See **text pages 783–784** for factors influencing the degree, onset, and duration of radiation-induced acute and chronic enteritis.
   c. **Table 33-23, text page 785,** gives dietary guidelines for enteritis.
   d. Management of severe diarrhea may include the use of opiates to decrease peristalsis, as well as administration of sandostatin.
   e. **Chronic radiation enteritis** can occur months to years after treatment, and its clinical features are often attributed to a recurrence of a malignancy.
   f. Conservative treatment of chronic radiation enteritis consists of decompression with a nasogastric tube and fluid support. It is the choice unless a patient presents with an acute problem requiring surgical intervention.
   g. **Chemotherapy-induced enteritis** results from destruction of rapidly proliferating cells of the intestinal mucosa by chemotherapy and can lead to diarrhea.
   h. Epithelial damage results in three stages: **initial injury, progressive injury, and regeneration.**
   i. The **diarrhea** is usually accompanied by **abdominal cramping and rectal urgency.** Severity is documented through the use of a grading scale.
   j. Since diarrhea can also be related to infection, stool cultures should be obtained and antidiarrheal drugs that inhibit gut motility should be used cautiously.
   k. **Antibiotic-associated colitis** is the overgrowth of *Clostridium difficile* in the colon, and almost all antibiotics can be responsible.

VIII. **ALTERATIONS OF THE GENITOURINARY MUCOUS MEMBRANES**

A. **RADIATION-INDUCED CYSTITIS AND URETHRITIS**

1. Temporary irritation of the bladder and/or urethra can result from radiation therapy for treatment of cancers of the prostate, cervix, and bladder.
2. See **Table 33-25, text page 789,** for radiation-induced genitourinary toxicities.
3. Treatment is directed at reducing irritation. Patients should increase fluid intake because dilute urine will cause less irritation.

B. **RADIATION-INDUCED VAGINITIS**

1. After high-dose pelvic irradiation for pelvic or colorectal cancer, vaginitis is characterized by **erythema, inflammation, mucosal atrophy, inelasticity,** and **ulceration.** Adhesion formation, stenosis, partial or total vaginal occlusion, and tissue necrosis may also occur.

2.   Patients with post-radiation vaginitis may report **vaginal discharge, spontaneous or contact bleeding, dyspareunia, pruritis, dysuria,** and **pain.**
3.   **Ulceration** of the vaginal mucosa can lead to the formation of **adhesions.** These are most likely to develop at sites of maximum irradiation. Adhesions must be broken soon after their formation, or permanent closure or stenosis can develop.
4.   **Early vaginal dilatation,** either by **frequent vaginal sexual intercourse** or use of a **dilator,** can prevent fibrosis and adhesions, maintaining vaginal patency for continued sexual intercourse and pelvic examination. If a dilator is used, a usual schedule is 15 minutes three times a week for the first year.
5.   Use of **estrogen cream** in the treatment of post-radiation vaginitis promotes epithelial regeneration and reduces bleeding, dyspareunia, and narrowing of the vaginal caliber. These creams are absorbed systemically, however, and are contraindicated in the case of estrogen-related cancers.
6.   Changes in the vaginal mucosa can alter distribution of normal vaginal flora and overgrowth of pathogenic organisms can develop. *Candida albicans, Trichanomas vaginalis,* and *Gardnerella vaginalis* are commonly associated with vaginitis.

C.   CHEMOTHERAPY-INDUCED VAGINITIS

1.   Symptoms may occur 3 to 5 days after chemotherapy and resolve 7 to 10 days later.
2.   **Proper hygiene,** use of a **water-based lubricant** during intercourse, use of **sitz baths,** and **cotton underpants** can help prevent and relieve vaginitis. **Topical medications** such as miconizole cream and suppositories are used for monilial vaginitis.

IX.   MALIGNANT WOUNDS

A.   DESCRIPTION

1.   Malignant wounds are uncommon; are characterized by excessive purulent drainage, odor, and infection; and **develop from local extension or tumor embolization** into the epithelium and its supporting structures.
2.   **Hyperthermia, radiation therapy, and cytotoxic drugs** have shown an effect on malignant wounds.

B.   NURSING CONSIDERATIONS

1.   Nursing care requires flexibility, creativity, and knowledge of normal wound healing and the pathophysiology of malignant wounds.
2.   Efforts are aimed at maintaining a wound environment conducive to healing, maintaining and promoting the integrity of the skin surrounding the wound, and preventing fluid and electrolyte imbalance resulting from excessive drainage.
3.   **Debridement**
     a.   **Chemical debridement** may be appropriate in the presence of a moderate amount of necrotic tissue or eschar.
     b.   Gentle **mechanical debridement** is the preferred choice and is done with vigorous wound irrigation with a large syringe.
4.   **Infection control**
     a.   Bacterial infiltration can lead to infection, so it is important to differentiate between normal wound inflammation and the presence of colonizing microorganisms.
5.   **Hemostasis**
     a.   **Anemia** can result from bleeding due to fragile vasculature and capillary oozing.
6.   **Cleansing**
     a.   Cleansing with a mild soap and water or nontoxic cleanser helps remove necrotic tissue with minimal trauma and assists in keeping the wound clean and free of debris.
7.   **Wound dressing**
     a.   Maintaining a **moist wound** environment is necessary in order to avoid trauma from drying and fissuring.
8.   **Odor management**
     a.   Patients often withdraw and avoid social situations because of odor.
     b.   **Frequent cleansing** will help eliminate bacteria and excessive drainage, as well as chlorophyll-containing ointments and solutions.
     c.   There are also **deodorizing sprays, solutions, and dressings** in case the odor cannot be eliminated.

PRACTICE QUESTIONS

1. Which characteristic of the skin and mucous membranes accounts for their sensitivity to the effects of chemotherapy and radiotherapy?
   - (A) the presence of glands for sweating and mucous production
   - (B) the large amount of skin and mucous membrane as a proportion of body weight
   - (C) the rapidly proliferating nature of the epithelial layer
   - (D) the presence of receptors for heat, cold, pain, and touch

2. Which of the following radiation-induced acute skin reactions may require an interruption in therapy?
   - (A) erythema
   - (B) hyperpigmentation
   - (C) dry desquamation
   - (D) moist desquamation

3. To help protect against the development of photosensitivity in the patient undergoing cancer therapy, the nurse teaches the patient to do all of the following **except**
   - (A) build up a base tan before prolonged sun exposure.
   - (B) use a sunscreen with a minimum sun protection factor of 15.
   - (C) cover irradiated skin with clothing or hat.
   - (D) check all medications for photosensitivity potential.

4. In teaching the patient about the potential side effects of chemotherapy on hair, the nurse would make all of the following points **except**
   - (A) Chemotherapy-related hair loss is essentially reversible and temporary.
   - (B) All chemotherapeutic agents result in alopecia.
   - (C) Hair that grows back may have a different color and texture.
   - (D) Hair preservation techniques may be ineffective and risk scalp metastases.

5. Your patient is experiencing stomatitis while receiving cancer therapy. Which of the following is **most** likely to be the result of the immunosuppressive effects of chemotherapy?
   - (A) taste changes
   - (B) soft-tissue necrosis
   - (C) infection of the gingiva
   - (D) xerostomia

6. The patient experiencing stomatitis should be counseled to do all of the following **except**
   - (A) alter food choices.
   - (B) suspend oral hygiene temporarily.
   - (C) use analgesics as needed.
   - (D) cleanse the mouth before using topical medications.

7. In addition to treatment for esophageal cancer, radiation-induced esophagitis can be expected with treatment for which of the following?
   - (A) Hodgkin's lymphoma
   - (B) bony metastasis of the lumbar spine
   - (C) nasopharyngeal cancer
   - (D) Ewing's sarcoma of the humerus

8. Surgery to relieve chronic radiation-induced enteritis symptoms is undertaken with all of the following considerations **except**
   - (A) conservative medical management with antidiarrheals and dietary modifications has failed.
   - (B) dehiscence of anastomosis can occur when the bowel end has been irradiated.
   - (C) bowel obstruction, intractable diarrhea, or abdominal pain are present.
   - (D) symptoms will always improve if surgery can be delayed.

9. Adhesions formed as a result of radiation-induced vaginal mucositis are a matter of concern for all of the following reasons **except**
   - (A) resultant changes in normal vaginal flora and overgrowth of pathogenic organisms.
   - (B) resultant loss of vaginal patency for sexual intercourse.

(C)   resultant loss of vaginal patency for continued pelvic examination.

(D)   resultant vaginal stenosis and shortening.

10.   Which of the following statements concerning malignant tumor wounds is correct?

(A)   They generally respond to systemic therapy with hormones or chemotherapeutic agents.

(B)   They have a physical impact but rarely a psychological impact on the patient and family.

(C)   They can be the source of electrolyte and protein loss.

(D)   They must be treated with surgery to ensure the patient's survival.

ANSWER EXPLANATIONS

1.   **The answer is (C).**   Chemotherapy and radiation therapy have their greatest effect on rapidly proliferating cells and tissues. The epithelial layer of the skin and mucous membranes display such a high rate of cell turnover. (737–738)

2.   **The answer is (D).**   Moist desquamation, the exposure of the dermis with serous exudate, is comparable to a second-degree burn. Therapy may be discontinued until reepithelialization occurs. (739)

3.   **The answer is (A).**   Sun exposure and tanning booths are to be avoided. Prevention of photosensitivity reactions focuses on knowledge of drugs that can result in photosensitivity and on protecting skin from ultraviolet light through clothing or the use of sunscreen. (748)

4.   **The answer is (B).**   The majority of antineoplastic agents do not cause hair loss. Chemotherapy-induced alopecia depends on the drug given, the dose, and the method of administration. When hair loss does occur, it is temporary and reversible, and regrown hair may be different from pre-therapy hair. Use of hair-preservation techniques is controversial due to incomplete studies and the risk for scalp metastases. (760–761)

5.   **The answer is (C).**   Chemotherapy can cause stomatotoxicity by its direct effect on cells or, indirectly, through myelosuppression. Taste changes and xerostomia are more likely due to effects at the cellular level; soft tissue necrosis is most often found as a chronic radiation side effect. Infection of an oral structure by a viral, fungal, or bacterial pathogen is most closely related to immunosuppression. (764–765)

6.   **The answer is (B).**   Diligent patient adherence to the selected oral hygiene program is an important factor in the treatment of stomatitis. The other choices are all appropriate for use by the patient experiencing stomatitis. (766)

7.   **The answer is (A).**   The mantle fields necessary for the radiotherapy of Hodgkin's disease include the esophagus, making the development of esophagitis likely. Radiation therapy to the mediastinum for the treatment of lung and breast cancer can also result in doses sufficient to cause esophagitis. (782)

8.   **The answer is (D).**   Chronic radiation-induced enteritis is a progressive, disabling disease of long duration. Surgery is required in 10%–20% of cases, with the indications being obstruction, intractable diarrhea, and pain. (787–788)

9.   **The answer is (A).**   Infection is a possibility with post-radiation vaginitis, but infection is not thought to be related to the development of adhesions and subsequent vaginal stenosis and occlusion. (789–790)

10.   **The answer is (C).**   Ulcerating skin lesions are the source of acute and chronic blood, protein, and electrolyte loss, and can serve as a portal for infection. Both physical and psychological impacts exist for the patient and family. Local treatment involving radiation and surgery may not improve survival, and systemic drug therapy may not lead to a response. (792–793)

34   Oncologic Emergencies

STUDY OUTLINE

I. INTRODUCTION

1. Individuals with cancer often experience medical emergencies as a result of their **disease process** or **treatment.** Prompt diagnosis and treatment are necessary to enable further treatment and to prolong life.

II. SEPTIC SHOCK

A. SCOPE OF THE PROBLEM

1. **Definition**
   a. **Septic shock** can result from **septicemia,** which is a **systemic invasion of the blood by microorganisms.**
   b. Septic shock is characterized by **hemodynamic instability, coagulopathies,** and **alterations in metabolism.**
2. **Incidence**
   a. The incidence of sepsis and septic shock has increased over the past 50 years due to the widespread use of invasive medical devices, corticosteroids, and chemotherapy and due to the enhanced longevity of persons who are susceptible to sepsis (e.g., diabetics).
   b. Usual sites of bloodstream microorganism invasion include the skin and the pulmonary, gastrointestinal, and genitourinary systems.
   c. Mortality rates are high (greater than 75%) for cancer patients in whom septic shock develops. Rapid and aggressive therapy is needed.
3. **Anatomy, physiology, and scientific principles**
   a. **Bacteria** produce **endodoxins** and **exotoxins;** both cause the release of chemical mediators and hormones that initiate various physiologic processes.
   b. Some of the cascade of events that occur in septic shock are **histamine release, vasodilation and increased capillary permeability,** and **activation of factor XII and the clotting process.**
   c. Septic shock is classified into two patterns: **early hyperdynamic shock** and **late hypodynamic shock.**
   d. The major events in **early hyperdynamic shock** include increased **cardiac output** and **vasodilation** that occur in an attempt by the body to maintain **tissue perfusion;** increased **respiratory rate;** development of **hypoxemia;** and a shift by cells to anaerobic metabolism, causing **metabolic acidosis.**
   e. In **late shock,** vasoconstriction of major vessels causes **organ ischemia, impaired alveolar gas exchange,** and **decreased urine output. Cardiac output, venous return,** and **blood pressure** decrease, and blood is trapped in vascular beds. Prolonged inadequate perfusion leads to **coma** and **cardiac death.**

B. PATHOPHYSIOLOGY

1. Cancer patients are at risk for infections that can lead to septic shock because of
   a. **Local effects** of tumor growth (e.g., disruption of normal mucocutaneous barriers).
   b. **Immunological effects of neoplastic disease** (e.g., impaired immunity that occurs with Hodgkin's, CLL, and multiple myeloma) or **treatment** (e.g., chemotherapy-induced neutropenia).

    c. **Iatrogenic/nosocomial** sources (e.g., invasive procedures or overgrowth of endogenous bacteria resulting from long-term antibiotic use).

C. CLINICAL MANIFESTATIONS

1. When caring for individuals with cancer, a high index of suspicion and close monitoring are essential to recognize persons at high risk of septic shock.
2. **Tachycardia, fever or hypothermia, tachypnea,** respiratory alkalosis, and evidence of inadequate tissue perfusion are usually the earliest signs of developing sepsis.
3. Refer to **Figure 34-1, text page 803,** for a list of the early and late signs of impending septic shock.
4. **Common signs of early hyperdynamic shock are fever, shaking chills, increased blood pressure and heart rate, and widened pulse pressure.**
    a. The **respiratory rate increases** because of capillary leakage into the lungs and hypoxia, and **bilateral rales** may be heard if pulmonary edema is present.
5. **In late hypodynamic or "cold" shock, vasoconstriction causes cool, clammy skin and cyanosis; rapid, thready pulse; and a fall in blood pressure.**
    a. Decreased venous return leads to **pulmonary edema, acute respiratory distress syndrome, coma,** and **death.**

D. ASSESSMENT

1. Patients with **total granulocyte counts less than 100/mm³** are at greatest risk for septic shock.
2. If **DIC** also occurs, thrombocytopenia and coagulation abnormalities are seen.

E. INTERVENTIONS

1. **Early identification** may prevent an episode of fever from becoming septic shock. A clinical pathway for the management of septic shock is given in **Figure 34-2, text page 804.**
2. After appropriate microbiology and blood cultures are taken, immediate administration of broad-spectrum **antibiotics** is initiated.
3. If shock develops in the presence of prolonged antibiotic therapy and persistent neutropenia, a **fungal source** is suspected and **amphotericin B** is started.
4. **Vigorous fluid replacement** is given to expand intravascular volume. It may include fluids, crystalloids, and colloids.
5. The patient is monitored for **signs of fluid overload. Vasopressors** may be necessary to maintain organ perfusion.
6. High-dose **corticosteroids** may be administered early in the course of shock (within the first 24 hours after septic shock is diagnosed) to produce anti-inflammatory activity and enhance survival. However, if steroids are given later in the course, they may delay death without effecting survival.
7. **Airway patency** is maintained, **oxygen therapy** may be initiated, and **arterial blood gases and electrolytes** are measured.
8. The effectiveness of therapies is evident in the patient's **vital signs, skin color, level of consciousness,** and **urinary output.**
9. The **mortality rate** associated with septic shock is estimated at between **50% and 90%.** The frequency of shock and the mortality rate increase if the patient does not mount an initial febrile response.

F. FUTURE TRENDS

1. Several new avenues for the treatment of sepsis are being explored.
    a. Anti-TNF and IL-1 receptor antagonists.
    b. Monoclonal antibodies against bacterial endotoxins.
    c. Agents that block or interfere with the cytokines responsible for many of the adverse effects that result in hypotension and the associated high mortality rate of septic shock.

III. **DISSEMINATED INTRAVASCULAR COAGULATION (DIC)**

    A. **SCOPE OF THE PROBLEM**

        1. **Definition**
           a. DIC, an abnormality of the coagulation system, is characterized by widespread clotting within the arterioles and capillaries, and simultaneous hemorrhage.
           b. DIC can be **acute** or **chronic.** Acute DIC must be treated as a medical emergency, whereas chronic DIC produces coagulation abnormalities, with or without clinical manifestations, that can be medically managed.
        2. **Incidence**
           a. **DIC is not a primary disorder: it is always a reflection of another event occurring in the body.**
           b. Refer to **Table 34-3, text page 805,** for an overview of the conditions associated with acute DIC.
           c. **Solid tumors** develop new vasculature with an abnormal endothelial lining that may activate the procoagulant system.
           d. **Necrotic tissue** or **tumor enzymes** may activate the coagulation system.
        3. **Anatomy, physiology, and scientific principles**
           a. Normally, the body maintains a steady state between clot formation **(thrombosis)** and clot dissolution **(fibrinolysis).**
           b. For clotting to be effective, **platelets** and 13 different **clotting factors** become involved in a chain reaction. The outcome of this **clotting cascade** is a thrombosis at the site, which stops leakage of fluids.
           c. Once healing has occurred, the **anticlotting system** is activated, and **plasmin** dissolves the clot.
           d. In DIC, the procoagulant and anticoagulant systems become unbalanced, and **microvascular thrombosis and bleeding occur simultaneously.**

    B. **PATHOPHYSIOLOGY**

        1. Low-grade chronic DIC may occur in patients with solid tumors but does not produce clinical manifestations.
        2. People with **acute promyelocytic leukemia (APL)** have a DIC rate of 85%. It is most likely caused by the release of procoagulant material from granules on the promyeolocytes.
        3. Complications of cancer therapy that cause **rapid cell lysis** and **endo-** and **exotoxin** release can also cause DIC. Thrombosis, manifested by deep venous thrombosis, phlebitis, or pulmonary embolism, is seen in 25% of persons with disseminated cancer.
        4. DIC sometimes results from **placement of foreign bodies** in a patient. **Ascitic fluid** may initiate the clotting cascade.

    C. **CLINICAL MANIFESTATIONS**

        1. DIC has been defined as the **presence of two or more of the following coagulation abnormalities:**
           a. **Prothrombin time (PT)** 3 or more seconds greater than control.
           b. **Activated partial thromboplastin time (APTT)** 5 or more seconds greater than the upper limit of normal.
           c. **Thrombin time (TT)** 3 or more seconds greater than control.
           d. **Fibrinogen (fib)** less than 150 mg/dl.
           e. **Fibrin split products (FSP)** equal to or greater than 40 ug/ml.
         2. Platelet count will be decreased as a result of consumption.
         3. Protamine sulfate or theanol gelatin tests will be positive.
         4. Red cell fragments called schistocytes can be seen on peripheral blood smears in all patients with chronic DIC, but in only 50% of patients with acute DIC.

    D. **ASSESSMENT**

        1. Persons with cancer who are considered at risk of DIC should be monitored closely. Observation and reporting of early signs of bleeding will aid in the diagnosis of DIC. Early and late signs of impending disseminated intravascular coagulation are listed in **Table 34-6, text page 808.**

2. Patients with acute DIC usually will have clinical evidence of bleeding from **at least three unrelated sites.**
3. Signs of **internal bleeding** include anxiety, restlessness, confusion, tachypnea, tachycardia, abdominal tenderness, and increased abdominal girth.
4. Headache, epistaxis, conjunctival hemorrhage, periorbital petechiae, bleeding gums, hemoptysis, diffuse ecchymosis, joint pains, and oozing of blood from wounds also may signal DIC.

E. **INTERVENTIONS**

1. **The only effective treatment for DIC is treating the underlying cause of the syndrome.**
2. Concomitant interventions to DIC include administering **platelets** and **fresh frozen plasma** to replace consumable factors, and **cryoprecipitate** to replace fibrinogen. A clinical pathway for the management of DIC is given in **Figure 34-4, text page 809.**
3. Use of **heparin** to inhibit factors IX and X is controversial. It may be used in certain cases of DIC.
4. **Anticoagulant therapy** is usually not indicated in septicemia-induced DIC.
5. During DIC, the patient is assessed for **signs of bleeding** (e.g., changes in vital signs and neurological status, and frank bleeding).
6. Other nursing interventions include **instituting bleeding precautions** and **protecting the patient from injury.**
7. A clinical pathway for the management of DIC is given in **Figure 34-4, text page 809.**

F. **PROGNOSIS**

1. Survival rate is 75% when the process that caused the DIC is removed and the patient is supported with blood products.

IV. **SUPERIOR VENA CAVA SYNDROME (SVCS)**

A. **SCOPE OF THE PROBLEM**

1. **Definition**
    a. SVCS, the result of compression of the superior vena cava by tumor, leads to a characteristic pattern of upper extremity manifestations. If untreated, SVCS can lead to airway obstruction.
2. **Incidence**
    a. SVCS is rarely an emergency, but it may be the presenting sign of a malignancy.
    b. SVCS occurs in approximately 3%–4% of the oncology population.
3. **Anatomy, physiology, and scientific principles**
    a. The **superior vena cava** is the main vessel for venous return from the upper thorax.
    b. The superior vena cava is a thin-walled vessel with relatively low intravascular pressure. It is surrounded by rigid structures, and thus the presence of an expanding mass in the mediastinum will compress the superior vena cava due to lack of room for expansion within the chest.

B. **PATHOPHYSIOLOGY**

1. Compression of the SVC can occur by
    a. **External compression** by tumor or lymph nodes.
    b. **Direct invasion** of the vessel wall by tumor.
    c. **Thrombosis** of the vessel.
2. **Lung cancer** and **lymphoma** are the two most frequent causes of SVCS.
3. A benign source of SVCS observed in the oncology population is **thrombus formation** around a central venous catheter.
4. SVCS can also be induced by radiation fibrosis, which can cause a narrowing of the SVCS.

C. **CLINICAL MANIFESTATIONS**

1. SVC obstruction causes **elevated venous pressure** and **congestion.**
2. The severity of symptoms of SVCS is related to the rapidity of onset and the adequacy of collateral circulation to help reduce venous congestion. The early and late signs of impending SVCS are listed in **Table 34-8, text page 810.**

3. **Clinical signs** include shortness of breath, facial edema, trunk and upper extremity edema, neck and chest vein distention, cough, hoarseness, and stidor.
4. **Increased intracranial pressure** may cause headache, dizziness, visual disturbances, and occasionally alterations in mental status.
5. A rapidly developing SVCS may be fatal, whereas gradual onset of SVCS allows the **collateral circulation** to shunt enough blood to minimize complications. Airway obstruction can occur with rapidly developing SVCS, leading to respiratory failure.

D. ASSESSMENT

1. In addition to clinical evidence, a **chest radiograph** will usually reveal a mediastinal mass or adenopathy.
2. **Biopsy** is performed if abnormal tissue (e.g., an enlarged lymph node) is readily accessible.
3. If the patient already has a diagnosis, then treatment for that particular malignancy should commence immediately to reverse SVCS.

E. INTERVENTIONS

1. In quickly progressing, acute SVCS with no tissue diagnosis, fractionated **irradiation of the mediastinum** is the treatment of choice. It should be noted that this scenario is the rare exception with SVCS, and every effort should be made to obtain a tissue diagnosis before initiating therapy.
2. With more slowly progressing SVCS, a tissue diagnosis is obtained and the **underlying disease is treated initially.**
3. **Chemotherapy** may be the most effective treatment for SVCS caused by chemosensitive tumors. The timing of systemic chemotherapy and/or mediastinal radiation is crucial: optimal therapy is administered with the **least amount of normal tissue damage** and **maximal tumor destruction.**
4. Radiation therapy is the treatment of choice for SVCS caused by radiosensitive tumors such as non–small-cell lung cancer; lymphomas; and for tumors that fail to respond to chemotherapy. It is also applied if SVCS continues to progress.
5. A new approach to the treatment of SVCS due to thrombosis is the use of tissue type plasminogen activator (rTPA) rather than traditional fibrinolytic agents.
6. **Catheter-induced SVCS,** most often the result of thrombosis, is treated with fibrinolytic therapy such as streptokinase or urokinase and possibly catheter removal. Urokinase is probably superior because it has fewer complications such as hemorrhage, pyrexia, and allergic reaction.
7. One of two **surgical approaches,** superior vena cava bypass graft and stent placement, may be performed for the patient with a good prognosis who has chronic or recurrent SVCS and has exhausted other treatment options.
8. **Figure 34-5, text page 812,** describes the clinical pathway for SVCS and highlights critical decisions and interventions for this syndrome.
9. Nursing care of the patient with SVCS includes **maintaining adequate cardiopulmonary status** and **monitoring the progression of SVCS.**
   a. **Positioning** the patient with head elevated may be helpful in allaying anxiety and maximizing breathing.
   b. **Invasive or constrictive procedures** involving the upper extremities should be avoided because of **impaired venous return** and the **potential for hemorrhage.**
10. The resolution of symptoms is evidence of effective treatment: this may occur within 1–3 days of the start of therapy.
11. More than 50% of patients with SVCS have either a partial or complete response to treatment of the syndrome.
12. Recurrence of SVCS is **infrequent among lymphoma patients** but **common among small-cell lung cancer patients.**

F. FUTURE TRENDS

1. The major trends in the management of SVCS are toward determining the underlying cause prior to treatment and evaluating new fibrinolytic therapies.
2. New and evolving therapies for the most prevalent underlying malignancies, lung cancer and lymphomas, will have the greatest impact on the resolution of SVCS.

V.   **CARDIAC TAMPONADE**

A.   **SCOPE OF THE PROBLEM**

1.   **Definition**
   a.   Cardiac tamponade occurs when excessive fluid accumulates in the pericardial space and creates pressure such that the heart's ability to fill and pump is severely compromised.

2.   **Incidence**
   a.   Neoplastic involvement of the heart is usually evident only on postmortem examination. Most patients whom autopsy reveals to have had cardiac or pericardial disease did not have clinically evident pericardial effusion, and even fewer had cardiac tamponade.

3.   **Anatomy, physiology, and scientific principles**
   a.   The heart is enclosed by a **pericardial sac,** which normally holds 25–35 ml of fluid.
   b.   Intracardial pressure results from the amount of fluid in the pericardial space and from the elasticity or flexibility of the pericardium.

B.   **PATHOPHYSIOLOGY**

1.   **Increased fluid** or **fibrosis and thickening of the pericardium** can raise the intrapericardial pressure to the point where the pressure interferes with the heart's function.

2.   Development of cardiac tamponade results from three pathophysiological changes: **disruption in pressure gradients, decreased diastolic filling, and decreased stroke volume and cardiac output.**

3.   **Figure 34-6, text page 814,** illustrates the cardiovascular effects of increased intrapleural pressure.

4.   **Compensatory mechanisms,** including increased heart rate and peripheral vasoconstriction, are activated in an effort to maintain adequate blood flow.

5.   If compensatory mechanisms fail and treatment is ineffective, coronary output falls, **coronary artery flow decreases,** and **myocardial ischemia and decline ensue.**

6.   Cardiac tamponade is most commonly caused by an abnormal **accumulation of fluid resulting from metastatic spread of tumor into the pericardium.**

7.   Patients with lung, breast, or gastrointestinal tumors, Hodgkin's disease, leukemia, lymphoma, melanoma, or sarcoma are at greatest risk for metastasis to the pericardium.

8.   **High-dose radiation therapy** (4,000 to 6,000 cGy) to the mediastinum may induce acute or chronic pericarditis, which can progress to cardiac tamponade.

9.   The rate of onset and severity of pericardial effusion and cardiac tamponade are determined by the rate of fluid accumulation, compliance of the pericardium, myocardial size, and intravascular volume.

10.   A rapidly occurring effusion will present dramatically due to the lack of time for compensatory mechanisms to impact on cardiac function.

C.   **CLINICAL MANIFESTATIONS**

1.   The primary clinical signs of cardiac tamponade are **venous distention, distant heart sounds,** and **paradoxical pulse,** which is defined as a pulse that is significantly weaker on inspiration than on expiration.

2.   The early and late symptoms of impending cardiac tamponade are listed in **Table 34-10, text page 814.**

D.   **ASSESSMENT**

1.   Assessment of the patient begins with a thorough history, a physical exam, and identification of risk factors and signs and symptoms associated with cardiac tamponade.

2.   On physical examination, **two key signs of cardiac tamponade are pulsus paradoxus and hepatojugular reflux.**

3.   The **echocardiogram** is the easiest, most sensitive, and most accurate tool with which to determine the presence of a pericardial effusion.

4.   **CT scan** and **radiograph of the chest** may be useful to illustrate certain aspects of an effusion.

E. **INTERVENTIONS**

1. Management of the patient with cardiac tamponade begins with early recognition and prompt diagnosis. Patients with cardiothoracic malignancies and widely disseminated disease (populations at risk for cardiac tamponade) should be assessed carefully, particularly if shortness of breath, fatigue, tachycardia, or hypotension is present.

2. The immediate goals in life-threatening tamponade include **hemodynamic stabilization** and **removal of fluid by pericardiocentesis.** Pericardiocentesis will immediately reverse tamponade and normalize vital signs, but systemic or local treatment is needed for a permanent resolution to the problem.

3. Stabilization of the patient awaiting pericardiocentesis is accomplished using volume expanders to improve cardiac filling pressures and to compensate for decreased cardiac output. Cardiac output can be further maximized by infusions of a vasoactive agent such as isoproterenol, epinephrine or dopamine.

4. During pericardiocentesis, the patient's hemodynamic status and EKG are monitored closely.

5. For palliation of recurrent effusions, three types of surgery are available: subxiphoid pericardotomy/pericardial window, pleuropericardial window, and total pericardectomy.

6. The postoperative monitoring of a patient following creation of a **pericardial window** is discussed on **text page 815.**

7. Some oncologists prefer drainage and sclerosing therapy by means of a catheter insertion similar to the approach for pleural effusions. Common sclerosing agents are tetracycline, quinacrine, thiotepa, nitrogen mustard, and 5-fluorouricil. Sclerosing is successful in about 50% of the attempts and causes transient chest pain, arrhythmias, nausea, and fever.

8. **Instilling cytotoxic agents into the pericardial space** to destroy cancer cells rather than sclerosing the cavity is another approach that is currently being evaluated.

9. **Corticosteroids** can help alleviate the inflammation of constrictive pericarditis as a short-term measure; however, the pericardial effusion frequently recurs.

10. **Figure 34-7, text page 817,** illustrates a clinical pathway for cardiac tamponade and highlights the critical decisions and interventions for this emergency.

11. **Pericardial effusion** usually occurs in patients with widely metastatic disease. In these patients, death is most often attributed to the cancer and not to cardiac complications.

12. Patients with a history of tamponade are monitored during frequent office visits.

13. Nurses need to help patients maximize their functional status and quality of life in the face of a potentially debilitating situation.

F. **FUTURE TRENDS**

1. The incidence of metastasis to the pericardium and cardiac complications of cancer treatment is increasing since effective treatments for cancer have prolonged overall survival.

2. Further research is needed to evaluate the use of intracavitary instillation therapy both compared to and in combination with creation of a pericardial window.

VI. **HYPERCALCEMIA**

A. **SCOPE OF THE PROBLEM**

1. **Definition**
   a. **Hypercalcemia is a metabolic disorder that, in cancer patients, results from increased bone resorption.**
   b. Increased bone resorption is a result of either **bone destruction by tumor** or **increased levels of parathyroid hormone (PTH), osteoclast-activating factor (OAF),** or **prostaglandin** produced by the cancer.
   c. If adequate renal clearance of calcium is not preserved, hypercalcemia can develop.
   d. Untreated or uncontrolled hypercalcemia can lead to life-threatening alterations in cardiac, neurologic, and renal function.

2. **Incidence**
   a. **Hypercalcemia** will occur in 10% of cancer patients. Its occurrence often heralds a lack of control of the malignant disease process.

3. **Anatomy, physiology, and scientific principles**
    a. Normal serum calcium levels are maintained by absorption of calcium from the gastrointestinal tract, secretion of PTH and calcitonin, effects of vitamin D, deposition or resorption of calcium from bone, renal clearance of calcium, and binding of calcium to serum proteins.
    b. **PTH** is released in response to low plasma calcium and in turn promotes the release of calcium from bone, increases gastrointestinal absorption of calcium, and stimulates renal tubular absorption of calcium.
    c. **Calcitonin** acts as a feedback mechanism to PTH; it lowers serum calcium by inhibiting bone resorption.
    d. Ninety-nine percent of body calcium is found in bones and teeth.
    e. When albumin is low, more calcium is ionized (free or unbound); ionized calcium is the critical component in clinical hypercalcemia.
    f. Prolonged **immobilization** is associated with increased resorption of calcium from the bones.
    g. **Dehydration** results in a decreased **glomerular filtration rate (GFR)** and an increased sodium resorption to conserve water, which then increases calcium reabsorption and decreases calcium excretion.

B. **PATHOPHYSIOLOGY**

1. Patients at greatest risk for hypercalcemia include those with **bony metastases** from primary tumors of the breast, lung, and kidney.
2. Hypercalcemia also occurs in persons with osteolytic lesions and hematologic cancers such as **multiple myeloma** and some **lymphoma.**
3. Other factors that contribute to hypercalcemia include **hyperparathyroidism, immobilization, anorexia, nausea/vomiting, dehydration,** and **renal failure.**
4. **Several humoral mediators** of cancer-related hypercalcemia have been identified, including a PTH-related protein (which may be produced by the tumor), IL-1, and tumor necrosis factor.
5. **Prostaglandin** has been associated with increased bone resorption following hormonal therapy.
6. Hypercalcemia associated with hematologic malignancy is due to the release of osteoclast activating factor by the malignant cells. In addition, several of the **cytokines** (e.g., IL-1 and tumor necrosis factor) appear to be potent simulators of bone resorption.

C. **CLINICAL MANIFESTATIONS**

1. Three categories of patients with hypercalcemia have been identified.
    a. Patients with serum calcium levels of 10.5–12.0 mg/dl (2.62–3.0 mm/l) who are asymptomatic should be observed carefully and may be given chronic therapy as outpatients.
    b. Patients with serum calcium levels of 12–13 mg/dl (3.0–3.25 mm/l) who are asymptomatic require specific but nonurgent therapy.
    c. Patients with serum calcium levels of 13 mg/dl (3.25 mm/l) or higher and any patients with symptoms require emergency treatment of hypercalcemia.
2. The clinical manifestations of hypercalcemia are often related to the **rapidity of onset.** Patients may develop symptomatic hypercalcemia when the serum calcium level is only marginally increased but the rise has occurred rapidly.
3. A **corrected total serum calcium (TSC)** needs to be calculated if albumin is low, according to the formula **"Corrected" TSC = Measured TSC + (4.0 – serum albumin) × 0.8.**

D. **ASSESSMENT**

1. The early and late symptoms of impending hypercalcemia are listed in **Table 34-13, text page 819.**
2. **Gastrointestinal manifestations** include anorexia, nausea/vomiting, constipation, abdominal pain, and dehydration.
3. **Neuromuscular signs** include lethargy, confusion, stupor, convulsions, and hyporeflexia.
4. **Cardiac abnormalities** may be bradycardia, tachycardia, and EKG abnormalities.
5. Signs of **renal compromise** include polyuria, polyolypsia, decreased renal concentrating ability, and progressive renal insufficiency.

E.   **INTERVENTIONS**

1.   Tumor control or reduction is the only long-term measure for reversing hypercalcemia.
2.   Cancer therapy and emergency medical intervention must be instituted for patients who have symptoms or who have a serum calcium level of 13 mg/dl or more.
3.   Vigorous hydration (4–6 liters/day) will restore the normal volume of extracellular compartment fluid, increase glomerular filtration, and promote urinary calcium excretion.
4.   **Intravenous furosemide** produces sodium diuresis, which in turn causes **calcium diuresis.**
5.   **Serum electrolytes** are monitored for hypokalemia, hyponatremia, hypocalcemia, and hypomagnesemia.
6.   **Intravenous mithramycin** inhibits bone resorption and can be given in a single dose, but it is used judiciously because of its many toxicities and side effects.
7.   **Calcitonin** also inhibits bone resorption, but the duration of response is limited, even with repeated administration. It also carries a risk of **anaphylaxis.**
8.   **Intravenous phosphate,** although extremely toxic, may be administered as a single injection if other measures fail to promote the precipitation of inorganic calcium phosphate.
9.   **Bisphosphonates** are potent inhibitors of osteoclastic bone resorption. They are well tolerated and relatively free of side effects. As with other interventions, however, these will not prevent recurrence of hypercalcemia within 2 to 4 weeks unless there has been successful treatment of the underlying tumor.
10. Five-day infusions of **gallium nitrate** have gained acceptance for the treatment of hypercalcemia.
11. **Oral phosphate** may be given to control chronic, mild hypercalcemia; however, diarrhea may be a dose-limiting side effect.
12. The use of **indomethacin and oral steroids** is considered controversial.
13. Recognition of early signs of hypercalcemia is an important nursing intervention.
14. Careful monitoring of patients taking thiazide diuretics (which inhibit calcium excretion) and digitalis preparations (the action of digitalis is potentiated in a hypercalcemic state) is indicated.
15. A clinical pathway for the assessment and management of the patient experiencing or at risk for hypercalcemia is provided in **Figure 34-8, text page 820.**

F.   **PROGNOSIS**

1.   Emergent hypercalcemia can be reversed in 80% of cases, but a lasting response is often difficult to achieve.

VII.   **TUMOR LYSIS SYNDROME**

A.   **SCOPE OF THE PROBLEM**

1.   **Definition**
     a.   **Acute tumor lysis syndrome (ATLS)** occurs when a large number of rapidly proliferating cells are lysed, releasing their intracellular minerals and uric acid into the blood.
     b.   It is characterized by the development of **acute hyperuricemia, hyperkalemia, hyperphosphatemia, and hypocalcemia with or without acute renal failure.**
2.   **Incidence**
     a.   ATLS is most commonly seen in cancer patients with high-grade lymphoma or acute lymphoblastic leukemia, since these cancer cells are particularly sensitive to treatment and will rapidly lyse.
     b.   In untreated persons with cancer, ATLS can also develop when there is a **rapidly growing, large tumor mass that undergoes profound cell destruction.**
     c.   Although rare, ATLS has been reported to occur in patients with solid tumors such as small-cell lung cancer, breast cancer, and medulloblastoma. However, the syndrome is usually milder since there is slower responsiveness to chemotherapy.
3.   **Anatomy, physiology, and scientific principles**
     a.   Intracellular components include potassium, phosphorus, and the nucleic acids that form DNA and RNA.
     b.   When the cell membrane is ruptured, released nucleic acids are converted by the liver into uric acid, while potassium and phosphorus are released into the bloodstream, causing abnormally high levels of these minerals and a decrease in calcium.

B. **PATHOPHYSIOLOGY**

1. Many chemotherapeutic agents destroy tumor cells while the cells are dividing; similarly, radiation therapy kills cells that are undergoing division. **Therefore, cancer patients with massive tumor burdens that are rapidly dividing are at risk for ATLS, particularly when treatment is initiated.**

2. When a large number of cells are lysed within a short period of time, the result is ATLS characterized by acute **hyperuricemia, hyperkalemia, hyperphosphatemia, hypocalcemia, and/or renal failure.**

3. The degree of metabolic abnormality depends on the adequacy of renal function, since uric acid, potassium, and phosphorus are excreted in the urine.

4. Precipitation of uric acid and/or crystallization of calcium phosphate in the renal tubules can cause acute renal failure.

C. **CLINICAL MANIFESTATIONS**

1. Pretreatment serum potassium levels may be elevated because of dehydration, compromised renal function, acidosis resulting from sepsis, adrenal insufficiency as steroids are tapered, or medications such as indomethacin and potassium-sparing diuretics.

2. Signs of **hyperkalemia** include weakness, paresthesia, muscle cramps, bradycardia, diarrhea, and nausea.

3. Clinical indicators of **hyperphosphatemia** include oliguria, anuria, and renal insufficiency.

4. Patients with **hypocalcemia** may experience muscle twitching, tetany, paresthesia, convulsions, hypotension, and ECG changes.

5. **Medications that may potentiate hyperphosphatemia and hypocalcemia** include phosphates, furosemide, mithramycin, gallium nitrate, and anticonvulsants.

6. **Signs of hyperuricemia and compromised renal function** include nausea, vomiting, diarrhea, lethargy, flank pain, hematuria, oliguria, and anuria.

D. **ASSESSMENT**

1. **When cancer patients with rapidly proliferating tumors are receiving cytoxic therapy, ATLS should be anticipated.** The early and late symptoms of impending tumor lysis syndrome are listed in **Table 34-15, text page 823.**

2. Patients with large tumor burdens in combination with high white blood cell counts, lymphadenopathy, splenomegaly, and elevated lactate dehydrogenase are at particularly high risk.

3. Patients should be assessed for **abnormalities in electrolyte levels** as well as clinical signs of hyperkalemia, hyperphosphatemia, hypocalcemia, hypomagnesmia, hyperuricemia, and compromised renal function.

4. **Baseline renal function** should be assessed prior to initiating therapy.

E. **INTERVENTIONS**

1. Electrolytes and blood chemistries should be monitored at frequent intervals.

2. **Adequate renal function** must be **preserved** during treatment for cancers associated with ATLS.

3. Avoiding uric acid crystallization can be accomplished by maintaining a urine pH of greater than 7 with the use of sodium bicarbonate and vigorous intravenous hydration to decrease the uric acid concentration in the urine. Sodium bicarbonate administration should be discontinued once serum uric acid has normalized, since overly vigorous alkalinization may accelerate phosphate precipitation in the renal tubules.

4. Simultaneous hydration and diuresis promote the excretion of phosphorus and potassium. Potassium and magnesium may need to be replaced if deficits in these electrolytes appear.

5. Urine output should be maintained at a minimum of 100 ml/hr. Diuretics may be administered as adjunctive therapy, particularly when the person has a coexisting condition (e.g., impaired cardiac function) that could potentiate the risk of fluid overload.

6. Fluid balance is assessed by monitoring of intake, output, and weight and by observing for edema of lower extremities or sacrum. Distended neck veins or shortness of breath should be noted, and the lungs should be auscultated for adventitious sounds.

7. **Allopurinol** is given as a prophylactic measure to decrease uric acid levels.

F.   **PROGNOSIS**

1.   The occurrence and resolution of ATLS is dependent on the **tumor's responsiveness to cytotoxic therapy.**
2.   **ATLS usually resolves** within 7 days following treatment, but it may recur.

VIII.   **SYNDROME OF INAPPROPRIATE ANTIDIURETIC HORMONE (SIADH)**

A.   **SCOPE OF THE PROBLEM**

1.   **Definition**
     a.   **SIADH** is a paraneoplastic disease that develops when excessive amounts of antidiuretic hormone (ADH) are present, exerting an effect on the kidney and causing water intoxication.
2.   **Incidence**
     a.   **SIADH** occurs in approximately 1%–2% of patients with cancer. It is most frequently associated with small-cell lung cancer and may even be one of the presenting symptoms of the disease.
3.   **Anatomy, physiology, and scientific principles**
     a.   **Antidiuretic hormone (ADH)** is secreted in response to either an **increase in plasma concentration** or a **decrease in plasma volume.**
     b.   **ADH** acts on the distal tubules of the kidney to **conserve and retain water.**

B.   **PATHOPHYSIOLOGY**

1.   With SIADH, excessive ADH is produced, resulting in **water intoxication** (excessive water retention).
2.   **Table 34-17, text page 826,** lists many of the etiologic factors in SIADH according to pathological mechanism, such as ectopic production of ADH, abnormal stimulation of ADH, and induced ADH effects on the kidneys.
3.   **Small-cell lung tumors** are those most frequently associated with ectopic production of ADH, although inappropriate levels of ADH can also occur with **GI and bladder cancers, thymoma, Hodgkin's disease,** and **sarcoma.**
4.   SIADH is sometimes induced by **drugs** (e.g., cyclophosphamide, vincristine, morphine, nicotine, and ethanol).

C.   **CLINICAL MANIFESTATIONS**

1.   Primary clinical characteristics of SIADH are those of water intoxication.
2.   Neurologic symptoms are attributed to the effects of **cerebral edema:** thirst, headache, anorexia, muscle cramps, and lethargy are seen with early or mild **hyponatremia.**

D.   **ASSESSMENT**

1.   Identification of patients at risk of SIADH and its manifestations aids in recognition and treatment of this emergency. Assessment of blood and urine chemistries and physical manifestations will help confirm the diagnosis of SIADH.
2.   **Hyponatremia (serum sodium less than 130 mEg/l) in conjunction** with **low serum osmolality, high urine sodium,** and **high urine osmolality** are indicative of SIADH. **Table 34-19, text page 826,** lists the laboratory values used to diagnose SIADH.

E.   **INTERVENTIONS**

1.   Management depends on the severity of the hyponatremia.
2.   Initial treatment consists of **water restriction** and **systemic chemotherapy** (if the patient's condition permits the latter).
3.   For moderate SIADH (serum sodium <125 mEq/l) **normal saline hydration, electrolyte replacement,** and **furosemide diuresis** are used as treatment.
4.   For severe SIADH (serum sodium <120 mEq/l) and severe hyponatremia, **hypertonic (3%) saline** and **furosemide diuresis** are used.
5.   Nursing interventions include ensuring **patient safety** in the face of **alterations in neurologic status.**

6. If **systemic chemotherapy** is used, weight, neurologic status, I/O balance, plasma and urine osmolality, and sodium levels are carefully monitored.
7. Some chemotherapy drugs can exacerbate SIADH. Patients should be taught about fluid restrictions, I/O measurements, symptoms of hyponatremia, and symptoms to report to the physician.
8. **Demeclocycline** may be used for chronic or resistant SIADH. It inhibits ADH action but induces a reversible diabetes insipidus.
9. Reversal of SIADH is evident when the serum sodium level approaches normal.
10. Untreated, SIADH can progress to seizure, coma, and death. The insidious onset of SIADH can delay early diagnosis. Awareness of the population at risk and the predisposing factors is crucial.
11. **Figure 34-11, text page 828,** provides a clinical pathway for SIADH and highlights the critical decisions and interventions for this syndrome.
12. Overall prognosis is determined by the underlying cause of the SIADH.
13. Neurologic impairment from water intoxication is usually reversible.

F. FUTURE TRENDS

1. Because of the increased incidence of small-cell lung cancer and other tumors associated with ectopic production of ADH, the incidence of SIADH is increasing.
2. Future research is geared toward better control of small-cell lung cancer and other cancers, prevention of lung cancer, and medications that reduce circulating ADH or its release from tumors.

IX.   SPINAL CORD COMPRESSION

A. SCOPE OF THE PROBLEM

1. **Definition**
    a. **Spinal cord compression (SCC)** refers to a malignant process in which tumor encroaches upon the spinal cord or cauda equina.
2. **Incidence**
    a. Spinal cord compression is an **aneurologic emergency** that requires prompt diagnosis and intervention so that neurologic function **can be preserved and maintained.**
    b. SCC develops in about 5% of patients with systemic cancer, and approximately 95% of these cases are due to metastasis to the vertebral column.
    c. As a result of prolonged survival and increased incidence of cancers with bone metastasis, the incidence of spinal cord compression may be rising.
3. **Anatomy, physiology, and scientific principles**
    a. The spinal cord is surrounded by three connective tissue membranes. **Figure 34-12, text page 829,** illustrates a cross-sectional view of the spinal cord showing the membranes surrounding the spinal cord and spaces between the membranes, as well as a cross section of vertebra and spinal cord.
    b. The vertebral column supports the body and provides flexibility and mobility.
    c. The vertebral column protects the spinal cord, which consists of ascending and descending nerve tracts that send impulses to the brain and the peripheral nerves transmitting sensory and motor signals.

B. PATHOPHYSIOLOGY

1. SCC can be classified according to the location of the tumor causing compression as intramedullary, intradural, extravertebral, or extradural.
2. Extradural compression of the spinal cord in any circumstance leads to edema of the cord and ischemia, which mechanically distort and damage neural tissue. Intramedullary metastatic involvement can destroy actual cord tissue. Extravertebral lesions extend through the foramina.
3. The **rate and degree of compression and resulting cord damage** are responsible for the clinical manifestations of SCC.
4. Epidural metastasis is most frequently associated with cancers that metastasize to bone, such as cancers of the **breast, lung, prostrate, and kidney and myeloma.** Lymphomas have a high correlation with spinal cord compression because of direct extension through the intervertebral foramina.

5. Lung and breast cancers most often cause **thoracic SCC,** whereas GI cancers most frequently metastasize to the **lumbosacral spine.**

C. CLINICAL MANIFESTATIONS

1. **Table 34-21, text page 831,** presents the relationship between symptoms/neurologic findings and significant spinal cord compression.
2. Over 95% of patients with spinal cord compression have **pain** as the presenting symptom. The pain is either **radicular or localized.** Thoracic radicular pain is most often described as a constrictive band around the chest or waist.
3. **The hallmark indicator to early detection of spinal cord compression is the pain changing location, intensity, or nature.**
4. **Motor weakness** is present in three-fourths of patients at the time of diagnosis of SCC, although it is rarely a presenting symptom.
5. The type and degree of sensory and motor loss will depend on the **level and degree of compression.**
6. **Autonomic dysfunction** caused by spinal cord compression includes various bladder and bowel disturbances, including incontinence, difficulty voiding, constipation, urinary retention, and overflow.
7. Sensory loss, autonomic dysfunction, and poor sphincter control are present in about half of the patients when the compression is diagnosed. They indicate progressive disease.

D. ASSESSMENT

1. The single critical prognosis factor in SCC is **neurologic status before initiation of treatment.** The less extensive the injury to the cord before treatment, the greater the likelihood of full ambulation, sensation, and bowel and bladder control after treatment.
2. The sooner the SCC is treated, the better the prognosis for neurologic recovery.
3. Even if back pain is the only symptom, spinal cord compression should be suspected in cancer patients. **Table 34-22, text page 831,** lists the early and late signs of impending spinal cord compression. Pain, sensory or motor changes, and autonomic dysfunction are typical signs.
4. **Spine radiographs** will demonstrate vertebral body collapse, pedicle erosion, osteolytic lesions, or vertebral paraspinal masses in more than 85% of epidural metastasis.
5. **Bone scans** may be helpful in identifying vertebral body metastasis.
6. **Myelography** can be used for diagnosis of SCC. A contrast is injected into the subarachnoid space, and the flow of contrast media is observed to identify defects or blockages.
7. **Magnetic resonance imaging (MRI)** has emerged as the safest and most definitive diagnostic tool for spinal cord compression. It provides better visualization of neural tissue and distinguishes extradural, intradural, and intramedullary and extravertebral masses.

E. INTERVENTIONS

1. Timely treatment of spinal cord compression is as important as rapid diagnosis.
2. Controversy exists over the initial treatment of choice: radiation therapy, surgical decompression, or a combined approach of surgery followed by irradiation.
3. Radiation therapy is the treatment most often used for patients with epidural metastasis and spinal cord compression.
4. In certain instances, surgical decompression with laminectomy or vertebral body resection can promptly relieve SCC.
5. Chemotherapy may be used with sensitive cancers, such as lymphoma or Hodgkin's disease.
6. Steroids are always used as part of the treatment for SCC to **reduce spinal cord edema and pain.** With certain tumors, steroids have an **oncolytic effect.**
7. Postoperative nursing care includes **turning, positioning, skin care, pain management, wound care, and rehabilitation.**
    a. Patient assessment includes **monitoring sensory and motor function** as well as **urinary and bowel sphincter control.**
    b. Assisting the patient in the **management of sensory and motor deficits and pain control** is an essential aspect of nursing care.
    c. **Patient education** includes managing the steroid taper, side effects, and conditions requiring medical care.

8. Evaluation of the treatment response for SCC consists of thorough **neurologic examination and assessment for pain, sphincter control, and motor function.**
9. **Figure 34-14, text page 833,** presents a clinical pathway for the assessment and management of spinal cord compression.
10. Rehabilitative potential is dependent on pretreatment status and response to treatment.
11. Nurses play a vital role in early recognition of SCC and can help ensure neurologic preservation and a higher quality of life for patients.

F. **FUTURE TRENDS**

1. Investigation is needed regarding the best treatment modality for the various tumor types, level, degree, and location of the compression, including the appropriate dosage and schedule for steroid administration.
2. **Newer surgical techniques and spinal stabilization materials** continue to evolve.
3. The development of MRI has begun to positively affect the speed and safety of diagnosing spinal cord compression.

PRACTICE QUESTIONS

1. The physiologic process responsible for the clinical picture observed in late shock is
   (A) hypoxemia.
   (B) vasoconstriction.
   (C) hypotension.
   (D) vasodilation.

2. The effectiveness of therapy for septic shock will be **most** evident in which of the following parameters?
   (A) vital signs and skin color
   (B) renal function tests, oxygen saturation, temperature, and blood pressure
   (C) vital signs, skin color, level of consciousness, and urinary output
   (D) arterial blood gases and vital signs

3. Which of the following statements about disseminated intravascular coagulation (DIC) is true?
   (A) DIC is an abnormality of the clotting system in which the major physiologic event is widespread clotting.
   (B) DIC is a primary disorder.
   (C) The clotting cascade may be initiated by necrotic tissue, tumor enzymes, and endo- and exotoxins.
   (D) The platelet count and the values of TT, PT, and APTT will increase in DIC.

4. The major and only effective treatment for DIC that occurs as a result of the cancer process is
   (A) management of its tumor- or therapy-related cause.
   (B) administration of platelets and fresh frozen plasma.
   (C) halting the clotting cascade by means of heparin administration.
   (D) medication to suppress the symptoms, along with a quiet environment.

5. Shortness of breath, facial edema, trunk and upper extremity edema, neck and chest vein distention, cough, hoarseness, and stridor are the major clinical signs indicative of which oncologic emergency?
   (A) cardiac tamponade
   (B) superior vena cava syndrome (SVCS)
   (C) DIC
   (D) These can be major clinical signs for any of the above.

6. What is the **most** likely initial treatment of choice for quickly-progressing superior vena cava syndrome (SVCS)?
   (A) radiation therapy
   (B) chemotherapy
   (C) surgical resection
   (D) administration of anticoagulants

7. Which of the following statements about cardiac tamponade is **false?**
   (A) The clinical picture in cardiac tamponade is caused by a buildup of pressure around the heart.

(B)   As cardiac output declines, compensatory mechanisms such as increased heart rate and peripheral vasoconstriction are activated.
(C)   A paradoxical pulse is defined as a pulse that is weaker on expiration than inspiration.
(D)   The echocardiogram is the most accurate tool for diagnosing cardiac tamponade.

8.   Nursing care of the patient with hypercalcemia includes all of the following **except**
(A)   monitoring the patient for polyuria and polydypsia.
(B)   restricting fluids and administering furosemide.
(C)   frequent electrolyte replacement.
(D)   monitoring blood protein levels.

9.   Which of the following is the **least** likely cause of acute tumor lysis syndrome (ATLS)?
(A)   high-grade lymphoma
(B)   liposarcoma
(C)   acute lymphocytic leukemia (ALL)
(D)   reinduction treatment for ALL

10.   Renal failure occurs in patients with uncontrolled ATLS because of high levels of
(A)   calcium phosphate.
(B)   nucleic acids and potassium.
(C)   potassium and calcium.
(D)   uric acid and phosphate.

11.   Which of the following is indicative of SIADH?
(A)   increased plasma sodium and decreased urine output
(B)   hyponatremia with high serum osmolality and high urine osmolality
(C)   hypernatremia with high serum osmolality and high urine osmolality
(D)   hyponatremia with low serum osmolality, high urine sodium, and high urine osmolality

12.   The single **most** critical prognostic factor in spinal cord compression is
(A)   location of the tumor within the spinal cord.
(B)   neurologic status before initiation of treatment.
(C)   type and histologic grade of tumor.
(D)   level of the tumor and degree of compression of the spinal cord.

ANSWER EXPLANATIONS

1.   **The answer is (B).**   In late shock, vasoconstriction causes the clinical picture of cold and clammy skin in addition to organ ischemia, impaired alveolar gas exchange, and decreased urine output. Cardiac output, venous return, and blood pressure decrease, and blood is trapped in vascular beds. Prolonged inadequate perfusion leads to coma and cardiac death. (802)

2.   **The answer is (C).**   Vital signs, skin color, level of consciousness, and urinary output are all good indicators of perfusion of tissues and vital organs, the best sign that septic shock is reversing. The other answers do not provide the clinician with as much information. (805)

3.   **The answer is (C).**   DIC is characterized by both widespread clotting within arterioles and capillaries and simultaneous hemorrhage. It is **not** a primary disorder but rather results from other abnormalities in the body (e.g., the disease process). The platelet count **decreases** in DIC as a result of consumption. (805–806)

4.   **The answer is (A).**   The only effective treatment for DIC is treating the underlying cause of the syndrome. DIC can be controlled by administering platelets and fresh frozen plasma to replace consumable factors, and cryoprecipitate to replace fibrinogen. During DIC, the patient is assessed for signs of bleeding, e.g., changes in vital signs and neurological status, and frank bleeding. Other nursing interventions include instituting bleeding precautions and protecting the patient from injury. (808).

5.   **The answer is (B).**   SVCS obstruction causes elevated venous pressure and congestion. Clinical signs include shortness of breath, facial edema, trunk and upper extremity edema, neck and chest vein disten-

tion, cough, hoarseness, and stridor. Increased intracranial pressure may cause headache, dizziness, visual disturbances, and occasionally alterations in mental status. Although some of these signs also may be present with cardiac tamponade, the clinical signs listed are the classic signs seen with SVCS. (810)

6.   **The answer is (A).**   In quickly progressing, acute SVCS with no tissue diagnosis, fractionated irradiation is the treatment of choice. With more slowly progressing SVCS, a tissue diagnosis is obtained and the underlying disease is treated. Combination chemotherapy may be preferred to reverse the SVCS if the tumor mass is so large that a significant portion of critical tissue would be irradiated. The timing of systemic chemotherapy and/or mediastinal radiation is crucial: optimal therapy is administered with the least amount of normal tissue damage and maximal tumor destruction. (811)

7.   **The answer is (C).**   A paradoxical pulse is weaker on inspiration than expiration, because the buildup of intrathoracic pressure is greater as the lungs are expanding. Increased intrathoracic pressure will put additional pressure on the heart and further inhibit its ability to pump. (814)

8.   **The answer is (B).**   Vigorous **hydration,** not restriction, and administration of furosemide are first-line therapy for hypercalcemia. Polyuria and polydipsia both occur in hypercalcemia. Electrolytes need to be replaced frequently because of the effects of hydration and furosemide, and albumin needs to be monitored to calculate total serum calcium levels. (819)

9.   **The answer is (B).**   Tumor lysis syndrome is caused by rapid cell kill in treatment-sensitive tumors like high-grade lymphomas and ALL. Liposarcoma is the least likely cause of TLS because it is not as chemosensitive as the others and because overall tumor bulk is likely to be smaller. (822)

10.   **The answer is (D).**   Acute tumor lysis syndrome (ATLS) occurs when a large number of rapidly proliferating cells are lysed, releasing their intracellular minerals and uric acid into the blood. Uric acid precipitates and calcium phosphate crystallizes in the renal tubules, causing renal failure. (822)

11.   **The answer is (D).**   Antidiuretic hormone (ADH) is secreted in response to either an increase in plasma concentration or a decrease in plasma volume. ADH acts on the kidney to conserve water, resulting in an increased plasma volume and a decreased plasma osmolality. In SIADH, excessive ADH is produced, resulting in water intoxication: fluid is conserved in the body and not excreted. Thus the clinical picture is one of hyponatremia and low serum osmolality, and high urine sodium and osmolality. (824)

12.   **The answer is (B).**   Neurologic status before treatment is the single most critical prognostic factor in SCC. This argues for prompt recognition and treatment of SCC. Rehabilitative potential is dependent on pretreatment status and response to treatment. Eighty percent of ambulatory patients remain ambulatory after treatment, whereas only 30% with significant pretreatment motor dysfunction are ambulatory after treatment. (831)

35   Late Effects of Cancer Treatment

STUDY OUTLINE

I.   INTRODUCTION

1.   More than 5 million Americans with a history of cancer are alive today; 3 million of these cases were diagnosed 5 or more years ago. At least half of these individuals can be considered **biologically cured,** meaning the patient
   a.   **Has no evidence of the disease.**
   b.   **Has the same life expectancy as a person who never had cancer.**
   c.   **Ultimately dies of unrelated causes.**
2.   **The consequence, or late effects, of biologic cure result from physiologic changes related to particular treatments or to the interactions among the treatment, the individual, and the disease. They are believed to progress over time and by different mechanisms from those of the acute side effects of chemotherapy and radiation.**
   a.   They can appear months to years after treatment.
   b.   They can be mild to severe to life-threatening.
   c.   They can be clinically obvious, clinically subtle, or subclinical.
   d.   Their impact depends on the **age** and **development stage** of the patient.
      (1)   The growing child may rebound from acute toxicities of treatment better than adults but also may be more vulnerable to the effects of delayed toxicities.
      (2)   A great unknown is what will happen to individuals who received intensive treatment in their youth as they age.
      (3)   For adults, we do not know how treatment toxicities, hereditary predispositions to particular health problems, and environmental exposure to pollutants will interact.

II.   CENTRAL NERVOUS SYSTEM

1.   **Neuropsychologic, neuroanatomic,** and **neurophysiologic** changes can occur as a result of CNS treatment.
2.   These late effects have been observed in children with **acute lymphoblastic leukemia (ALL)** and **brain tumors** and in adult **small-cell carcinoma of the lung (SCCL)** patients, all of whom received CNS treatment for the primary tumor or as prophylaxis against meningeal disease.

A.   NEUROPSYCHOLOGIC EFFECTS

1.   Neuropsychologic effects do not become apparent until 24 to 36 months following treatment.
2.   The most frequently described neuropsychologic effects include **decrements in general intellectual performance and academic achievement scores,** as well as specific deficits in visual-motor integration, attention, memory, and visuomotor skills.
   a.   Nonverbal, or performance, skills are particularly vulnerable.
3.   These effects appear to be related to **cranial radiation alone** or **in combination with intrathecal (IT) methotrexate.**
   a.   There may be a synergistic effect between cranial radiation and chemotherapy that increases the magnitude of toxicity.
   b.   **Higher doses of radiation** (>2400 cGy) also tend to result in more severe impairments.

4. **Age** at the time of CNS treatment is an important risk factor for neurologic sequelae; children under the age of 5 who receive high doses of radiation are at greatest risk. Recent evidence also suggests that girls are more severely affected than boys in terms of general cognitive performance such as IQ scores.

B. **NEUROANATOMIC EFFECTS**

1. Brain **atrophy** and **decreased subcortical white matter** are the most frequent abnormalities.
2. Effects appear to be **age and dose-related.** Evidence suggests that children under 3 and adults over 60 are at greatest risk for abnormalities.

C. **MECHANISMS OF PATHOGENESIS**

1. A synergistic relationship between radiation and methotrexate may account for **progressive demyelination** (disruption of the myelin sheath that insulates axons). This may account for degenerative changes during the early stage of delayed injury following CNS treatment. Antigens released from the damaged glial cells initiate an autoimmune response that can also contribute to the pathogenesis of delayed tissue damage.
2. Later effects appear to be due to progressive **ischemia** and **loss of parenchymal tissue function** caused by damage to the endothelial cells of the microvasculature. These cells may be particularly vulnerable to the effects of radiation because of their replicating capacity.

D. **VISION AND HEARING**

1. **Enucleation,** which may be necessary in the treatment of ocular tumors such as retinoblastoma, is the most disabling visual defect.
2. **Cataracts** may result from cranial irradiation and long-term corticosteroid treatment.
3. **Hearing loss** in the high-tone range is most closely associated with the chemotherapeutic agent **cisplatin,** especially when treatment is combined with cranial irradiation.

III. **ENDOCRINE SYSTEM**

1. Cancer treatment can adversely affect a number of endocrine functions, including **metabolism, growth, secondary sexual development,** and **reproduction.**
2. These late effects result from damage to the **target organ** (i.e., thyroid, ovary, and testis) and/or the **hypothalamic pituitary axis.**
3. **Table 35-1, text page 844,** summarizes the major endocrine sequelae, related risk factors, and recommendations for evaluation and treatment.

A. **THYROID**

1. Review **Table 35-1, text page 844,** under **Thyroid** for a summary of the major sequelae, related risk factors, and recommendations for evaluation and treatment.
2. Direct radiation damage to the thyroid causes **primary hypothyroidism** with a decreased production of thyroxine (T_4) and triiodothyronine (T_3).
    a. These hormones affect oxygen consumption, the central and peripheral nervous systems, skeletal and cardiac muscle, carbohydrate and cholesterol metabolism, and growth and development.
    b. Undamaged tissue may become overstimulated to compensate for primary hypothyroidism. This chronic overstimulation may increase the risk of malignant transformation in previously undamaged cells.
3. **Secondary hypothyroidism** can occur when the hypothalamic pituitary axis is in the field of radiation to the nasopharynx or the CNS.

B. **GROWTH**

1. Review **Table 35-1, text page 844,** under **Hypothalamic-pituitary axis** for a summary of the major sequelae, related risk factors, and recommendations for evaluation and treatment.

C. **SECONDARY SEXUAL DEVELOPMENT AND REPRODUCTION**

1. Review **Table 35-1, text page 844,** under **Ovaries** and **Testes** for a summary of the major sequelae, related risk factors, and recommendations for evaluation and treatment.

IV. **IMMUNE SYSTEM**

1. **Immunosuppression** is one of the most serious acute toxic effects of chemotherapy and radiation. Certain aspects of the immune system also can be adversely affected for years after the completion of treatment.
2. These immunologic late effects have been studied most thoroughly in patients treated for **leukemia (ALL), Hodgkin's disease,** and **breast cancer.**
3. Radiation and chemotherapy may result in an **inversion of the ratio of helper T-cells to suppressor T-cells.**
   a. Helper T-cells seem to be particularly radiosensitive.
   b. This inversion can persist for as long as 10 years following treatment for breast cancer and Hodgkin's disease and total body irradiation prior to bone marrow transplantation.
4. **Bone marrow regeneration** can also be affected by high doses of radiation.
5. The clinical significance of these long-term alterations in immune function is not well understood.
   a. There is no evidence that patients with persistent immunologic abnormalities are at increased risk for infections.
   b. The exception is patients who have undergone **splenectomy,** who are at greater risk of bacterial infection because of the protective role of the spleen.

V. **CARDIOVASCULAR SYSTEM**

1. Review **Table 35-2, text page 847,** for a summary of biologic late effects on the cardiovascular system, including methods of assessment and suggestions for intervention.
2. One of the most serious late effects of anthracyclines used for many cancers is **cardiac toxicity,** which typically presents as **cardiomyopathy,** with or without clinical signs of congestive heart failure.

VI. **PULMONARY SYSTEM**

1. Review **Table 35-2, text page 847,** for a summary of biologic late effects on the pulmonary (respiratory) system, including methods of assessment and suggestions for intervention.
2. **Pneumonitis** and **pulmonary fibrosis** are the major biologic late effects of treatment to the pulmonary system.

VII. **GASTROINTESTINAL SYSTEM**

1. Review **Table 35-2, text page 847,** for a summary of biologic late effects on the gastrointestinal system, including methods of assessment and suggestions for intervention.
2. Late effects on the **liver** are most common and include **hepatic fibrosis, cirrhosis,** and **portal hypertension.**

VIII. **RENAL SYSTEM**

1. Review **Table 35-2, text page 847 (Kidney and urinary tract),** for a summary of biologic late effects on the renal system, including methods of assessment and suggestions for intervention.
2. **Nephritis** and **cystitis** are the major long-term renal toxicities that result from cancer treatment.

IX. **MUSCULOSKELETAL SYSTEM**

1. Review **Table 35-2, text page 847,** for a summary of biologic late effects on the musculoskeletal system, including methods of assessment and suggestions for intervention.
2. Most late effects are associated with **radiation.**
3. Skeletal abnormalities become more apparent during periods of rapid growth such as the adolescent growth spurt. Factors associated with the occurrence of significant late orthopedic problems include **higher radiation dose and larger irradiated field.**

X.   **SECOND MALIGNANT NEOPLASMS**

    1.   Adults and children who have received chemotherapy or radiation therapy, or both, for a primary malignancy are at **increased risk for the development of a second malignant neoplasm.**

    2.   **Alkylating agents** and **ionizing radiation** are the treatments most closely linked to a second malignant neoplasm.

    3.   The risk of developing a second cancer depends on several predisposing factors, including

       a.   Type and dose of treatment received.

       b.   An underlying etiologic factor linking two or more cancers, e.g., smoking and lung and bladder cancer.

       c.   Genetic susceptibility, e.g., genetic retinoblastoma in children.

A.   **SECOND MALIGNANCIES FOLLOWING CHEMOTHERAPY**

    1.   **Acute nonlymphocytic leukemia (ANL)** following treatment with **alkylating agents** is the most common chemotherapy-related neoplasm.

    2.   The disease can occur as early as 1.3 years following initiation of chemotherapy for primary malignancy. It peaks at 5 years and plateaus at 10 years following treatment.

    3.   Occurrence of a second malignancy appears to be related to the **dose of the alkylating agent.**

    4.   Incidence of ANL appears to be highest following **Hodgkin's disease** and **multiple myeloma,** although it also appears following other cancers.

B.   **SECOND MALIGNANCIES FOLLOWING RADIATION**

    1.   **Sarcomas of the bone and soft tissue** are the most common second malignant neoplasm after radiation therapy.

    2.   The incidence has been found to peak at 15 to 20 years following radiation.

    3.   Malignant transformation of normal cells can occur in doses ranging from 1000 to 8000 cGy.

    4.   In one study the risk was highest among children treated for **retinoblastoma** and **Ewing's sarcoma** but also increased significantly in patients treated for rhabdomyosarcoma, Wilms' tumor, and Hodgkin's disease.

    5.   In addition to sarcomas and leukemia, a variety of solid tumors have been linked to treatment with radiation.

    6.   **Table 35-3, text page 851,** summarizes the findings from selected studies on the risk of ANL in patients treated for various types of cancer.

PRACTICE QUESTIONS

1.   Which of the following statements about the late effects of cancer treatment is **incorrect?**
    (A)   Late effects are believed to progress over time.
    (B)   Late effects are believed to involve different mechanisms from those of the acute side effects of chemotherapy and radiation.
    (C)   Late effects are severe but clinically subtle.
    (D)   Late effects are the consequence of biologic cure.

2.   Late effects involving the central nervous system (CNS) are **most** likely to occur in which of the following individuals?
    (A)   a child treated for Hodgkin's disease
    (B)   a child treated for bone sarcoma
    (C)   an adult treated for small-cell carcinoma of the lung
    (D)   an adult treated for primary hypothyroidism

3.   The most frequently described neuropsychologic late effects of CNS treatment for cancer include a deterioration in general intellectual performance. If we can assume that neuropsychologic changes in the brain are related to **neuroanatomic** abnormalities that result from cranial radiation, then one plausible explanation for the deterioration of intellectual performance is
    (A)   a decrease in subcortical white matter.
    (B)   destruction of the hypothalamus.

(C)   the formation of myelin membranes on nerve axons.
(D)   the overstimulation of thyroid tissue.

4.   Which of the following treatments is **most** closely associated with progressive demyelination, which may be important in the early stage of delayed injury to the brain?
(A)   methotrexate alone
(B)   radiation alone
(C)   methotrexate combined with radiation
(D)   methotrexate combined with both radiation and surgery

5.   The late effects of cancer treatment on the endocrine system result from damage to the hypothalamus pituitary axis and/or to
(A)   target organs, e.g., the thyroid.
(B)   the cortical areas of the brain.
(C)   the chemical structure of key hormones, e.g., insulin.
(D)   epithelial tissue, e.g., blood vessel linings.

6.   Growth impairment as a late effect of treatment for cancer occurs as the result of
(A)   overproduction of thyroxine by the thyroid gland.
(B)   deficient growth hormone release by the hypothalamus.
(C)   primary hypothyroidism.
(D)   a disruption in pituitary control of several target organs.

7.   Damage to ovaries and testes resulting in gonadal failure is **most** likely to be a late effect associated with which of the following malignancies?
(A)   brain cancer
(B)   bone sarcomas
(C)   acute nonlymphocytic leukemia
(D)   Hodgkin's disease

8.   Which of the following statements **best** summarizes the late effects of cancer treatment on the immune system?
(A)   There is no evidence that patients with persistent immunologic abnormalities are at increased risk for infections.
(B)   Immunologic late effects have been studied most thoroughly in patients treated for hypothyroidism, liver cancer, and splenectomy.
(C)   Radiation and chemotherapy are more destructive of suppressor T-cells than of helper T-cells.
(D)   There is no evidence that persistent immunologic impairment follows radiation and chemotherapy.

9.   An individual is admitted with congestive heart failure. Medical records indicate a history of acute leukemia, which was treated 10 years earlier with anthracyclines. The **most** likely late effect of this treatment is
(A)   angina.
(B)   pulmonary fibrosis.
(C)   pericarditis.
(D)   cardiomyopathy.

10.   Scoliosis and kyphosis are **most** likely to develop as late effects of the treatment of intra-abdominal tumors with
(A)   combination MOPP therapy.
(B)   radiation to one side of the body.
(C)   pelvic irradiation combined with alkylating agents.
(D)   prolonged use of corticosteroids.

11.   The risk of developing a second malignant neoplasm after treatment for a primary malignancy depends on several factors, including all of the following **except**
(A)   the type and dose of treatment received, e.g., radiation and alkylating agents.
(B)   a common underlying etiologic factor, e.g., smoking.
(C)   genetic susceptibility, e.g., genetic retinoblastoma.
(D)   the timing of withdrawal of chemotherapeutic agents, e.g., MOPP latency.

12. The most common second malignancy neoplasms following radiation therapy are
    (A) breast carcinomas and gynecologic tumors.
    (B) cancers of the gastrointestinal tract.
    (C) sarcomas of the bone and soft tissue.
    (D) tumors of the bladder and lung.

ANSWER EXPLANATIONS

1. **The answer is (C).** The late effects of biologic cure result from physiologic changes related to particular treatments or to the interactions among the treatment, the individual, and the disease. Unlike the acute side effects of chemotherapy and radiation, however, late effects are believed to progress over time and by different mechanisms. They can appear months to years after treatment, can be mild to severe to life-threatening, and can be clinically obvious, clinically subtle, or subclinical. Their impact appears to depend on the age and development stage of the patient. (841)

2. **The answer is (C).** The late effects of CNS treatment, including neuropsychologic, neuroanatomic, and neurophysiologic changes, have been observed most commonly in children with acute lymphoblastic leukemia (ALL) and brain tumors and in adult small-cell carcinoma of the lung (SCCL) patients, all of whom received CNS treatment for the primary tumor or as prophylaxis against meningeal disease. (841–842)

3. **The answer is (C).** Brain atrophy and decreased subcortical white matter are the most frequent abnormalities that have been observed in long-term survivors who received whole brain radiation. Because both abnormalities affect brain function, it is reasonable to see a connection between these neuroanatomic late effects and a deterioration in general intellectual performance. Other treatment-related changes in the brain, including demyelination of nerves, calcifications, and thickening of capillary walls, no doubt also are associated with intellectual deterioration. (843)

4. **The answer is (C).** Progressive demyelination (disruption of the myelin membrane that insulates nerve axons) may be due to a synergistic relationship between radiation and methotrexate. The myelin-producing glial cells in the CNS are proliferative during early childhood and therefore radiosensitive. Damage to or a reproductive loss of glial cells from radiation can disrupt the myelin membrane. Methotrexate appears to contribute to this effect. (842–843)

5. **The answer is (A).** The target organs most commonly affected are the thyroid, ovaries, and testes. Late effects can include alterations in metabolism, growth, secondary sexual characteristics, and reproduction. (843)

6. **The answer is (B).** High doses of radiation to the hypothalamic pituitary axis can damage the hypothalamus and disrupt the production of growth hormone. Growth hormone deficiency with short stature is one of the most common long-term endocrine consequences of radiation to the CNS in children. (844–845)

7. **The answer is (D).** Those at highest risk for late effects involving the gonads, including gonadal failure, are women treated for Hodgkin's disease, breast cancer, and ovarian germ cell tumors, and men treated for Hodgkin's disease, pelvic and testicular tumors, and testicular leukemia. Damage occurs both with radiation and alkylating agents. (845)

8. **The answer is (A).** Although persistent immunologic impairment appears to follow radiation and chemotherapy, there is no evidence that patients with persistent immunologic abnormalities are at increased risk for infections. The exception is patients who have undergone splenectomy, who are at greater risk of bacterial infection because of the protective role of the spleen against encapsulated organisms. Immunologic late effects have been studied most thoroughly in patients treated for leukemia (ALL), Hodgkin's disease, and breast cancer. Helper T-cells, and not suppressor T-cells, are particularly radiosensitive. (846)

9. **The answer is (D).** One of the most serious side effects of anthracyclines is cardiac toxicity which typically presents as cardiomyopathy, with clinical signs of congestive heart failure. Recent evidence, however, indicates that structural damage can occur in the absence of clinical signs, and that cardiac failure may occur many years following completion of therapy. (846)

10. **The answer is (B).** Uneven radiation to vertebrae, soft tissue, and muscles for the treatment of intra-abdominal tumors frequently results in scoliosis or kyphosis, or both. Although recent therapies have been modified to minimize this problem, it may still occur in some children and tends to become most apparent during periods of rapid growth such as the adolescent growth spurt. (850)

11. **The answer is (D).** Adults and children who have received chemotherapy or radiation therapy, or both, for a primary malignancy are at increased risk for the development of a second malignant neoplasm. Alkylating agents and ionizing radiation are the treatments most closely linked to a second malignant neoplasm. In addition to the type and dose of treatment received, the risk of the development of a secondary cancer depends on several predisposing factors, including choices (B) and (C). (850–851)

12. **The answer is (C).** Sarcomas of the bone and soft tissue are the most common second malignant neoplasms after radiation therapy, with the incidence peaking at 15 to 20 years following radiation. In a large study of survivors of childhood cancer, risk of bone cancer was highest among children treated for retinoblastoma and Ewing's sarcoma but also increased significantly in patients treated for rhabdomyosarcoma, Wilms' tumor, and Hodgkin's disease. In addition to sarcomas and leukemia, a variety of solid tumors have been linked to treatment with radiation, including carcinomas of the breast and tumors of the bladder, rectum, and uterus. (851–852)

36   AIDS-Related Malignancies

STUDY OUTLINE

I. **INTRODUCTION**

1. **Human immunodeficiency virus (HIV)** appears to provide further evidence supporting the theory of immune surveillance and the evolution of cancer.
    a. Malignancy is diagnosed in approximately 70% of those whose immune systems have been destroyed by the HIV virus and who have acquired immunodeficiency syndrome (AIDS).
2. The three most common malignancies in AIDS are **Kaposi's sarcoma (KS), non-Hodgkin's lymphoma (NHL),** and **primary central nervous system (CNS) lymphoma.**
    a. These diseases are referred to as **opportunistic** malignancies because they occur in patients with preexisting immunodeficiency.
    b. Because these individuals are immunosuppressed, the above cancers proliferate rapidly.

II. **KAPOSI'S SARCOMA**

1. **Kaposi's sarcoma (KS)** was a rare skin cancer until the 1970s, when it began to appear in patients who were chemically immunosuppressed to prevent rejection of transplanted organs.
2. In 1981 outbreaks were reported in scattered populations of previously healthy, young, homosexual men who were neither receiving chemotherapy nor undergoing organ transplantation.
    a. Other opportunistic infections, e.g., *Pneumocystis carinii* pneumonia, were diagnosed in the same population.
    b. All individuals were found to have some degree of immunosuppression.
    c. These findings led to the clinical definition of AIDS, in which the **underlying immunodeficiency resulted in the appearance of indicator diseases.**
    d. In 1987, the diagnosis of AIDS was expanded to include the advent of KS in a person of any age who is seropositive for HIV antibody.

A. **EPIDEMIOLOGY**

1. **Classic KS (non-African)** is predictably a chronic, fairly benign malignancy that is rarely fatal.
    a. It occurs primarily in men of Mediterranean or Jewish ancestry in the fifth to eighth decades of life.
    b. It is characterized as an indolent, slow-growing cutaneous nodule or plaquelike lesion. Most lesions are confined to the lower extremities.
    c. Typically, it is not invasive and does not disseminate.
2. **African KS,** in contrast, is a malignant disease that affects persons of all ages and is found almost exclusively in black Africans.
    a. Twice as many men as women are affected.
    b. Clinical presentations range from one similar to that observed in classic KS to a **florid, infiltrative, and highly aggressive lymphadenopathic form that progresses rapidly and is frequently fatal.**
3. **KS in transplant recipients** affects men at a higher incidence than women. Presentations range from localized skin lesions to disseminated visceral and mucocutaneous disease.
    a. The more depressed the immune system, the greater the incidence of KS.
    b. Spontaneous remissions have been documented in transplantation patients whose immunosuppression has been reversed.

4. **AIDS-related KS** is distinctly different from the other categories of KS.
   a. Clinical presentation ranges from **localized skin lesions to disseminated disease that involves multiple body organs.**
   b. KS that occurs with AIDS tends to be **highly aggressive,** although patients rarely die as a direct result of KS.
   c. The cause of death is usually from **concomitant opportunistic infections** or the **pathologic effects of HIV itself.**
5. See **Table 33-1, text page 691,** for a summary of the clinical features and response to therapy of the four types of KS.

B. **ETIOLOGY**

1. **Early reports indicated KS was the initial diagnosis in only 30%–35% of all AIDS cases. However, a steady decline has been noted.**
2. Infection by a **cytomegalovirus (CMV)** may be the cause of KS.
   a. CMV is found in a large percentage of homosexual men and AIDS patients, which may offer an explanation for the diagnosis of KS predominantly in homosexual men.
3. It appears that in the gay population, a decline of 20% per year has been noted; in other populations with AIDS-related KS, a 10% decline per year has been reported.

C. **DETECTION**

1. Detection of KS is typically by **self-observation of cutaneous lesions.** Patient education in lesion identification is therefore important.
2. Nurses also should routinely perform a careful visual examination of cutaneous surfaces of all persons who are **seropositive for HIV** or who are at **high risk for AIDS.**
3. Biopsy specimens of suspicious lesions are then examined.

D. **PATHOPHYSIOLOGY**

1. After histologic examination the pathologist has the responsibility of diagnosis.
2. In the early, or **macular,** stage of the disease changes are subtle, and only abnormally dilated vessels surrounding normal superficial vasculature may be observed.
3. As the lesion matures and becomes a plaque, it demonstrates **more extensive neoplastic involvement,** with proliferation through many layers.
   a. Marked **inflammation** occurs at this stage, with a corresponding **increase in numbers of spindle cells** and **extravasation of red cells.**
   b. **Hemosiderin deposits** are also noted at this time.
4. These effects become exaggerated as the lesion advances toward nodular formation. Spindle cells are dense, with considerable reticulum deposits.

E. **CLINICAL MANIFESTATIONS**

1. Lesions can be found on almost any skin surface.
   a. They do not metastasize; instead they are **multicentric** (i.e., each lesion is a primary lesion unto itself).
   b. **Pigmentation** ranges from brown, brown-red, purple, dark red, to violet or deep blue-purple.
   c. Lesions may be **raised bullous nodules** or **flat plaquelike lesions.**
   d. They **do not blanch when touched** and are **not painful** unless they are responsible for structural damage or impinge on vital organs or nerves.
2. The tumor also can involve various **mucocutaneous surfaces** as well as the sclera of the eyes.
3. Involvement of one or more organ systems is frequent at the time of initial diagnosis.
   a. **Lymph nodes, GI tract,** and **lungs** are the internal organs most often affected.
   b. KS in these organ systems can cause severe morbidity.
4. As HIV infection progresses, the immune system becomes increasingly suppressed.
   a. Involvement of the lymph nodes may compromise lymphatic drainage and blood circulation, resulting in **edema** and **stasis ulcers.**
   b. The patient may succumb to **anascara,** which is due to internal coalesced lesions and a decreased total serum protein/albumin resulting from the shift of fluid.

5. When the GI tract is involved, the patient may have a **protein-losing enteropathy,** in which protein is not absorbed from the GI tract. This also decreases serum protein/albumin level.
6. Involvement of the lung may cause **dyspnea** and **shortness of breath,** eventually culminating in fatal respiratory distress.

F. **STAGING**

1. See **Table 36-2, text page 865,** for two proposed staging systems for AIDS-related KS.
2. Poorer prognosis may be associated with several factors, including
    a. A **low T4-lymphocyte count** and **reduced helper/suppressor ratio.**
    b. Involvement with the **head and neck.**
    c. Prior or concomitant **opportunistic infections.**
    d. **Presence of "B" symptoms,** including weight loss, fever, chills, night sweats, and diarrhea.
3. With the exception of the lung, organ involvement does not seem to influence prognosis, nor does tumor burden correlate with prognosis.
4. A new recommended staging classification has been developed for uniform evaluation, response, and staging criteria for KS. Patients are assigned to either a good risk or a poor risk category, depending upon the extent of the tumor, immune system status, and other systemic illnesses. See **Table 36-3, text page 866.**

G. **ASSESSMENT**

1. Assessment begins with a **complete history** and **physical examination,** including
    a. The patient's past history of drug use, sexual practice, and ethnic ancestry.
    b. Close examination of the sclera, oral cavity, and integumentary system.
2. Suspicious lesions are **biopsied** before a diagnosis can be established.
3. Suspected KS involvement of the lung requires **bronchoscopic examination;** suspected involvement of the GI tract requires **endoscopic examination.**
    a. Because bleeding and increased morbidity may result from biopsy of these sites, visual inspection and identification may be adequate.
4. Other abnormalities related more to **HIV infection** than to KS may also be detected, e.g., elevated erythrocyte sedimentation rate (ESR), mild anemia, and leukopenia.

H. **TREATMENT**

1. **Medical**
    a. See **Table 36-4, text page 868,** for a summary of guidelines for therapy in AIDS-related Kaposi's sarcoma.
    b. In AIDS-related KS, treatment provides only temporary remission or stabilization of disease and **does not improve survival rate.**
    c. Treatment options include surgery, radiation therapy, and chemotherapy.
        (1) Except in diagnosis, **surgery** has almost no role in KS treatment.
        (2) **Radiation therapy** is highly effective and plays a role in local control of lesions and in cosmetic effect.
        (3) **Chemotherapeutic agents** are useful when a systemic effect is necessary and the benefits of treatment outweigh the risks to the patient. Although the response of lesions to chemotherapy can be dramatic, the lesions do not go away.
    d. Interferon has also shown efficacy in treatment of AIDS-related KS.
2. **Nursing**
    a. Consideration is given to the **psychosocial aspects** of the disease, as well as to the **physical status** of the patient.
    b. A determination of the patient's **risk group** and whether the KS is the patient's first diagnosis or one of a succession of indicator diseases will help the nurse establish a plan of care.
    c. Nurses should be particularly sensitive to the issues of **sexual preference** and **drug use.**
        (1) The patient may be disclosing his homosexuality to his family. Emotional support is crucial.
        (2) The patient may be a drug user. Realistic goals are necessary in this patient population because of both drug-seeking and manipulative behavior.
    d. Side effects of chemotherapy tend to be **more severe in the AIDS population.** For this reason the nurse should

      (1)   Be aggressive in the assessment of potential complications.

      (2)   Alert the physician promptly when complications occur.

      (3)   Implement appropriate nursing interventions.

      (4)   Remember that these patients have an underlying illness that predisposes them to other opportunistic infections and malignancies.

    e.   Treatment with **vinca alkaloids** should be discontinued in patients who experience severe jaw pain. They may cause irreversible nerve damage.

III.   NON-HODGKIN'S LYMPHOMA

A.   EPIDEMIOLOGY

1.   NHL in a person who is also **seropositive for HIV antibody** or has **positive culture results** is considered to affirm a diagnosis of AIDS.

2.   It has been estimated that NHL has been diagnosed in 4% to 10% of patients with AIDS, although some underreporting may occur.

3.   It is generally recognized that the increased survival attributed to azidothymidine (AZT) increases the likelihood of developing NHL.

B.   ETIOLOGY

1.   The DNA-containing **herpes virus known as EBV** has been suggested as an important etiologic agent in AIDS-NHL.

    a.   This virus has been associated with Burkitt's lymphoma, a type of high-grade NHL, and is suspected of playing a similar role in AIDS-NHL.

    b.   One possibility is that once HIV infection occurs, EBV may **trigger lymphocyte proliferation** that remains unchecked as a result of HIV-induced immune dysfunction.

    c.   This proliferation, in turn, may **allow the expression of two oncogenes,** resulting in a polyclonal or monoclonal NHL.

C.   PATHOPHYSIOLOGY

1.   AIDS-associated NHLs are typically **intermediate- to high-grade B-cell malignancies** and may arise from a **polyclonal B-cell lymphoproliferation** that results from EBV and HIV infection.

    a.   AIDS-NHL has been associated with persistent generalized **lymphadenopathy,** suggesting polyclonal B-cell activation.

2.   Lymph node invasion of a tumor may cause structural damage to the node as well as extension of cellular proliferations beyond the node.

3.   All organs have lymphocytes within their boundaries that are capable of transforming and forming tumors.

D.   CLINICAL MANIFESTATIONS

1.   Presentation of non-AIDS NHL is diffuse, with no symptoms apparent in most patients in the early stages.

2.   In contrast, patients with HIV-related NHL have **very advanced disease,** which frequently involves **extranodal sites,** including the CNS, bone marrow, bowel, and anorectum.

    a.   These extranodal sites may be the only site of the disease; that is, peripheral lymphadenopathy may be absent.

    b.   Patients may also exhibit signs and symptoms of HIV infection, AIDS-related complex, or AIDS, which makes diagnosis difficult.

E.   ASSESSMENT

1.   The diagnosis and classification of lymphoma can be made only by means of a **biopsy specimen** that is examined by a pathologist.

2.   The patient's status must first be **staged** and **graded.**

    a.   It is unusual for patients with HIV-related NHL to present at a stage **lower than stage III.**

    b.   Staging is accomplished by means of the Ann Arbor staging classification system.

  c. The staging work-up includes
      (1) A careful **history,** which notes the presence or absence of "B" symptoms.
      (2) A complete **physical examination** with special attention to Waldeyer's ring, the liver, and the spleen.
      (3) **Laboratory tests** that assess the overall wellness of the patient and screen for other conditions.
      (4) A **chest film** and **CT scans** of the chest, abdomen, and pelvis.
      (5) A **bilateral bone marrow biopsy and aspiration** and a **lumbar puncture.**
3. If AIDS has not been previously diagnosed, then an **HIV antibody test** is indicated.
    a. Not all swollen lymph nodes are malignant; benign reactive lymphadenopathy is common in this HIV-seropositive population.
    b. Abdominal masses or swollen lymph nodes may be related to infection. Thus it is essential to obtain a biopsy specimen and compare it with normal tissue before a diagnosis is made.

F. **TREATMENT**

1. **Medical**
    a. Treatment options can be determined on the basis of **method,** as well as by **grade of tumor.**
    b. Intermediate-grade tumors can be treated with either **chemotherapy** or **radiation therapy,** depending on the stage at presentation.
    c. Advanced intermediate/high-grade lymphoma is treated with **combination chemotherapy,** with **cyclophosphamide** the most active and effective agent.
        (1) Initial responses are usually dramatic but are not long-lived.
        (2) Relapse typically occurs in 4 to 6 weeks following discontinuation of chemotherapy.
        (3) Treatment-related **neutropenia** is severe and sometimes precipitates an opportunistic infection.
        (4) Regardless of outcome, patients still have HIV infection and AIDS.
    d. **Radiation therapy** may be useful for
        (1) Patients with limited bulky disease.
        (2) Patients who are unable to tolerate chemotherapy either because of poor health or low blood counts.
        (3) Local control or CNS prophylaxis.
2. **Results and prognosis**
    a. As with other types of cancer, a group of patients can be identified who will respond better than others to treatment.
    b. Indicators of a "good" prognosis include prior AIDS diagnosis, Karnofsky performance status, site of disease, and CD4 count.
3. **Nursing**
    a. Nursing care is no different from that for non-AIDS-related NHL, except that additional **emotional support** is needed.
    b. Patients with big, bulky, high-grade disease are at high risk for **tumor lysis syndrome.**
        (1) It generally occurs when the patient is initially treated.
        (2) Tumor cells spill their contents into the general circulation, causing a metabolic disturbance.
        (3) Renal failure and death may occur.
        (4) The treatment of choice is **prevention,** including **hydration, sodium bicarbonate,** and intravenous or oral **allopurinol** to prevent hyperuricemia nephropathy.
        (5) The patient's urine output is monitored hourly, and the physician is alerted to any sign of urinary insufficiency.
        (6) Serum chemistry levels are monitored every 6 hours in high-risk patients.
        (7) Dialysis is administered if electrolyte levels continue to rise and renal function deteriorates.
    c. All patients with HIV-related NHL should be observed for a full 72 hours for any sign of tumor lysis syndrome. Signs and symptoms include a **decreased urine output** and **increased lethargy.**
    d. Some cell tumor lysis prior to treatment may occur.
        (1) Complications are the same as those experienced by all patients with NHL: **neutropenia sepsis, thrombocytopenia,** and untreated **tumor lysis syndrome.**

IV.   **PRIMARY CENTRAL NERVOUS SYSTEM LYMPHOMA**

   A.   **EPIDEMIOLOGY**

   1.   **Primary CNS lymphoma** is rare. Most of those diagnosed are immunocompromised, as with HIV infection.
   2.   Patients with AIDS are also at risk for the development of opportunistic infections of the CNS, including **cryptococcosis** and **toxoplasmosis,** which complicates the diagnosis process.
   3.   The cell of origin for primary CNS lymphoma is the same as that causing NHL elsewhere in the body.
      a.   The transformed cell, which multiplies in an area that does not allow expansion (i.e., inside the cranium), is the cause of most presenting symptoms.
      b.   In some cases the neoplasm will be multicentric, arising in several areas of the brain at the same time.

   B.   **CLINICAL MANIFESTATIONS**

   1.   The most frequently observed symptoms of HIV-associated CNS lymphomas include **confusion, lethargy, memory loss,** and **alterations in personality or behavior. Seizures** may also develop.
   2.   Symptoms are very similar to those caused by other mass lesions in the CNS, for which **toxoplasmosis** is the usual explanation.
      a.   Primary CNS lymphoma is usually a diagnosis of **exclusion:** if the patient fails to respond to treatment for toxoplasmosis, primary CNS lymphoma is the presumptive diagnosis.
   3.   Primary CNS lymphoma usually appears on CT scans and MRI images as **single or multiple discrete lesions** and exhibits a characteristic pre- and postcontrast appearance.
      a.   A diagnosis cannot be determined by scans alone, however.
   4.   Tests on **cerebral spinal fluid (CSF)** may reveal some abnormalities and can help rule out certain diagnoses, including toxoplasmosis and syphilis.

   C.   **TREATMENT**

   1.   **Medical**
      a.   Most AIDS-associated CNS lymphoma patients die of concomitant opportunistic infections whether or not they are treated.
   2.   **Nursing**
      a.   Nursing responsibility includes a thorough assessment, paying particular attention to any focal findings, motor incoordination, and cognitive deficits.
      b.   Safety and provisions for daily living in the home must be considered.
      c.   Providing emotional support to the patient and family is essential.
      d.   Ethical questions may arise over the patient's mental competence to make decisions.
         (1)   If the patient is not thought to be competent, the next of kin or a legal guardian will need to make decisions for the patient.

   D.   **COMPLICATIONS**

   1.   The most frequent complication is the patient's mental deterioration to the point of becoming **moribund** and **comatose.**
   2.   This may be the result of the HIV virus and its effect on the brain, by the treatment itself, or by some combination of these, or some other factor.

V.   **OTHER MALIGNANCIES AND HUMAN IMMUNODEFICIENCY VIRUS**

   1.   Although other cancers may be seen in AIDS patients, no epidemiologic link or direct causal relationship has been established for these malignancies.
   2.   It is useful to know, however, the HIV status of a patient with a malignancy because response to therapy is typically poor in the person with HIV infection.
   3.   It is reasonable to expect an increasing incidence of virally linked malignancies (e.g., hepatomas and cervical cancer) as the incidence of AIDS and HIV infection continues to rise.

PRACTICE QUESTIONS

1. Diseases such as Kaposi's sarcoma that are common in AIDS are referred to as **opportunistic.** This is because they
    (A) affect any or all organs and tissues in the body.
    (B) normally occur in a benign state in most individuals.
    (C) occur in patients with preexisting immunodeficiency.
    (D) affect only HIV-infected individuals who have other diseases.

2. AIDS-related Kaposi's sarcoma (KS) is distinctly different from the other categories of KS in several ways. One of these differences is that it
    (A) often presents as a disseminated disease that involves multiple body organs.
    (B) occurs most often in the extremities, especially in the legs distal to the knee.
    (C) typically appears as an indolent, slow-growing cutaneous nodule or plaquelike lesion.
    (D) affects many more men than women.

3. Evidence that Kaposi's sarcoma may be linked to infection by cytomegalovirus (CMV), as well as by HIV, is that
    (A) CMV is found in a large percentage of homosexual men and AIDS patients.
    (B) the genetic makeup of CMV is almost identical to that of HIV.
    (C) CMV has been demonstrated to produce immunodeficiency in non-AIDS patients, including those receiving organ transplants.
    (D) CMV has been found only in the fluids and organs of AIDS patients.

4. Which of the following would **not** be a typical clinical manifestation of Kaposi's sarcoma?
    (A) a lesion that does not blanch when touched
    (B) a dark red lesion
    (C) a lesion that is painful when touched
    (D) a raised bullous nodule

5. Some KS patients have a shorter life expectancy than others. This poorer prognosis appears to be associated with several factors, including all of the following **except**
    (A) the presence of "B" symptoms such as fever and diarrhea.
    (B) a low absolute T4-lymphocyte count.
    (C) involvement of the disease with the head and neck.
    (D) the extent of organ involvement and tumor burden.

6. The main goal of treatment in AIDS-related Kaposi's sarcoma (KS) is
    (A) improving survival rate.
    (B) lessening morbidity.
    (C) raising levels of immune response.
    (D) reducing infection.

7. In caring for patients with AIDS-related Kaposi's sarcoma, nurses should be aware of both the special psychosocial (e.g., homosexuality, drug use) and physical aspects of the disease. For example, regarding physical aspects of the disease it is important to remember that
    (A) tumor lysis syndrome is a common side effect that requires immediate attention.
    (B) confusion, lethargy, and memory loss occur frequently in KS patients.
    (C) side effects of chemotherapy tend to be more severe in the AIDS population.
    (D) risk must be established before effective care can begin.

8. The occurrence of non-Hodgkin's lymphoma (NHL) in AIDS patients appears to be related to
    (A) the destruction of helper T-cells as a result of infection by cytomegalovirus (CMV).
    (B) decreased levels of serum protein/albumin as a result of internal coalesced lesions.
    (C) opportunistic infections of the CNS related to toxoplasmosis.
    (D) the proliferation of B-lymphocytes as a result of EBV and HIV infection.

9. In contrast to patients with non-AIDS NHL, those with HIV-related NHL are more likely to
    (A) have a history of lymphadenopathy that has been present for several months.
    (B) present with a painless, enlarged, discrete lymph node located in the neck.

    (C)   have no symptoms.
    (D)   have very advanced disease involving extranodal sites.

10.   Which of the following would typically **not** be part of the assessment of HIV-related non-Hodgkin's lymphoma (NHL)?
    (A)   CT and MRI examination of the head and neck
    (B)   a physical examination with special attention to Waldeyer's ring, the liver, and the spleen
    (C)   a bilateral bone marrow biopsy and aspiration
    (D)   laboratory tests that screen for hypercalcemia and other conditions not directly related to NHL

11.   Treatment of an advanced intermediate/high-grade NHL is **most** likely to involve
    (A)   invasive surgery.
    (B)   high doses of topical radiation.
    (C)   combination chemotherapy.
    (D)   cyclophosphamide combined with radiation.

12.   NHL patients with big, bulky, high-grade disease are at high risk for tumor lysis syndrome. One important aspect of the nursing care for such patients is
    (A)   looking for signs of motor incoordination and cognitive deficits.
    (B)   monitoring urine output for signs of renal failure.
    (C)   discontinuing vinca alkaloid treatment if signs of severe jaw pain occur.
    (D)   providing oral or intravenous agents that keep blood and urine acidic.

13.   The most frequently observed symptoms of HIV-associated CNS lymphomas include
    (A)   nerve inflammation and fever resulting from cryptococcosis or toxoplasmosis.
    (B)   increased metabolism and pulse due to decreased serum protein/albumin levels.
    (C)   "B" symptoms, including fever, chills, weight loss, and diarrhea.
    (D)   confusion, lethargy, memory loss, and alterations in personality or behavior.

14.   Although cancers other than KS, NHL, and primary CNS lymphomas may be seen in AIDS patients, no epidemiologic link or direct causal relationship has been established for these malignancies. Nevertheless, it is useful to know the HIV status of a patient with a malignancy because
    (A)   response to therapy is typically poor in HIV-infected patients.
    (B)   most malignancies are affected by the overall condition of the body's immune system.
    (C)   this knowledge may give clues to the etiology of the malignancy.
    (D)   HIV tends to convey some level of protection against the rapid spread of most other malignancies.

ANSWER EXPLANATIONS

1.   **The answer is (C).**   AIDS-related diseases such as Kaposi's sarcoma, non-Hodgkin's lymphoma (NHL), and primary CNS lymphoma are referred to as opportunistic because they occur in patients with preexisting immunodeficiency. This immunodeficiency can be the result of HIV infection (which destroys the immune system), therapeutic immunosuppression (e.g., chemotherapeutic agents used in organ transplantation), or primary immunodeficiency (e.g., as the result of a genetic defect). Normally these malignancies occur at a low incidence and in a more benign form. An AIDS-related opportunistic disease that is not a malignancy is *Pneumocystis carinii* pneumonia. (862)

2.   **The answer is (A).**   Choices (B) and (C) describe classic KS. Choice (D) is true of both classic and African KS as well as AIDS-related KS. Probably the most striking features of AIDS-related KS are that it is (1) highly aggressive and (2) invasive and disseminates to multiple body organs. (862–863)

3.   **The answer is (A).**   One study found the DNA of cytomegalovirus in the nucleus of cells of KS lesions, which suggests a viral cause of KS. Serologic testing demonstrates that as many as 94% of all homosexual men have been infected by CMV, as evidenced by antibodies to CMV. CMV has also been isolated from the body fluids and organs of patients with AIDS, which suggests the possible role of latent CMV infection in AIDS-related KS. CMV indeed may produce a similar effect in patients receiving immunosuppressing drugs, but it has not been demonstrated. CMV may be found in the fluids and organs of individuals who do not have AIDS. (863–864)

4. **The answer is (C).** The skin lesions of KS may appear as raised bullous nodules or as flat, plaquelike lesions. In either presentation they do not blanch when pressure is applied and are not painful unless they are responsible for structural damage or impinge on vital organs or nerves. Lesions are multicentric (each lesion is a primary lesion unto itself) and may be pigmented brown, brown-red, purple, violet, or rarely deep blue-purple. (864)

5. **The answer is (D).** With the exception of the lung, organ involvement does not seem to influence prognosis, nor does tumor burden correlate with prognosis. In addition to the above factors, a helper/suppressor T-cell ratio of less than 0.5 (<1:2) and prior or concomitant opportunistic infections are associated with poor prognosis. (865–866)

6. **The answer is (B).** In AIDS-related KS, treatment of the malignancy provides only temporary remission or stabilization of disease and does not improve survival rate. The main goal of treatment is to lessen the morbidity associated with the disease. This is accomplished by radiation therapy or chemotherapy, or both. (867)

7. **The answer is (C).** Because side effects of chemotherapy tend to be more severe in the AIDS population, the nurse should be aggressive in the assessment of potential complications, should alert the physician promptly when complications occur, should implement appropriate nursing interventions, and should remember that these patients have an underlying illness that predisposes them to other opportunistic infections and malignancies. (867)

8. **The answer is (D).** AIDS-associated NHLs are typically intermediate- to high-grade B-cell malignancies. They appear to be associated with a rise in polyclonal B-cell lymphoproliferation that results from EBV and HIV infection. AIDS-NHL has been associated with persistent generalized lymphadenopathy, suggesting polyclonal B-cell activation. One possibility is that once HIV infection occurs, EBV may trigger lymphocyte proliferation that remains unchecked as a result of HIV-induced immune dysfunction. This proliferation, in turn, may allow the expression of two oncogenes, resulting in a polyclonal or monoclonal NHL. (868–869)

9. **The answer is (D).** Choices (A)–(C) are more likely to refer to patients with non-AIDS NHL. In contrast, patients with HIV-related NHL have very advanced disease, which frequently involves extranodal sites, including the CNS, bone marrow, bowel, and anorectum. These extranodal sites may be the only site of the disease; that is, peripheral lymphadenopathy may be absent. Patients may also exhibit signs and symptoms of HIV infection, AIDS-related complex, or AIDS, which makes diagnosis difficult. (869)

10. **The answer is (A).** The patient's status must first be staged and graded before the diagnosis and classification of lymphoma can be made by examination of a biopsy specimen. Staging is accomplished by means of the Ann Arbor staging classification system and includes a careful history, which notes the presence or absence of "B" symptoms; a complete physical examination with special attention to Waldeyer's ring, the liver, and the spleen; laboratory tests that assess the overall wellness of the patient and screen for conditions not directly related to lymphoma; a chest film and CT scans of the chest, abdomen, and pelvis; and a bilateral bone marrow biopsy and aspiration and a lumbar puncture. If AIDS has not been previously diagnosed, then an HIV antibody test is indicated. (870)

11. **The answer is (C).** Whereas intermediate-grade tumors can be treated with either chemotherapy or radiation therapy, depending on the stage at presentation, advanced intermediate/high-grade lymphoma is treated with combination chemotherapy. Cyclophosphamide, the most active and effective agent, commonly is used in combination with other agents. Initial responses are usually dramatic but are not long-lived; relapse typically occurs in 4 to 6 weeks following discontinuation of chemotherapy. In addition, treatment-related neutropenia is severe and sometimes precipitates an opportunistic infection. Regardless of outcome, patients still have HIV infection and AIDS. (870)

12. **The answer is (B).** Tumor lysis syndrome generally occurs when the patient is initially treated. Tumor cells spill their contents into the general circulation, causing a metabolic disturbance. Renal failure and death may occur. The treatment of choice is prevention, including hydration, sodium bicarbonate, and intravenous or oral allopurinol to prevent hyperuricemia nephropathy. The patient's urine output is monitored hourly, and the physician is alerted to any sign of urinary insufficiency. Serum chemistry levels are monitored every 6 hours in high-risk patients. Dialysis is administered if electrolyte levels continue to rise and renal function deteriorates. All patients with HIV-related NHL should be observed for a full 72 hours

for any sign of tumor lysis syndrome. Signs and symptoms include a decreased urine output and increased lethargy.   (872)

13. **The answer is (D).**   The cell of origin for primary CNS lymphoma is the same as that causing NHL elsewhere in the body. The transformed cell, which multiplies in an area that does not allow expansion (i.e., the brain), is the cause of most presenting symptoms, including confusion, lethargy, memory loss, and alterations in personality or behavior. Seizures may also develop. Symptoms are very similar to those caused by other mass lesions in the CNS, for which toxoplasmosis is the usual explanation. (872–873)

14. **The answer is (A).**   There is a significantly greater incidence of indicator malignancies such as KS in individuals who are seropositive for HIV. The same is **not** true for the other malignancies described in AIDS patients, nor does HIV positivity prevent the development of any other cancer at the same rate seen in those who are seronegative. Choice (C) is a reasonable answer, though probably not as important as choice (A). (874)

37 Bone and Soft Tissue Sarcoma

STUDY OUTLINE

I.   **INTRODUCTION**

1.   The diagnosis and treatment of bone and soft tissue malignancies, which are rare, are complex and require a multidisciplinary approach.

II. **EPIDEMIOLOGY**

1.   **Primary malignant bone tumors** comprise only a small percent of all malignant tumors diagnosed in the United States.
2.   Incidence is slightly higher for men and white persons.

III. **ETIOLOGY**

1.   Little is known regarding the etiology of primary bone tumors, making prevention and detection difficult.
2.   There is evidence of a **familial tendency** in certain types of bone tumors (osteosarcoma, Ewing's sarcoma, chondrosarcoma), suggesting that **common susceptibility** may be the critical factor.
3.   Malignant bone neoplasms have been associated with a number of preexisting bone conditions, such as **Paget's disease** and **chronic osteomyelitis;** the mechanisms responsible for this relationship may be **prolonged growth or overstimulated metabolism.**
4.   Individual tumors have a predilection for certain locations. Soft tissue sarcomas arise in the **extremities** but can involve head and neck, and retroperitoneum areas.

IV. **PATHOPHYSIOLOGY**

1.   The three groups of primary bone tumors are classified according to **cells of origin.**
     a.   One group is produced by cells characterized by their **ability to produce collagen,** and includes **osteogenic, chondrogenic,** and **fibrogenic tumors.**
     b.   A second group originates in the **bone marrow reticulum,** and includes **Ewing's sarcoma** and **reticulum cell sarcoma.**
     c.   A third group arises in the **blood vessels of the bone,** and includes **angiosarcomas.**
2.   Primary bone tumors differ in cellular characteristics and progression of disease. Bone tumors tend to involve contiguous tissue and muscle and metastasize early to the lungs.

V.   **ASSESSMENT**

A.   **PATIENT HISTORY**

1.   The **evaluation of pain** assumes a major focus in the patient interview; knowledge of **location, onset,** and **duration** of pain assists in the differential diagnosis.
2.   Bone tumor pain often has a **gradual onset,** being present for months before the person seeks medical attention, and is **local,** although it may be **radiating** if the tumor involves nerves.
3.   The **character of the pain** helps to differentiate the site of origin and extent of tumor growth; bone pain is usually described as **dull, deep, and having a quality of boring into the bone.**

342

    4. The pain evaluation should also include a description of **frequency** and **course.**
       a. Pain resulting from a bone tumor is often **constant** and **worse at night.**
       b. The severity of the pain steadily increases as the tumor enlarges.
       c. The relationship of the pain to rest and activity must be determined.
    5. Attention is given to **symptoms of pulmonary metastasis,** including a history of hemoptysis, chest pain, cough, fever, and weight loss.
    6. To determine potential problems and needs, a **psychosocial assessment** is included in the initial interview.
    7. Soft tissue sarcomas present as **painless masses,** unless they are impinging upon other structures such as nerves, blood vessels, or viscera.
    8. Attention is given to symptoms of **pulmonary metastasis,** and note is made of hemoptysis, chest pain, cough, fever, chills, weight loss, malaise, exposure to toxic substances, radiation, or travel out of the country.

  B. **PHYSICAL EXAMINATION**

    1. The physical examination involves **inspection and palpation of the affected area.**
       a. A **firm, nontender enlargement** may be present, although malignant bone tumors are not always visible or palpable.
    2. Evaluation for **adenopathy** and **hepatomegaly** is performed.

  C. **DIAGNOSTIC STUDIES**

    1. **Radiographs,** even though they often do not yield a specific diagnosis, provide the opportunity to view the **location** and the **anatomy of the lesion,** as well as the status of surrounding tissue.
    2. Three basic **patterns of tumor destruction,** often correlated with the pathologic aggressiveness of the tumor, may be viewed radiographically.
       a. The **geographic pattern,** indicating a slow rate of growth, is characterized by a **large well-defined hole in which the edge of completely destroyed bone interfaces with the edge of bone that is completely intact.**
       b. The **moth-eaten pattern,** indicating a moderately aggressive tumor and implying severe cortical destruction, is characterized by **multiple holes that tend to coalesce.**
       c. The **permeative pattern,** suggestive of an aggressive tumor with a strong capacity for infiltration, demonstrates **multiple tiny holes in cortical bone which tend to diminish in size and number in the peripheral area of the lesion.**
       d. **Figure 37-2, text page 880,** illustrates these radiographic patterns of tumor destruction.
    3. Several other radiographic methods may be useful in evaluating primary bone tumors, including bone scans, arteriography, CT, fluoroscopy, and MRI.
    4. **Biopsy** is important both for diagnosis and to determine the best treatment for a particular lesion.
    5. **Incisional biopsy** is the most common type of biopsy for bone lesions, although **percutaneous needle biopsy** may be performed.

VI. **CLASSIFICATION AND STAGING**

    1. The **World Health Organization** scheme of classification (**Table 37-1, text page 882**) is based on the **type of differentiation shown by the tumor cells** and the **type of intracellular material they produce.**
       a. The main types of primary bone tumors in this classification scheme are **bone-forming, cartilage-forming,** and **marrow-forming.**
    2. The **surgical staging system for musculoskeletal sarcomas** (**Table 37-2, text page 882**) includes **surgical grade, surgical site, and presence of metastases.**

VII. **TREATMENT/NURSING CARE**

    1. The goals of treatment of primary malignant bone cancer include **eradication of the tumor, avoidance of amputation** when possible, and **preservation of maximum function.**
    2. Treatment, utilizing surgery, radiotherapy, and/or chemotherapy, is highly individualized, because an optimal treatment program has not been identified.

A. **SURGERY**

1. Surgical management of primary neoplasia of the bone is influenced by the **histopathologic features of the lesion,** the **anatomic site of the lesion,** and the **physical size of the lesion.**
2. In 1984, the same disease-free survival rate was reported for individuals who underwent limb-sparing surgery as for those who underwent amputation.
3. The traditional contraindications for limb salvage are an **inability to attain adequate surgical margins, tumor involvement of neurovascular bundle,** and **age group** (e.g., children younger than 10 years old due to resultant limb length discrepancy).
4. Limb salvage is indicated for **late metastasizing lesions** (periosteal osteosarcoma) and **locally aggressive chondrosarcomas** or **fibrosarcomas that have not invaded soft tissue.**
5. The **Van Nes rotationplasty** is a procedure utilized for distal femur lesions that would otherwise require an above-the-knee amputation.
6. **Radical resection with reconstruction**
   a. Postoperatively, the nurse conducts a **baseline assessment of neuromuscular function** distal to the surgical site, and observes for signs of **hemorrhage** because of the bone vascularity.
   b. Nursing care involves continuous attention to **position** and **alignment** of the involved extremity.
   c. **Independence and an adapted body image are the goals of rehabilitation.**
      (1) Physical therapy regimens are indicated to improve and develop muscle tone.
      (2) Gait retraining may be necessary.
      (3) The importance of safety within the home environment cannot be overemphasized.
   d. The three most common methods of **reconstruction** following sarcoma resections are
      (1) **Arthrodesis,** or fusion, which results in a stiff joint.
      (2) **Arthroplasty,** or construction of an artificial joint, which allows maintenance of joint function.
      (3) **Intercalary allograft reconstruction,** in which the allograft actually heals to the host bone, which provides joint mobility.
   e. The role of **surgery in the management of disseminated disease** has gained support.
      (1) Individuals in whom lung metastases develop are good candidates for resection, provided
         (a) The primary tumor is controlled.
         (b) There is no indication of other visceral metastases.
         (c) The lung nodules are resectable.
      (2) **Wedge excision** is the preferred procedure for lung nodules.
   f. **Anemia** from blood loss can result from extensive tumor resection and reconstruction, and some patients may elect to have their family and friends donate the 4–6 units of blood that may be necessary.
   g. **Hip flexion** is restricted for approximately 6 weeks after the surgery, in order to avoid a hip dislocation.
   h. **Wound necrosis** can occur if large flaps are used to close the wound.
   i. **Broad-spectrum antibiotics** are used for 48 hours or longer after surgery. Prophylactic oral antibiotics may be prescribed to help prevent infection postoperatively.
   j. **Postoperative care** includes assessment for signs and symptoms of pneumonia, pulmonary embolism, and deep vein thrombosis.
   k. Independence, observance of safety measures, and a gradual adaptation to changes in body image are **rehabilitation** goals.
7. **Allografts**
   a. Allograft bone used in **limb reconstruction** provides improved joint stability and function by suturing allograft soft tissue attachments to host tissue.
   b. Bone allograft recipients do not require immunosuppressive agents, and tissue typing is not performed.
   c. **Osteoconduction** describes the growth of capillaries and osteoprogenitor cells of the host into the allograft.
   d. Long-term **activity restrictions** for individuals undergoing allografts are the same as for those receiving metallic implants. They include limiting weight bearing and wearing a cast or brace for up to 6–12 months.
8. **Metastatic sarcoma**
   a. Patients with untreated pulmonary metastasis die within 18 months, but if they are good candidates for resection with good primary tumor control and no indication of other visceral metastatic disease, the pulmonary nodules are resected.

9. **Radical resection without reconstruction**
   a. Resections without reconstruction are performed in patients with soft tissue sarcomas and bone sarcomas in **expendable** bones such as a fibula, a clavicle, or sections of the pelvis.
10. **Amputation preparation**
    a. The **psychologic needs** of the individual who is undergoing amputation should be considered during the preoperative period, since this person may have fears regarding disability and deformity.
    b. The plan of care includes interventions aimed at **minimizing fear, decreasing anxiety, and promoting realistic optimism.**
    c. **The goal for the individual is independent function with the use of prostheses.**
    d. In evaluating **rehabilitation potential,** factors such as age, effects of adjuvant therapy, the existence of unrelated disease, and the person's attitude must be considered.
    e. Phantom limb phenomenon
       (1) Preoperative teaching should include a discussion of phantom limb sensation and phantom limb pain that otherwise can be frightening for the patient.
       (2) **All individuals who have an amputation can expect to feel some phantom limb sensation, whereas only 35% of those experience phantom limb pain.**
       (3) **Phantom limb sensation** is an awareness of the position or existence of the limb, as well as itching, tingling, or pressure.
       (4) **Phantom limb pain** may be cramping, throbbing, or burning pain and is a poorly understood phenomenon.
       (5) A variety of measures may be used to alleviate phantom limb pain, including application of **heat or pressure to the stump, distraction/diversion techniques,** and **tranquilizers or muscle relaxants.**
    f. **Amputation of the lower extremity**
       (1) General **strengthening measures** and **mobility training,** as well as training in transfers and ambulation with assistive devices, should be initiated preoperatively for all individuals undergoing amputation.
       (2) The goals of postoperative care are to
          (a) Maintain the individual's general health status.
          (b) Use modern prostheses.
          (c) Achieve the highest level of function possible.
          (d) Minimize the negative psychosocial consequences of amputation.
       (3) Postoperative care varies according to whether the individual has an **immediate prosthetic fitting** or a **conventional delayed prosthetic fitting.**
          (a) The relative advantages and disadvantages for immediate and delayed prosthesis fitting are summarized in **Table 37-4, text page 889.**
          (b) The stump is usually **elevated for 24 hours** after surgery to prevent edema and to promote venous return.
          (c) Hip contractures are prevented through **frequent position changes** and **exercises.**
          (d) Stump care involves **frequent wrapping with elastic bandages** or **stump shrinkers** to facilitate stump shrinking.
       (4) Most individuals with amputated limbs are capable of returning to work with restrictions.
       (5) Teaching the person how to care for the stump and the prosthesis is an essential element of the rehabilitation program.
       (6) In **designing the prosthesis,** consideration is given to the person's age, ability, endurance, financial status, occupation, and factors such as comfort, fit, safety, ease of application, and appearance.
       (7) After discharge, the individual should be seen by the prosthetist every 4 to 6 weeks for the first postoperative year.
       (8) The rehabilitation process is complete when the person has attained an **optimal level of independence** and has successfully **incorporated the prosthesis into his/her body image.**
    g. **Amputation of the upper extremity**
       (1) **Upper limb prostheses are far less satisfactory** in both appearance and function than those created for lower extremities; power and motion are supplied in only comparatively gross fashion.
       (2) The most functional terminal (hand) device is a **hook,** which may have negative social stigma attached to it.

(3) Adequate cosmetic appearance can be obtained at the expense of function.

(4) The reality is that the inadequacy of upper limb prostheses can be disappointing for the person with an upper limb amputation.

(5) **Rehabilitation goals emphasize use of the remaining arm for activities of daily living.**

(6) **Vocational rehabilitation** assumes particular importance for the individual with an upper extremity amputation.

B. **RADIOTHERAPY**

1. The use of radiotherapy in the management of primary or metastatic bone tumors depends on the **radiosensitivity** of the particular tumor type.

    a. **Most bone tumors are relatively unresponsive to radiation;** therefore, radiation is reserved for **palliation** or in conjunction with surgery or chemotherapy.

    b. Radiotherapy plays an integral role in the management of **Ewing's sarcoma,** a highly radiosensitive tumor.

2. Complications of treatment include **tendon contractures, edema of the extremity, cessation of growth,** and **nonhealing fractures.**

C. **CHEMOTHERAPY AND IMMUNOTHERAPY**

1. The addition of chemotherapy to the treatment of sarcomas has **increased survival rates from 20% to more than 50%.**

2. The rationale for **preoperative chemotherapy** is to

    a. **Treat micrometastasis.**

    b. **Decrease the size of the primary tumor,** thereby increasing the likelihood of limb-salvage surgery.

    c. **Assess the effectiveness of the chemotherapeutic agents** for 2 to 3 months.

3. The duration of chemotherapy treatment ranges from **6 to 12 months.**

VIII. **SARCOMAS**

A. **OSTEOSARCOMA**

1. **Epidemiology and etiology**

    a. **Osteosarcoma** is the most common osseous malignant bone tumor, accounting for **20%** of such lesions.

    b. The incidence is greatest in persons **between 10 and 25 years of age.** The increased incidence of osteosarcoma during adolescence has been correlated with **skeletal growth patterns.**

    c. **Males** are affected twice as often as females.

2. **Pathophysiology**

    a. The histologic pattern of osteosarcoma is so variable that no two specimens are exactly alike.

    b. Whatever the pattern, the essential criteria for the **diagnosis** of osteosarcoma includes the **presence of frankly sarcomatous stroma** and the **formation of tumor osteoid and bone by malignant connective tissue.**

    c. The most frequent sites of osteosarcoma include the **distal end of the femur,** the **proximal end of the tibia,** and the **proximal end of the humerus.**

    d. **Metastatic spread** occurs primarily to the lungs by the hematogenous route.

    e. Evidence of bone or pulmonary metastases usually appears **within 24 months** of definitive treatment.

3. **Assessment**

    a. The individual with osteosarcoma typically has **pain,** which is worse at night and becomes more severe as the tumor grows in size.

    b. **Weight loss** and **moderately severe anemia** may be seen in persons with rapidly growing tumors.

    c. The **duration of symptoms varies from weeks to six months** before medical attention is sought.

    d. Half of the individuals with osteosarcoma have an **elevated alkaline phosphatase level,** which declines with treatment.

4. **Treatment**
   a. **Chemotherapy protocols** have included doxorubicin, high-dose cyclophosphamide, high-dose methotrexate, or a combination of these and other drugs.
   b. When preoperative chemotherapy is used, effectiveness is assessed at the time of tumor resection; if there is **90% tumor necrosis,** the chemotherapy is continued postoperatively for 9 to 12 months.
      (1) The greater the necrosis, the greater the survival.
      (2) If tumor necrosis is less, the chemotherapy is changed to **cisplatin.**
   c. The improved results of chemotherapy have increased interest in **limb-salvage resections,** since the chemotherapy can result in decreased tumor size.
      (1) Resumption of chemotherapy after definitive surgery is delayed for 1 to 3 weeks.
   d. Development of **pulmonary metastases** requires surgical resection, often followed by chemotherapy.

B. **CHONDROSARCOMA**

1. **Epidemiology and etiology**
   a. **Chondrosarcoma** accounts for approximately **13%** of malignant bone tumors.
   b. The incidence is greatest **between 30 and 60 years** of age and among **males.**
2. **Pathophysiology**
   a. Chondrosarcoma arises from **cartilage,** and may be of either a **central** or **peripheral** type.
   b. Diagnosis is based on **cytologic changes of the cartilage cells.**
   c. The most frequent sites of chondrosarcomas include the **pelvic bones, long bones, scapula,** and **ribs.**
   d. Most chondrosarcomas do not tend to metastasize early, but remain **slow growing and locally invasive.**
   e. Regional lymph nodes may occasionally be involved.
3. **Assessment**
   a. Persons with chondrosarcoma often seek advice for **a slow-growing mass with intermittent dull, aching pain at the tumor site.**
   b. Physical examination reveals a **firm enlargement over the affected area.**
4. **Treatment**
   a. When the diagnosis of chondrosarcoma has been made, **surgery,** either **amputation** or **limb salvage,** is indicated.
   b. Chondrosarcoma remains **nearly totally refractory to chemotherapy,** since chondrosarcomas have such a poor blood supply that intravenous drugs do not reach the tumor in high enough concentrations to be effective.
   c. **Radiotherapy** is reserved for palliation.
   d. The overall **survival rate** of individuals treated with wide resection or amputation has been reported to be **67% at 5 years** and **50% at 10 years.**
   e. Survival correlates well with **histologic grade of the lesion.**

C. **FIBROSARCOMA**

1. **Epidemiology and etiology**
   a. **Fibrosarcoma** accounts for **fewer than 4%** of primary malignant bone tumors.
   b. Although rare in children, this tumor may occur at any age.
   c. Predisposing factors for fibrosarcoma may include **Paget's disease, therapeutic radiation, chronic osteomyelitis,** or **fibrous dysplasia.**
2. **Pathophysiology**
   a. Fibrosarcoma is a **malignant fibroblastic tumor** that usually **originates in the medullary cavity,** eventually penetrating the overlying cortex and extending into the periosteum and muscle.
   b. Fibrosarcomas range from well-differentiated to poorly differentiated tumors, with the latter being more aggressive.
   c. Some fibrosarcomas are surprisingly indolent in their growth patterns and **may change little over a period of years.**
   d. The **femur** and the **tibia** are the most common sites of occurrence and account for **50%** of all fibrosarcomas.

3. **Assessment**
   a. The person with a fibrosarcoma usually has **pain** and **swelling of the affected area.**
   b. The diagnosis is based on histologic study.
4. **Treatment**
   a. **Radical surgery is indicated for fibrosarcoma.**
   b. Fibrosarcoma is considered to be **radioresistant,** and radiotherapy is reserved for inoperable tumors.
   c. Adjuvant chemotherapy is being evaluated.
   d. The 5- and 10-year survival rates after surgery are 21.8% and 28%, respectively.
   e. **Individuals with poorly differentiated lesions have an extremely poor prognosis.**

D. **EWING'S SARCOMA**

1. **Epidemiology and etiology**
   a. **Ewing's sarcoma** accounts for 5% of all malignant bone tumors.
   b. Eighty percent of such tumors are in individuals **younger than 30 years.**
   c. Sixty-six percent **more males** are affected than females.
   d. No specific etiologic factor has been linked to Ewing's sarcoma.
2. **Pathophysiology**
   a. Ewing's sarcoma appears to be derived from the **mesenchymal connective tissue framework of bone marrow,** and usually arises in the **shaft of long bones.**
   b. No one site seems to predominate; the tumor is commonly situated in the **pelvis** and the **diaphyseal or metadiaphyseal regions of the long bones.**
   c. Ewing's sarcomas **metastasize early** and frequently involve the **lungs,** although the lymph nodes and skull are also frequent sites of metastasis.
   d. Metastasis may be present in nearly 20% of individuals at the time of diagnosis.
3. **Assessment**
   a. The individual with Ewing's sarcoma frequently has a **history of pain** that has become increasingly severe and persistent.
   b. Many individuals have **initial fever, anemia, high erythrocyte sedimentation rates,** and **leukocytosis.**
   c. The physical examination usually reveals a **tender and palpable mass.**
   d. **Radiographs** show **bone destruction that involves the shaft.**
4. **Treatment**
   a. **Integrated therapy with radiation and/or surgery in combination with chemotherapy is the treatment of choice for Ewing's sarcoma.**
   b. The tumor is **extremely radiosensitive** and is capable of being cured locally with 5000 cGy.
   c. Surgery combined with radiotherapy improves the local control rate.
   d. Surgery or radiation alone will not prevent the appearance of tumor foci elsewhere; therefore, **chemotherapy,** as prophylactic therapy for micrometastases, is used as part of the initial treatment for all patients.
      (1) Chemotherapy treatment duration is usually 6 to 12 months, with local treatment beginning approximately 3 months after chemotherapy starts.

E. **SOFT TISSUE SARCOMAS**

1. **Epidemiology and etiology**
   a. Histologic subtypes of soft tissue sarcomas include **malignant fibrous histiocytoma, liposarcoma, fibrosarcoma, synovial sarcoma, rhabdomyosarcoma,** and **leiomyosarcoma.**
   b. Half of the time, soft tissue sarcomas occur in the **extremities.** The remainder of the time they occur in the head and neck and the retroperitoneum.
2. **Pathophysiology**
   a. **Lymph node involvement** is a poor prognostic sign.
   b. A tumor **smaller than 5 cm** has a better prognosis.
   c. **High-grade** soft tissue sarcomas have a poor prognosis with detectable pulmonary metastasis being more common. Local recurrences and metastasis usually occur in the first 2 years.
   d. Depending upon the subtype, survival rates are 30%–95%.

3. **Treatment/nursing care**
   a. **Surgery** with complete tumor removal, and wide excision with no evidence of microscopic tumor cells at the site, is necessary.
   b. **Postoperative external beam radiation** allows for thorough histological grading and diagnosis without surgical delay, and wound healing is uncomplicated.
   c. **Preoperative radiation** has a smaller treatment area with fewer complications, and the patient may be a candidate for limb-salvage surgery if the tumor has regressed.
   d. **Chemotherapy** has shown improved local control but frequent distant metastases. Its role in the adjuvant setting is still being studied.

IX. **METASTATIC BONE TUMORS**

1. **Metastasis to bone** occurs by one of three mechanisms.
   a. **Direct extension of the tumor** to adjacent bone.
   b. **Arterial embolization** after passage through the right cardiopulmonary circulation.
   c. **Direct venous spread** through the pelvic and vertebral veins.
2. A number of primary tumors, including **lung, breast, prostate, kidney,** and **thyroid,** have a particular predilection for metastasizing to the bone.
3. The individual with a metastatic bone lesion typically has **dull, aching bone pain which increases as the day progresses and peaks in the night hours.**
4. Weight-bearing may become intolerable and **pathologic fractures** may occur if a sufficient amount of bone is involved.
5. Diagnostic evaluation includes **conventional radiography** and **bone scanning techniques.**
   a. **Biopsy** is indicated in the absence of a known or suspected primary.
6. Treatment may include **surgery, radiotherapy,** and **chemotherapy.**
   a. The goals of surgery include **augmenting the material strength of the bone, improving functional use,** and **resuming ambulatory status.**
   b. Radiotherapy may be used to **shrink the tumor,** to **facilitate surgical intervention,** or for **palliation of pain.**
   c. Chemotherapy is used to **reduce the tumor cell mass.**

PRACTICE QUESTIONS

1. Incidence of bone cancer is most common in people older than 65 years of age and also in those between the ages of
   (A) 5–10 years.
   (B) 15–19 years.
   (C) 25–35 years.
   (D) 40–45 years.

2. Malignant bone neoplasms are associated with the preexistence of other bone conditions. An example of one of these conditions is
   (A) fetal alcohol syndrome.
   (B) Paget's disease.
   (C) vitamin D deficiency.
   (D) Fanconi's anemia.

3. Bone tumors originate in the blood vessels of the bone, in the bone marrow, or in collagen-producing cells. An example of a bone tumor that originates in the bone marrow is
   (A) Ewing's sarcoma.
   (B) osteogenic sarcoma.
   (C) chondrosarcoma.
   (D) angiosarcoma.

4. One characteristic of the pain associated with the presence of a bone tumor is that it
   (A) has a sudden, unexplainable onset.
   (B) is exacerbated with activity.
   (C) is worse upon awakening.
   (D) has a gradual onset.

5. In the presence of a known bone tumor, symptoms such as hemoptysis, cough, fever, weight loss, and malaise may indicate
   (A) pulmonary metastases.
   (B) pernicious anemia.
   (C) radiotherapy toxicity.
   (D) infection.

6. The rationale for the use of preoperative chemotherapy in patients with osteogenic sarcoma includes all of the following aspects **except**
   (A) It treats micrometastases.
   (B) It decreases the size of the primary tumor, possibly facilitating limb-salvage surgery.
   (C) It enhances the effect of postoperative radiation.
   (D) It evaluates the effectiveness of the chemotherapy.

7. All of the following are goals in the treatment of primary malignant bone cancer **except**
   (A) preservation of maximum function.
   (B) early detection and intervention in children felt to be at high risk.
   (C) eradication of tumor.
   (D) avoidance of amputation.

8. All of the following are considered to be indications for limb-salvage surgery **except**
   (A) a locally aggressive chondrosarcoma.
   (B) the absence of soft tissue invasion.
   (C) a tumor that typically metastasizes late.
   (D) a child younger than 10 years of age.

9. Phantom limb pain occasionally occurs following amputation. When it does occur, the nurse should be aware that it
   (A) generally resolves in several months.
   (B) is likely to worsen with aging.
   (C) indicates a patient's inability to cope with loss.
   (D) usually occurs immediately following surgery.

10. Most bone tumors are relatively unresponsive to radiation therapy. An exception is
    (A) chondrosarcoma.
    (B) Ewing's sarcoma.
    (C) fibrosarcoma.
    (D) angiosarcoma.

11. The most common sites of occurrence for chondrosarcoma are the
    (A) femur, tibia, patella, and metatarsal.
    (B) vertebrae and scapula.
    (C) ribs, scapula, long bones, and pelvic bones.
    (D) mandible and maxilla.

12. The **most** effective modality currently being used to treat chondrosarcoma is
    (A) surgery.
    (B) chemotherapy.
    (C) radiotherapy.
    (D) hormone therapy.

13. The most common site of metastasis for tumors of the bone is the
    (A) lymph nodes.
    (B) central nervous system.
    (C) liver.
    (D) lungs.

14. Treatment of metastases to the bone may include surgery, chemotherapy, and/or radiotherapy. When radiation therapy is used, the primary goal often is to
    (A) eliminate the need for surgical intervention.

(B)   palliate pain.
(C)   decrease the likelihood of further metastases.
(D)   treat the primary cancer.

ANSWER EXPLANATIONS

1.   **The answer is (B).**   The bimodal pattern of occurrence in bone cancer reveals peak incidence at the ages of 15–19 years and again after age 65. Incidence is also slightly higher for men and for white persons. (878)

2.   **The answer is (B).**   Paget's disease primarily predisposes individuals to osteosarcoma, but occasionally to fibrosarcoma, chondrosarcoma, and giant cell tumor as well. Incidence of sarcomas in patients with symptoms of Paget's disease is 0.8%. Other conditions associated with increased incidence of bone tumors include hyperparathyroidism, chronic osteomyelitis, old bone infarct, and fracture callus. (878)

3.   **The answer is (A).**   Ewing's sarcoma is an example of a bone tumor which originates in the bone marrow reticulum. Other examples in this category are reticulosarcoma and lymphosarcoma. (878, 881)

4.   **The answer is (D).**   The most common presenting symptom in bone cancer is pain (sometimes described as "dull" or "aching") which has had a gradual onset and may have been present for several months before evaluation is sought. Abrupt onset of pain is **possible,** although not common, and would most likely indicate a pathologic fracture. (878)

5.   **The answer is (A).**   Metastatic spread in bone cancer occurs primarily to the lungs by the hematogenous route. Symptoms of pulmonary metastases include weight loss, malaise, hemoptysis, cough, chest pain and fever. (880)

6.   **The answer is (C).**   Currently chemotherapy is given preoperatively. The rationale for preoperative chemotherapy is to treat micrometastasis, decrease the size of the primary tumor, thereby increasing the likelihood of limb-salvage surgery, and assess the effectiveness of the chemotherapeutic agents for 2 to 3 months. The route of the chemotherapy is either intravenous or intra-arterial. (893–894)

7.   **The answer is (B).**   Avoidance of amputation, preservation of maximum function, and eradication of tumor are all goals in the treatment of primary malignant bone cancer. Although there is evidence of a familial tendency in some of the bone cancers, early intervention in these cases is not common practice. (878, 881–882)

8.   **The answer is (D).**   Three scenarios in which limb salvage is not a treatment option are (1) if the surgeon is unable to attain adequate surgical margin, (2) if the neurovascular bundle is involved, and (3) if the patient is younger than 10 years old. In the latter case limb salvage is contraindicated because of the resultant limb length discrepancy, although recent advances in expandable prostheses are making it possible for more children afflicted with bone cancer to retain their limbs during surgery. (881–882)

9.   **The answer is (A).**   Although phantom limb **sensations** (i.e., itching, pressure, tingling) are often experienced shortly after surgery, phantom limb **pain** (i.e., cramping, throbbing, burning) usually does not occur until one to four weeks after surgery. For most individuals, phantom limb pain resolves in a few months; 5–10% of those who have limbs amputated have a worsening of pain over the years. This worsening may be a sign of a neuroma or of locally recurrent cancer in the stump. (888)

10.   **The answer is (B).**   Radiotherapy is mainly used palliatively and in conjunction with chemotherapy for inoperable tumors in the treatment of bone cancer. It plays an integral role, however, in the management of Ewing's sarcoma, which is one of the only bone tumors that is radiosensitive. (893)

11.   **The answer is (C).**   Chondrosarcoma is a tumor arising from either the interior medullary cavity of the cartilage (central chondrosarcoma) or from the bone through malignant changes in benign cartilage tumors (peripheral chondrosarcoma). The most frequent sites for this cancer are the pelvic bones, long bones, scapula, and ribs. Less common sites include the bones of the hands and feet. (895)

12.   **The answer is (A).**   Chondrosarcoma is primarily treated surgically. This form of bone cancer is almost totally refractory to chemotherapy because of its poor blood supply. Likewise, radiation therapy has limited effectiveness and is usually reserved for palliation. In terms of surgery, limb-salvage surgery as well as amputation are both options. (895)

13.   **The answer is (D).**   Although some bone tumors metastasize to the lymph nodes (e.g., Ewing's sarcoma), few, if any, seem to metastasize to the CNS or liver. Most of the more common bone tumors metastasize to the lungs. Whether or not these metastases develop, and when, depends on the stage and aggressiveness of the disease process. (893, 895–896)

14.   **The answer is (B).**   In the treatment of bone metastases, radiotherapy may be used **preoperatively** to shrink the tumor in order to better facilitate surgical intervention, or **postoperatively** as adjuvant therapy. Radiotherapy may also be used alone to treat bone metastases in cases where surgical intervention clearly would not provide any benefits. (899–900)

38 Breast Cancer

STUDY OUTLINE

I. INTRODUCTION

1. Breast cancer is the most common cancer in women and the leading cause of death for women age **40–44 years old, and over 70% of all breast cancer occurs in women who are 50 years or older.**
2. Breast cancer incidence **increases rapidly with age** until menopause, and then increases more slowly.
3. Breast cancer **occurs** in approximately 1 in every 9 women.
4. Despite the increased incidence over the past 30 years, the **mortality rate** has remained stable.

II. ETIOLOGY

A. RISK ASSESSMENT

1. See **Table 38-1, text page 905,** for risk factors and their importance in the development of breast cancer.

B. HORMONAL FACTORS

1. The link of breast cancer development and **endogenous hormones** is demonstrated by the facts that women are 100 times more likely to develop breast cancer than men; early menarche, late menopause, and nulliparity or parity after 35 are considered risk factors, and the relationship of the tumor estrogen receptor with the response to hormonal manipulation.
2. The role that endogenous estrogens may play in the development of breast cancer suggest that **exogenous therapy** may be instrumental in breast cancer development.
3. The connection between breast cancer development and oral contraceptives is not established since the studies are contradictory.
4. Current studies suggest either no effect on breast cancer risk from **estrogen replacement therapy (ERT)** or an elevation in risk of less than twofold.

C. FAMILY HISTORY

1. In **combination with age and gender,** family history of breast cancer is a primary indicator of the potential risk of developing the disease.
2. The majority of breast cancer cases are **sporadic,** where the patient has no history of breast cancer through two generations.
3. **Familial or polygenic** breast cancer is defined as a positive family history, often with related cancers, consistent with an autosomal dominant factor that includes onset at an early age, an excess of bilaterality, and other multiple cancers.

D. DIET

1. The **risk** of breast cancer is the greatest in developed countries, especially in North America, and is lowest in third-world countries. It is thought to be linked to diet.
2. **High-fat diets** have been implicated in countries showing sudden increases in breast cancer incidence.

3. The assumption of a relationship between dietary fats and breast cancer is based on animal studies. **Breast tissue proliferation** may be altered by changes in estrogen and in pituitary and thyroid function, which are sensitive to dietary changes.

E. **OBESITY**

1. A slightly **increased risk** is associated with obesity but is more significant for women who are **postmenopausal** than other groups.

F. **ALCOHOL**

1. There is a possible association between alcohol and breast cancer risk.

G. **RADIATION**

1. There is a **risk** associated with radiation therapy for a broad spectrum of health problems such as chronic mastitis, tuberculosis, tinea capitis, thymus disorders, and cancers at any age.

H. **PROLIFERATIVE DISEASE**

1. The presence of proliferative breast disease as documented by **histology** may demonstrate an increased risk of subsequent carcinoma.
    a. A **slight** risk is 1½ to 2 times the normal risk.
    b. A **moderate** risk is 4 to 5 times the normal risk.
    c. A **marked** risk is 8 to 10 times the normal risk.
2. **Carcinoma in situ** refers to a localized process that is confined to a duct or lobule and is incapable of spreading.

I. **NONPROLIFERATIVE DISEASE**

1. Approximately 70% of biopsies reflect **cellular changes** that impart no risk or a very small risk to the patient.

III. **PREVENTION OF BREAST CANCER**

A. **CHEMOPREVENTION**

1. The most promising such attempt to prevent breast cancer is a study using **tamoxifen** in high-risk women.
2. See **text page 910,** column 1, for a review of Tamoxifen.

B. **EXERCISE**

1. Exercise may reduce the breast cancer risk by **reducing** the amount of body fat and hence the amount of free estrogen stored in the fat.

C. **PROPHYLACTIC MASTECTOMY**

1. Removal of the majority of breast tissue for a prophylactic mastectomy has been indicated under some conditions. See **text page 910,** column 2, for the conditions.

IV. **SCREENING AND DETECTION**

1. Early detection reduces the mortality rate of breast cancer and provides a **90% survival** rate for 5 years.

A. **BSE**

1. Trained professionals should teach BSE to women beginning at the age of 20, since 90% of breast lumps are found by women or their partner.
2. See **Figure 38-1, text page 912,** for BSE instructions.

B. **MAMMOGRAPHY**

1. Annual mammograms are recommended for asymptomatic women at 40 years of age. They are generally not recommended for women under 35 years old since younger breasts are difficult to image due to their density.
2. It is an NCI goal to have 80% of women by the year 2000 use mammograms. The present **utilization rate** is approximately **15%–20%.**
3. The risk of harmful radiation from mammography is **minimal,** and the **cost** may vary from $50 to $200.

V. **DIAGNOSTIC EVALUATION**

1. See **Figures 38-2 and 38-3, text pages 914 and 915,** for the steps involved in the diagnostic evaluation of a nonpalpable and a palpable breast mass, respectively.

A. **CHARACTERISTICS OF BENIGN VERSUS MALIGNANT BREAST DISEASE**

1. Eight out of ten lumps biopsied are benign. A **benign** lesion is usually a mobile encapsulated mass with a distinct barrier, soft and smooth with regular borders, associated with bilateral diffuse pain and tenderness that is more prominent during the menstrual period, and clear on transillumination.
2. Clinical signs of **malignant disease** include nipple retraction or elevation, skin dimpling or retraction, inflammation, skin edema, and peau d'orange.

B. **MAMMOGRAMS**

1. **Screening mammograms**
   a. **Routine screening mammograms** provide a highly sensitive study at the lowest cost since the goal of screening is to detect a malignancy before it becomes clinically apparent.
   b. A screening mammogram allows the radiologist to detect characteristic benign and malignant masses.
2. **Diagnostic mammograms**
   a. When specific symptoms or suspicious clinical findings exist, or an abnormality on a screening mammogram is found, a **diagnostic mammogram** with additional views of the affected breast is done.

C. **SONOGRAM**

1. Determination of a lesion to be **solid or cystic** is done by sonogram or ultrasound.

D. **MRI**

1. An MRI evaluates the rate at which the contrast initially enters the breast tissue and may allow for earlier detection based on the ability to determine smaller lesions.

E. **FINE-NEEDLE ASPIRATION**

1. FNA utilizes a needle aspiration to determine if a lump in question is a cyst, in which case the lump will resolve after aspiration.

F. **STEREOTACTIC NEEDLE-GUIDED BIOPSY**

1. This permits diagnosis of benign disease without the trauma or scarring of an open biopsy by immobilizing the breast from fixed horizontal and vertical coordinates to calculate the exact position of the lesion within a three-dimensional field.

G. **WIRE LOCALIZATION BIOPSY**

1. The goal of this biopsy is to assist the surgeon in locating the nonpalpable lesion for the purpose of excisional biopsy.

H. **OPEN BIOPSY**

1. An excisional biopsy may be recommended for the following reasons:
    a. **The sonogram shows the lesion to be solid.**
    b. **The cytology or histology results are insufficient.**
    c. **The clinical or mammographic findings are suspicious.**
    d. **The patient requests a biopsy to allay her anxiety.**
2. An excisional biopsy involves removal of the lump along with a small amount of surrounding tissue using curvilinear incision over the lesion.

VI. **MULTIDISCIPLINARY BREAST CENTERS**

1. See **text page 921,** column 2, for the purpose and goals of a multidisciplinary breast center.
2. The coordinator of the breast center is often an oncology **clinical nurse specialist** who arranges a woman's visit and evaluation, facilitates decision making and informed consent, provides education, and may follow the patient postoperatively.

VII. **PATHOPHYSIOLOGY–CELLULAR CHARACTERISTICS**

1. **Adenocarcinomas** comprise the majority of primary breast cancers, located in the upper outer quadrant of the breast.
2. See **Table 38-3, text page 922,** for common types of breast tumors.
    a. **Infiltrating ductal carcinoma** has an overall survival rate of 50%–60%.
    b. **Invasive lobular carcinoma,** which constitutes 5%–10% of all breast cancers, has a 50%–60% 10-year survival rate.
    c. **Tubular carcinoma** is uncommon and represents a well-differentiated adenocarcinoma of the breast.
    d. **Medullary carcinomas** account for 5%–7% of all breast cancers and occur commonly in women under 50 years of age.
    e. **Mucinous or colloid carcinoma** is uncommon, occurring in women 60–70 years of age, with metastasis to axillary nodes in one-third of cases.
    f. **Other** breast cancers include sarcomas, papillary carcinoma, apocrine, invasive cribriform, and Paget's disease.

VIII. **PROGNOSTIC INDICATORS**

1. Identification of prognostic indicators helps identify subsets of women who might benefit from more aggressive therapies and assists in establishing prognosis.

A. **AXILLARY LYMPH NODE STATUS**

1. A key feature in determining prognosis is the presence or absence of **positive axillary nodes** upon pathological staging.
2. See **Figure 38-14, text page 924,** for a diagram of the lymphatics.
3. The metastases need to be identified as **microscopic or macroscopic, and the number of nodes involved, the levels of involvement, and whether the lymph node capsule has been invaded must be determined.**

B. **TUMOR SIZE**

1. Tumors measuring 1–3 cm tend to lead to a 5-year survival rate of 91%, while tumors measuring more than 3 cm have an 85% 5-year survival rate.

C. **CELL PROLIFERATIVE INDICES AND DNA PLOIDY**

1. Tumors with positive estrogen receptor protein tend to demonstrate a low proliferative activity, (low S-phase fraction), whereas tumors that are estrogen receptor negative reflect a more aggressive metastatic potential (high S-phase fraction).
2. Patients whose tumors have an abnormal amount of DNA (aneuploidy) have a worse prognosis compared to those with normal DNA content (diploid).

D. **HISTOLOGICAL GRADE**

    1. According to the degree of anaplasia, tumors are classified as **well differentiated, poorly differentiated,** or **moderately differentiated.**

E. **EPIDERMAL GROWTH FACTOR RECEPTOR**

    1. The fact that some breast cells develop estrogen independence accounts for variance in clinical behavior and treatment response in **estrogen dependent** and **estrogen independent** breast cancer.
    2. Breast cancer tissue that stained positive for epidermal growth factor tends to be estrogen receptor negative, suggesting that **estrogen may exert inhibitory action on epidermal growth factor receptor (EGFR).**
    3. EGFR may actually increase proliferation of breast cancer cells.

F. **c-erb B-2 ONCOGENE**

    1. An overexposure of the c-erb B-2 oncogene has been **found in 10%–35% of breast cancers.**
    2. The presence of this oncogene is correlated with a poor prognosis in node-positive women.

G. **CATHEPSIN D**

    1. Cathepsin D is a lysosomal enzyme that may be overexpressed and secreted in certain breast cancers, correlating with tissue invasion and metastasis.

IX. **CLASSIFICATION AND STAGING**

    1. See **Table 38-6, text pages 928–929,** for the pathologic staging recommended by the American Joint Committee on Cancer, which is used along with work-up and diagnostic tests for planning the treatment regimen.

X. **TREATMENT ALTERNATIVES**

A. **LOCAL-REGIONAL MANAGEMENT**

    1. **Invasive breast cancer** is a systemic disease, and patients who die have distant occult metastases at the time of local therapy or metastases from inadequately treated local or regional disease.
    2. Women with **stage I or II disease** are commonly treated by breast conservation procedures plus breast radiation.
    3. **Axillary node dissection** is performed to determine the presence of involved nodes.
    4. **Modified radical mastectomy** is indicated for larger, multicentric disease and involves removal of all breast tissue and nipple areola complex, along with level I and II axillary node dissection.
    5. **Carcinoma in situ** does not present in any discernible manner but is usually discovered by the pathologist during removal of a benign condition. It is treated by frequent physical examination, ipsilateral mastectomy with contralateral biopsy, or bilateral mastectomy with reconstruction.
    6. **Intraductal carcinoma** can be treated with total mastectomy with low axillary dissection, wide excision followed by radiation, or wide excision alone.
    7. The cosmetic result following **partial mastectomy and radiation therapy** is considered good, with survival rates equivalent to those of total mastectomy. The major criteria for choosing partial mastectomy over total mastectomy are feasibility of resecting the primary tumor without causing major cosmetic deformity and the likelihood of tumor recurrence in the breast.

B. **ADJUVANT SYSTEMIC THERAPY**

    1. **Early stage I and II breast cancer**
      a. See **Table 38-7, text page 931,** for factors influencing the design of adjuvant chemotherapy trials in curable breast cancer.

     b.   The majority of patients with node-negative breast cancer are cured following breast conserving treatment or total mastectomy and axillary node dissection. The rate of local and distant **relapse** following local therapy for node-negative breast cancer is decreased both by combination cytotoxic chemotherapy and by tamoxifen.

     c.   In stage I node-negative breast cancer, **combination chemotherapy** can reduce the odds of recurrence to almost 20%, but in order to achieve this, the majority of women will undergo unnecessary therapy because they will have been cured by surgery alone.

     d.   See **Table 38-9, text page 932,** for studies of adjuvant systemic therapy in node-negative disease.

     e.   In stage II node-positive breast cancer, women with **lymph node involvement** are identified as being likelier to have distant metastasis and recurrence.

     f.   In a study involving 1200 postmenopausal women, **tamoxifen plus chemotherapy** proved more effective than tamoxifen alone.

     g.   Efforts to **improve outcome in node-positive patients** have focused on giving available drugs more effectively with dose intensification, giving optimal doses at regular intervals, and avoiding dose reductions or treatment delays.

  2. **Locally advanced breast cancer (stage III)**

     a.   The larger the **tumor size and the greater the number of positive nodes,** the greater the risk of metastasis and death.

     b.   **High-dose chemotherapy with autologous bone marrow rescue** is currently being studied for women with high-risk advanced disease.

C. **NURSING CONSIDERATIONS IN THE CARE OF THE WOMAN WITH LOCALIZED BREAST CANCER**

  1. Since most women actively participate in the decision-making process, the nurse in the role of **supportive advocate** needs to be knowledgeable concerning the options for therapy, the goals of therapy, measures to minimize complications of treatment, and the various resources that may need to be mobilized.

  2. **Surgical considerations**

     a.   The cosmetic result of breast-preserving surgery utilized in the surgical management of stage I and II breast cancer requires **education before surgery** with information that the breast will appear different from the other breast; scar tissue may form, causing contractures over time; and complications of arm edema, seroma formation and wound infection, shoulder dysfunction, upper extremity weakness, fatigue, and limitations in mobility may occur.

     b.   Care of the **postmastectomy patient** involves maintaining drain patency, providing exercises, and being sure the patient has clear instructions regarding wound care upon discharge.

  3. **Chemotherapy**

     a.   There is high probability that premenopausal women receiving chemotherapy will experience **ovarian failure and early menopause,** and all women receiving chemotherapy will be at risk for experiencing decreased frequency and quality of sexual relations.

     b.   Weight gain is a troublesome side effect of therapy. **Increased caloric intake** is due to prednisone, oral cyclophosphamide, taste changes, increased appetite, depression, psychological distress, and mild nausea that is relieved by eating.

     c.   **Fatigue** (characterized by total body tiredness, forgetfulness, and wanting to rest) increases through the course of treatment and is a common, troublesome symptom.

     d.   **Nausea and vomiting** occur in response to the chemotherapy drugs used in the treatment regimen.

  4. **Radiation**

     a.   Radiation usually begins 3–4 weeks after surgery and is associated with fatigue, nausea, and skin changes. **Breast swelling** is associated with more extensive axillary node dissection.

XI. **BREAST RECONSTRUCTION**

  1. **Breast reconstruction** with silicone implants, and autologous transplants with procedures such as latissimus dorsi flap, TRAM flap, and free transfer of abdominal or gluteal tissue, are used for women who choose not to have a breast-preserving procedure or who for other reasons cannot preserve the breast.

A.   **SILICONE IMPLANTS**

    1.   **Silicone implants** are used for reconstruction when there is adequate skin postmastectomy.

B.   **SALINE TISSUE EXPANDERS**

    1.   **Saline expanders, the most common reconstructive procedure,** are placed behind the chest wall, often along the mastectomy incision, and are used when there is inadequate skin supply.

C.   **LATISSIMUS DORSI FLAP**

    1.   An **ellipse of skin along the latissimus dorsi muscle** is rotated onto the mastectomy site when inadequate skin is available or when tissue is needed to fill the supraclavicular hollow.

D.   **TRAM FLAP**

    1.   The **transverse rectus abdominous muscle flap** involves a low transverse ellipse incision, and abdominal muscle and fat are tunneled under abdominal skin to the mastectomy site. See **Figures 38-18 and 38-19, text pages 943 and 944.**

E.   **FREE FLAP**

    1.   A portion of **skin and fat from the buttocks or lower abdomen is removed and grafted to the mastectomy site along with microvascular anastomoses.** The success of this procedure is dependent upon the viability of the flap and on maintenance of the blood supply.

F.   **NIPPLE-AREOLAR CONSTRUCTION**

    1.   The nipple-areolar complex is the final phase of reconstruction. See **Figure 38-20, text page 945.**

XII.   **METASTATIC BREAST CANCER**

    1.   Thirty to forty percent of women diagnosed with potentially curable disease will have metastatic disease and eventually die, and approximately **10%** of women will be diagnosed with metastatic disease at presentation.
    2.   The lymphatics is the most common mode of metastasis. Breast cancer most commonly metastasizes to bone **(the spine, ribs, and long bones) liver, lung, and brain.**
    3.   Management is aimed at judicious use of radiation and systemic therapy (chemotherapy and hormone therapy) to **palliate symptoms and improve quality of life.**

A.   **DEFINING EXTENT OF DISEASE**

    1.   Chest films, liver scan, bone scan, MRI, and cytologic analysis of the cerebral spinal fluid are performed based on a woman's symptoms in order to **assess the extent of disease.**

B.   **CHEMOTHERAPY**

    1.   See **Table 38-14, text page 946,** for commonly used regimens in women who have a disease-free interval of less than 2 years, have hormone receptor negative disease, are refractory to hormone therapy, or have aggressive disease in the liver or pulmonary system.
    2.   **Combination agents** result in higher response rates than single agents, and individuals with slow growing disease and those with rapidly progressive disease will benefit the most.

C.   **ENDOCRINE THERAPY**

    1.   **Estrogens**
        a.   Women who have estrogen receptor-positive breast cancer demonstrate a consistently superior survival after recurrence, compared to women who are estrogen receptor negative.
        b.   **Receptor-negative breast cancer** is usually associated with a short disease-free interval and more aggressive disease.

2. **Androgens**
   a. A **response rate of 20%** is seen in women who are 5 years or more after menopause and utilize androgens, which exert their therapeutic effect by opposing endogenous estrogens.
3. **Progestins**
   a. Megestrol acetate has a response rate of 26%–36%, the major side effect being weight gain.
4. **Corticosteroids**
   a. Corticosteroids can result in responses of 30%, and the response generally lasts only 3 months.
5. **Antiestrogens**
   a. **Tamoxifen** is indicated for both primary and metastatic breast cancer. Tamoxifen blocks the effect of estrogen on target tissues.
6. **Oophorectomy**
   a. Oophorectomy is effective in removing **endogenous sources of estrogens** in premenopausal and some perimenopausal women but is not indicated in women with estrogen receptor-negative tumors.
7. **Secondary ablative procedures**
   a. **Medical adrenalectomy** is equivalent to surgical ablation without the risks of surgery and permanent adrenal suppression.
   b. See **Figure 38-21, text page 948,** for treatment options for women with metastatic breast cancer.
8. **Research in hormone therapy for metastatic breast cancer**
   a. Some **new antiestrogens** showing promise in breast cancer include Mifepristone, which is being used for women who have not benefited from conventional hormone manipulation; Fenretinide, which has chemopreventive and therapeutic benefit in animals; and Fadrozole, which has a good therapeutic effect as a second-line treatment in postmenopausal women with metastatic breast cancer.

XIII. **MALE BREAST CANCER**

1. Male breast cancer accounts for **less than 1%** of all breast cancers. The incidence increases in men who have undergone sex-change operations.
2. Due to small numbers, it is difficult to conduct clinical trials to determine appropriate therapies, but treatment is based primarily on the treatment of female breast cancer.

XIV. **COMPLICATIONS OF METASTATIC DISEASE**

A. **BONE METASTASIS**

1. Bone scans are indicated when patients report pain over the rib cage, pain when rising from a sitting position, and any pain that worsens with time.
2. Destructive lesions involving the femur or humerus are at risk for fracture and may require irradiation for pain relief and recalcification of bone.

B. **SPINAL CORD COMPRESSION**

1. Cord compression may result from epidural tumor or altered bone alignment due to pathologic fractures with initially subtle signs and symptoms.
2. **Pain** occurs weeks before **neurologic symptoms,** and imminent compression should be suspected in people who have known bone metastases, progressive back pain associated with weakness, paresthesia, bowel or bladder dysfunction, or gait disturbances.
3. **Radiotherapy combined with corticosteroids** is a common treatment modality, but decompression laminectomy may be indicated for individuals who develop compression.

C. **BRAIN METASTASIS AND LEPTOMENINGEAL CARCINOMATOSIS**

1. Brain metastasis occurs in 30% of people with breast cancer and is often associated with devastating physical and emotional problems, the most frequent signs and symptoms being **headaches, seizures, visual defects, motor weakness, and mental changes.**
2. Since most chemotherapeutic agents do not cross the blood-brain barrier, treatment generally involves **total brain irradiation.**

D. **CHRONIC LYMPHEDEMA**

1. Lymphedema occurs in women with breast cancer approximately 8% of the time and is most common in women with axillary node dissection followed by radiation.
2. Common **causes** include infection, tumor recurrence, and tumor enlargement.

XV. **PREGNANCY AND BREAST CANCER AS A SIMULTANEOUS EVENT**

1. The **incidence** of concurrent pregnancy or lactation and breast cancer is 0.2%–3.8%.
2. Treatment in this particular population is determined by the extent of the disease and the term of pregnancy and lactation. Previous poor survival rates may have been due to delayed diagnosis and/or treatment.
3. Radiation is not recommended, and chemotherapy, if indicated, should not be administered during the first trimester.
4. A more advanced disease stage may call for urgent palliation and possibly a therapeutic abortion.

PRACTICE QUESTIONS

1. One of the conditions that may increase a woman's risk for the development of breast cancer is
    (A) exposure to DES.
    (B) pregnancy before the age of 20.
    (C) menarche before the age of 12.
    (D) early menopause.

2. Women with a history of breast cancer are considered at increased risk for the development of
    (A) ovarian cancer.
    (B) Hodgkin's disease.
    (C) strokes.
    (D) superior vena cava syndrome.

3. One drug that may eventually be used prophylactically by women considered at high risk for breast cancer is
    (A) ifosfamide.
    (B) megace.
    (C) estrogen.
    (D) tamoxifen.

4. The majority of breast cancers are detected
    (A) on self-examination.
    (B) during pregnancy.
    (C) during yearly physical exam by a physician.
    (D) using mammography.

5. The current recommendation of the American Cancer Society and the National Cancer Institute is that all women begin screening mammography at age
    (A) 25.
    (B) 30.
    (C) 35.
    (D) 40.

6. The majority of primary breast cancers are
    (A) inflammatory carcinomas.
    (B) adenocarcinomas.
    (C) cystosarcoma phyllodes.
    (D) rhabdomyosarcomas.

7. A peau d'orange (skin of the orange) appearance of the breast is characteristic of
    (A) medullary carcinoma.
    (B) infiltrating lobular carcinoma.
    (C) inflammatory carcinoma.
    (D) cystosarcoma phyllodes.

8. The three most common sites of metastasis from breast cancer are the
    (A) liver, bone, and lungs.
    (B) adrenal glands, liver, and bone.
    (C) brain, bone, and diaphragm.
    (D) lungs, brain, and bone marrow.

9. Benign breast tumors are more likely to be _____ than malignant breast tumors.
    (A) painful
    (B) unilateral
    (C) immobile
    (D) opaque on transillumination

10. The procedure or test that is used to make a positive diagnosis of breast cancer is the
    (A) mammogram.
    (B) biopsy.
    (C) CT scan.
    (D) modified mastectomy.

11. The single **most** important prognosticator of survival and recurrence of breast cancer is
    (A) the woman's age at diagnosis.
    (B) how quickly treatment is initiated once diagnosis is made.
    (C) the number of axillary nodes involved.
    (D) how sensitive the tumor is to conventional chemotherapy.

12. The treatment of choice for women with stage II or stage III breast cancer is
    (A) modified radical mastectomy.
    (B) lumpectomy followed by radiotherapy.
    (C) chemotherapy.
    (D) hormone therapy.

13. Receptor-negative breast cancer is usually associated with
    (A) a good long-term prognosis.
    (B) tumor resistance to chemotherapy.
    (C) an aggressive disease process.
    (D) positive axillary lymph nodes at diagnosis.

14. Male breast cancers are **most** likely to
    (A) be estrogen receptor negative.
    (B) occur in men who have undergone sex-change procedures.
    (C) occur in young men, aged 18–25.
    (D) be treated primarily with radiation therapy.

15. An individual with breast cancer who complains of back pain associated with weakness, parasthesias, and/or bowel or bladder dysfunction may be exhibiting symptoms of
    (A) spinal cord compression.
    (B) chemotherapy toxicity.
    (C) disease progression.
    (D) bone metastases.

16. Treatment for the chronic lymphedema associated with axillary node dissection for breast cancer includes
    (A) keeping the affected arm below the level of the heart.
    (B) a high-protein diet.
    (C) radiation therapy.
    (D) intermittent compression with a pump.

ANSWER EXPLANATIONS

1. **The answer is (C).** Women who have an adverse hormonal milieu (e.g., 40 or more years of ovarian function) are considered at high risk for the development of breast cancer. Women who have 40 or more

years of ovarian function include those who have a late natural menopause and those who began menstruating before the age of 12. (905)

2. **The answer is (A).** Women with breast cancer are at risk for subsequent development of cancer of the endometrium, ovary, and colon. (907)

3. **The answer is (D).** Prophylactic use of the antiestrogen drug tamoxifen by women who are considered at high risk for the development of breast cancer has been proposed and is currently being studied. This type of prophylactic treatment is known as chemoprevention. (909–910)

4. **The answer is (A).** Ninety percent of breast cancers are self-detected, although they are for the most part found accidentally. Only one-third of women surveyed stated that they perform regular monthly breast self-examinations. (911)

5. **The answer is (D).** Screening mammography is recommended for women beginning at age 40. After age 50 a mammogram should be done yearly; between ages 39 and 50 it should be done yearly for high-risk women or according to physician recommendation. (911–912)

6. **The answer is (B).** The majority of primary breast cancers are adenocarcinomas, specifically infiltrating intraductal and infiltrating lobular carcinomas. Other, less common types of breast cancer include colloid, medullary, and inflammatory carcinomas and cystosarcoma phyllodes. (922)

7. **The answer is (C).** A peau d'orange appearance to the skin over the breast is typical of inflammatory carcinoma. In this condition subdermal lymphatic spread causes skin edema and lymph stasis, which leads to congestion of prominent pores in the skin. (916)

8. **The answer is (A).** The pulmonary system, bone, and liver are the three most common sites of metastasis in breast cancer. Other sites include the pleura; the pituitary, adrenal, and thyroid glands; the kidneys; and the ovaries. (944)

9. **The answer is (A).** Benign breast disease is frequently associated with diffuse, bilateral breast pain and tenderness that is more prominent at the time of menstruation. A benign mass is usually clear on transillumination, encapsulated with a distinct barrier from adjacent tissues, and mobile. (914–915)

10. **The answer is (B).** The positive diagnosis of breast cancer can be made only by histologic examination following an open or closed biopsy. Noninvasive tests should be done before proceeding with any invasive diagnostic procedures. (921)

11. **The answer is (C).** The **most** important prognostic indicators for the woman with breast cancer are tumor size, the tumor's degree of invasiveness, and axillary node status. The presence of cancer in any of the axillary lymph nodes reduces the overall survival rate, and the actual number of nodes involved is the single most important prognosticator of disease recurrence. (923–924)

12. **The answer is (A).** For women with stage II and stage III disease, modified radical mastectomy (including removal of the breast, pectoralis minor muscles, intervening lymphatics, and a sampling of axillary lymph nodes) is the treatment of choice. At times it may also be advocated for those with minimal disease. (933–934)

13. **The answer is (C).** Receptor-negative tumors are usually associated with a shorter disease-free period and more aggressive disease; the opposite holds true for receptor-positive tumors. (947)

14. **The answer is (B).** The incidence of breast cancer is increased in men who have undergone sex-change procedures secondary to the administration of estrogen, which results in lobular development and breast enlargement. (950)

15. **The answer is (A).** The pain related to spinal cord compression is usually present for several weeks before the development of neurologic symptoms; however, when these symptoms are present, imminent compression should be suspected, and the situation should be treated as a medical emergency. (951)

16.   **The answer is (D).**   Intermittent compression with a pump may be necessary for those individuals with massive edema who have no evidence of infection. When the arm has decreased somewhat in size, the treatment is discontinued and the individual is measured for a support or encouraged to use an elastic stockinette to aid in venous flow. (952)

39 Central Nervous System Cancers

STUDY OUTLINE

I. INTRODUCTION

1. Tumor involvement within the central nervous system (CNS) is associated with a high degree of morbidity and mortality.
2. The CNS is a common site for metastatic disease, and therefore CNS tumor involvement often reflects advanced systemic disease.

II. ANATOMY AND PHYSIOLOGY

1. The figures and accompanying text discussion on **text pages 960–962** provide a comprehensive review of the structures and physiologic functioning of the human brain.

III. EPIDEMIOLOGY

1. The most prevalent malignant CNS tumor is the tumor within the cranium, or **brain tumor.**
   a. More than 50% of primary brain tumors are malignant and infiltrate the brain substance.
   b. Malignant brain tumors account for **1.4%** of all cancer in the United States.
2. The death rate from brain and nervous system tumors is **slightly higher for males** than for females.
3. Five-year survival rates for brain and nervous system cancer are **23% for white persons** and **31% for blacks.**
4. **Most malignant CNS tumors are metastatic from a distant site, most commonly including the lung, the breast, and the colon.** The **lung** is considered the primary site with the greatest propensity for brain metastasis.
5. The incidence of primary malignant brain tumors is smaller, estimated at 5 per 100,000 persons.
6. A **familial tendency** is implicated for some brain tumors, particularly **glioblastoma.**

IV. ETIOLOGY

1. Specific causes of the various CNS tumors remain speculative.
2. **Prophylactic radiation therapy** of the brain and the use of **immunosuppressive therapy** have been linked with the increased incidence of both primary and metastatic brain tumors.
3. Some evidence suggests that certain **occupational exposures,** such as vinyl chloride and petroleum, may predispose an individual to the development of CNS tumors.

V. PATHOPHYSIOLOGY

1. Classification of primary CNS tumors is based on the presumed **cell type of the tumor.** The universally accepted histologic classification of CNS tumors is listed in **Table 39-1, text page 964.**
2. Primary brain tumors arise from **neuroepithelial cells (glial cells),** which are among the few neural cells capable of division.
   a. Neuroepithelial tumor cells are often found diffusely in the perivascular spaces and subpial region of the cortex, and such tumors may appear to be **multicentric.**

      b.   These tumors, called **gliomas,** may spread via the cerebrospinal fluid (CSF) to distant parts of the nervous system, although metastases outside the CNS are rare.

      c.   Gliomas include **astrocytic tumors** (the most common type), **oligodendroglial tumors, ependymal and choroid plexus tumors,** and **poorly differentiated embryonal tumors.**

A. ASTROCYTOMA

1. **Astrocytomas** make up the largest group of primary brain tumors of one cell type.
2. The incidence of astrocytomas is highest in the fifth and sixth decades of life.
3. Astrocytomas generally arise in the **cerebral hemispheres** and develop in the central and subcortical white matter.
4. **Grade I astrocytomas** consist of well-differentiated astrocytes, whereas **grade IV tumors** demonstrate pleomorphism, cellularity, numerous mitoses, and necrosis.
5. **Grade III** and **grade IV astrocytomas,** known as **glioblastoma multiforme,** are considered highly malignant because of their **infiltrative nature and lack of capsulation.**

B. OLIGODENDROGLIOMA

1. Fewer than 5% of all primary brain tumors are **oligodendrogliomas.**
2. These tumors, usually **located in the frontal lobes,** are typically circumscribed, spongy, and vascular masses.
3. **Cellular pleomorphism** in the form of multinucleated giant cells of the Langhans type is a feature of the oligodendroglioma.
4. This is a **slow-growing tumor** that is most commonly manifested as a seizure disorder.

C. GLIOBLASTOMA

1. **Glioblastomas are the most common (60%) of the primary adult brain tumors,** and arise in the cerebral hemisphere with a predilection for the **frontal lobe.**
2. Glioblastoma is characterized by necrosis, vascular endothelium proliferation, and areas of old and fresh hemorrhages.
3. This is typically a **grade IV tumor.**

D. PRIMARY MALIGNANT LYMPHOMA

1. Since 1980, the number of cases of this formerly rare neoplasm has tripled, due to the increasing incidence of these tumors in **immunosuppressed** (inherited or acquired) patients. Approximately **3% of patients with AIDS** develop CNS lymphoma.
2. Studies suggest that the **Epstein-Barr virus** plays a role in the development of this non-Hodgkin's lymphoma.
3. CNS lymphoma appears in various ways, including **neurologic dysfunction, apathy, confusion,** or **personality changes.**

E. SPINAL CORD TUMORS

1. **Intraspinal tumors** may be primary (approximately 15% of primary CNS tumors) or metastatic. Regardless of type, intraspinal tumors may result in **spinal cord compression,** considered an oncologic emergency, which can rapidly lead to irreversible neurologic changes.
2. Spinal cord tumors typically become clinically manifest in one of three ways.
    a.   **Sensorimotor spinal tract syndromes** compress the cord and cause destruction of cord tracts, resulting in initial asymmetric motor disturbance.
    b.   **Radicular-spinal cord syndrome** results in pain in the distribution of a sensory nerve root, with pain radiating away from the spine.
    c.   A **syringomyelic syndrome** results from an intramedullary tumor and produces a mixed sensorimotor tract syndrome.

F. METASTATIC TUMORS

1. **The incidence of metastatic brain tumors is estimated at 24% of persons who die of cancer.**
2. Intracranial metastases occur at three main sites.

a. The **skull and dura** are infiltrated by tumors that metastasize to the bone, such as breast and prostate cancers.

b. Metastases to the **brain** occur by hematogenous spread, primarily via the arterial pathway, and most commonly occur in the **cortex.** The major symptoms of metastatic brain tumors are a result of **increased intracranial pressure (ICP).**

c. **Meningeal carcinomatosis** is rare, involving widespread dissemination of tumor cells throughout the meninges and ventricles.

VI. CLINICAL MANIFESTATIONS

1. The clinical manifestations of brain tumors vary depending on **site, size,** and **method of expansion. Figure 39-7, text page 967,** illustrates the interacting mechanisms responsible for the clinical manifestations of intracranial tumors.

A. INCREASED INTRACRANIAL PRESSURE

1. In adults the skull acts as a rigid sphere, encasing the three normal components of the intracranial cavity: **brain, CSF,** and **blood.**
   a. To maintain normal ICP, an increase in the volume of one component must be accompanied by a proportional decrease in the volume of one or both of the other components.
   b. The compensatory changes are limited, especially when a volume increase is too large or too sudden.

2. **Brain tumors increase ICP by their size, cerebral edema, or obstruction of CSF pathways; a combination of tumor bulk and peritumoral edema is usually responsible for an increase in ICP.**
   a. Clinical manifestations are produced by the effects of increasing ICP on nerve cells, blood vessels, and dura.
   b. **An expanding tumor mass can create a vicious cycle of intracranial hypertension,** as illustrated in **Figure 39-8, text page 968.**
   c. When ICP rises to very high levels, the autoregulatory system of cerebral blood flow fails, and the cerebral blood flow drops.

3. **Generalized increased ICP causes mental changes, papilledema, headache, vomiting, and changes in vital signs, as well as secondary effects due to the displacement of brain tissue.**
   a. **Changes in mental status** include alterations in the level of consciousness, confusion, short-term memory loss, and personality changes, which can initially be quite subtle in nature.
   b. **Papilledema** is considered a cardinal sign of increased ICP, and is due to an increase in CSF pressure around the optic nerve, impairing the outflow of venous blood with swelling of the optic disc.
   c. **Headaches** are reported as an early symptom in approximately one-third of persons with a brain tumor.
      (1) The headache that accompanies increased ICP usually is **bilateral** and **located in the frontal or occipital regions.**
      (2) Individuals may give a history of early morning headache that subsides on arising and that may be aggravated by coughing, bending over, or initiating the Valsalva maneuver.
      (3) The headache increases in severity, frequency, and duration over time.
   d. **Vomiting,** apparently unrelated to food ingestion and often projectile in nature, is part of the **classic triad** (with papilledema and headache) of increased ICP.
   e. **Changes in vital signs,** resulting from increased pressure on the vasomotor centers of the medulla, are a late finding in cases of increased ICP.

B. SECONDARY EFFECTS: DISPLACEMENT OF BRAIN STRUCTURES

1. Pressure normally is distributed equally throughout the compartments of the cranial cavity (see **Figure 39-9a, text page 969).**

2. A growing tumor mass and the edema associated with it cause increased pressure within a compartment, which in turn may cause brain tissue to **shift** or **herniate** from the high-pressure compartment into the lower-pressure compartment.

    a. **Herniation** is a neurologic emergency, since shifting brain tissue causes compression damage, cerebral edema, ischemia, damage to blood vessels, and obstructed flow of blood and CSF.

3. There are two major classifications of herniation: **supratentorial brain shifts** and **infratentorial brain shifts,** with differing clinical manifestations.

    a. **Supratentorial tumors,** lesions above the tentorium cerebelli, displace brain structures in the anterior and middle fossae, causing **changes in the level of consciousness** and **ocular, motor, and respiratory signs.**

        (1) **Central** or **transtentorial herniation** occurs when the cerebral hemispheres, basal ganglia, diencephalon, and adjacent midbrain are forced downward (see **Figure 39-9b, text page 969).** The signs include changes in level of consciousness, reduction in pupil size, and alterations in eye movements.

        (2) **Uncal herniation** occurs when the medial part of one of the temporal lobes is forced toward the midline and downward through the tentorial opening (see **Figure 39-9c, text page 969).** The early signs of uncal herniation include sluggish contraction of the pupil in response to light, due to compression of the third cranial nerve.

        (3) **Contralateral hemiparesis** occurs when the motor pathways of the cerebral peduncle are compressed.

        (4) Both central and uncal herniations cause **changes in respiratory pattern,** including irregular depth and rhythm, as well as rate.

    b. **Infratentorial herniations** involve displacement of the cerebellum (see **Figure 39-10, text page 970).**

        (1) **Downward cerebellar herniation** (or **foramen magnum herniation**) results in medullary compression that may lead to respiratory or circulatory collapse as the vasomotor centers of the medulla are compressed.

            (a) Frequently, individuals with cerebellar-foramen magnum herniation have a **sudden loss of consciousness followed by respiratory arrest.**

            (b) Other early signs include suboccipital headache, neck pain, an arched neck, vomiting, and cranial nerve palsies.

        (2) **Upward transtentorial herniation** compresses the midbrain. Signs include the loss of consciousness and altered respiratory, pupillary, ocular, and motor signs.

C. FOCAL EFFECTS

1. **The focal effects of brain tumors are caused by direct compression of nerve tissue or destruction and invasion of brain tissue through infiltration.**

2. Neurologic deficits are related directly to the damaged area of the brain, and the accompanying signs and symptoms may help to locate the tumor. **Table 39-2, text page 971,** lists some of the clinical manifestations of intracranial tumors according to location.

3. **Cranial nerve function** may be affected by tumors that are located in intracranial compartments through which the cranial nerves pass.

4. **Seizures** are a major manifestation of cerebral brain tumors, and **in many adults they are the first clinical manifestation.**

    a. Nerve tumor cells are abnormal, epileptogenic cells that are highly excitable and fire repetitively, resulting in focal or generalized seizures.

    b. A careful description of the onset of a seizure, the seizure activity, and the postictal phase may have tumor-localizing value.

VII. ASSESSMENT

1. **Patient assessment** includes documentation of the presence and severity of both focal and generalized symptoms. A baseline measurement of neurologic dysfunction is made.

2. **Metastatic brain tumors** often present with symptoms in the following order: headache, focal weakness, mental disturbances, seizures, aphasia, and visual abnormalities.

3. The evaluation of headaches and any seizure activity are of major importance.

4. A thorough neurologic examination includes an evaluation of the cranial nerves (see **Table 39-3, text page 972),** the motor nervous system, the sensory nervous system, and cerebellar function.

VIII.   **DIAGNOSTIC STUDIES**

     1.   **Pneumoencephalography,** the study of the ventricular and cisternal systems, permits the determination of the shape and positions of the ventricles and whether any abnormal masses exist in this area.

     2.   **CT scanning** offers advantages other than detection and diagnosis of brain tumors. It demonstrates the precise location of lytic metastases, as well as the extent of accompanying soft tissue masses, both intracranially and beneath the scalp. Edema surrounding a tumor may also be discerned.

     3.   **MRI** provides information about the chemical composition of tissue, and also has a higher soft tissue contrast than does CT scan.

     4.   **PET (positron-emission tomography) scanning** is a noninvasive nuclear imaging technique capable of quantifying metabolic processes, which may be useful in evaluating low-grade gliomas.

     5.   While innovations in neuroradiology have contributed greatly to the diagnosis and precise localization of brain tumors, the ultimate diagnosis and subsequent treatment arise from **histopathologic findings.**

IX.   **CLASSIFICATION AND STAGING**

     1.   Staging of CNS tumors, particularly intracranial tumors, has clinical and prognostic implications.
         a.   **Anatomic staging** includes primary site, regional lymph nodes, and metastatic site.
         b.   **Clinical staging** is based on neurologic signs and symptoms, as well as on diagnostic tests.

     2.   **The most critical feature in classification of CNS tumors is histopathology.** The histologic staging of brain tumors is found in **Table 39-4, text page 974.**

X.   **TREATMENT**

     1.   The treatment of CNS malignancies is determined by factors such as **primary site, tumor grade, overall condition of the patient,** and **specific tumor type.**

A.   **SURGERY**

     1.   The individual with a primary brain tumor usually is a candidate for **surgical excision as the initial treatment.** The surgical treatment of brain tumors has improved with the use of the operating microscope and medical treatment to minimize cerebral edema.

     2.   Several factors are considered in the evaluation of the individual for surgery: **tumor location, size, method of spread, general condition of the patient,** and **neurologic status.**

     3.   There are several approaches to the surgical management of the individual with a brain tumor.
         a.   **Surgery as the primary treatment in which the aim is the complete removal of the tumor.**
            (1)   Partial debulking may also improve the person's neurologic condition by decreasing local compression and decreasing ICP.
            (2)   The advantage of surgical therapy in carefully selected cases is increased survival time and an improved quality of survival.
         b.   **Surgery to facilitate nonsurgical therapy.**
            (1)   Postoperative radiotherapy/chemotherapy is considered when recurrence is likely or when the excision is only partial.
            (2)   Surgery may be used to place radioactive substances within the tumor mass or to confirm the identification of a mass by biopsy.
         c.   **No surgery at all.**

     4.   **Factors favorable for surgery** include
         a.   A long interval between treatment of primary extracranial neoplasm and diagnosis of an intracranial tumor.
         b.   A single brain metastasis with no other metastases to other parts of the body.
         c.   An extracranial tumor that is responsive to therapy.
         d.   A significant improvement in neurologic status with the administration of steroids.
         e.   Minimal neurologic deficit, with increased ICP the major problem.

5. **Factors unfavorable for surgery** include
    a. The presence of multiple small intracranial tumors.
    b. A major neurologic deficit that is unresponsive to steroid therapy.
    c. A rapidly growing or disseminated tumor.
6. The most serious **postoperative complications** of neurosurgery are intracranial bleeding, cerebral edema, and water intoxication.
7. Surgery generally is the immediate treatment choice for tumors that cause spinal cord compression.

B. **RADIOSURGERY**

1. **Stereotactic radiosurgery** is a noninvasive technique delivering a single, large fraction of ionizing radiation to a small, well-defined target.

C. **RADIOTHERAPY**

1. The use of radiotherapy in the treatment of primary malignant brain tumors depends on the **radiosensitivity** of the particular tumor type.
2. Radiotherapy is used in the treatment of metastatic brain tumors, since individuals typically have multiple cerebral metastases and are not candidates for surgery.
3. **Radiation dosages** to the brain vary according to tumor type and bulk and the individual's general condition.
4. **Hypoxia** is believed to be a factor that limits the effectiveness of radiation, since malignant brain tumors contain a large proportion of hypoxic cells that are radioresistant.
5. Response to radiotherapy treatment is measured in part by the degree to which the person is able to perform activities of daily living.
6. **Irreversible radiation necrosis** may develop after cranial therapy.
7. Experimental radiotherapy techniques include intraoperative radiotherapy and stereotactic radiosurgery with a gamma knife.

D. **CHEMOTHERAPY AND RELATED DRUGS**

1. Chemotherapy is indicated for patients who have a histologic **grade III or grade IV tumor.** However, chemotherapy for most brain tumors is a limited approach, since most chemotherapeutic agents do not cross the blood-brain barrier.
    a. The **blood-brain barrier (BBB)** consists of a continuous lining of endothelial cells that are connected by tight junctions (see **Figure 39-12, text page 977).**
2. The group of drugs classified as **nitrosoureas,** including carmustine (BCNU) and lomustine (CCNU), are successful in penetrating the BBB because they are lipid soluble.
3. Other means that are being investigated to break down or penetrate the BBB, thereby allowing chemotherapy to reach the tumor, include
    a. Transitory osmotic disruption of the BBB with mannitol.
    b. The use of liposomes as drug carriers.
    c. **Intra-arterial or intrathecal administration,** which has been used for regionally confined malignancies, including intracranial tumors. Problems with this approach include the drugs' direct toxic effects to the ipsilateral eye and leukoencephalopathy.

XI. **GENERAL SUPPORTIVE MEASURES**

1. Symptoms of metastatic brain tumors are ameliorated in 60% to 75% of individuals treated with **adrenocorticosteroids.**
    a. Dexamethasone is used frequently in neurologic settings to decrease cerebral edema.
    b. Individuals receiving steroids should be observed for
        (1) Acute adrenal insufficiency.
        (2) Cardiovascular and renal problems.
        (3) Gastrointestinal disturbances.
        (4) Metabolic problems such as hyperglycemia.
        (5) Musculoskeletal problems.

    c.   Individuals who receive high doses of steroids for a prolonged period of time may develop a **steroid psychosis,** manifested by personality changes and paranoid behavior, which develops suddenly.

  2. **Nursing measures** involve the performance of activities that affect ICP, including turning and positioning the patient, and pulmonary hygiene and suctioning.

    a.   The outflow of venous blood from the cranial cavity should be unimpeded by head rotation, neck flexion, neck extension, and lowering the head of the patient's bed.

    b.   Increases in the patient's intra-abdominal and intrathoracic pressures caused by coughing, straining, and the Valsalva maneuver should be avoided.

    c.   Efforts to prevent seizures are important, since seizure activity may produce local brain tissue ischemia and permanent neurologic disability.

  3. **Discharge goals** include helping the patient attain realistic goals and directing the family to appropriate resources.

    a.   A **safe home environment** is required, regardless of activity level.

    b.   **Reality-orientation devices** (clocks, calendars) should be readily available.

    c.   The patient with progressive CNS involvement generally is in a terminal state, and death at home may occur slowly, through progression of disease and complications of immobility.

PRACTICE QUESTIONS

1.   The majority of central nervous system tumors are metastatic from a distant site. The type of tumor **most** likely to metastasize to the brain is
  (A)   renal cell cancer.
  (B)   prostate cancer.
  (C)   lung cancer.
  (D)   multiple myeloma.

2.   Primary brain tumors arise from _____ cells, which are among the few neural cells capable of division.
  (A)   medullary
  (B)   pituitary
  (C)   dural
  (D)   glial

3.   Since 1980 the number of cases of primary malignant central nervous system (CNS) lymphoma has tripled due to the increasing incidence of
  (A)   lung cancer.
  (B)   bone marrow transplantation procedures.
  (C)   radiation exposure.
  (D)   AIDS.

4.   A common manifestation of CNS lymphoma is
  (A)   a change in personality.
  (B)   syndrome of inappropriate antidiuretic hormone (SIADH).
  (C)   frontal headache.
  (D)   spinal cord compression.

5.   Most of the symptoms of metastatic brain tumors occur as a result of
  (A)   displacement of brain structures.
  (B)   inadequate transmission of nerve impulses.
  (C)   increased intracranial pressure.
  (D)   brain cell destruction and subsequent replacement with tumor cells.

6.   A supratentorial brain shift, involving structures in the anterior and middle fossae, are **most** likely to cause
  (A)   acute renal failure.

    (B)   a coagulation disorder.
    (C)   metabolic changes.
    (D)   changes in respiratory status.

7.   The headache that accompanies an increase in intracranial pressure is usually _____ and located in the _____ region of the brain.
    (A)   bilateral; frontal or occipital
    (B)   unilateral; temporal
    (C)   bilateral; temporal
    (D)   unilateral; parietal or occipital

8.   One of the classic signs of increased intracranial pressure is
    (A)   papilledema.
    (B)   facial droop.
    (C)   frequent nosebleeds.
    (D)   shortness of breath.

9.   The **most** effective treatment for the majority of individuals with a primary brain tumor is
    (A)   surgery.
    (B)   intravenous chemotherapy.
    (C)   radiation therapy.
    (D)   hyperthermia.

10.   Surgery is indicated for the individual with a brain tumor for all of the following reasons **except**
    (A)   to confirm the identification of a mass by biopsy.
    (B)   to shrink the tumor.
    (C)   to remove large numbers of metastases.
    (D)   to place radioactive substances within the tumor mass.

11.   The most common treatment for the individual with multiple metastatic brain tumors is
    (A)   intra-arterial chemotherapy.
    (B)   intravenous chemotherapy.
    (C)   local excision.
    (D)   radiotherapy.

12.   One of the reasons chemotherapy is **not** used in the treatment of primary brain tumors is that
    (A)   chemotherapeutic agents are known to destroy healthy brain tissue.
    (B)   most chemotherapeutic agents do not cross the blood-brain barrier.
    (C)   chemotherapy predisposes brain tumor patients to cerebral hemorrhage.
    (D)   the only effective chemotherapeutic agents produce severe side effects.

13.   One category of chemotherapeutic drugs that can cross the blood-brain barrier are the
    (A)   antimetabolites.
    (B)   alkylators.
    (C)   nitrosoureas.
    (D)   vinca alkaloids.

14.   Individuals receiving adrenocorticosteroids for the treatment of cerebral edema should be monitored for the presence of
    (A)   hyperglycemia.
    (B)   hypokalemia.
    (C)   petechiae.
    (D)   pain.

ANSWER EXPLANATIONS

1. **The answer is (C).**   The lung is considered the primary tumor site with the greatest propensity for brain metastases. From the lungs cancer cells may enter the pulmonary veins and reach the left atrium and ventricle; from there they can enter the arterial circulation via the capillaries. (962–965)

2. **The answer is (D).**   Primary brain tumors, or gliomas, arise from neuroepithelial or glial cells, which are among the few neural cells capable of division. Astrocytomas, oligodendrogliomas, ependymal and choroid plexus tumors, pineal cell tumors, neuronal tumors, and poorly differentiated and embryonal tumors are all examples of gliomas. (964)

3. **The answer is (D).**   The populations at greatest risk for the development of primary central nervous system (CNS) lymphoma include transplant recipients, those with congenital immunodeficiencies, and those with AIDS. Three percent of patients with AIDS will develop CNS lymphoma. (965)

4. **The answer is (A).**   CNS lymphoma commonly causes neurologic dysfunction, apathy, confusion, and/or personality changes. It does not typically cause the headaches that are common to brain tumors, spinal cord compression, or SIADH. (965)

5. **The answer is (C).**   The clinical manifestations of metastatic brain tumors (i.e., papilledema, headache, and/or vomiting) are all related to an increase in intracranial pressure. Papilledema is caused by an increase in cerebrospinal fluid pressure around the optic nerve, which causes swelling of the optic disk. Headaches are believed to be the result of pressure on the pain-sensitive structures of the dura, venous sinuses, surface blood vessels, and cranial nerves. Vomiting, often projectile in nature, may be caused by increased pressure on the vomiting center of the medulla. (968)

6. **The answer is (D).**   Both central and uncal herniations cause changes in respiratory pattern. Initially, respirations may become irregular with occasional pauses; later, total respiratory arrest may occur. (969)

7. **The answer is (A).**   The headache that accompanies an increase in intracranial pressure is usually bilateral and located in the frontal or occipital regions of the brain. The pain may be described as dull, sharp, or throbbing and may be initiated or aggravated by performing certain activities. Over time, the headaches generally increase in severity, frequency, and duration. (968)

8. **The answer is (A).**   The most common symptoms of a generalized increase in intracranial pressure include papilledema, headache, vomiting, change in mental status, and change in vital signs. (968)

9. **The answer is (A).**   The initial treatment for an individual with a primary brain tumor usually is surgical excision of that tumor. In addition, surgery may be performed palliatively on metastatic brain tumors or to extend life. (975)

10. **The answer is (C).**   Surgery is used to relieve the symptoms of local compression and increased intracranial pressure through debulking. It is also used to place radioactive substances within the tumor to confirm the histologic or cytologic identification of a mass by biopsy. In general, individuals with **multiple** cerebral metastases are not considered to be candidates for surgical resection. (975–976)

11. **The answer is (D).**   The treatment of choice for individuals with multiple metastatic brain tumors is radiotherapy; as stated above, these individuals are not likely to be surgical candidates. Response of the metastases to radiotherapy depends on the histologic characteristics of the primary tumor. In general, metastases from breast and lung tumors respond better to irradiation than do metastases from melanoma or sarcoma. (976)

12. **The answer is (B).**   Most chemotherapeutic agents are water-soluble and therefore do not cross the blood-brain barrier. The use of liposomes to transport chemotherapy represents a recent, encouraging approach to the administration of these drugs. (977–978)

13. **The answer is (C).**   The group of drugs classified as nitrosoureas successfully penetrate the blood-brain barrier. These drugs include carmustine (BCNU), lomustine (CCNU), and semustine (methyl-CCNU), all of which are lipid-soluble. (977)

14. **The answer is (A).**   Steroids are often used to ameliorate the symptoms of metastatic brain cancer. Individuals receiving steroids need to be monitored for multiple side effects, including acute adrenal insufficiency, cardiovascular and renal problems, gastrointestinal disturbances, musculoskeletal problems, and metabolic disturbances as evidenced by gluconeogenesis that leads to hyperglycemia. (980)

40   Endocrine Cancers

STUDY OUTLINE

I. **INTRODUCTION**

    1. The clinical presentation of endocrine tumors depends on their **anatomic location** and their **ability to produce excess hormone secretion.**

        a. Depending on the location of the tumor, **local growth** can cause compression of vital structures.

        b. **Hyperplasia,** in which the number of hormone-secreting cells increases, can result in excess secretion of hormones.

            (1) These cells are not subject to the normal regulatory feedback processes that control hormonal secretion.

    2. Even some endocrine tumors that are not histologically malignant can result in morbidity or death through expansion and hyperplasia.

II. **THYROID CANCER**

    A. **EPIDEMIOLOGY**

        1. Thyroid cancer remains relatively **rare,** accounting for just over 1% of the total cancer incidence and approximately 0.2% of all cancer deaths.

        2. Women are more than twice as likely as men to have a thyroid malignancy, with a majority of cases occurring between the ages of 25 and 65.

    B. **ETIOLOGY**

        1. The only well-documented etiologic factor in the development of thyroid cancer is **head and neck irradiation given during early childhood and adolescence.**

        2. Other factors that have been investigated include **thyroid-stimulating hormone (TSH)** and **genetics.**

            a. TSH may function as a growth factor for well-differentiated thyroid malignancies but may not actually induce neoplasia.

            b. Approximately 25% of medullary thyroid cancer cases occur as part of the genetically transmitted **multiple endocrine neoplasm (MEN) syndromes.**

    C. **PATHOPHYSIOLOGY**

        1. Four types of primary thyroid carcinoma—**papillary, follicular, medullary, and anaplastic**—account for 95% of all thyroid neoplasms.

            a. The majority of thyroid tumors arise from the **follicular** and **parafollicular (C cells)** of the gland. These tumors are usually well differentiated.

            b. Papillary, follicular, and anaplastic tumors arise from **follicular cells.** Medullary carcinoma of the thyroid (**MCT**) is the only tumor of **parafollicular** origin.

            c. Anaplastic tumors are **undifferentiated.** They bear little resemblance to their tissue of origin and lack the functional and histologic characteristics of normal thyroid tissue.

        2. Thyroid tumors vary in their ability to **concentrate iodine.**

            a. This has therapeutic implications, in that treatment with ^{131}I is effective only for tumors that are able to concentrate iodine.

3. **Table 40-1, text page 986,** outlines the clinical characteristics, including the incidence, survival rate, and metastatic pattern, of each of these four tumor types.
   a. **Papillary tumors** have both a higher incidence rate and a higher survival rate than those of the other tumor types. Cervical lymph nodes are involved early in the disease; metastasis is to the lungs and less frequently to bone.
   b. **Follicular tumors** are more locally invasive than are papillary tumors but are less likely to have lymph node involvement. These tumors have a propensity for hematogenous spread to bone and, occasionally, to the lung.
   c. **Anaplastic tumors** have both the lowest incidence and the lowest survival rates among the tumor types. Invasion is rapid and compresses adjacent structures early in the disease. The lung is the most common site of metastases.
   d. **Medullary tumors** are relatively rare; 10-year survival is 61%. Half of these tumors have lymph node involvement at diagnosis. Metastasis is to bone, liver, and lung.
4. **Papillary carcinoma**
   a. Papillary carcinoma generally follows an indolent course and survival is measured in decades, even when distant metastases occur.
   b. Poorer prognosis is associated with
      (1) **Age of patient:** older patients have a lower rate of survival.
      (2) **Sex:** men have a poorer prognosis than women.
      (3) **Extent of disease at the time of diagnosis:** symptoms of advanced disease (e.g., dysphagia, dyspnea, dysphonia) confer a worse prognosis.
   c. Approximately 25% of cases are small, nonpalpable lesions that are benign and highly curable.
5. **Follicular carcinomas**
   a. Follicular carcinomas tend to be more locally invasive than papillary carcinoma but are less likely to metastasize to regional lymph nodes.
   b. They are more likely to concentrate iodine and to cause hyperthyroidism.
6. **Medullary carcinoma**
   a. Approximately 20% of the cases occur as part of the genetically transmitted MEN syndromes. The remainder develop spontaneously.
   b. The best prognosis is for women younger than 40 years with an early stage of disease.
7. **Anaplastic carcinoma**
   a. These are among the most rapidly growing, lethal neoplasms. Death usually occurs within months of diagnosis, regardless of therapy.
   b. The majority of patients are **elderly women** and individuals with a **history of goiter.**
   c. Death usually occurs as a result of local invasion and tracheal encroachment.

D. **CLINICAL MANIFESTATIONS**

1. The most common clinical presentation includes an otherwise **asymptomatic thyroid mass** on routine physical presentation and **cervical lymphadenopathy.**
2. Other symptoms, including dyspnea or stridor and dysphagia, are more commonly associated with an anaplastic tumor and relate to **compressive effects of the tumor mass on adjacent structures.**

E. **DIAGNOSTIC EVALUATION**

1. **Assessment** includes
   a. A **patient history and physical examination,** focusing on evidence of thyroid masses or dysfunction.
   b. **Fine-needle aspiration,** for the evaluation of discrete thyroid nodules.
   c. **TSH suppression** by thyroxine, to reduce the size of nodules.
   d. **Radionuclide imaging,** for information regarding the ability of nodules to concentrate iodine.
   e. **Laboratory tests,** focusing on general thyroid dysfunction and evidence of elevated thyroid hormone levels.
      (1) **Serum calcitonin** is an important tumor marker used in screening for the familial forms of medullary thyroid cancer.

2. **Staging** of thyroid cancer is done according to the system proposed by the American Joint Committee of Cancer (see **Table 40-2, text page 989**). It incorporates the important prognostic factors of **age** and **histologic type** into the classification.

F. TREATMENT

1. **Surgery**
   a. The selection of type of surgical procedure depends on the **histologic findings** and the **extent of the disease.**
   b. **Near-total** or **total thyroidectomy** is widely used as the initial treatment for all differentiated thyroid cancers.
      (1) Total thyroidectomy decreases local recurrences and increases effectiveness of ^{131}I treatment but has a higher incidence of postoperative complications.
      (2) Near-total thyroidectomy has fewer complications and comparable rates of recurrence and survival.
   c. **Lobectomy** is more commonly used with anaplastic (undifferentiated) carcinoma.
2. **Postoperative complications**
   a. Postoperative complications include **hemorrhage, damage to parathyroid glands** with associated hypercalcemia, **damage to laryngeal nerves** with associated vocal paralysis, and **hypothyroidism.**
      (1) Exogenous **thyroid hormone** may be required to prevent hypothyroidism and suppress endogenous TSH that may serve as a growth factor for differentiated thyroid tumors.
3. **Radiotherapy**
   a. ^{131}I is used to
      (1) **Treat residual and metastatic disease** in certain patients with well-differentiated cancer after surgical resection of the thyroid.
      (2) **Ablate any remaining thyroid tissue** left in the neck following surgery, which optimizes the effectiveness of ^{131}I treatment so that the isotope will be concentrated in functional tumor tissue.
   b. Thyroid hormone is discontinued prior to ^{131}I therapy, which begins **6 months following ablation** and continues at 4- to 6-month intervals until whole body imaging studies reveal no evidence of functioning tumor.
   c. Inpatient admission in a **private room** is required since radiation precautions are instituted. **No children or pregnant women** are allowed in the patient's room after the isotope is administered.
   d. ^{131}I is administered orally and is present in all body secretions.
   e. Patients may be discharged when radiation dose emission readings are sufficiently low (after 72 hours).
   f. **Complications** include nausea and vomiting, fatigue, headache, inflammation of the salivary glands (sialadenitis), bone marrow suppression, and, rarely, pulmonary radiation fibrosis and leukemia.
      (1) **Fatigue, headache,** and **nausea and vomiting** may be related to radiation sickness and can occur within 12 hours of ^{131}I administration. Premedication with antiemetics may be helpful.
      (2) **Sialadenitis** occurs within 24 hours and may be due to concentration of radioisotope in the salivary glands. Stimulation of salivary flow with hard candy may avert this problem.
   g. **External-beam irradiation** may be used, either alone or with ^{131}I, for patients with incompletely excised tumors. It may also be helpful in the palliation of painful bone metastases.
4. **Chemotherapy** has been disappointing in the treatment of thyroid cancer. As a single agent, only doxorubicin has demonstrated any significant antitumor activity.
5. **Follow-up**
   a. Due to the incidence of late recurrences, long-term follow-up should occur with **serum thyroglobulin measurements and serial isotope scanning.**

III. PITUITARY TUMORS

A. EPIDEMIOLOGY

1. Pituitary carcinoma is extremely rare. Most pituitary tumors are **benign adenomas** that arise in the adenohypophyseal cells of the anterior portion of the gland.

B. **ETIOLOGY**

1. No definitive causative factors have been established for pituitary tumors, but **changes in hormonal equilibrium** within the pituitary may play a role.
    a. **Hyperplasia of adenohypophyseal cells** can result from prolonged stimulation of pituitary hormones, i.e., when target glands are not secreting sufficient hormone to provide negative feedback for the pituitary gland. However, hyperplastic cells may or may not be more susceptible to neoplastic transformation.
    b. Adenomas of the prolactin-secreting cells may result from disorders of dopamine synthesis and secretion.

C. **CLASSIFICATION**

1. Pituitary adenomas are categorized according to **hormone secretion.** The hormonal classification of pituitary adenomas, their relative incidence, and associated clinical syndromes are listed in **Table 40-3, text page 993.**
2. Adenomas are also classified according to their **size** and **extension outside the sella turcica.**
    a. Those smaller than 10 mm in diameter are classified as **microadenomas.** These tumors have a better overall prognosis because they are generally confined to the sella turcica and are **more easily resected.**
    b. Those larger than 10 mm in diameter are classified as **macroadenomas.**

D. **PATHOPHYSIOLOGY**

1. Pituitary adenomas are "malignant" by virtue of their ability to produce morbidity through **growth in a confined space** and **mediation of hormonal dysfunction.**
    a. The majority of adenomas are well differentiated and the cells retain their hormone-producing capabilities.
    b. They are, however, **not subject to the normal regulatory mechanisms of the body** and produce hormones, regardless of feedback from target organs.
2. Adenomas may be slow-growing and noninvasive or more aggressive, exhibiting rapid growth rates, invading adjacent tissues, and causing symptoms indicative of compression of vital structures.

E. **CLINICAL PRESENTATION**

1. The most common manifestations of pituitary adenoma are **alterations in hormonal patterns** and **pressure symptoms from a growing tumor.**
    a. Functional tumors will produce symptoms of **hormonal excess.**
    b. Expanding tumors will result in **headache, visual disturbances,** and **functional** impairment of cranial nerves.

F. **DIAGNOSTIC EVALUATION**

1. The **anatomic extent of the pituitary mass** and its **functional status** can be determined with appropriate endocrine and neuroradiologic studies.
    a. Hypersecretion of pituitary hormones can be determined by means of **radioimmunoassay,** although elevated levels do not necessarily confirm the diagnosis of a pituitary adenoma.
    b. **Magnetic resonance imaging (MRI)** and **CT scans** provide more precise information regarding
        (1) Tumor margins.
        (2) Effect of tumor on adjacent structures.
        (3) Location of vascular structures.
        (4) The optic apparatus and cavernous sinus.
        (5) Consistency of the tumor.
        (6) Presence of normal pituitary tissue.
2. Information obtained by diagnostic tests may aid in the selection of therapeutic approach, as well as provide baseline data for assessment of response to therapy.
3. Diagnostic tests are repeated after initial therapy to assess treatment effectiveness.

G. **TREATMENT**

1. The goals of treatment are **removal or eradication of the tumor, restoration of normal hormonal function,** and **elimination of mass effects without residual morbidity.**
2. **Surgery**
    a. Surgery remains the most effective treatment for **microadenomas.**
    b. Surgery also is indicated in patients with **pituitary apoplexy** (hemorrhage into the tumor and precipitous deterioration of neurologic status).
    c. With **macroadenomas,** hormones may be used to shrink the tumor to resectable size. Subtotal resection followed by postoperative radiation then can be curative.
    d. **Diabetes insipidus, cerebrospinal fluid (CSF) leak,** and **meningitis** are the most frequently reported complications following surgery.
    e. Additional nursing considerations pertain to the operative site.
        (1) **Sneezing and nose-blowing** are contraindicated to minimize pressure on the site.
        (2) **Oral inspection and mouth care** are instituted to maintain integrity of mucous membranes and to prevent infection.
    f. **Postoperative measurement** of pituitary hormone levels is done to assess the effectiveness of surgery in removing hypersecreting tissue.
3. **Radiotherapy**
    a. **External-beam radiation** normally is used only in combination with surgery to treat adenomas.
        (1) It is most effective in controlling regrowth of tissue rather than in controlling hypersecretion.
        (2) Full effects on normalizing hormone levels may not be seen for months to years after treatment.
        (3) The major complication is **hypothyroidism,** which may become evident years after treatment.
4. **Pharmacotherapy**
    a. The focus of medical management of pituitary adenomas has been **hormone manipulation** of pituitary secretions.
    b. **Bromocriptine,** a dopamine antagonist, has been used to treat patients with prolactin-secreting tumors but may affect the outcome of surgery because of an increase in interstitial fibrosis.

IV. **ADRENAL TUMORS**

1. Tumors may arise from either the **cortex** or the **medulla** of the adrenal gland.
    a. The majority of cancers of the cortex are **adenocarcinomas.**
    b. The majority of cancers of the medulla are either **pheochromocytomas** or **neuroblastomas.**

A. **ADRENOCORTICAL CARCINOMAS**

1. **Epidemiology**
    a. Incidence is **rare** and equal between sexes, although women appear to have a higher proportion of functional neoplasms.
        (1) Functional tumors are those that produce excess amounts of **corticosteroids.**
        (2) Nonfunctional tumors occur more often in men and in patients 40 to 70 years of age.
2. **Pathophysiology**
    a. These tumors are **aggressive,** with most patients having either advanced or metastatic disease.
        (1) Tumors are difficult to detect and symptoms are gradual and often nonspecific.
        (2) Survival with treatment ranges from 1 month to 5 years.
    b. The most common sites of metastasis are **lung, liver,** and **lymph nodes.** More than 50% of patients die from **pulmonary insufficiency** and **sepsis.**
3. **Clinical presentation**
    a. Patients with **nonfunctional tumors** commonly have a **palpable abdominal mass** with associated abdominal or back pain. **Fever, weight loss, weakness,** and **lethargy** are symptoms of advanced disease.

    b. Patients with **functional tumors** will have **hypersecretion of one or more of the adrenal cortex secretions**—cortisol, aldosterone, progesterone, testosterone, and estradiol.

        (1) The majority of functional tumors result in **Cushing's disease, virilization and feminization syndromes,** and **hyperaldosteronism.**

  4. **Diagnostic evaluation**

    a. **Immunoassays** of hormones, their precursors, or their metabolites detect the presence of functional adrenal tumors.

    b. **CT** and **MRI** are used to localize tumors, assess hepatic, renal, and vena caval involvement, and distinguish benign adenomas from adrenocortical carcinomas and pheochromocytomas. MRI may be particular useful in the screening of asymptomatic masses.

  5. **Treatment**

    a. **Surgery** is the major treatment for adrenocortical carcinoma. It can be curative for patients with small, localized tumors.

    b. Locally advanced and invasive tumors are first **surgically debulked** before additional radiation therapy and chemotherapy is initiated.

    c. **Glucocorticoids** are administered before and after surgery until normal function of the adrenal cortex returns.

    d. **Permanent replacement therapy of mineralocorticoids and glucocorticoids** may be needed for patients undergoing ablation of both adrenals.

    e. The adrenocorticolytic drug, **o,p'-DDD (mitotane),** may be used after surgical debulking. It causes selective necrosis of the cortex.

    f. **Radiation therapy** after surgical resection does not improve survival but can be effective in palliation of painful bone metastases.

B. PHEOCHROMOCYTOMA

  1. **Epidemiology**

    a. These tumors are extremely rare and can be differentiated from benign tumors only by their invasiveness and distant metastases.

    b. They are **catecholamine-secreting tumors** that arise from chromaffin cells of the sympathoadrenal system. Chromaffin cells synthesize amine hormones.

  2. **Clinical presentation** usually involves excess production of catecholamines. Symptoms include hypertension, headache, sweating, nausea and vomiting, palpitations, and anxiety.

  3. **Diagnostic evaluation** is by measurement of urinary and circulating catecholamines or their metabolites.

    a. **CT** and the **metaiodobenylguanidine scan (MIBG)** are used to localize tumors before surgery.

  4. **Treatment** involves **surgery** to remove all accessible disease and metastases.

    a. Patients are pretreated with **a-adrenergic blocking agents** to minimize possible catecholamine release during surgery.

    b. Postoperatively, patients are monitored for shock related to the profound decrease in available catecholamines.

V. PARATHYROID TUMORS

A. EPIDEMIOLOGY

  1. These are rare tumors found equally in men and women, typically between the ages of 30 and 60 years.

  2. There is some evidence that **irradiation of the head and neck** may induce neoplastic transformation in hyperplastic glands.

B. PATHOPHYSIOLOGY

  1. Most parathyroid tumors are **biochemically functional,** causing clinical effects of **hypercalcemia** from hypersecretion of parathyroid hormone (PTH). Death frequently results from hypercalcemia.

  2. Generally, these tumors are **indolent and noninvasive.** Metastases to regional nodes, liver, and lung occur late in the disease. The 5-year survival rate is only 50%, but prolonged survival has been observed.

C.   **CLINICAL PRESENTATION**

1. Tumors are frequently detected by the **finding of hypercalcemia** during routine laboratory examination. On X-ray examination, over one-half of the patients show evidence of bony disease caused by increased bone resorption, which occurs with elevations in PTH levels.
2. Diagnosis is difficult because of the similarity of the presentation to that of benign parathyroid disorders.

D.   **DIAGNOSIS**

1. **Hypercalcemia** usually is present and leads to detection of a parathyroid tumor.
2. **Nuclear scanning, CT, and ultrasound** are the most useful methods in localizing a parathyroid mass.

E.   **TREATMENT**

1. Treatment consists of **en bloc resection** of abnormal parathyroid tissue and **ipsilateral neck dissection** if cervical nodes are involved. Recurrence is common.
2. Postoperative complications include **hypoparathyroidism, recurrent laryngeal nerve damage,** and **hemorrhage.** Temporary administration of calcium may be necessary to prevent tetany from hypoparathyroidism.

VI.   **MULTIPLE ENDOCRINE NEOPLASIA SYNDROMES**

1. Multiple endocrine neoplasia (MEN) is used to describe development of hyperplasia or neoplasia in multiple different endocrine glands or tissues. These disorders occur in distinct clinical patterns and are **characterized by familial inheritance of specific endocrine tumors.**
2. Identification of specific genetic abnormalities provides the basis for **screening family members.** Early detection and intervention minimize morbidity and mortality associated with these syndromes.

PRACTICE QUESTIONS

1. The clinical presentation of endocrine tumors depends on two factors. One is their anatomic location. The other is their
   (A) size and extension.
   (B) ability to produce excess hormone secretion.
   (C) origin in the embryonic tissue.
   (D) ability to concentrate iodine or other activating substances.

An elderly woman presents with a thyroid mass and symptoms of dyspnea and dysphagia. There is a history of goiter. Assessment indicates tumor invasion with metastases to the lung. **Answer questions 2–4 with this information in mind.**

2. What is the **most** likely diagnosis?
   (A) papillary carcinoma
   (B) follicular carcinoma
   (C) medullary carcinoma
   (D) anaplastic carcinoma

3. Assuming the primary tumor is resectable, what is the **most** likely treatment?
   (A) thyroid lobectomy
   (B) near-total thyroidectomy
   (C) total thyroidectomy
   (D) radiotherapy with ^{131}I

4. Symptoms of dyspnea and dysphagia in this patient are **most** likely to be the result of
   (A) involvement of the parathyroid gland and associated hypercalcemia.
   (B) compressive effects of the tumor on the larynx and esophagus.
   (C) infection caused by irritation of the oral mucosa.
   (D) a high concentration of iodine in the follicular cells of the thyroid.

5. ^{131}I radiotherapy is used to treat residual and metastatic disease in certain patients with well-differentiated thyroid cancer after surgical resection of the thyroid. It is also used in the treatment of thyroid tumors to
   (A) prevent hemorrhage that often occurs as a complication of thyroid surgery.
   (B) prevent damage to the parathyroid glands associated with hypoparathyroidism.
   (C) confirm a diagnosis of malignancy in papillary and medullary forms of thyroid carcinoma.
   (D) eradicate any remaining thyroid tissue left in the neck following surgery.

6. Which of the following statements about pituitary tumors is **incorrect?**
   (A) The cells of functional pituitary tumors typically fail to secrete their usual hormone(s).
   (B) Most pituitary tumors are histologically benign.
   (C) The most common manifestations of pituitary tumors are alterations in hormonal patterns and pressure symptoms from a growing tumor.
   (D) Microadenomas are more easily resected than macroadenomas.

7. A patient is being evaluated for a possible pituitary adenoma. In addition to the use of CT and MRI to help localize the suspected tumor and to determine its effect on adjacent structures, the diagnostician is **most** likely to use
   (A) fine-needle aspiration for the evaluation of discrete pituitary nodules.
   (B) radionuclide imaging for information regarding the ability of the tumor to concentrate iodine.
   (C) radioimmunoassay to determine if there is hypersecretion of pituitary hormones.
   (D) laboratory tests that allow determination of calcium levels in the blood and urine.

8. An important nursing intervention during the postoperative period following surgery for pituitary adenoma pertains to the operative site and involves
   (A) stimulation of salivary flow with hard candy to avert the problem of sialadenitis.
   (B) the administration of antiemetics to counteract the effects of radioisotopes.
   (C) oral inspection and meticulous mouth care to maintain integrity of the mucous membranes.
   (D) monitoring for signs of shock related to the profound decrease in available catecholamines.

9. Evidence of a functional tumor in the adrenal cortex comes from abnormally high levels of
   (A) catecholamines.
   (B) parathyroid hormone (PTH).
   (C) prolactin.
   (D) corticosteroids.

10. Detection of parathyroid tumors frequently occurs by the finding of
   (A) hoarseness and/or dysphagia during diagnostic evaluation.
   (B) high levels of glucocorticoids in blood immunoassays.
   (C) multicentric lesions in the bladder, bowel, and spleen.
   (D) hypercalcemia during routine laboratory examination.

ANSWER EXPLANATIONS

1. **The answer is (B).**   When tumors arise in endocrine tissue, the ability of these cells to perform their specific endocrine functions is altered. Even if they are not histologically malignant, they can produce significant morbidity and mortality by hyperplasia, in which the number of hormone-secreting cells increases, resulting in excess secretion of hormones, or by expansion, which may cause compression of vital structures. (985)

2. **The answer is (D).**   All evidence—age and sex of the patient, history of goiter, dyspnea and dysphagia as symptoms, presence of metastasis—point to anaplastic carcinoma of the thyroid as the likely disease. These carcinomas are among the most rapidly growing, lethal neoplasms, with death occurring within months

of diagnosis, regardless of therapy. Advanced papillary, follicular, or medullary carcinoma may also produce these signs and symptoms. (987)

3. **The answer is (A).** Patients with anaplastic carcinoma who have resectable lesions generally are treated with lobectomy, because more radical surgery results in increased complications and does not alter the outcome of the disease. In patients with unresectable lesions, palliative surgery is performed to debulk the tumor locally. Near-total and total thyroidectomy are more likely to be used in the treatment of well-differentiated thyroid carcinomas such as papillary and follicular carcinomas. (989–990)

4. **The answer is (B).** Because anaplastic carcinomas rapidly invade surrounding structures, symptoms may occur that are related to compressive effects of the enlarging mass on adjacent structures. Patients may experience dyspnea or stridor when the trachea is compressed or infiltrated. Compression of the esophagus may cause dysphagia. Hoarseness can result from malignant infiltration or destruction of the recurrent laryngeal or vagus nerves. (987)

5. **The answer is (D).** ^{131}I can be given for treatment and/or ablation after surgical resection. Ablation is done before treatment for the purpose of totally eradicating any remaining normal thyroid tissue left in the neck after near-total thyroidectomy. Even after total thyroidectomy, ablation optimizes the effectiveness of ^{131}I treatment so that the isotope will be concentrated in functional tumor tissue. (991)

6. **The answer is (A).** Pituitary adenomas are "malignant" by virtue of their ability to produce morbidity through growth in a confined space and mediation of hormonal dysfunction. Functional tumors will produce symptoms of hormonal excess, not hormonal deficit. The majority of these adenomas are well differentiated, and the cells retain their hormone-producing capabilities. They are, however, not subject to the normal regulatory mechanisms of the body and continue to produce hormones regardless of negative feedback from target organs. Expanding tumors will result in headache, visual disturbances, and functional impairment of cranial nerves. (992)

7. **The answer is (C).** The anatomic extent of the pituitary mass and its functional status can be determined with appropriate endocrine and neuroradiologic studies. Hypersecretion of pituitary hormones can be determined by means of radioimmunoassay, although elevated levels do not necessarily confirm the diagnosis of a pituitary adenoma. Magnetic resonance imaging (MRI) and CT scans provide more precise information regarding the physical location and characteristics of the tumor. (992–993)

8. **The answer is (C).** Because the incision in surgery for a pituitary adenoma is located in the upper gingiva, oral inspection and meticulous mouth care are instituted to maintain integrity of the mucous membranes and to prevent infection. In addition, sneezing and nose-blowing are contraindicated during this period to minimize pressure on the operative site. (994–995)

9. **The answer is (D).** The majority of cancers of the adrenal cortex are aggressive adenocarcinomas, with up to 90% of the patients having either locally advanced or metastatic disease. Patients with functional tumors will have hypersecretion of one or more of the adrenal cortex secretions—cortisol, aldosterone, progesterone, testosterone, and estradiol. The majority of functional tumors result in Cushing's disease, virilization and feminization syndromes, and hyperaldosteronism. Patients with nonfunctional tumors commonly have a palpable abdominal mass with associated abdominal or back pain. (996)

10. **The answer is (D).** Most parathyroid tumors are biochemically functional, causing clinical effects of hypercalcemia, with frequent mortality, from hypersecretion of parathyroid hormone (PTH). Parathyroid tumors are most frequently detected by the finding of hypercalcemia during routine laboratory examination. On X-ray examination, approximately one-half of the patients have evidence of bony disease caused by increased bone resorption, which occurs with elevations of PTH levels. (998)

41 Gastrointestinal Cancer: Esophagus, Stomach, Liver, and Pancreas

STUDY OUTLINE

I. INTRODUCTION

1. **The gastrointestinal (GI) system accounts for the highest incidence of malignant tumors, with the colorectal area the most frequent site.**
2. **Table 41-1, text page 1006,** demonstrates the percentage distribution of gastrointestinal tumors by sex; there is a bidirectional pattern in which incidence increases in men from the esophagus to the colon, whereas the opposite is true for women.
3. Tumors of the gastrointestinal tract are often **insidious in onset.** Early detection and diagnosis are difficult; many etiologic risk factors are nonspecific, making it difficult to identify individuals at high risk.
4. Most GI tumors are **adenocarcinomas,** with the exception of the esophagus and anus, where squamous cell carcinomas predominate.
5. The **metastatic spread** of GI tumors typically occurs by local spread, blood vessel invasion, and dissemination via the lymphatic system.
6. **Prognosis** depends on tumor site, tumor size, degree of cellular differentiation, extent of metastases, treatment efficacy, and the individual's general health status.

II. ESOPHAGEAL TUMORS

1. Esophageal tumors are often diagnosed late because the patient had mistakenly attributed the symptoms to indigestion or heartburn.
2. Accordingly, aggressive therapy is often too risky, and survival rates are poor.

III. EPIDEMIOLOGY

1. Esophageal cancer is uncommon, accounting for only **1%** of all forms of cancer. However, it has one of the poorest survival rates among malignant diseases, with **only 7% alive five years after diagnosis.**
2. Black men and women are affected more frequently than whites in the United States.
3. The **average age** of onset is 62 years, with most persons with the disease between 50 and 70 years of age.
4. No other tumor demonstrates such a marked difference according to **geographic location;** there are countries with 400 to 500 times the incidence of that in the United States.

IV. ETIOLOGY

1. Incidence by geographic location points to **nutritional and environmental factors.**
2. Individuals with esophageal cancer typically have a history of **heavy alcohol intake, heavy tobacco use,** and **poor nutrition.**
3. Conditions of **chronic irritation** have been cited as possible etiologic agents, including hiatal hernia, reflux esophagitis, and diverticula.
4. Persons with **untreated achalasia** have a sevenfold to eightfold greater risk of esophageal cancer.

5. Dietary deficiencies of certain mineral elements, including selenium, are considered risk factors for esophageal cancer.

V. PATHOPHYSIOLOGY

A. CELLULAR CHARACTERISTICS

1. **Squamous cell carcinoma (>85%) and adenocarcinoma (<10%) are the two major histologic types of esophageal cancer;** this distribution is reasonable in an organ lined almost entirely with squamous epithelium.
2. The **site** of esophageal tumors is an important factor in detection and prognosis. The distribution of esophageal cancer according to site is as follows:
   a. Cervical esophagus: 25%
   b. Upper thoracic esophagus: 50%
   c. Lower thoracic esophagus: 25%
3. Carcinoma of the esophagus may be grossly classified as **polypoid, ulcerative,** or **infiltrative.** Any of these types can compromise the patency of the esophagus.

B. PROGRESSION OF DISEASE

   a. **Squamous cell carcinomas often extend beyond the lumen wall to invade contiguous structures,** in about 60% of cases, preventing resection and negating surgical cure.
   b. Tumors of the esophagus **metastasize principally via the lymphatic system,** since the rich intramural plexus of lymphatic vessels and the lack of a serosal barrier permit early regional extension and dissemination before clinical signs appear.
   c. **Distant metastases by hematogenous spread** to the lungs, liver, adrenal glands, bone, brain, and kidney are common in advanced disease.

VI. CLINICAL MANIFESTATIONS

1. **The initial symptoms are often nonspecific,** including a vague sense of pressure, fullness, indigestion, and occasional substernal distress.
2. **Progressive dysphagia becomes a dominant symptom in almost 90% of cases.**
3. When tumor size exceeds a critical luminal circumference, saliva, food, and liquids may spill over into the lungs, causing **aspiration pneumonitis,** signalled by coughing and fever.
4. **Pain on swallowing** occurs in about 50% of patients with esophageal cancer.
5. A **weight loss** of 10%–20% of initial body weight is common.
6. Tumor involvement of the **recurrent laryngeal nerve** results in laryngeal paralysis and **hoarseness.**

VII. ASSESSMENT

1. The **diagnosis** of esophageal cancer depends on a thorough patient history with particular attention to the sequelae of symptoms and nutritional alterations.
2. The most definitive diagnostic procedures are routine and include special **radiologic examinations, endoscopic examinations, endoluminal ultrasound biopsy, cytologic examinations,** and **exploratory surgery.**

A. PHYSICAL EXAMINATION

1. Physical examination reveals few findings for the definitive diagnosis.

B. DIAGNOSTIC STUDIES

1. **Radiologic examination**
   a. **The double-contrast barium study** is useful for diagnosis, showing typical changes such as mucosal irregularity, displacement, narrowing, and stricture. The nurse should be certain that laxatives or an enema are given after the test to prevent a barium impaction.
   b. **CT scan** of the mediastinum and abdomen, liver scan, bone scan, and skeletal survey are usually indicated for staging.

2. **Endoscopy and biopsy**
   a. **Endoscopic visualization** plays an important role in the differential diagnosis of esophageal tumors.
   b. A diagnosis can be made by **cytologic study,** with brushings obtained during endoscopy, with an accuracy rate of 90%.
   c. Endoscopic ultrasound makes possible direct visualization of the tumor and determination of the depth of invasion and the presence of adenopathy.

VIII.   **CLASSIFICATION AND STAGING**

1. The aggressiveness of the therapeutic approach is based on an **evaluation of the individual** and the **extent to which the disease has progressed.**
2. **Table 41-2, text page 1009,** presents a standard classification system for esophageal tumors.

IX.   **TREATMENT**

A.   **TREATMENT PLANNING**

1. **Selection of the treatment plan**
   a. Careful **interdisciplinary planning** is needed to define the extent of the disease, to assess the individual's physiologic status, and to discuss alternatives completely with the individual.
   b. The most effective combination or sequence of therapies for esophageal cancer has yet to be established.
   c. In light of the nature of this disease and its poor prognosis, efforts are aimed at cure or palliation dependent on the extent of the disease.
   d. The optimal candidate for **curative treatment** should be free of concomitant renal, cardiac, and pulmonary disease; be relatively well nourished; and have a tumor that is localized, responsive, and accessible to treatment.
   e. **In cases of advanced disease, restoration or maintenance of a patent alimentary tract is the aim of therapy.**
   f. Certain findings usually preclude an individual from consideration for curative treatment, including fixed lymph nodes, a fixed tumor mass, extension of the tumor outside the esophagus, and recurrent laryngeal nerve involvement.
2. **Preparation for treatment**
   a. If an aggressive treatment plan has been selected, ideally the patient will undergo **supportive treatment** to improve general health and nutrition before the initiation of therapy.
   b. The degree of weight loss can be correlated with prognosis.
   c. Because of the high incidence of aspiration that occurs with esophageal cancer, **pulmonary hygiene** is a priority in pretreatment care. Expectorants, antibiotics, and bronchodilators can be used to facilitate pulmonary hygiene.
   d. The individual with a large esophageal tumor usually **cannot swallow saliva** and will drool or spit frequently, which may have a strong psychological impact. An acceptable method to control drooling (e.g., nearby basin, oral suction equipment) should be established.

B.   **RADIOTHERAPY**

1. **Esophageal squamous cell carcinoma is more responsive than adenocarcinoma to radiotherapy,** which can result in rapid relief of an obstruction and, used alone, is an excellent therapeutic alternative for a person who is debilitated or has advanced disease.
2. The most important factor in determining the appropriateness of radiotherapy is whether the patient is potentially curable or palliation is the only option.
   a. About 60% of cancers are beyond potential curability at diagnosis because of distant spread.
3. Radiotherapy is the treatment favored by many clinicians for stages I and II cervical esophageal lesions because surgical mortality with this location is so high and radiotherapy allows preservation of the larynx.
4. **Complications and side effects of radiotherapy** relate to tissue tolerance, site and amount of radiation, and adjuvant therapy but may include esophageal fistula, stricture, radiation pneumonitis, and skin reactions.

5. **Nursing management** should be aimed at
   a. Anticipating and preventing complications of the radiation therapy.
   b. Maintaining adequate nutritional intake.
   c. Minimizing the discomfort of esophageal and skin irritation.
6. **Preoperative radiotherapy**
   a. **Preoperative radiotherapy** can decrease tumor bulk, increase resectability rates, and permit individuals to swallow, leading to improved nutritional status and less surgical risk; it also can potentially eradicate local microscopic disease.
7. **Postoperative radiotherapy**
   a. **Postoperative radiotherapy** is administered to eradicate residual tumor cells in the area of the surgical site, as well as for local control in the case of unresectable tumors.
8. **Intracavity radiation**
   a. Intraluminal brachytherapy provides a therapeutic boost to the local area involved.

C. SURGERY

1. **Surgery is employed selectively for lesions at all three levels of the esophagus.**
2. **Curative surgery** attempts to eradicate the tumor and reestablish esophageal continuity, whereas **palliative surgery** may aim at maintaining esophageal patency.
3. **Indications for curative surgery** include satisfactory nutritional state, a resectable tumor without evidence of invasion of contiguous structures, no distant metastases, and no serious concomitant disease.
4. Surgery can be used alone or in combination with chemotherapy or radiotherapy.
5. Improved perioperative care measures have significantly reduced operative mortality.
6. **Surgical approaches**
   a. The surgical technique and approach to esophageal resection depend on the location of the tumor.
   b. Surgical approaches and reconstruction techniques used in curative surgery are illustrated in **Figures 41-2, 41-3,** and **41-4, text pages 1012–1014.**
   c. **Esophagectomy,** with complete removal of the adjacent lymph nodes, is the most widely accepted procedure for surgical resection aimed at cure.
7. **Special considerations: cervical esophagus**
   a. Tumors of the cervical esophagus are the least common.
   b. Resection of cervical esophagus lesions involves removing all or part of the pharynx, larynx, thyroid, and proximal esophagus, and **pharyngogastrostomy** is the reconstructive procedure of choice.
   c. Postoperative mortality ranges from 3% to 26%.
8. **Postoperative care**
   a. **Respiratory complications** (severe atelectasis, pneumonia, respiratory failure, and pulmonary edema), fistulae, and **anastomotic leaks** comprise the bulk of complications after surgical resection for esophageal cancer.
      (1) Because the esophagus is thin-walled and drawn upward with each swallow, an **anastomosis** involving the esophagus has more of a tendency toward dehiscence and anastomotic leak than any other area of the GI tract.
      (2) Fever or pain is usually the earliest sign of dehiscence and leak.
      (3) Six or seven days after surgery a limited barium swallow is done to evaluate anastomotic healing.
   b. Virulent mouth organisms and overgrowth of pathogenic bacteria on ulcerating lesions may be the source of wound and intracavitary **infections.**
   c. The **postoperative nursing care** of the person with an esophagogastrectomy includes anticipation and prevention of reflux aspiration. **Suture lines** should be monitored for signs of inflammation, edema, and fistula formation.

D. CHEMOTHERAPY

1. Chemotherapy in the treatment of esophageal tumor has assumed an increasingly important role.
2. Combination regimens are more effective than single-agent therapy.
3. **Preoperative chemoradiation,** using combination chemotherapy (5-FU, cisplatin) and radiation of 3000 cGy to 5000 cGy, allows an attack on both local and systemic disease simultaneously.

E.   **PALLIATIVE THERAPY**

1.   The objective of palliative therapy, usually radiation therapy, is to relieve the distressing symptoms of esophageal cancer, particularly **progressive dysphagia,** which occurs in about 90% of patients with advanced disease.

2.   A number of **synthetic endoesophageal prosthetic tubes** have been designed to create an open passage for swallowing when the esophagus is obstructed by tumor.
     a.   **Esophageal perforation** is a complication that occurs in about 5% to 10% of patients.
     b.   **Increased food intake** occurs in about 80% of patients after tube placement.
     c.   With the prosthesis in place, reflux of gastric contents can lead to **aspiration pneumonia.**

3.   **Laser therapy** is used to reduce esophageal stricture caused by tumor.

4.   **Gastrostomy** and **jejunostomy** are alternative palliative procedures, but while allowing nutritional maintenance, they do not relieve the debilitating problem of inability to swallow saliva.

X.   **STOMACH TUMORS**

1.   In the United States, the incidence of gastric cancer has declined progressively since 1930, when it was the leading cause of cancer mortality.

2.   Stomach cancer is **insidious in onset and development,** and can be disseminated widely before overt signs are manifested.

3.   Overall **5-year survival rates** range from 16% to 92%.

4.   Inappropriate use of home remedies and self-medication for GI maladies and misdiagnosis are major hurdles to overcome in early detection.

XI.   **EPIDEMIOLOGY**

1.   Japan has the highest incidence of gastric cancer in the world.

2.   U.S. statistics reflect a 65% decrease in incidence within the past 35 years, with the greatest decline occurring among white persons.

XII.   **ETIOLOGY**

1.   Factors that are believed to contribute to or that are associated with gastric cancer are largely **environmental** and **genetic.** The various possible risk factors for gastric cancer are listed on **text page 1017,** column 2, and include **nutrition, pernicious anemia, achlorhydria, polyps, and family history.**

XIII.   **PATHOPHYSIOLOGY**

A.   **CELLULAR CHARACTERISTICS**

1.   Ninety percent of all gastric cancers are predominantly adenocarcinomas.

2.   Most gastric cancers arise in the antrum, the lower third of the stomach.

B.   **PROGRESSION OF DISEASE**

1.   **Gastric cancer is usually advanced when symptoms appear.**

2.   Gastric cancer **metastasizes** by several routes.
     a.   By extension and infiltration along the mucosal surface and stomach wall or lymphatic vessels.
     b.   Via lymphatic or vascular embolism.
     c.   By direct extension into adjacent structures such as the pancreas, liver, or esophagus.
     d.   By hematogenous spread.

3.   The pattern of metastatic spread correlates with the size and location of the tumor.

4.   Distant metastatic sites are the lung, adrenal glands, bone, liver, and peritoneal cavity.

XIV.   **CLINICAL MANIFESTATIONS**

1.   The **early symptoms** of gastric cancer include a vague, uneasy sense of fullness, a feeling of heaviness, and moderate distention after meals. **Pain in the epigastric, back, or retrosternal area** is often an early symptom that is ignored.

2.   As the disease advances, **progressive weight loss** results from anorexia, nausea, and vomiting.

XV.   **ASSESSMENT**

      A.   **PATIENT AND FAMILY HISTORY**

           1.   Areas to be included in a **nutritional history/assessment** include **food patterns, symptoms associated with eating, dietary changes, weight, bowel habits, medications, and previous/ concurrent illnesses.**

      B.   **PHYSICAL EXAMINATION**

           1.   The physical examination includes palpation of the abdomen and lymph nodes, particularly the supraclavicular and axillary lymph nodes because they are possible metastatic sites.
           2.   Englarged lymph nodes and hepatomegaly indicate the need for a biopsy.
           3.   Advanced gastric cancer can result in **anemia** and **jaundice.**

      C.   **DIAGNOSTIC STUDIES**

           1.   An **upper gastrointestinal series** will reveal the mucosal pattern, character of mobility, distensibility, and flexibility of the walls.
           2.   **CT scan** is useful in defining metastases and tumor extension.
           3.   Accuracy of diagnosis is enhanced by **endoscopic gastroscopy** to view the lesion directly and to obtain washings for cytologic examination.
           4.   Laboratory analyses may reveal anemia resulting from gradual blood loss.

XVI.   **CLASSIFICATION AND STAGING**

           1.   **Table 41-3, text page 1019,** illustrates the TNM classification system for staging gastric cancer.
           2.   The prognosis and treatment plan depend on the stage of the disease and on the general well-being of the individual.

XVII.   **TREATMENT**

           1.   **Localized gastric carcinomas** are treated with curative intent with aggressive surgery alone or in combination with chemotherapy or radiotherapy. Approximately 50% of patients are candidates for curative resection.
           2.   **Advanced tumors** are treated with combination therapy, including palliative surgery.

      A.   **SURGERY**

           1.   Operability rates are high, usually around 80%, whereas resectability rates are lower, around 60%.
           2.   **Total gastrectomy**
               a.   If the lesion is located in the midportion of the stomach, the entire stomach is removed en bloc, along with supporting mesentery and lymph nodes, and the esophagus is anastomosed to the jejunum.
               b.   Overall mortality rates are 10% to 15%.
           3.   **Radical subtotal gastrectomy**
               a.   Lesions located in the middle and distal half of the stomach are treated preferentially with a **Billroth II** resection, which involves removal of the antrum, pylorus, first portion of the duodenum, and all visible and palpable lymph nodes; the remaining stomach is anastomosed end-to-side to the jejunum.
               b.   **Gastric emptying** is altered by this procedure, resulting in dumping syndrome, steatorrhea, vitamin deficiency, diarrhea, nausea, and vomiting.
           4.   **Subtotal esophagogastrectomy**
               a.   If a resectable tumor is located in the proximal portion of the stomach, cardia, or fundus, a subtotal esophagogastrectomy is performed and the esophagus is anastomosed to the duodenum or jejunum.
           5.   **Postoperative care**
               a.   **Pneumonia, infection, anastomotic leak, hemorrhage, and reflux aspiration are frequent complications of radical gastric surgery.**

      b. **Dumping syndrome** may occur and requires small, frequent feedings of low carbohydrate, high-fat, high-protein foods and fluid restriction for 30 to 40 minutes before and after meals.

      c. **Vitamin B12 deficiency** usually occurs with monthly parenteral replacement required.

B. RADIATION THERAPY

1. Since gastric adenocarcinomas are **radiosensitive,** radiotherapy is useful for the treatment of locally advanced, recurrent, or unresectable disease.
2. In the abdomen there are dose-limiting organs such as the liver, kidney, and spinal cord which may restrict the use of radiotherapy.
3. Intraoperative radiotherapy has been used most extensively in Japan.

C. CHEMOTHERAPY

1. No one specific chemotherapeutic regimen for gastric cancer has had a clear impact on survival, and objective response rates are low.
2. The combination regimens used most commonly are 5-FU, doxorubicin, and mitomycin C and etopside, doxorubicin, and asplatin.

D. SUPPORTIVE THERAPY

1. As gastric cancer progresses, **nutrition** becomes a serious problem, either because of disruption of gastric continuity or gastric dysfunction; nutritional maintenance is a high nursing priority.
2. Individuals with gastric cancer commonly die of **bronchopneumonia** as a result of malnutrition or immobility.

XVIII. LIVER CANCER

1. Liver cancer is one of the leading causes of death from cancer in Africa and Asia. It is also frequently associated with **cirrhosis.**

XIX. EPIDEMIOLOGY

1. An unusual epidemiologic aspect of liver cancer is its geographic distribution.
2. The average age of onset is 60 to 70 years.

XX. ETIOLOGY

1. Hepatocellular carcinomas are associated with alcohol-induced, nutritional, and posthepatitic **cirrhosis** of the liver, possibly due to the chronic liver injury and continuous regeneration involved in that condition.
2. **Malnutrition** has been cited as an etiologic factor.
3. **Aflatoxins** and mycotoxins derived from the fungi *Aspergillus flavus* and *A. parasiticus*, are thought to be etiologic agents.
4. An increased incidence of liver damage and liver tumors has been reported among industrial employees who work with **vinyl chloride.**

XXI. PATHOPHYSIOLOGY

A. CELLULAR CHARACTERISTICS

1. **Primary liver carcinoma**
   a. Most primary malignant tumors of the liver are adenocarcinomas of two major cell types.
      (1) Ninety percent are **hepatocellular** carcinomas arising from liver cells.
      (2) Seven percent are **cholangiocarcinomas** arising from the bile duct cells.
   b. Hepatocellular tumors originate mainly in the right lobe, and infiltration of the diaphragm and invasion of the portal and hepatic veins may occur.
   c. Cholangiocarcinoma tends to invade surrounding parenchyma and metastasizes late.

        d. **Liver tumors often are well-differentiated tumors that resemble the tissue of origin.**

        e. About 50% of patients with primary liver cancer will not develop extrahepatic spread of tumor.

     2. **Secondary liver carcinoma**

        a. A tumor in the liver is 20 times more likely to be a metastatic deposit than a primary liver cancer and usually indicates that the primary tumor is incurable.

        b. Two patterns of secondary liver carcinoma predominate:

           (1) Invasive growth from neighboring organs or structures.

           (2) Metastasis through the portal veins.

B. PROGRESSION OF DISEASE

1. Liver cancer advances by **direct extension** within and around the liver.
2. About 50% of persons with liver cancer will have **distant metastases** to lungs, regional lymph nodes, bone, adrenal glands, and brain.
3. **Portal vein occlusion is common.**
4. **Liver failure and hemorrhage** have been cited as the cause of death in about 50% of individuals with liver cancer.
5. Esophageal varices and unrelenting ascites are common sequelae of liver cancer.
6. Overall 5-year survival is about 5%; death usually occurs within 6–8 weeks following diagnosis if the disease is not treated.

XXII. CLINICAL MANIFESTATIONS

1. The most common clinical manifestation is **dull, aching pain** which is confined to the **right upper quadrant,** although pain may radiate to the right scapula.
2. Other symptoms include **profound, progressive weakness, fullness in the epigastrium, fatigue, constipation or diarrhea,** and anorexia and weight loss.
3. Mild **jaundice** is present is some cases.
4. **Cirrhosis** is found in 30% to 70% of persons with hepatocellular carcinoma.

XXIII. ASSESSMENT

1. Since the only definitive diagnostic tool is tissue diagnosis and the risk of hemorrhage following needle biopsy is significant, noninvasive measures are relied on heavily.

A. PHYSICAL EXAMINATION

1. A physical examination usually reveals a painful, enlarged liver, ascites, edema, esophageal varices, jaundice, circulatory disorders, or hematemesis.

B. DIAGNOSTIC STUDIES

1. A simple **radiograph** of the abdomen may establish hepatomegaly and displacement deformity of contiguous structures.
2. Ultrasound can detect masses and help determine the extent of invasion of the vasculature of the liver.
3. **CT,** particularly with contrast, is able to demonstrate small lesions and vascular rearrangements.
4. **Radionuclide scanning** is an effective noninvasive technique for outlining primary and metastatic lesions of the liver.
5. **Selective hepatic arteriography** is the single most useful procedure for identifying the tumor's vasculature prior to hepatic resection.
6. **Laboratory studies**

        a. In the absence of cirrhosis, tumor growth can extensively involve parenchyma before liver function is impaired.

        b. Liver enzyme levels and liver function tests are not definitive diagnostic tests but can alert the clinician to a possible liver tumor.

        c. **Alpha-fetoprotein** is a tumor marker that is elevated in the serum of 70% to 90% of persons with primary hepatocellular carcinoma.

        d. Serum alpha-L-fucosidose is a new serum marker being investigated with liver cancer.

7. **Biopsy**
    a. Biopsy, commonly ultrasound-guided **percutaneous needle biopsy,** is required to establish a histologically verified diagnosis.
    b. Because most liver tumors are highly vascular, the individual must be monitored closely for intra-abdominal hemorrhage after needle biopsy.

XXIV. **STAGING**

1. **Table 41-4, text page 1025,** presents a staging system for liver cancer that incorporates tumor size, location within the liver, extent of disease within and external to the liver, and metastatic sites.

XXV. **TREATMENT**

A. **TREATMENT PLANNING**

1. For individuals with solitary localized liver cancer, advances in surgery, radiotherapy, and chemotherapy offer hope of cure or extended control.
2. The **choice of treatment** depends on such factors as type and extent of the tumor, concomitant diseases, liver function and reserve, age, hematologic status, nutritional status, and patient and family preference.
3. **Pretreatment therapy**
    a. **Anemia** is common and must be addressed.
    b. **Deficits in clotting mechanisms** may exist and vitamin K may be administered.
    c. The **pruritus** which frequently accompanies jaundice may be treated with local measures such as meticulous skin hygiene, application of oil-based lotions, and administration of antihistamines.
    d. **Nutritional status** must be corrected. Individuals can benefit from a diet high in proteins and carbohydrates and low in fats.
4. **Objectives of treatment**
    a. **Primary liver cancer**
        (1) **Cure is the objective if the tumor is a localized, solitary mass without evidence of regional lymph node involvement, or distant metastasis.**
        (2) Only about 25% of patients are candidates for radical resection. In other cases, **control** or **palliation** are the treatment objectives.
    b. **Secondary liver tumors**
        (1) **Aggressive therapy** is employed if the metastatic deposit is a solitary or well-defined mass in a single lobe of the liver.
        (2) The aim of aggressive treatment of metastatic tumors in the liver is to control the tumor, increase survival time, and palliate debilitating symptoms such as jaundice, anemia, and pain.

B. **SURGERY**

1. **Surgical excision is the most definitive treatment for primary liver tumors;** from 80% to 85% of the noncirrhotic liver can be safely removed.
2. **Contraindications to major hepatic resection** include
    a. Severe cirrhosis.
    b. Distant metastases.
    c. Multiple discrete tumor nodules throughout both lobes.
    d. Ascites, which usually indicates liver failure.
    e. Jaundice, which may indicate obstruction of the common bile duct.
    f. Poor visualization on angiographic studies.
    g. Involvement of the inferior vena cava.
    h. Biochemical changes that indicate poor liver function.
3. **Postoperative care**
    a. Overall surgical mortality (individuals who do not survive the hospitalization period) is less than 15% with hepatic resection.
    b. The **major complications after liver resection** include hemorrhage, biliary fistula, infection, subphrenic abscess, pneumonia and atelectasis, transient metabolic consequences, portal hypertension, and clotting defects.

4. **Postoperative complications**
   a. **Hemorrhage**
      (1) Hemorrhage will usually appear in the first 24 hours following surgery.
      (2) Nursing observations and assessments should include CVP monitoring; examination of the skin and extremities for perfusion; accurate measurement of abdominal girth; frequent checks for bleeding from incision sites, urine, and stool; and close attention to fluid and electrolyte levels and blood profiles.
   b. **Biliary fistula**
      (1) An **excessive drainage of bile** through the subhepatic drain placed in the area of the surgical resection could indicate a biliary fistula pouring large amounts of bile into the subhepatic space.
   c. **Subphrenic abscess**
      (1) Incomplete or **insufficient drainage** of the surgical defect can precipitate a subphrenic abscess.
      (2) Development of sharp, piercing, right upper quadrant **pain** later in the postoperative course and a low-grade fever are other warning signs.
   d. **Infection**
      (1) Individuals with cirrhosis are more prone to infection following hepatic resection than individuals without cirrhosis.
      (2) Frequent monitoring of vital signs and assessment of the wound and drainage will provide early clues of impending infection.
   e. **Pneumonia and atelectasis**
      (1) Early ambulation, administration of analgesics prior to pulmonary exercise, incisional support, and avoidance of contact with persons with respiratory infections are important nursing care measures.
   f. **Transient metabolic consequences**
      (1) Jaundice is common during the first postoperative week, possibly resulting from temporary inability of the remaining liver to handle bile, but the condition usually subsides by the third week.

C. CHEMOTHERAPY

1. Chemotherapy may be used as the treatment of choice for unresectable liver tumors.
2. **Systemic administration** of chemotherapy has utilized combinations of agents, including doxorubicin, mitomycin C, and 5-FU.
3. **Regional infusion of chemotherapy via the hepatic artery or portal vein is considered superior to systemic chemotherapy.**
   a. The premise on which regional therapy is based is **the ability to provide a high concentration of drug to the tumor with minimal systemic exposure.**
   b. In regional therapy, catheters are placed into specifically defined vessels that have been identified as the major source of blood supply to the tumor, and drug is delivered by totally implantable pumps or continuous infusion pumps.

D. RADIOTHERAPY

1. A recent development to enhance the effectiveness of radiation therapy without damage to the normal parenchyma is the use of ^{131}I-Lipidiol, a radiolabeled iodinated contrast medium.
2. In conjunction with surgery or chemotherapy, radiotherapy is used to **palliate symptoms** or to **eradicate micrometastases.**
3. The major side effects of radiotherapy to the liver are nausea, vomiting, anorexia, and fatigue.

E. SUPPORTIVE THERAPY

1. **Pain** is one of the most difficult problems to manage; in later stages, it is severe, worsens at night, and radiates to the right scapular area.
2. Palliative measures for **ascites** include fluid and sodium restriction, diuretic therapy, paracentesis, or albumin administration.
3. **Anticipatory management** of the rapidly developing symptoms and patient and family support are the major goals of nursing care in advanced disease.

XXVI. **PANCREATIC CANCER**

1. **The onset of pancreatic cancer is insidious, with signs and symptoms that occur late, are vague and misleading, and mimic other diseases.**
2. Fewer than 5% of individuals with pancreatic cancer are alive at 5 years.

XXVII. **EPIDEMIOLOGY**

1. Pancreatic cancer comprises approximately **2%** of all cancers in American men and women. Peak incidence occurs between the ages of 60 to 70 years.
2. In the United States extensive studies have been done to correlate incidence with geography, with some evidence for **clustering.**

XXVIII. **ETIOLOGY**

1. Possible factors implicated in pancreatic cancer include **tobacco smoking, certain industrial pollutants, high-fat diets, alcohol abuse, diabetes, chronic pancreatitis, and a history of peptic ulcer surgery.**

XXIX. **PATHOPHYSIOLOGY**

1. Tumors in the pancreas develop in both the exocrine and endocrine parenchyma.
2. Approximately 95% of pancreatic tumors arise from the exocrine parenchyma, and adenocarcinoma of ductal cell origin is the predominant morphologic type.

A. **CELLULAR CHARACTERISTICS**

1. Cancer most commonly arises in the proximal areas of the gland, which includes the head, neck, and uncinate process.
2. Adenocarcinomas commonly invade the entire pancreas, obliterate the lobulated tissue, and obstruct the common bile duct and Wirsung's canal.
3. Although uncommon (<5% of pancreatic tumors), **islet cell tumors** can arise from the **endocrine parenchyma** and are usually well vascularized, encapsulated, and compress adjacent parenchyma.

B. **PROGRESSION OF DISEASE**

1. At the time of diagnosis, pancreatic tumors have invaded locally or metastasized in 90% of patients. Tumor growth frequently extends to the common bile duct and celiac nerve plexus.
2. **Metastatic spread** involves regional lymph nodes, the liver, peritoneal seeding, the lung, pleura, adrenal glands, and bone.
3. Individuals with advanced pancreatic cancer usually die in a short time of **cachexia, infection,** or **liver failure. Eighty-five percent of those diagnosed with pancreatic cancer die within 1 year of diagnosis.**

XXX. **CLINICAL MANIFESTATIONS**

1. Manifestations of the disease differ according to the location of the tumor in the pancreas.

A. **HEAD OF THE PANCREAS**

1. A **classic triad of symptoms** is apparent with cancer of the head of the pancreas: **pain, profound weight loss,** and **progressive jaundice.**
   a. The **pain** is usually in the epigastric region. It is dull and intermittent in nature, and may be attributed to indigestion. Often, however, it is continuous and radiates to the right upper quadrant of the abdomen or to the dorsolumbar area. The intensity of the pain is affected by eating, activity, and posture.
   b. As the disease advances, **weight loss** of 20 to 30 pounds in a few weeks is common.
      (1) Tumor involvement prevents the secretion of digestive enzymes and diminishes insulin production.
      (2) Malabsorption can lead to diarrhea, steatorrhea, and weakness.

      c. **Jaundice,** which is precipitated by common bile duct obstruction, is the presenting symptom in 80% to 90% of cases of cancer of the head of the pancreas. The evolution of jaundice in pancreatic cancer follows a distinctive pattern.

B. BODY OF THE PANCREAS

1. Severe **epigastric pain** usually is the first and predominant symptom, occurring 3 to 4 hours after a meal, and is often accompanied by **vomiting.**
2. Relief of the pain is brought about by assuming certain positions.
3. Jaundice rarely occurs.

C. TAIL OF THE PANCREAS

1. Metastases may cause the first symptoms.
2. Although pain is not encountered as often as with tumors of the head and body of the pancreas, upper abdominal pain may occur, radiating to the back left hypochondrial area.

XXXI. ASSESSMENT

A. PHYSICAL EXAMINATION

1. In many persons with cancer of the head of the pancreas, physical examination may demonstrate an **enlarged gall bladder** and a **palpable, smooth liver.**
2. With tumors of the body and tail, a **hard, well-defined mass** may be palpated in the subumbilical or left hypochondrial region.

B. DIAGNOSTIC STUDIES

1. **Radiologic examination**
   a. **Abdominal ultrasonographic examination** or **CT scans** are useful initial diagnostic tests.
   b. **Endoscopic retrograde cholangiopancreatography** allows specimens for biopsy and cytologic examination to be obtained.
2. **Laboratory tests**
   a. The use of laboratory tests is limited because early disease produces few alterations that laboratory tests definitively demonstrate.
   b. Some useful laboratory tests include bilirubin, transaminase levels, serum and urine amylase levels, prothrombin time, plasma insulin immunoassay, and fasting blood glucose levels.
   c. The DNA content of pancreatic tumors is being studied to determine if the ploidy characteristics could be used as prognostic indicators to guide the aggressiveness of therapeutic interventions.
3. **Tumor markers**
   a. **CEA,** the carbohydrate **CA 19-9,** and **pancreatic oncofetal antigen (POA)** are the tumor-associated antigens being studied in relation to pancreatic cancer.

XXXII. CLASSIFICATION AND STAGING

1. **Table 41-5, text page 1033,** illustrates the stage and classification system being used by the Cancer of the Pancreas Task Force of the American Joint Committee on Cancer.

XXXIII. TREATMENT

A. TREATMENT PLANNING

1. **Surgery** offers the only hope for cure, and is used if the tumor is localized and not fixed to other structures, and if there is no evidence of regional or distant metastases.
2. Approximately 40% to 70% of all cases of pancreatic cancer are diagnosed when the tumor is unresectable; **palliation** will be the goal with surgical bypass procedures, radiotherapy, or chemotherapy.

B. **SURGERY**

1. In recent years, reports of increasing survival periods following resection have been encouraging, particularly when the patients are stratified according to extent of disease.
2. The surgical approaches most used for pancreatic cancer when cure is the objective are **total pancreatectomy** and **pancreatoduodenectomy (Whipple procedure).**
3. **Table 41-6, text page 1034,** provides a comparison of the various types of pancreatic resections used for pancreatic malignancies.
4. **Overall surgical mortality rates range from 10% to 50%.**
5. **Total pancreatectomy**
   a. **The total pancreatectomy** is an extensive en bloc resection and is illustrated in **Figure 39-6, text page 838.**
6. **Pancreatoduodenal resection**
   a. The **pancreatoduodenectomy (Whipple procedure)** is illustrated in **Figure 39-7, text page 838.**
7. **Regional pancreatectomy**
   a. This is an extensive en bloc surgery that includes the entire pancreas; duodenum; gastric antrum, bile duct, gallbladder, spleen, the parapancreatic celiac, and mesenteric nodes; and a sleeve resection of the portal vein.
8. **Distal pancreatectomy**
   a. In rare cases, tumors of the body or tail of the pancreas are detected early enough to be considered curable, and a **distal pancreatectomy** is performed.
9. **Palliative surgical procedures**
   a. **Palliative surgical procedures** are used to remove tumor, relieve jaundice and obstruction, and decompress or bypass involved organs such as the duodenum or biliary tract.
10. **Postoperative care**
    a. In the immediate postoperative period, **hemorrhage, hypovolemia** (due to fluid loss and third spacing), **hypotension** (due to severance of the sympathetic nerve fibers of the mesenteric complex), **fistula, infections,** and **anastomotic leak** pose the greatest threats.
    b. **Endocrine function** most often is altered by resection of the head of the pancreas; most individuals can be controlled with a daily dose of NPH insulin and a sliding scale of insulin dosages.
    c. Alteration of the **exocrine function** results in a **malabsorption syndrome** that is characterized by an inability to use ingested forms of fat and protein.
       (1) **Pancreatic enzymes are replaced with oral enzyme supplements** such as pancreatin or pancrelipase, containing lipase, amylase, and trypsin.
       (2) After a pancreatectomy, patients are placed on a **diet of bland, low-fat foods that are high in carbohydrate and protein.**
       (3) Several small feedings are better tolerated than large meals.
       (4) Restrictions include overindulgence, caffeine, and alcohol.
       (5) The **stool** should be examined daily for the characteristic signs of **steatorrhea:** frothy, foul-smelling stool with fat particles floating on the water.

C. **CHEMOTHERAPY**

1. The high rate of mortality associated with metastatic disease indicates that systemic therapy is needed, but current applications of chemotherapy have failed to produce significant results.
2. The combination regimens most often used include streptozocin, mitomycin C, 5-FU, and doxorubicin.
3. Chemotherapy alone has made no significant difference in survival, although it has provided **palliation of pain** in some cases.

D. **RADIOTHERAPY**

1. External radiation has been used for both palliative and curative therapy of pancreatic cancer. **Local control of tumor growth** and **relief of debilitating symptoms** are accomplished in about 40% of individuals.
2. The **major limitation to radiotherapy** appears to be the large volume of tumor that is usually present at diagnosis.

3. The average survival time with radiotherapy alone is 6 months, but with combination radio-therapy and chemotherapy it is 11 months.
4. It is postulated that chemotherapy may reduce tumor burden and act as a radiation sensitizer, increasing the impact of radiotherapy.

E. **SUPPORTIVE THERAPY**

1. **Relief of pain** is a primary objective since pancreatic tumors usually invade the celiac plexus and cause excruciating pain.
2. As a result of obstruction, **nutritional support** is a serious problem.
3. **Jaundice** can cause pruritus and dry, friable skin. **Cholestyramine,** which combines with and promotes excretion of excess bile acids, may provide some relief of pruritus.
4. Nonsurgical procedures, such as percutaneous transhepatic biliary drainage or endoscopic endoprosthesis placement, may be used to relieve obstructive jaundice.

PRACTICE QUESTIONS

1. In the United States, the highest incidence of esophageal cancer is found among
    (A) women aged 29 to 39 years.
    (B) black men.
    (C) perimenopausal women.
    (D) men aged 30 to 40 years.

2. Individuals with esophageal cancer typically have a history of
    (A) occupational exposure to radiation.
    (B) obesity.
    (C) oral contraceptive use.
    (D) heavy alcohol intake.

3. Which of the following conditions usually precludes an individual with esophageal cancer from consideration for curative treatment?
    (A) extension of the tumor outside of the esophagus
    (B) excessive weight loss (i.e., >25% of ideal body weight)
    (C) age greater than 65 years
    (D) tumor location in the cervical esophagus

4. Individuals with esophageal cancer are considered at high risk for the development of
    (A) other gastrointestinal cancers.
    (B) superior vena cava syndrome.
    (C) aspiration pneumonia.
    (D) xerostomia.

5. Complications and side effects of radiotherapy for esophageal cancer include all of the following **except**
    (A) esophageal stricture.
    (B) radiation pneumonitis.
    (C) skin reaction.
    (D) diarrhea.

6. Approximately a week after surgery for esophageal cancer, a modified barium swallow is likely to be done to check for
    (A) local edema.
    (B) any signs of residual tumor.
    (C) anastomotic leaks.
    (D) swallowing ability.

7. Early detection of gastric cancer is unlikely because
    (A) the cancer metastasizes readily.
    (B) people tend to self-medicate themselves for gastrointestinal distress.
    (C) risk factors for the disease have not yet been identified.
    (D) none of the diagnostic tests or procedures currently available accurately detect gastric cancer in its early stages.

8. The country with the highest incidence of gastric cancer is
    (A)   Japan.
    (B)   China.
    (C)   England.
    (D)   the United States.

9. The use of radiotherapy in the treatment of gastric cancer is limited by the
    (A)   radiosensitivity of the tumor.
    (B)   close proximity of the liver, kidneys, and spinal cord.
    (C)   severity of the side effects experienced.
    (D)   size of the tumor mass.

10. Liver cancer is often associated with
    (A)   a long smoking history.
    (B)   obesity.
    (C)   cirrhosis.
    (D)   a bacterial infection.

11. The majority of tumors of the liver are
    (A)   nodular hepatocellular tumors.
    (B)   cholangiocarcinomas.
    (C)   hepatoblastomas.
    (D)   metastases from other malignancies.

12. One of the common sequela of liver cancer is
    (A)   esophageal varices.
    (B)   visual disturbances.
    (C)   fat intolerance.
    (D)   urinary retention.

13. A liver tumor may be suspected if laboratory tests reveal elevated levels of
    (A)   gastrin.
    (B)   cholesterol.
    (C)   alpha-fetoprotein.
    (D)   amylase.

14. The individual who has recently had an ultrasound-guided percutaneous needle biopsy of the liver must be monitored closely for symptoms of
    (A)   spinal cord compression.
    (B)   hematemesis.
    (C)   headache.
    (D)   hemorrhage.

15. Nursing care of the client with liver cancer involves
    (A)   meticulous skin care for pruritis.
    (B)   providing a low-protein, high-fat diet.
    (C)   continuous administration of anticoagulants.
    (D)   assistance with an abdominal binder.

16. All of the following are possible contraindications to hepatic resection for liver cancer **except**
    (A)   jaundice.
    (B)   severe cirrhosis.
    (C)   chemotherapy failure.
    (D)   ascites.

17. Ideally, chemotherapy for liver cancer is administered via hepatic artery or
    (A)   portal vein.
    (B)   subclavian artery.
    (C)   inferior vena cava.
    (D)   jugular vein.

18. Peak incidence for the occurrence of pancreatic cancer is between the ages of
    (A) 20 and 30.
    (B) 30 and 40.
    (C) 50 and 60.
    (D) 60 and 70.

19. Individuals with pancreatic cancer generally die within _____ year(s) of _____ .
    (A) one; hemorrhage or infection
    (B) two; liver failure or hemorrhage
    (C) one; cachexia, infection or liver failure
    (D) three; infection or renal failure

20. The three classic signs of a pancreatic tumor located in the head of the pancreas are progressive jaundice, profound weight loss, and
    (A) pain.
    (B) projectile vomiting.
    (C) confusion.
    (D) hyperkalemia.

21. The treatment of choice of pancreatic cancer, and the treatment presently offering the only hope for cure, is
    (A) systemic chemotherapy.
    (B) intra-arterial chemotherapy.
    (C) surgery.
    (D) radiotherapy.

22. Postoperative care of an individual who has undergone palliative surgery for pancreatic cancer includes all of the following **except**
    (A) administration of pancreatic enzyme supplements.
    (B) providing a diet that is low in fat, high in protein, and includes a glass of red wine with lunch and dinner.
    (C) observing for hemorrhage, hypovolemia, and hypotension.
    (D) examining stools for steatorrhea.

ANSWER EXPLANATIONS

1. **The answer is (B).**   In the United States, black men have a significantly higher incidence of esophageal cancer than white men; similarly, black women have a higher incidence of the disease than white women. This type of cancer also seems to develop at a younger age in black persons than it does in white persons. (1006)

2. **The answer is (D).**   Esophageal cancer appears to be associated with heavy alcohol intake, heavy tobacco use, and poor nutrition; cirrhosis, vitamin deficiency, anemia, and poor oral hygiene may be contributing factors. (1006)

3. **The answer is (A).**   The findings that usually preclude an individual from consideration for curative treatment are: (1) fixed lymph nodes; (2) fixed tumor mass; (3) extension of the tumor outside of the esophagus; and (4) recurrent laryngeal nerve involvement. A combination of surgery, radiotherapy, and/or chemotherapy appears to offer the greatest hope of cure, although the most effective combination or sequence has yet to be established. (1009)

4. **The answer is (C).**   When an esophageal tumor gets so large that it causes saliva, food, and liquids to spill over into the lungs, affected individuals are at high risk for the development of aspiration pneumonia. Because of this potential, pulmonary hygiene and aspiration precautions should be a focus of nursing care for the person with esophageal cancer. (1007, 1010)

5. **The answer is (D).**   Esophageal fistula, stricture, hemorrhage, radiation pneumonitis, and pericarditis are all possible complications of radiotherapy for esophageal cancer. Side effects to be expected are swallowing difficulties, including burning, pain, dryness, and skin reactions. (1010)

6. **The answer is (C).**   Because the esophagus is thin-walled and draws upward with each swallow, an anastomosis involving the esophagus has more of a tendency to leak than any other area of the gastrointestinal tract. It is for this reason that a barium swallow is performed 6 to 7 days after surgery to check for patency of the anastomosis. Small leaks usually close spontaneously; larger leaks often require surgical approximation. (1013)

7. **The answer is (B).**   The earliest symptoms of gastric cancer, such as a sense of fullness or heaviness and moderate distention after meals, are usually vague in nature. Home remedies and self-medication are often employed successfully for a while until other symptoms appear. Because of the elusive nature of gastric disorders, this type of cancer is usually quite advanced by the time medical attention is sought out. (1018)

8. **The answer is (A).**   Japan has the highest incidence of gastric cancer in the world, and stomach cancer is the major cause of death in that country. The incidence of gastric cancer is low in the United States. The dramatic differences in geographic distribution of the disease remain an enigma to epidemiologists. (1017)

9. **The answer is (B).**   Gastric adenocarcinomas are generally radiosensitive; however, the close proximity to dose-limiting organs in the abdomen (i.e., the liver, kidney, and spinal cord) restricts the use of radiotherapy as a treatment modality. (1021)

10. **The answer is (C).**   Hepatocellular cancers are associated with alcohol-induced, nutritional, and posthepatitic cirrhosis of the liver. It is thought that chronic liver injury and subsequent continuous liver regeneration associated with cirrhosis may precipitate a loss of normal cellular control and lead to neoplasia. (1022)

11. **The answer is (D).**   Most **primary** malignant tumors of the liver are adenocarcinomas of two major cell types: about 90% are hepatocellular carcinomas arising from liver cells and about 7% are cholangiocarcinomas arising from bile duct cells. A very small proportion are hepatoblastomas, angiosarcomas, or sarcomas. However, a tumor is **20 times** more likely to be a metastatic deposit than a primary liver cancer. Tumors of the lung, breast, kidney, and the intestinal tract metastasize to the liver. (1023)

12. **The answer is (A).**   As liver cancer advances, serious complications, usually involving many body systems, arise. Portal vein obstruction many lead to necrosis, rupture, and hemorrhage. Esophageal varices and unrelenting ascites are also common sequela of either primary or secondary liver cancer. (1023–1024)

13. **The answer is (C).**   Elevated base levels of bilirubin, alkaline phosphatase, aspartate transaminase (SGOT), and lactic dehydrogenase (LDH) may alert a clinician to the possible presence of a liver tumor, although in the absence of cirrhosis, tumor growth can be extensive before liver function is impaired and laboratory findings become abnormal. **Alpha-fetoprotein** is a tumor marker that is elevated in the serum of 70% to 90% of individuals with primary hepatocellular carcinoma, but because levels of alpha-fetoprotein are not specific for liver cancer, histologic diagnosis is required. (1025)

14. **The answer is (D).**   Because most liver tumors are highly vascular, the person having an ultrasound-guided percutaneous needle biopsy of the liver performed must be monitored closely for intra-abdominal hemorrhage. In general, this procedure is rapid, safe, and commonly used; however, there are those clinicians who strongly believe that needle biopsies should be avoided at all cost if there is any potential for curative resection, because of the potential for seeding and spreading the cancer during the procedure. (1025)

15. **The answer is (A).**   Pruritus, which frequently accompanies jaundice, is precipitated by irritation of the cutaneous sensory nerve fibers by accumulated bile salts. Therefore, an individual with liver cancer must have meticulous skin hygiene and efforts to reduce itching should be implemented. Depending on the extent of liver dysfunction, deficits in clotting mechanisms may exist, occasionally necessitating the use of vitamin K to prevent bleeding. Most individuals with liver cancer are in a poor nutritional state and benefit greatly from a diet high in proteins and carbohydrates and low in fats. (1026)

16. **The answer is (C).**   Possible contraindications to major hepatic resection for liver cancer include: (1) severe cirrhosis; (2) distant metastases in the lung, bone, or lymph nodes; (3) jaundice which is often indicative of obstruction of the common bile duct; (4) ascites which is usually indicative of liver failure and an

inability to tolerate a surgical procedure; (5) poor visualization on angiographic studies, which may jeopardize the certainty with which the surgeon resects the tumor; (6) certain biochemical changes which indicate poor liver function and lower the probability of survival; and, (7) involvement of the inferior vena cava or portal vein which would make surgical intervention hazardous. (1026–1027)

17. **The answer is (A).** Chemotherapeutic agents can be administered systemically, either in single or combination drug regimens, or regionally, via hepatic artery or portal vein. Regional therapy allows a higher concentration of the drug to reach the tumor directly and continuously with minimal systemic exposure. (1028–1029)

18. **The answer is (D).** Cancer of the pancreas occurs at all ages, but peak incidence of the disease is between the ages of 60 to 70 years. It is rare before the age of 40, and although predominantly a disease that affects adults, cases of children with pancreatic cancer have been reported. (1030)

19. **The answer is (C).** Of those diagnosed with cancer of the pancreas, 85% will die within one year of diagnosis, and the cause of death will usually be cachexia, infection, or liver failure. (1031)

20. **The answer is (A).** A classic triad is apparent with cancer of the head of the pancreas: progressive jaundice, profound weight loss, and pain. Jaundice, which is precipitated by common bile duct obstruction, is the presenting symptom in 80% to 90% of all cases of cancer of the head of the pancreas, and is the symptom that inevitably leads individuals to seek medical attention. The weight loss that occurs with this disease can be as much as 20 to 30 pounds in just a few weeks, and is often accelerated by pain, anorexia, flatulence, nausea, and/or vomiting. The pain is initially dull and intermittent in nature, but eventually becomes continuous and much more distinctive. (1031)

21. **The answer is (C).** In general, **palliative** procedures are the mainstay of therapy for cancer of the pancreas because the disease is usually far advanced, with both local and distant metastases, by the time it is diagnosed. For a few individuals whose disease is detected early, the goal of surgery will be to obtain a cure. Current applications of chemotherapy have failed to produce significant results in the treatment of pancreatic cancer. If the cancer is unresectable, many clinicians advocate use of a combination of chemotherapy and radiotherapy, which occasionally controls local tumor growth and relieves the patient of some debilitating symptoms. (1036)

22. **The answer is (B).** Hemorrhage, hypovolemia, and hypotension pose the greatest threats to the individual who has just undergone surgery for cancer of the pancreas. As soon as possible after pancreatectomy, small feedings will be started with a diet that is usually bland, low in fat, and high in carbohydrates and protein. Restrictions will include caffeine, alcohol, and overindulgence. The stool should be examined daily for the characteristic signs of steatorrhea: frothy, foul-smelling stool with fat particles floating in the water. (1036–1037)

42 Gastrointestinal Cancer: Colon, Rectum, and Anus

STUDY OUTLINE

I. **INTRODUCTION**

   1. It is estimated that there were a total of 152,000 new cases of colorectal cancers in the United States in 1993.

II. **EPIDEMIOLOGY**

   A. **INCIDENCE**

   1. Colorectal cancer accounts for 15% of all malignancies in the United States.

   B. **DEATH RATE**

   1. Approximately 11% of total cancer deaths are due to colorectal malignancies.

   C. **SEX AND AGE**

   1. Colorectal cancer incidence increases after age 40, with a mean time of diagnosis of 63 years for men and 62 years for women. A decline is seen after age 75.

   D. **RACE AND RELIGION**

   1. Similar patterns of occurrence of colorectal cancer exist for white Americans and African Americans, whereas the occurrence rate for native Americans is less than half that for white Americans.
   2. Studies have demonstrated that some religious groups have lower cancer mortality than that of the general population, which is felt to be related to diet and restrictions on alcohol, tobacco, and caffeine-containing products.

III. **ETIOLOGY**

   A. **DIET**

   1. There are several reasons for suggesting diet as a factor in colorectal cancer.
      a. Ingested foods come into contact with the bowel mucosa. Thus certain foods and/or the time that they are in contact with a specific bowel area may be the initiating factor for a malignancy by altering the environment of the gut.
      b. Incidence rates differ in various populations throughout the world whose diets differ greatly.
      c. Selenium has been found to inhibit carcinogenesis.
   2. **Fat and protein**
      a. Dietary fat increases the risk of colon cancer through several mechanisms.
         (1) Large amounts of dietary fat result in increasing amounts of fecal bile acid coming into contact with the GI mucosa.
         (2) Metabolites of fecal bile acid may be carcinogenic.

402

        (3)   Transit time through the GI tract is slowed with fat present, thus extending the time interval that the bile acid or any other carcinogenic substance is in direct contact with the bowel lining.

        b.   People who ingest large amounts of beef are reported to have a higher incidence of colorectal cancer.

  3.   **Fiber**

        a.   Fiber acts as a **protective agent** against colon cancer by increasing defecation frequency and thus limiting the contact time that carcinogenic agents have with the bowel; altering the colonic pH, binding potentially of cancer-causing agents, and decreasing the concentration of ammonia in the gut.

        b.   High fiber intake may be protective only when fat content remains low.

  4.   **Calcium**

        a.   Calcium may decrease the risk of colon cancer in general or in individuals who are asymptomatic yet kindreds of someone with hereditary colon cancer.

        b.   The protective role of calcium is derived from its effect on the proliferative activity on the colonic mucosa.

            (1)   While the mechanism for reduction in cellular proliferation is not completely known, it is suggested that the calcium binds to free, ionized fatty acids and bile salts and then converts these acids and salts into calcium soaps, thus reducing their possible toxicity and cancer-promoting tendencies.

B.   **BACTERIA, VIRUSES, AND PARASITES**

  1.   It is theorized that fecal bacteria act on bile salts to produce metabolites that initiate malignant changes, and there is evidence that increased amounts of secondary bile acids are present in people with cancer.

C.   **CHEMOPROTECTIVE AGENTS**

  1.   These agents are potential inhibitors of carcinogenesis. They include ascorbic acid, flavones and indoles.

  2.   The incidence of colon cancer is inversely related to the intake of **cruciferous vegetables,** which contain ascorbic acid, flavones, and indoles.

D.   **PREDISPOSING CONDITIONS**

  1.   **Familial adenomatous polyposis (FAP)** is an inherited disease that is characterized by multiple colorectal adenomatous polyps. The polyps are at an extremely high risk for developing into carcinoma.

  2.   **Gardner's syndrome** is similar to FAP but also results in osteomas of the long bones, mandible and skull; polyps of the gastric and duodenal areas; and cysts, keloids, cutaneous fibromas, peritoneal adhesions, and retroperitoneal fibrosis.

  3.   **Peutz-Jeghers syndrome,** also a polyposis syndrome, is associated with multiple hematomas within the GI tract, mucocutaneous pigmentation, and an increased cancer risk.

  4.   **Hereditary nonpolyposis colorectal carcinoma (HNPCC)**

        a.   Originally called **"cancer family syndrome,"** HNPCC accounts for 4%–6% of all colorectal cancers. Despite the name, it is characterized by polyps.

        b.   HNPCC accounts for 7% of all colon cancers.

  5.   Family history of colon cancer in a first-degree relative increases risk to three times normal.

E.   **INFLAMMATORY BOWEL DISEASE**

  1.   **Ulcerative colitis**

        a.   Patients with IBD, particularly ulcerative colitis (UC), have **higher rates** of colorectal cancer than the general population.

        b.   Indications for **colectomy** in patients with UC include active disease unresponsive to treatment, massive hemorrhage, toxic megacolon, and the development of dysplasia or carcinoma.

2. **Crohn's colitis**
   a. Although the risk of colorectal cancer development is less for the person with Crohn's colitis than for the person with UC, the **risk is still 4–20 times higher** than for the general population.
   b. **Mucosal dysplasia** is present in 25% of cases prior to finding cancer.

F.   OTHER FACTORS

1. Prior pelvic irradiation, previous appendectomy or cholecystectomy, and possibly nulliparity are also risk factors for colorectal cancer.
2. See **Table 42-1, text page 1048,** for clinical risk factors of colorectal cancer.

IV.   PATHOPHYSIOLOGY

A.   CELLULAR CHARACTERISTICS

1. See **Table 42-2, text page 1048,** for histologic classification of cancer of the large bowel and anus.
2. Ninety-four percent of cancers of the colorectal area are adenocarcinomas, which extend into the adjacent organs or spread via lymphatics to regional lymph nodes and then into the bloodstream.
3. **Mucinous tumors,** which comprise 7.8% of the adenocarcinomas, produce large amounts of mucus, differ both epidemiologically and clinically, appear in persons under 30 years old, occur frequently in blacks, and have a poor prognosis.
4. **Tumor types**
   a. Adenocarcinomas may be characterized as polypoid or annular constricting lesions. **Polypoid tumors,** the second most frequent type, appear more on the right side and are usually a large mass.
   b. **Annular constricting lesions** present as nodular infiltrating lesions that may ulcerate; are more common on the left side, sigmoid, or rectum; and have a characteristic "apple core" appearance on barium enema.
5. **Anal cancer**
   a. Anal cancer is rare, accounting for 4% of distal GI tumors. The incidence of anal cancer increases with age. It occurs more commonly in females, but its incidence has been increasing in men, particularly those who are homosexual or bisexual or have a history of anal condylomata acuminata.
   b. Squamous cell is the most common (63%) histologic type.
   c. Lesions can occur in the anal canal and on the perianal skin, perineum, and vulvar area.

B.   PROGRESSION OF DISEASE

1. **Table 42-3, text page 1049,** details arguments for an adenomatous polyp-to-cancer transition.
2. **Disease progression** depends upon histological classification, degree of differentiation, and local and distant metastases.
3. Survival times usually vary according to stage: 81% to 32%. Primary colon cancers grow slowly. However, once metastases occur, the doubling rate increases.
4. Lymph node involvement may be present in 50% of individuals at diagnosis.
5. Venous invasion is an indicator of poor prognosis. Venous invasion leads to widespread dissemination, and thus surgical resection becomes ineffective.
6. Sites of **metastasis** are the liver, lungs, bones, and brain.
7. **Peritoneal implants** develop in 10% of people with colon cancer, with or without vascular or lymphatic spread.

V.   CLINICAL MANIFESTATIONS

1. **Early symptoms** such as rectal bleeding are infrequent and usually can be interrupted through dietary changes, but as the tumor grows, symptoms develop that reflect **characteristics of the lesion of a particular anatomical site.**
2. Carcinomas of the **right side of the colon** may become large and fungating tumors prior to producing symptoms.
   a. At the time of diagnosis, as many as 75% of patients will have a **palpable abdominal mass.**

      b. **Pain** experienced prior to the identification of this mass is described as a vague cramping or an aching-pressure sensation.

      c. Even though gross GI **bleeding** is not present, there can be chronic blood loss resulting in fatigue and shortness of breath secondary to the development of an iron deficiency anemia.

      d. Tumors of the right colon may **obstruct** the cecal and ascending colon and cause appendicitis-like symptoms.

3. Cancers of the transverse colon may cause blood in the stool and changes in bowel patterns or possibly a bowel obstruction.

      a. The increasing **consistency** of the stool versus the liquid content found in the ascending and cecal area also contributes to the potential for obstruction.

4. Cancer on the **left side of the colon** tends to be constricting due to lesions that can progressively reduce the lumen of the bowel.

      a. Initially, sensations of **fullness or cramping** are identified, progressing to changes in bowel habits as the tumor increases in size.

      b. **Obstipation** and **constipation** result, and acute abdominal **pain** is experienced from either an intestinal obstruction or a perforation.

      c. **Bleeding** with bright-red blood is more common with a carcinoma of the left side.

5. Cancer of the **rectum** manifests as changes in bowel habits, particularly in increased frequency of evacuation in the morning.

      a. As the tumor grows, a sense of **incomplete evacuation** and **tenesmus** develop, along with rectal pressure and/or fullness.

      b. Stool caliber decreases and is described as "pencil-like" by the patient.

      c. There will be frequent **GI bleeding** that is bright red, either mixed with or on the surface of the stool.

      d. As the tumor enlarges and invades perirectal tissues, a sensation of rectal fullness develops and may progress to dull, aching, perineal or sacral pain that can radiate down the legs.

      e. A patient may complain of mucus-laden diarrhea, since some tumors produce large amounts of mucus.

6. **Less common symptoms** of colorectal cancer include weight loss and fever.

7. **Nonmetastatic cutaneous manifestations** of colorectal cancer can develop, such as acanthas nigrisams, dermatomyositis, and pemphigoid.

VI. ASSESSMENT

A. PHYSICAL EXAMINATION

1. Physical examination involves inspection for obvious masses, distension, or enlarged veins, followed by auscultation for peristaltic sounds and then palpation and percussion to determine masses, liver enlargement, and occurrence and location of pain.

2. Examination of the rectal area includes visual and manual inspection of the anal and perianal area.

B. DIAGNOSTIC STUDIES

1. Endoscopic exam is achieved with a rigid **proctosigmoidoscope, a flexible fiberoptic sigmoidoscope, or a colonoscope.**

2. **Colonoscopy** is highly sensitive and allows visualization of the entire large bowel in 85%–95% of patients.

3. A **barium enema** is diagnostic in only 70% of cases, so it is often combined with sigmoidoscopy or colonoscopy.

4. Although **fecal occult blood testing** has been used for years as an indicator of GI malignancies, there are false-positive and false-negative tests.

5. **Carcinoembryonic antigen (CEA)** may be useful as a prognostic tool in the pretreatment phase for evaluating the effectiveness of various treatment protocols, surgery, chemotherapy, or radiation and to determine the presence of residual tumor or recurrence.

6. **The CA 19-9 test** is a radioimmunoassay measuring a carbohydrate determinant of circulating antigen. It has become useful in predicting recurrence among persons who have undergone curative resection of a colorectal tumor.

7. **Routine abdominal films,** both flat and upright, are suggested to evaluate those with an intestinal obstruction. The films may facilitate distinguishing between large- and small-bowel involvement.

C. **STAGING STUDIES**

1. **CT scanning** is used to determine tumor spread to adjacent organs, to assess lymph node involvement, and to detect liver, lung, or other distant metastasis.
2. **MRI** is used more in staging of rectal cancer than in that of colon cancer since it identifies tumor spread to structures of the pelvis and distinguishes postoperative fibrosis from tumor.
3. **Endoluminal ultrasonography** evaluates the penetration depth of tumor into the bowel wall and confirms impressions originating from the rectal examination.
4. In addition to **biopsy** of suspicious lesions, testing for **HIV** is indicated with anal cancers since they are associated with AIDS.

VII. **CLASSIFICATION AND STAGING**

1. See **Figure 42-2, text page 1053,** for colon and rectum staging criteria.

VIII. **TREATMENT**

A. **SURGERY**

1. Surgery is the treatment of choice for colorectal carcinoma. The extent of the resection is determined by location, vascular supply, and distribution of the lymph nodes. See **Figure 42-3, text page 1056,** for illustrations of surgeries.
2. **Right hemicolectomy**
   a. A right hemicolectomy is indicated for neoplasms of the appendix, cecum, ascending colon, and hepatic flexure.
   b. A right hemicolectomy involves removal of the terminal ileum, cecum, ascending colon, and right transverse colon with end-to-side anastomosis of the remaining large bowel to the ileum.
3. **Transverse colectomy**
   a. Tumors in the transverse colon are resected based on their location, the blood supply involved, and the ability to create an adequate anastomosis.
4. **Left hemicolectomy, left partial colectomy**
   a. A left hemicolectomy is the treatment of choice if the splenic flexure and descending colon are involved. A left partial hemicolectomy is preferred for tumors of the distal transverse colon, splenic flexure, and descending colon.
5. **Sigmoid colectomy**
   a. Sigmoid colectomy involves anastomosis of the colon end to the upper rectum.
6. **Subtotal or total colectomy**
   a. These procedures, which are indicated for large tumors found in either the left or the right colon, involve removal of the majority of, or the entire, colon.

B. **SURGICAL PROCEDURES FOR RECTAL CANCER**

1. The surgical procedure for a rectal tumor is based on **tumor location and on the probability of preserving bowel continuity.** Since the procedures are aimed for cure, an external ostomy may be required.
2. **Low anterior resection (LAR)**
   a. Tumors lying in the distal sigmoid and upper rectum result in a LAR and either a temporary or a permanent colostomy.
   b. Complications associated with LAR include hemorrhage, anastomotic leak, stricture, abscess, irregular bowel function, and wound infection.
3. **Abdominal perineal resection (APR)**
   a. An APR is performed when a rectal cancer or anal cancer is adjacent to the sphincter, requiring a **combined surgical approach through the abdomen and the perineum and a permanent colostomy.**

    b. **Complications** of an APR include possible injury to the ureters, urinary dysfunction, perineal and abdominal wound infections, and stomal complications.

    c. The **perineal wound** may be closed immediately following the removal of the rectum, anus, muscle, and fatty tissue, or it may be left open for healing by secondary intention, with primary closure being the preferred method.

    d. Sexual dysfunction

      (1) The wide excision required for an APR includes anatomical structures related to sexual functioning. The pelvic resection is **extensive,** and injury results to the parasympathetic and sympathetic nerves.

      (2) There may be **preexisting medical conditions** or medications that have already affected sexual functioning and resulted in the loss of erectile capacity for the male.

      (3) Presurgery treatment with **radiation** is damaging to the blood vessels needed for erection.

      (4) The APR can **impair erectile function,** but recovery rates of erectile function are higher than those associated with radical prostatectomy or cystectomy.

        (a) **Dry ejaculations** will occur due to damage of presacral parasympathetic nerves; however, the sensation of orgasm with mild loss of intensity remains.

      (5) Female sexual functioning following an APR remains relatively unchanged, because the sexual response is controlled by different and higher nerve centers not subject to dissection during APR.

        (a) Reproductive status can be affected if the uterus, cervix, ovaries, or fallopian tubes are removed.

      (6) A negative emotional response to the cancer diagnosis, the surgery, the stoma, or the appliance that contains the effluent from the bowel may cause problems requiring professional counseling.

4. **Colostomy**

    a. A colostomy can be created in any anatomic segment of the bowel, being thus identified as cecal, ascending, transverse, descending, or sigmoid colostomy.

    b. The **stoma** may be identified by the type of surgical construction: end, loop, or double barrel.

    c. **Anatomic location** is indicative of the type of effluent, either liquid or semiformed.

      (1) Stomas on the right side of the colon produce a stool that is more liquid in content, while the consistency of the stool becomes more formed from the left transverse and descending colon toward the rectal area.

    d. The **end stoma** is created by dividing the bowel and suturing the proximal colon segment onto the abdominal surface.

      (1) When the segment used for the end stoma is located in the low descending or sigmoid area, the oversewn rectal segment often is referred to as "Hartmann's pouch."

    e. A **loop colostomy** is created in the transverse bowel, and a segment of bowel is exteriorized and secured to the abdomen over some type of supporting device in order to prevent it from recessing into the abdominal cavity.

      (1) Once the bowel adheres to the abdominal wall, usually in 7–10 days, the device is removed.

    f. A **double-barrel colostomy** indicates two stomas side by side or apart from one another, with the distal stoma referred to as a mucous fistula when they are apart from one another.

    g. **Stoma site selection**

      (1) **Stoma sites need to be selected** prior to surgery following examination of the patient's abdomen in the sitting, lying, and standing positions.

      (2) The selected site should be within the rectus muscle and in an area that can physically support ostomy equipment, should be visible for the patient to see, and (if possible) should not include any scars, skin folds, bony prominences, belt and waist lines that might interfere with the appliance seal.

      (3) The anatomical location of the stoma influences the abdominal quadrant placement as well as the surgical techniques.

    h. **Colostomy management**

      (1) In the immediate postoperative period the stoma needs to be evaluated for viability, condition, size, and shape and to ensure that all sutures holding the everted stoma onto the abdomen are secure.

        (a)   An **inadequate** blood supply or tension on the bowel segment may cause the stoma to appear pale, dusky, or even black in color.

      (2)   The first time the patient views the stoma usually is emotionally painful.

      (3)   The time when the stoma will begin to function is variable. Usually, the more proximal a stoma is in the bowel, the sooner it functions and the more liquid the stool content.

      (4)   Peristomal skin should resemble the skin on the abdominal surface.

   i. **Appliance selection**

      (1)   Pouches are specifically evaluated and selected to accommodate the consistency of the stool output, to provide peristomal skin protection, to enable ease of client use and lifestyle, and to minimize profile beneath clothing.

      (2)   **Equipment costs** vary but are reimbursable to some degree by Medicare and most private insurers.

   j. **Teaching patients**

      (1)   **Preoperatively,** the patient needs to understand the surgery and its rationale, to understand the planned creation of a stoma and its function, and to see and handle the containment equipment.

      (2)   Postoperative teaching begins immediately with early activities progressing from small areas, such as removing or applying the pouch closure clamp, to looking at and cleansing the stoma to applying and emptying the appliance.

          (a)   See **Figure 42-5, text page 1059,** for patient instructions regarding fecal pouch application.

      (3)   **Discharge preparation** includes providing educational materials that the patient can consult at home and referring the patient to home health agencies and to nurses who are sensitive to the needs of the ostomy patient.

      (4)   Patients need to leave the hospital not only with detailed instructions but also with ostomy supplies adequate for 2–3 weeks, the names of the items to be used, and the name of the community vendors as well as a catalog from a mail order vendor.

C. **SURGICAL PROCEDURES FOR ANAL CANCER**

   1. The tumor size, stage, and depth of penetration determine the treatment approach.

   2. An **APR** has been the standard therapy for anal cancer; however, other therapies such as radiation are now being incorporated or used alone (radiation therapy), with similar or improved 5-year survival rates.

      a. The inability of surgery alone to cure is due in part to the anatomy of the anal region, which makes it difficult to remove adequately the lateral and distal zones of the lymphatic spread.

D. **RADIATION THERAPY**

   1. The primary reason for failure of disease control after surgery alone is a result of both local and regional recurrence.

   2. **Preoperative radiation**

      a. Radiation therapy prior to surgery is proposed as advantageous for the following reasons:

         (1)   The **rate of surgical resectability would improve.**

         (2)   **There would be a reduction in the viability of malignant cells.**

         (3)   **The number of positive lymph nodes would be reduced.**

         (4)   **The chance of local recurrence would be lessened without compromising cure rate.**

      b. Also noted are disadvantages with the use of preoperative RT.

         (1)   Some patients may be treated unnecessarily with radiotherapy if they have early-stage disease that could have been removed with surgery alone.

         (2)   The histopathology of the tumor can be altered by preoperative radiation, thus making comparisons of treatment outcomes difficult.

   3. **Combined pre- and postoperative radiotherapy**

      a. Use of pre- and postoperative adjuvant treatments is referred to as the **"sandwich"** technique, resulting in a decrease in tumor dissemination prior to surgery.

         (1)   There also would not be an alteration in the ability to stage the tumor histologically at surgery.

    (2) A suggested disadvantage of the sandwich approach is the potential for repopulation by residual malignant cells if slow wound healing occurs following the surgical procedure and delays the delivery of postoperative RT.

  4. **Postoperative radiation**
    a. Postoperative radiation is used primarily for those individuals at **high risk** of local recurrence. Local recurrence is decreased by radiation, but **distant metastasis** remains a problem.
    b. Patients with colon cancer are less likely to have locoregional disease than those with a rectal malignancy.
    c. Treatment techniques for colon cancer may involve therapy to the whole pelvis and a boost to the tumor bed and/or the draining lymphatics.

  5. **Palliative radiation**
    a. Palliative radiotherapy is effective in treating symptoms of advanced rectal cancer.

  6. **Other radiotherapy techniques**
    a. **Endocavitary radiation** by placement of an endoscope directly against the lesion, followed by the administration of a minimally penetrating dose of high-intensity irradiation, is used as a local treatment for rectal tumors.
    b. **Intraoperative radiation** can treat locally advanced, recurrent, or inoperable rectal cancer.
    c. **Brachytherapy** is accomplished by inserting radioactive sources into a body cavity or implanting sources into a tumor.
     (1) This therapy may be selected for pelvic recurrence of rectal cancer, local tumor control, palliation of symptoms, and treatment of liver metastases.
    d. Hyperthermia may be used as adjunct therapy with RT and chemotherapy. It enhances the cytotoxic effects of the other modalities by interfering with the repair of intracellular damage caused by radiation and chemotherapy.

  7. **Laser therapy**
    a. Laser therapy may be useful for treating inoperable rectal and descending colon tumors in selected patients.
    b. Benefits include relief of bleeding, diarrhea, mucus drainage, and tenesmus.

E. **CHEMOTHERAPY**

  1. Chemotherapy is used as adjunct therapy for colorectal cancer that is residual, advanced, or metastatic.
  2. Colorectal cancers are resistant to most chemotherapeutic agents.
  3. 5-FU, the most researched single agent, has been used to treat different stages of the disease with various dosage schedules and by different routes.
    a. Studies using continuous infusions of 5-FU for protracted times have shown response rates of 17%–40%.
  4. Other single agents have been tested for use with colorectal tumors, and none of these has demonstrated a response rate greater than 20% in any of the reported studies.
  5. Due to its immunorestorative activity, **levamisole** has been included with 5-FU and other agents for treatment of advanced colorectal carcinoma. After several extensive trials, it now appears that the drug plays a limited role in the treatment of colorectal cancer.
  6. Trials are now in progress to explore the effectiveness of various chemotherapy agents, radiation, and surgical combinations for rectal cancer.
  7. Intra-arterial or intraportal chemotherapy has been developed based on the knowledge that hepatic metastasis from colorectal tumors occurs via the portal circulation.
    a. A major factor affecting intra-arterial administration of chemotherapy is the high incidence of chemical hepatitis.
  8. A multimodal treatment approach has been shown to improve cure rates and lessen the number of patients with anal cancer undergoing radical surgical procedures.
  9. **Side effects** from chemotherapeutic agents are drug-specific and may include bone marrow suppression, gastrointestinal changes, and radiation-induced skin reactions.

F. **ALTERNATIVE THERAPIES**

  1. Biologic response modifiers have also received attention in treating colorectal carcinomas. Studies using **alpha-interferon, interleukin-2,** and **monoclonal antibodies** have demonstrated varying degrees of activity and response rates.
  2. Treatment of solid tumors with autologous bone marrow transplant is being examined.

PRACTICE QUESTIONS

1. Fat and fiber are two dietary factors that appear to be correlated with the occurrence of colorectal cancer. It is thought that they operate by affecting, in opposite ways, the
    (A)   conversion of ionized bile salts into insoluble compounds.
    (B)   rate of uptake of calcium by the GI tract.
    (C)   breakdown of carcinogenic compounds by digestive enzymes.
    (D)   exposure of the GI tract to promoters of carcinogenesis.

2. Which of the following conditions is commonly associated with colorectal carcinoma?
    (A)   appendicitis or gallbladder disease
    (B)   hemorrhoids
    (C)   anal condylomata acuminata
    (D)   chronic ulcerative colitis

3. The prognosis for a patient with colorectal cancer is probably **poorest** if which of the following exists?
    (A)   venous invasion
    (B)   high blood pressure
    (C)   location of the tumor above the peritoneal reflection
    (D)   squamous cell involvement

4. Which of the following clinical manifestations is **most** likely to exist in patients with a cancer of the transverse, descending, or sigmoid colon?
    (A)   anemia and a vague, dull, persistent pain in the upper right quadrant
    (B)   a change in bowel habits and blood in the stool
    (C)   sensations of incomplete evacuation and tenesmus
    (D)   bright-red bleeding through the rectum

5. Physical examination and diagnostic studies of a patient with cancer of the right colon are **most** likely to find which of the following?
    (A)   a palpable mass
    (B)   polyps in the rectum
    (C)   anemia
    (D)   high levels of carcinoembryonic antigen (CEA)

6. Which of the following procedures is the surgeon **most** likely to perform when a colorectal lesion is obstructing the bowel?
    (A)   a right hemicolectomy that includes the related lymphatic and circulatory channels
    (B)   a one-stage procedure involving resection of the lesion and a primary anastomosis
    (C)   a two-stage procedure involving a temporary colostomy or ileostomy
    (D)   a three-stage procedure involving a diverting colostomy, a resection of the tumor, and takedown of the colostomy

7. The type of colostomy that is **most** likely to be performed when the resected tumor is in the transverse colon is the
    (A)   single-barrel colostomy.
    (B)   double-barrel colostomy.
    (C)   loop colostomy using an external supporting device.
    (D)   loop colostomy using a fascial bridge.

8. Placement of a stoma following colorectal surgery is **least** likely to be
    (A)   on smooth skin large enough in area to allow the appliance to be secured to the abdomen.
    (B)   in a location that the patient can see without difficulty.
    (C)   outside the borders of the rectus muscle to avert accidental dislodgement of the appliance.
    (D)   on a site close to the transverse colon.

9. Which of the following postoperative assessments of stoma viability is a matter of concern that should be brought to the surgeon's attention?
    (A)   persistent peristalsis in the bowel
    (B)   bleeding of the stoma when rubbed

(C)   a dusky or gray stoma
(D)   protrusion of the stoma

10.   Postoperative care and teaching of the patient undergoing abdominoperineal resection (APR) for rectal cancer is **most** likely to be influenced by which of the following?
(A)   the type of colostomy to be performed
(B)   the patient's age, sex, and physical condition
(C)   the extent of hepatic invasion
(D)   the type of closure of the perineal wound to be used

11.   Chemotherapy is used in combination with other treatment modalities because
(A)   surgery is always the primary treatment modality with any solid tumor.
(B)   colorectal carcinomas are extremely resistant to antineoplastic agents.
(C)   higher doses of drugs can be administered when given in combination with radiation therapy.
(D)   intra-arterial drug administration can be achieved only after tumor resection and bowel anastomosis.

ANSWER EXPLANATIONS

1.   **The answer is (D).**   It is believed that dietary factors affect the exposure of the GI tract to promoters of carcinogenesis. Fats to promote cellular changes in the bowel mucosa; fiber is thought to reduce the carcinogenic process. A diet high in unsaturated fat may promote carcinogenesis by increasing the level of fecal bile acids, which have also been implicated as a promoter. It is thought that low-fiber, high-fat foods work synergistically to increase the risk of colorectal cancer. In addition, a diet high in fiber may actually protect against the disease even in the presence of a high-fat diet. Fiber may limit the time the colon is exposed to cancer promoters by speeding intestinal transit time. (1045–1046)

2.   **The answer is (D).**   A number of predisposing conditions have been associated with an increased risk of colorectal cancer. These include chronic ulcerative colitis; Crohn's disease; familial polyposis; and a strong family history of predisposition to colon cancer and familial adenamatous polyposis. (1048)

3.   **The answer is (A).**   Overall prognosis depends on early detection. The diagnosis of colorectal cancer in asymptomatic individuals has been shown to be related to improved survival. Poor prognosis has been associated with obstructing or perforating carcinomas, occurrence in young people, location of the tumor below the peritoneal reflection, lymph node involvement, venous invasion, hepatic metastasis, and invasion of the bowel wall. Metastasis to the liver is most common. (1050)

4.   **The answer is (B).**   Cancers of the transverse, descending, and sigmoid colon are manifested by a change in bowel habits and blood in the stool. Obstruction of the bowel is more common in the transverse colon than in the ascending colon because of a decrease in bowel lumen, an increase in the consistency of the stool, and a narrowing of the lumen at the hepatic and splenic fixtures. The manifestations in choice (A) are those of a tumor of the right colon; manifestations in choices (C) and (D) are those of rectal cancer. (1050)

5.   **The answer is (A).**   Because the transverse colon is the most anterior and movable part of the colon, tumors here are more accessible to detection by palpation. Other possible symptoms that might have been determined by inspection, auscultation, palpation, and percussion of the abdomen include distention of the abdomen, enlarged and visible abdominal veins, occult blood in the stool, and enlarged lymph nodes or organs (especially the liver). Diagnostic examination by fiberoptic colonoscopy would confirm the presence of the tumor. Anemia is more likely to occur with cancer of the right colon. Polyps in the rectum might be present and might indicate the patient was at high risk for colorectal cancer. CEA, while useful in evaluating the efficacy of treatment, is of limited value in the detection of colon cancer. (1050)

6.   **The answer is (B).**   When a malignant lesion results in an obstruction, the standard procedure involves resection of the lesion and a primary anastomosis. The two- and three-step procedures are riskier and less often performed. A right hemicolectomy is performed on the cecum or ascending colon. (1054)

7.   **The answer is (D).**   A loop colostomy, in which a colon loop is exteriorized and secured over some device to prevent it from recessing back into the abdominal cavity, is used most often in the transverse colon, frequently as a temporary procedure to allow healing of an anastomosis site or a diseased distal colon.

A fascial bridge is preferred as a substitute for the external supporting device. A layer of fascia is stitched to the loop and supports it. (1055)

8.   **The answer is (C).**   Preoperative selection and marking of a stoma site is critical to postoperative management. The stoma site should be located within the borders of the rectus muscle. Bringing the bowel through this muscle sheath prevents later complications of peristomal hernia and prolapse. To determine the ideal location of the stoma, the patient's abdomen is observed in the sitting, standing, bending, and lying positions. (1058)

9.   **The answer is (C).**   An important postoperative nursing function is the assessment of stoma viability to identify early signs of compromised circulation to the stoma. A stoma that is dusky, gray, or black indicates an inadequate blood supply and is documented and brought to the surgeons's attention. A stoma that necroses will slough and generally lead to stomal stenosis. The postoperative occurrences in choices (A), (B), and (D) all are normal. (1058)

10.   **The answer is (D).**   Because APR requires a combined surgical approach through the abdomen and perineum, a major complication of APR is the occurrence of perineal and abdominal wound infections. The type of closure employed—primary closure, partial closure with an incisional drain, or leaving the wound open and packing it—will determine the necessary postoperative care and teaching. (1055)

11.   **The answer is (B).**   Colorectal carcinomas are extremely resistant to most antineoplastic agents. When chemotherapy is used as the only therapy for colorectal tumors, it has been found to be inadequate. Chemotherapy may be used with surgery or combined with surgery and radiation therapy. (1061)

43   Gynecologic Cancers

STUDY OUTLINE

I.   INTRODUCTION

1. Gynecologic cancers account for approximately 13% of all cancers in women. See **Table 43-1, text page 1066,** for specific site statistics and estimated new cases.

II.   ENDOMETRIAL CANCER

A.   EPIDEMIOLOGY

1. Endometrial cancer is the predominant cancer of the female genital tract, occurring mainly in postmenopausal women.
2. The median age at diagnosis is 61 years, with the majority of women diagnosed between 50 and 59 years of age.
3. The low mortality rate reflects the fact that 79% are diagnosed with localized disease.
   a. Survival rates by stage are 76% for stage I, 50% for stage II, 30% for stage III, and 9% for stage IV.

B.   ETIOLOGY

1. **Risk factors** associated with endometrial cancer are: obesity, nulliparity, late menopause, diabetes, hypertension, infertility, irregular menses, failure of ovulation, a history of breast or ovarian cancer, adenomatous hyperplasia, and prolonged use of exogenous estrogen therapy.
2. **Excessive endogenous estrogen** metabolism or production has been implicated in endometrial cancer development.
3. Several **hormonal aberrations** can be linked to obesity, and increased body size plays a role in androgen conversion to estrogen.
4. **Obese women** with an **upper body fat** pattern have a 5.8-fold increase in risk over women who are nonobese or have a lower body fat pattern.
   a. Fat cells are an excellent storage depot for estrogen, and the chronic slow release of estrogen from these cells may account for the increased risk.
   b. In obese postmenopausal women, secretion of serum sex hormone-binding globulin (SHBG) is depressed, leaving higher concentrations of free estradiol in the blood.
   c. Obese women also have endocrine malfunctions that cause anovulatory cycles with irregular menses, resulting in failure of progesterone to oppose chronic estrogen effects on the endometrium.
5. Oral contraceptives and cigarette smoking appear to have a **protective effect** in preventing the development of endometrial cancer, but the risks of smoking outweigh any protection gained.

C.   PATHOPHYSIOLOGY AND CELLULAR CHARACTERISTICS

1. Endometrial cancer develops in the **epithelial layer of the uterine corpus.**
   a. Tumors that arise in the lower uterine segment involve the cervix sooner and have a higher incidence of pelvic and para-aortic lymph node involvement.
   b. Tumors that have deep myometrial invasion tend to be more aggressive and have a poorer survival rate.
2. Over 90% of endometrial cancers are **adenocarcinomas.**

D. **NATURAL HISTORY**

1. Histologic type and differentiation, uterine size, stage of disease, myometrial invasion, peritoneal cytology, lymph node metastasis, and adnexal metastasis affect the **natural history and prognosis** of endometrial cancer.
2. Endometrial cancer **originates in the fundus** and may spread to involve the entire endometrium. Through direct extension and infiltration, the cancer **spreads to the myometrium, endocervix, cervix, fallopian tubes, and ovaries.**
3. **Adnexal spread** is infrequent but is found at surgery in about 10% of women with clinical stage I.
4. **Recurrence** appears in 38% of women with adnexal spread versus 11% of those without such involvement.
5. Metastasis is usually to the pelvis and para-aortic lymph nodes and has been correlated with tumor differentiation, stage of disease, and amount of myometrial invasion.
6. See **Figure 43-1, text page 1068,** for the spread pattern of endometrial cancer.
7. **Less common sites of metastases** include the vagina, peritoneal cavity, omentum, and inguinal lymph nodes.
8. Hematogenous spread often involves the lung, liver, bone, and brain.
9. Histologic differentiation is one of the most sensitive indicators of metastases and prognosis. The **less differentiated the tumor,** the poorer the prognosis.
10. Another prognostic indicator, the **degree of myometrial invasion,** is generally classified as none (localized to the endometrium), superficial, or deep.
    a. The greater the invasion, the poorer the prognosis.
11. **The grade of the tumor is combined with the degree of myometrial invasion to estimate survival.**
12. **Women with positive peritoneal fluid washings, taken during laparotomy, are at a higher risk for pelvic recurrence.**

E. **CLINICAL MANIFESTATIONS**

1. **Abnormal vaginal bleeding** associated with endometrial cancer causes women to seek medical attention promptly.
2. Other more **infrequent symptoms** are pyometria and hematometria, particularly in the older woman, and lumbosacral, hypogastric, or pelvic pain in women with more advanced disease.

F. **ASSESSMENT**

1. In women suspected of having endometrial cancer, a thorough pelvic examination, including Pap smear, is performed.
2. **Endometrial biopsy** is the most reliable test for endometrial cancer, which allows histologic rather than cytologic examination. If that test result is negative and symptoms persist, a fractional dilation and curettage (D&C) is performed.
3. The American Cancer Society recommends endometrial sampling every 1–2 years for women taking exogenous estrogens and at high risk for the development of endometrial cancer at menopause.
4. Chest X ray, intravenous pyelogram, complete blood count, and blood chemistry profiles are other diagnostic tests.
5. Cystoscopy, barium enema, and proctoscopy are performed if bladder or rectal involvement is suspected.
    a. Other studies that may be used to evaluate pelvic, abdominal, and nodal disease status include hysterography, hysteroscopy, lymphangiography, CT scan, and MRI.

G. **TREATMENT, RESULTS, AND PROGNOSIS**

1. **Primary**
    a. Endometrial cancer is **staged surgically in patients who are surgical candidates, that is, if medical condition and intra-abdominal disease permit.** See **Table 43-2, text page 1069,** for corpus cancer staging.
    b. Surgical staging assists in defining tumor size and location as well as extent of spread beyond the uterus.

    c. Surgical staging and treatment involve an extensive evaluation of the abdomino-pelvic cavity and the following procedures: **bimanual examination under anesthesia, peritoneal cytology, inspection and palpation of all peritoneal surfaces, biopsy of suspicious areas, selective pelvic and para-aortic lymphadenectomy, total abdominal hysterectomy (TAH), bilateral salpingo-oophorectomy (BSO),** and **possible omentectomy and resection of tumor implants.**

    d. Tissue from the primary tumor is obtained for analysis of estrogen and progesterone receptors.

    e. Surgical staging **prior** to any **r**adiation therapy is advantageous since more women with early-stage disease will not need additional postoperative therapy and thus can avoid the time, effort, and morbidity associated with pelvic radiation therapy.

    f. Selection of adjuvant radiation therapy for early endometrial cancer is determined by stage, histology, and cytopathology.

    g. Patients with **stage I, grade 1** disease and no myometrial invasion require only a TAH-BSO; whereas patients with **stage I, grade 2** disease with less than 50% myometrial invasion require intravaginal radiation to reduce the risk of central recurrence.

    h. Indications for **pelvic external beam radiation** therapy include disease localized to the pelvis, a high-grade tumor, or greater than 50% myometrial invasion.

    i. Whole-pelvis radiation, in contrast to intravaginal radiation, allows treatment of all pelvic tissue including nodes and lymphatics.

  2. **Advanced or recurrent disease**

    a. Endometrial cancer is one of the most difficult cancers to treat if metastasis or recurrence has occurred.

    b. Women with **vaginal recurrences** can be treated successfully with surgery or radiation.

    c. Recurrences **outside the upper vagina** are not easily treated, but hormonal therapy and chemotherapy are used.

    d. **Hormonal therapy**

      (1) Synthetic **progestational agents** are the most common systemic therapy for recurrent endometrial cancer with response rates ranging from 30% to 37%.

      (2) Response seems to be related to histologic grade of the tumor, length of the disease-free interval, the woman's age, and presence of areas of squamous metaplasia within the primary tumor.

      (3) Positive estrogen and progesterone receptor status correlates with a better response to progestin therapy regardless of the grade of the tumor.

      (4) **Side effects of progestational agents** include fluid retention, phlebitis, and thrombosis.

      (5) Oral preparation of megace or intramuscular medroxyprogesterone acetate are effective agents against endometrial cancer.

      (6) The use of tamofixen is still experimental.

    e. **Chemotherapy**

      (1) Cytotoxic agents have a limited role in advanced endometrial cancer since only a few agents have demonstrated activity equal to or greater than progestin therapy, i.e., doxorubicin, cisplatin, and cyclophosphamide.

H. **NURSING MANAGEMENT**

  1. See **Table 43-4, text page 1071,** for information needs related to endometrial cancer, including health maintenance issues, therapeutic interventions, and psychosexual concerns.

I. **FUTURE TRENDS**

  1. The role of **whole-abdominal radiation therapy** in preventing or treating recurrences is not yet defined; however, prospective clinical trials are in progress.

  2. Clinical trials aimed at **identifying cytotoxic drugs** and drug regimens with improved response and survival rates continue.

  3. The **role** of estrogen and progesterone receptor status in the choice of therapy and as a predictor of response needs to be defined.

  4. Estrogen replacement therapy (ERT), while historically contraindicated in women with endometrial cancer, also needs further investigation in order to identify the appropriate candidate for ERT.

III. **OVARIAN CANCER**

A. **EPIDEMIOLOGY**

1. Ovarian cancer is the fifth leading cause of cancer death and the most common cause of death from gynecologic cancers in women in the United States.
2. Most cases are seen in women between 55 and 59 years of age. Only 7%–8% of ovarian cancers occur in women under 35 years of age.
3. The overall 5-year survival rate for women with ovarian cancer is between 30% and 35% and has not changed over the past 30 years.
4. The **poor survival rate** is due in part to: (1) the difficulty diagnosing ovarian cancer early; (2) the treatment, although intensive, has not been curative; (3) a high-risk population has not been clearly defined; and (4) the etiology is essentially unknown.

B. **ETIOLOGY**

1. **Multiple risk factors** that have been identified include environmental, hormonal, menstrual, reproductive, dietary, and hereditary.
2. Increased risk has been identified in nulliparous women, and to a lesser degree in women who first became pregnant after 35. Risk seems inversely related to the cumulative time that ovulation is suppressed during the childbearing years due to pregnancy, lactation, or oral contraceptives.
   a. The use of oral contraceptives not only has a protective effect against ovarian cancer, but this effect seems to persist for at least 15 years after use has stopped.
3. Early menarche, late menopause, and hormonal therapy have also been identified as impacting the risk for ovarian cancer.
4. Although only 5%–10% of women with ovarian cancer have a genetic predisposition, women with a **family history** of ovarian, breast, or colon cancer have an increased risk of developing the disease.

C. **PATHOPHYSIOLOGY AND CELLULAR CHARACTERISTICS**

1. Epithelial ovarian cancers arise from a malignant transformation of the ovarian surface epithelium.
2. Study of **cytogenetics, oncogenes, and growth factor regulation** has occurred in cultured tissue from patients with advanced ovarian cancer, but information about the early phases of the malignant transformation of the ovarian surface epithelium is not defined.
3. Epithelial, stromal, and germinal cells give rise to the major subsets of ovarian cancer: epithelial, germ cells, and stromal tumors.

D. **NATURAL HISTORY**

1. Most ovarian tumors originate from the **epithelial surface of the ovary and grow to invade the stromal tissue and penetrate the capsule of the ovary.**
2. The most common mechanisms of spread are by direct extension and peritoneal seeding.
   a. **Direct extension** occurs when tumor cells on the surface of the ovary invade the adjacent structures of the fallopian tubes, uterus, bladder, and rectosigmoid and pelvic peritoneum.
   b. **Peritoneal seeding** occurs when cells exfoliate into the peritoneal cavity where they move within the fluid to other surfaces such as the liver, diaphragm, bladder, and large and small bowel, with intraperitoneal seeding being the most common method of dissemination.
3. Ovarian lymphatics may have a role in dissemination. The most frequently encountered distant sites are the liver, lung, and pleura.
4. **Death is usually secondary to intra-abdominal tumor dissemination,** which can lead to obstruction, pulmonary emboli, electrolyte imbalance, sepsis, or cardiovascular collapse.

E. **CLINICAL MANIFESTATIONS**

1. There are typically no early manifestations of ovarian cancer that could identify localized disease, but instead, as the mass enlarges, the woman may experience abdominal discomfort, dyspepsia, indigestion, flatulence, eructation, anorexia, pelvic pressure, or urinary frequency.

F. **ASSESSMENT**

1. Although routine **pelvic examinations** only detect one ovarian carcinoma in 10,000 exams, they are the most usual method for detecting early disease.
    a. The use of transvaginal ultrasound in conjunction with CA-125, a tumor-associated antigen, is gaining popularity but needs further investigation as a screening method.
2. The staging of ovarian cancer is based on surgical evaluation and forms the basis for planning subsequent therapy.
3. The initial surgical exploration enables the surgeon to determine the precise diagnosis and accurate stage and to perform optimal debulking.
4. Unfortunately, accurate surgical staging is not obtained in all patients presenting with early ovarian cancer.

G. **TREATMENT, RESULTS, AND PROGNOSIS**

1. Initial ovarian therapy includes thorough evaluation, staging and cytoreduction.
2. A TAH-BSO, omentectomy, selected pelvic and para-aortic lymph node sampling, and maximal cytoreduction are performed when surgically feasible.
3. Selection of additional therapy for women diagnosed in late stages is decided on by reviewing **stage, grade, size, and location of residual tumor,** and presence of ascites or malignant peritoneal washings.
4. See **Table 43-4, text page 1075,** for staging classification of malignant ovarian tumors.
5. **Stage I**
    a. Surgery alone provides a 90% survival rate for women with stage I, grade 1 ovarian cancer.
    b. There is **no standard adjuvant therapy** for other stage I ovarian cancers, and the therapies used include no therapy, chemotherapy, intraperitoneal radioisotopes, and external radiotherapy.
    c. A **platinum-based chemotherapy regimen** is considered beneficial for patients with stage I, grade 3 tumors who are at high risk for recurrence.
6. **Stage II**
    a. Following the surgical staging and cytoreduction, intraperitoneal ^{32}P, whole-abdominal radiation, single-agent chemotherapy, or platinum-based combination chemotherapy may be employed.
    b. Treatment options vary because few women are diagnosed in this early stage.
7. **Stages III, IV**
    a. When the patient is a surgical candidate, aggressive staging with cytoreductive surgery is advocated to reduce the tumor burden and amount of residual disease.
    b. If the tumor is cytoreduced and the patient has no area of residual disease greater than 1 cm in diameter, she may be treated with platinum-based chemotherapy or whole-abdominal and pelvic radiation.
    c. Platinum-based combination chemotherapy is administered for stage III with residual disease greater than 1 cm and for stage IV disease.
8. **Recurrent or persistent disease**
    a. The benefits of salvage therapy is limited in the person with persistent or recurrent disease following initial therapy.
    b. **Second-look surgery**
        (1) A second-look operation is performed on patients who have a complete clinical response following the full course of chemotherapy as evidenced by negative tumor markers (CA-125), and negative CT scan or ultrasound.
        (2) Second-look surgery is **advocated** for the following reasons: (1) to determine whether the patient had a complete remission and therapy can be stopped, (2) to assess the response and determine whether a change in therapy is indicated, and (3) to perform secondary cytoreductive surgery to attempt to prolong survival.
    c. **Tumor-associated antigens**
        (1) One monoclonal antibody that reacts with epithelial ovarian cancer cells has been developed and studied extensively because it can detect an **antigen (CA-125)** in the blood of women with ovarian cancer.
        (2) **CA-125** is not specific for ovarian cancer alone and can be elevated in the blood of women with ovarian cancer.
        (3) **CA-19-9** is another tumor marker used in combination with CA-125, but it remains controversial.

9. **Chemotherapy**
   a. **Single-agent therapy**
      (1) The mainstay of adjuvant therapy for stages III and IV epithelial ovarian cancer is chemotherapy.
         (a) Response rates seen with alkylating agents varied from 33%–65% but because of the risk of leukemia from alkylating agents, other drugs were evaluated.
      (2) Cisplatin is the single most effective cytotoxic agent used in the treatment of ovarian cancer with response rates as high as 55%, depending on dose.
   b. **Combination chemotherapy**
      (1) The **overall response rates** for combination chemotherapy vary, with clinical complete remission seen in up to 40%–50% of women.
      (2) See **Table 43-6, text page 1079,** for selected combination chemotherapy regimens.
      (3) The addition of **cisplatin** into combination chemotherapy regimens markedly improved response rates; moreover, cisplatin given without dose modification offers the best chance for response (up to 80%) and for achieving a complete remission (20%–50%) in women with advanced ovarian carcinoma.
      (4) Carboplatin, like cisplatin, has a significant dose-response relationship and can be given to patients who are not platinum refractory yet can no longer tolerate the neurotoxicity or nephrotoxicity associated with cisplatin.
      (5) Colony stimulating factors (CSF) may allow higher doses of myelosuppressive drugs and are currently being incorporated into treatment regimens.
      (6) Another approach to enable high doses of myelosuppressive drugs is the use of autologous bone marrow rescue. Taxol has demonstrated a 30% response in previously treated patients and is under investigation in phase III trials.
   c. **Drug resistance**
      (1) Due to the development of multidrug resistance, the effectiveness of chemotherapy is limited, and patients with ovarian cancer die from chemotherapy-refractory disease.
      (2) Drug resistance is likely due to multiple factors.
      (3) Debulking surgery to reduce tumor burden to aggregates of 1 cm or less improves the response to postoperative chemotherapy by reducing the potentially refractory disease.
   d. **Intraperitoneal chemotherapy**
      (1) Intraperitoneal chemotherapy (IP) is used to increase cytotoxic drug levels to the tumor sites, because ovarian cancer usually remains confined to the abdominal cavity.
      (2) Patients benefitting the most from IP therapy are women with minimal residual disease following systemic therapy with or without surgical reduction, high-grade tumors with a surgically defined complete response, high-grade stage I/II with the risk of covert disease in the upper abdomen, advanced disease with all or some drugs administered IP, and advanced disease with IP therapy following a limited course of intravenous therapy with or without secondary surgical debulking.
      (3) See **text page 1080,** column 2, for the techniques of IP administration.
10. **Hormone therapy**
    a. Hormone therapy for ovarian cancer has resulted in uneven responses, and further clinical trials are needed to define the role of hormonal therapy.
11. **Radiotherapy**
    a. **Radioactive chromic phosphate (^{32}P)** and **radioactive gold (Au)** have been used as adjuvant therapy in women with stage I ovarian cancer.
       (1) Complications of ^{32}P can include small bowel obstruction and stenosis and are higher in women who have uneven distribution of the radioactive material in the peritoneal cavity.
       (2) See **Figure 43-3, text page 1081,** for the administration method of radioactive colloidal chromic phosphate into the peritoneal cavity.
    b. The effectiveness of **external beam radiation therapy** in advanced cancer is directly related to the volume of disease at the time of radiation.
    c. Whole-abdominal radiation (WAR) appears most effective in those selected individuals with little or no gross residual disease.
12. **Biologic therapy**
    a. **Immunotherapy,** including monoclonal antibodies, adoptive cellular immunotherapy, and interferon, may soon become the fourth modality of therapy for ovarian cancer.
    b. Further study is needed to more clearly define the role of biologics in the treatment of ovarian cancer.

H.   **NURSING MANAGEMENT**

   1.   See **Tables 43-7 and 43-8, text pages 1082 and 1083,** for common nursing management issues.

I.   **FUTURE TRENDS**

   1.   One area of ongoing research is new drug development and testing.
   2.   In addition to taxol, topotecan and tetraplatin are being tested to determine their activity in treating ovarian cancer.
   3.   **Another investigational approach is to define methods of overcoming intrinsic or acquired drug resistance.**
   4.   **Efforts need to continue to define sensitive and specific screening methods that can be widely applied.**

IV.   **CERVICAL CANCER**

A.   **EPIDEMIOLOGY**

   1.   Invasive cervical cancer has steadily decreased as a result of the **Pap smear,** which can diagnose the disease in a preinvasive state.
   2.   Twenty-four percent of new cases and 40% of deaths from cervical cancer occur in **women age 65 years** and older.
   3.   The **number of deaths** from cervical cancer has decreased in women over age 45, whereas mortality in women under 35 years has increased.
   4.   While the incidence of invasive cancer has decreased by nearly 50%, the incidence of new cases of **carcinoma in situ (CIS)** has steadily increased.

B.   **ETIOLOGY**

   1.   See **Table 43-9, text page 1085,** for risk factors and preventive measures associated with cervical cancer.
   2.   A **higher incidence** of cervical cancer occurs in women who are from lower socioeconomic groups, smokers, blacks, or Hispanics; have many sexual partners; became sexually active prior to age 17; or are multiparous.
       a.   Conversely, cervical carcinoma is infrequent in women who are nulliparous and those who are lifetime celibates or lifetime monogamous.
   3.   Some types of human papillomavirus (HPV) are associated with genital warts, precancerous lesions, or invasive cervical carcinoma.
       a.   Both **HPV 16 and 18** are associated with high-grade cervical intraepithelial lesions or invasive cancer.
   4.   The **male** plays a role in the etiology of cervical cancer.
       a.   Women married to men whose previous spouses had cervical cancer seem to be at a higher risk of developing cervical cancer.
       b.   The male partner's age at first coitus, smoking habits, visitation of prostitutes, and number of sexual partners also may affect relative risk.
   5.   Factors **lowering a woman's risk** include barrier-type contraception, vasectomy, recommended daily allowances of vitamin A, beta carotene, and vitamin C, limiting the number of sexual partners, and initiating sexual activity at a later age.

C.   **PATHOPHYSIOLOGY**

   1.   Cancer of the cervix is the culmination of a **progressive** disease that begins as a neoplastic alteration of the squamocolumnar junction. These abnormal cells can progress to involve the full thickness of epithelium and invade into the stromal tissue of the cervix.
   2.   **Cervical intraepithelial neoplasia (CIN)** defines epithelial cervical abnormalities. The CIN classification demonstrates the progression of the disease process rather than delineating distinctly different abnormalities.
       a.   **CIN I** is dysplasia in **less than one-third** the thickness of the cervical epithelium.
       b.   **CIN II** is neoplastic changes in **two-thirds the thickness** of the cervical epithelium.
       c.   **CIN III or carcinoma in situ** is a lesion that has **full thickness neoplastic changes** and there is no evidence of stromal invasion or metastases.

3. See **Table 43-10, text page 1087,** for the Bethesda System for reporting cervical/vaginal cytological diagnoses.
4. Cervical cancer develops into either an **exophytic, excavating (ulcerative), or endophytic lesion.** See **Figure 43-4, text page 1086.**
   a. **Exophytic lesions** are the most common and appear as cauliflowerlike, fungating cancers that are friable and bleed easily.
   b. The **excavating or ulcerative** lesion is a necrotic lesion that replaces the cervix and upper vagina with an ulcer or crater that bleeds easily and is often associated with local infection and purulent drainage.
   c. The **endophytic** lesion is located within the endocervical canal and is without visible tumor or ulceration. The cervix appears normal or enlarged and barrel-shaped but is hard to the touch.

D. **CELLULAR CHARACTERISTICS**

1. Historically, 80%–90% of cervical tumors are **squamous,** and 10%–20% are adenocarcinomas.
2. Adenocarcinomas, generally in younger women, impose a **greater risk** because the tumor is within the cervix and can become quite bulky before becoming clinically evident.

E. **NATURAL HISTORY**

1. Each type of CIN lesion can regress, persist, progress, and become invasive.
   a. CIN III is more likely to progress than the milder forms, which may regress spontaneously to normal.
2. Once invasive, cervical cancer spreads by **direct extension, via lymphatics, and by hematogenous spread.**
   a. Direct extension is the most common route. The lesion begins on the endocervix and spreads throughout the entire cervix, into the parametrium, and through the vesicovaginal, the bladder, and the rectum.

F. **CLINICAL MANIFESTATIONS**

1. In the majority of cases, the disease is discovered by **Pap smear** during routine examination.
2. Cervical cancer is usually asymptomatic in the preinvasive and early stage, although women may notice a watery vaginal discharge.
3. **Postcoital bleeding, intermenstrual bleeding, or heavy menstrual flow** are later symptoms that prompt women to seek medical attention.
   a. Chronic bleeding may lead the woman to complain of symptoms related to anemia.
   b. A common complaint in advanced cervical malignancy is foul-smelling vaginal discharge.
4. **Other late symptoms that are indicative of advanced disease** include pelvic pain, hypogastrium, flank, or leg pain.
5. End-stage disease can be characterized by edema of the lower extremities due to lymphatic and venous obstruction.

G. **ASSESSMENT—CIN**

1. The **Pap smear** is an effective, accurate, and economical screening technique to detect cervical neoplasia.
2. The American Cancer Society recommends an annual Pap test and pelvic examination for women who are or have been sexually active or are 18 years or older.
3. Women who have any pelvic symptoms such as pain, vaginal discharge, or abnormal bleeding should be evaluated by their physician promptly.

H. **TREATMENT, RESULTS, PROGNOSIS—CIN**

1. **Pap smear, colposcopy, and biopsy** determine the extent and severity of a lesion, differentiating between CIN and invasive cervical cancer.
2. Treatment for CIN may include a direct cervical **biopsy, electrocautery/cryosurgery, laser surgery, electrosurgery, cone biopsy, or hysterectomy.**

3. **Cryosurgery,** which involves placement of a probe on the lesion to induce freezing, is the most common method used. It is cost-effective, is painless, and can be performed in the office.

4. **Laser** mounted on the colposcope can eradicate 80%–90% of CIN, while removing less disease-free tissue.

5. The **loop electrosurgical excision procedure (LEEP)** is an increasingly popular alternative and allows for diagnosis and treatment of CIN by utilizing a thin wire loop electrode that excises lesions with minimal tissue ablation.

6. See **Figure 43-6, text page 1090,** for a diagram of the cone biopsy for endocervical disease, which can be used as a **diagnostic** or **therapeutic** technique.

7. **Complications** of the conization procedure are related to the amount of endocervix removed.
   a. Major immediate complications include hemorrhage, uterine perforation, and anesthetic complications. Delayed complications include bleeding, cervical stenosis, infertility, cervical incompetence, and increased chances of preterm delivery.

8. **Total vaginal hysterectomy (TVH)** may be employed for treatment of individuals with CIS, whereas total abdominal hysterectomy (TAH) is appropriate for women with CIN who have completed childbearing.

9. Therapy is selected based on the extent of the disease, the physician's experience, and the woman's wishes to preserve reproductive and ovarian function.

10. See **Figure 43-7, text page 1090,** for an evaluation and management schema for an individual with an abnormal Pap smear.

I. **NURSING MANAGEMENT—CIN**

1. Educating the patient includes defining the disease, explaining the treatment, stressing the importance of follow-up, and clarifying that CIN is not invasive cancer.

2. See **Table 43-12, text page 1091,** for issues related to the management of women diagnosed with cervical, vulvar, or vaginal cancer.

J. **ASSESSMENT—INVASIVE DISEASE**

1. Cervical cancer is staged **clinically,** with the initial staging being the best prognostic indicator, and is confirmed by examination under anesthesia.
   a. When clinical and surgical stages are compared, 30%–40% are **understaged.**

2. A thorough **clinical work-up** includes cervical biopsies, endocervical curettage, cystoscopy, and proctosigmoidoscopy with additional tests including chest X ray, IVP, barium enema, CBC, blood chemistries, liver scan, CT scan, MRI, and node biopsy if nodes are palpable.

3. Clinical staging is **not changed** on the basis of surgical findings, but treatment may be altered.

K. **TREATMENT, RESULTS, PROGNOSIS—INVASIVE DISEASE**

1. Therapy is chosen on the basis of the woman's age, medical condition, extent of cancer, and any complicating abnormalities.

2. **Stage Ia**
   a. **Stage Ia1 (microinvasive carcinoma)** is treated by TAH or TVH, conization, or intracavity radiation.
   b. **Stage Ia2** is treated by TAH or TVH if invasion is less than 3 mm in depth and there is no lymphovascular space involvement.

3. **Stage Ib and IIa**
   a. Although choice of therapy may differ among some physicians, these stages can be treated with radical abdominal hysterectomy and pelvic lymphadenectomy or with external beam radiation with one or two intracavitary insertions of radiation.
   b. Surgery is preferred to radiotherapy by some gynecologic oncologists because ovarian function can be preserved and the vagina usually remains more pliable.
   c. Patients with bulky disease (barrel-shaped cervix) have a higher incidence of central recurrence, pelvic and para-aortic lymph node metastases, and distant dissemination.
      (1) An increased dose of radiation to the central pelvis or radical hysterectomy or both has been advocated.

4. **Stages IIb, III, and IV**
   a. In these stages, women are usually treated with high doses of external pelvic radiation, with parametrial boosts, or with intracavitary radiation.

b. Pelvic exenteration is only employed as primary therapy in a select group of advanced disease patients wherein the disease is not adherent to pelvic side walls and does not involve lymph nodes, and the patient is able to adjust to the major body changes.

c. Surgical staging of advanced disease before initiating treatment is being advocated in an attempt to gain a more precise evaluation of the extent of the disease.

d. **Complications of surgery**
   (1) The major complications of radical hysterectomy include ureteral fistulas, bladder dysfunction, pulmonary embolus, lymphocysts, pelvic infection, bowel obstruction, rectovaginal fistulas, and hemorrhage.

e. **Complications of radiotherapy**
   (1) The higher the **dose** of radiation, the greater the rate of complications. Major complications include vaginal stenosis, fistula formation, sigmoid perforation or stricture, rectal ulcer or proctitis, intestinal obstruction, fistula, ureteral stricture, severe cystitis, pelvic hemorrhage, pelvic abscess, and sexual dysfunction secondary to vaginal atrophy and stenosis.

5. **Recurrent or persistent disease**
   a. Approximately **35% of women** with invasive cervical cancer will have recurrent or persistent disease.
   b. Histologic confirmation of recurrence is essential because cells and cervical configuration are altered from prior radiation therapy.
   c. Most recurrences occur within 2 years following therapy.
      (1) Signs and symptoms include unexplained weight loss, leg edema, pelvic pain (a prognostically poor triad of symptoms), vaginal discharge, ureteral obstruction, lymph node enlargement, cough, hemoptysis, and chest pain.
      (2) Twenty-five percent of recurrences involve distant metastases (lung, liver, bone, mediastinal or supraclavicular lymph nodes), and 75% of recurrences are local (cervix, uterus, vagina, parametrium, and regional lymph nodes).
   d. One-year survival rates of women with persistent or recurrent carcinoma are low, at 10%–15%.
   e. **Surgery**
      (1) See **Figure 43-8, text page 1096,** for a diagram of total pelvic exenteration, which might be considered if cervical cancer recurs centrally.
      (2) It is reserved only for women who are good surgical candidates and do not have disease outside the pelvis or do not have the triad of unilateral leg edema, sciatic pain, and ureteral obstruction.
      (3) Immediate **postoperative problems** include pulmonary embolism, pulmonary edema, cardiovascular accident, myocardial infarction, hemorrhage, sepsis, and small bowel obstruction.
      (4) **Long-term problems** include fistula formation, urinary obstruction, infection, and sepsis.
   f. **Chemotherapy**
      (1) Due to decreased pelvic vascular perfusion, a limited bone marrow reserve, poor renal function, and possible ureteral obstruction, cytotoxic drug administration is complicated.
      (2) Response rates for patients with recurrent squamous cell cervical cancer treated with single-agent and investigational chemotherapy range from 10%–40%. See **Table 43-14, text page 1097,** for agents used.
      (3) Combination chemotherapy has not been proven more effective than single agents.
      (4) Chemotherapy can be used as a radiation **sensitizer,** particularly hydroxyurea and cisplatin.
         (a) Improved survival rates from the concurrent administration of radiation and hydroxyurea have been shown.
   g. **Radiotherapy**
      (1) The role of radiation therapy in metastatic disease is variable depending on previous treatment, sites of recurrent disease, presence of symptoms, and intent to cure or palliate.

L. **NURSING MANAGEMENT—INVASIVE DISEASE**

   1. See **Table 43-12, text pages 1091–1092,** for issues related to the nursing management of women with malignancies of the lower genital tract.

M. **FUTURE TRENDS**

1. Chemotherapy as part of the initial treatment regimen is being investigated.
   a. Because radiotherapy is more effective with a smaller tumor volume, induction chemotherapy can be given to debulk the tumor before other therapies are started, which might also reduce the incidence of pelvic recurrence.
2. Little is known about the efficacy of biologic response modifiers in the treatment of cervical cancer.
3. **Growth factors** may allow for higher and more frequent doses of chemotherapy, while reducing myelosuppressive effects of therapy.

V. **VULVAR CANCER**

A. **EPIDEMIOLOGY**

1. Vulvar cancer is a disease of the elderly, with peak incidence occurring in the seventh decade of life, and accounts for only 3%–4% of all gynecologic malignancies.
2. **Vulvar intraepithelial neoplasia (VIN)** describes epithelial abnormalities of the vulva and is divided into three grades that differentiate the degree of epithelial invasion by neoplastic cells.
3. Peak incidence is between 48 and 51 years of age, but vulvar cancer appears to be increasing in younger women.

B. **ETIOLOGY**

1. Although the causes are not clear, there is some connection with venereal disease, including herpes simplex virus type 2 and condylomata acuminatum.
2. Clinical characteristics of the woman with vulvar carcinoma are advanced age (>60 years), chronic vulvar disease, previous malignancy of lower genital tract, history of breast cancer, HPV, HSV2, chronic irritation, and exposure to coal tar derivatives.

C. **PATHOPHYSIOLOGY AND CELLULAR CHARACTERISTICS**

1. The **labia** is the site of vulvar cancer in 70% of cases, with the labia majora involved three times more often than the labia minora.
2. **Squamous cancer** accounts for about 90% of vulvar malignancies; melanoma accounts for 5%. The remaining 10% are Bartholin's gland, sarcoma, basal cell, Paget's, and verrucous cancer.

D. **NATURAL HISTORY**

1. Common routes of **metastasis** are through direct extension, lymphatic dissemination to regional lymph nodes, and, rarely, hematogenous spread to distant sites (lung, liver, bone).

E. **CLINICAL MANIFESTATIONS**

1. Symptoms of both VIN and invasive vulvar carcinoma are variable and insidious.
   a. With VIN, 50% of women experience vulvar pruritus or burning; 50% are asymptomatic.
2. The most common complaint associated with vulvar cancer is the presence of a mass or growth in the vulvar area.
   a. Other symptoms include vulvar bleeding and pain.
3. The woman with vulvar cancer may delay seeking assistance because she is embarrassed due to the intimate area of the body that is involved.

F. **ASSESSMENT—VIN**

1. Methodical **inspection** is the most important diagnostic tool; colposcopy and multiple vulvar biopsies should be done when lesions are noted.

G. **TREATMENT—VIN**

1. Currently, **wide local excision** using either primary-closure skin flaps or skin graft is recommended, with close follow-up for localized lesions.

2.   For multicentric disease, a **skinning vulvectomy** is performed in which the vulvar skin is excised while conserving the fat, muscle, and glands below the skin.
3.   Lesions may be treated locally by electrocautery, cryosurgery, or laser, resulting in the possibility of requiring 3 months to heal.
4.   Other local therapies include topical 5% 5-FU and dinitrochlorobenzene (DNCB) and bleomycin.

H.   **ASSESSMENT–INVASIVE DISEASE**

1.   Vulvar cancer is diagnosed by local excisional biopsy of the lesions and careful physical examination with attention to the inguinal lymph nodes.
2.   Colposcopy is useful for defining areas to biopsy. Pap smear of the cervix is essential because 10% of women with vulvar neoplasia also have cervical CIN or invasive cancer.
3.   EUA may be needed to fully evaluate the cervix, vagina, and pelvis.
4.   Metastatic evaluation includes chest radiograph, proctosigmoidoscopy, cystoscopy, arium enema, IVP, and biochemical profile.
5.   See **Table 43-17, text page 1101,** for FIGO staging of vulvar cancer.

I.   **TREATMENT–INVASIVE DISEASE**

1.   **Surgery** is the treatment of choice with en bloc dissection of tumor, contiguous skin, subcutaneous fat, regional inguinal and femoral nodes, and vulva.
2.   See **Figure 43-9, text page 1101,** for a diagram of surgical incisions for groin dissection.
3.   See **Table 43-18, text page 1102,** for a list of reported complications following radical surgery for vulvar carcinoma. The major complications include:
     a.   **Wound breakdown** occurs in nearly 50% of patients.
     b.   Varying degrees of **lymphedema** of the lower extremities occur in about 30% of patients.
     c.   Other complications include **femoral nerve damage during surgery, causing paresthesia of the anterior thigh, lymphocyst formation in the groin area, stress incontinence, genital prolapse,** and **femoral vessel rupture.**

J.   **NURSING MANAGEMENT–VIN AND INVASIVE DISEASE**

1.   Nursing management issues related to VIN and invasive vulvar cancer are seen in **Table 43-12, text pages 1091–1092.**

K.   **RESULTS AND PROGNOSIS**

1.   The **5-year survival rate can be correlated with stage and nodal involvement,** and the overall 5-year survival rate for all stages is between 70% and 75%; for women with stage I and II disease, the survival rate is about 90%.

L.   **RECURRENCE**

1.   High recurrence rates correlate with more than three positive nodes, and 80% of recurrences occur within the first 2 years after initial treatment.

M.   **FUTURE TRENDS**

1.   Interferon has been utilized in the treatment of condylomatous vulvitis and HPV-associated VIN.
2.   Investigation is required in order to determine the population for whom a conservative surgical approach will not compromise cure.
3.   **Studies defining microinvasive carcinoma and those investigating methods to reduce the radical extent of surgical procedures are especially important.**

VI.   **VAGINAL CANCER**

A.   **EPIDEMIOLOGY**

1.   Carcinoma of the vagina, a rare malignancy, accounts for **1%–2% of gynecologic malignancies.**
2.   Vaginal tumors are secondary sites of malignant dissemination from primary cancers of the cervix or other sites.

3. Peak incidence occurs in women between 50 and 70 years of age.
4. **Vaginal intraepithelial neoplasia (VAIN)** is usually seen in women who have been treated for CIN or after radiotherapy for invasive cervical cancer.

B. **ETIOLOGY**

1. Incidence of squamous cell cancer of the vagina increases with age.
2. **Rates are higher** in the black population and persons with limited education and income.
3. Other related risk factors include a history of HPV, vaginal trauma, previous abdominal hysterectomy for benign disease, and absence of regular Pap smears.
4. The risk of developing vaginal cancer is 1 in 1000 for women who were exposed to **diethylstilbestrol (DES)** in utero.

C. **PATHOPHYSIOLOGY AND CELLULAR CHARACTERISTICS**

1. Vaginal cancers occur most commonly on the posterior wall of the upper-third of the vagina, and the second most common site is the anterior wall in the lower one-third of the vagina.
2. **Squamous cell carcinoma** comprises 75%–95% of the vaginal cancer cases.

D. **NATURAL HISTORY**

1. Tumor spreads by **direct extension** into the obturator fossa, cardinal ligaments, lateral pelvic walls, and uterosacral ligament.
2. The incidence of lymph node metastasis is directly proportional to the stage of the vaginal cancer.

E. **CLINICAL MANIFESTATIONS**

1. An abnormal Pap smear is usually the event that initiates the search for a definitive diagnosis since many lesions are asymptomatic.
2. The most common initial symptoms of invasive vaginal cancer are **abnormal vaginal bleeding, foul-smelling discharge,** and **dysuria.**

F. **ASSESSMENT**

1. **Clinical diagnosis of a vaginal neoplasm is made by careful visual examination and palpation** of the vagina.
2. Pap smears and colposcopy are useful for directed biopsies.
3. Women with invasive vaginal cancer should have a history and physical exam, chest radiograph, biochemical profile, IVP, barium enema, cytoscopy, and proctosigmoidoscopy.

G. **TREATMENT—VAIN**

1. Location, size, and whether single focus or multiple foci lesion are considered in determining the treatment option.
2. **Local excision** is used for single lesions or several clustered in a single portion of the vagina.
3. Surgery for diffuse multiple lesions may result in shortened or absent vagina.
4. Local application of 5-FU cream can be effective.
5. Laser therapy can cure between 69% and 80% of patients with vaginal intraepithelial lesions.

H. **TREATMENT—INVASIVE DISEASE**

1. **Radiation therapy** is the treatment of choice for most invasive vaginal cancers, especially stages I and II disease.
2. Surgery may be used in early-stage adenocarcinoma and may involve partial or total vaginectomy, radical hysterectomy, and upper vaginectomy plus pelvic lymphadenectomy, depending on the tumor location.
3. A combination of surgery and radiation may be useful for stages I and II disease.
4. Depending on the extent of disease, **surgery** for recurrence may range from wide local excision to total pelvic exenteration.

I.   NURSING MANAGEMENT—VAIN AND INVASIVE DISEASE

1. See **Table 43-12, text pages 1091–1092,** for nursing management issues.

J.   **RESULTS AND PROGNOSIS**

1. The overall 5-year survival rate for all stages of squamous cell vaginal carcinoma is 40%–50% and is as high as 80% for patients with stage I disease.
2. Clinical stage is the most important **prognostic indicator** in vaginal cancer.
3. Eighty percent of pelvic recurrences occur within 2 years of treatment.

PRACTICE QUESTIONS

1. Stage III cervical intraepithelial neoplasia is characterized by dysplasia that is severe but without areas of invasion. Stage III CIN is also known as
    (A) preclinical invasive carcinoma.
    (B) carcinoma in situ.
    (C) adenocarcinoma.
    (D) verrucous carcinoma.

2. The most effective method of detecting cervical neoplasia is with
    (A) X rays.
    (B) routine visual examination/inspection.
    (C) biopsy.
    (D) a Pap smear.

3. One of the factors that seems to put a woman at higher risk for developing cervical dysplasia is
    (A) DES exposure.
    (B) hypertension.
    (C) diabetes.
    (D) human papillomavirus.

4. The American Cancer Society recommends that all women who are sexually active or who are 18 years of age or older have a Pap smear performed
    (A) every three years.
    (B) every two years.
    (C) annually.
    (D) biannually.

5. Vulvar intraepithelial neoplasia is **usually** discovered by means of
    (A) intravenous pyelography (IVP).
    (B) inspection.
    (C) a Pap smear.
    (D) a patient history.

6. Incidence of cervical cancer is highest in women aged
    (A) 20–25.
    (B) 20–35.
    (C) 35–50.
    (D) 65 or older.

7. One of the first symptoms of cervical cancer is
    (A) pelvic pain.
    (B) malaise.
    (C) regional lymphedema.
    (D) watery vaginal discharge.

8. All of the following are commonly used in the diagnosing/staging of cervical cancer **except**
    - (A) serum chemistries.
    - (B) proctosigmoidoscopy.
    - (C) chest radiograph.
    - (D) laparoscopy.

9. The treatment(s) of choice for advanced cervical cancer is
    - (A) local surgery.
    - (B) chemotherapy and surgery.
    - (C) internal or external radiotherapy.
    - (D) chemotherapy.

10. The chemotherapeutic agent felt to have the greatest antineoplastic activity in the treatment of recurrent cervical cancer is
    - (A) ifosfamide.
    - (B) cisplatin.
    - (C) cyclophosphamide.
    - (D) methotrexate.

11. One of the primary risk factors associated with the development of endometrial cancer is
    - (A) late menopause.
    - (B) oral contraceptive use.
    - (C) radiation exposure.
    - (D) sex at an early age.

12. Endometrial cancer is known to spread to
    - (A) local lymph nodes only.
    - (B) the lungs, liver, bone, and brain only.
    - (C) local lymph nodes as well as distant sites, e.g., lungs and bone.
    - (D) It does not readily metastasize.

13. The most effective method of detecting endometrial cancer is with a(n)
    - (A) Pap smear.
    - (B) endometrial biopsy.
    - (C) laparotomy.
    - (D) blood test.

14. The primary systemic agent used in the treatment of recurrent endometrial cancer is
    - (A) synthetic progestin.
    - (B) cyclophosphamide.
    - (C) alpha-interferon.
    - (D) tumor necrosis factor.

15. One of the factors that seems to place a woman at higher risk for the development of ovarian cancer is
    - (A) occupational exposure.
    - (B) a great many sexual partners.
    - (C) DES use by the mother.
    - (D) a history of breast cancer.

16. One of the early signs of ovarian cancer is
    - (A) frequent urinary tract infections.
    - (B) thin, bloody vaginal discharge.
    - (C) heavy and painful menstruation.
    - (D) There are usually no early signs of ovarian cancer.

17. A common site of metastasis for ovarian cancer is the
    - (A) lung.
    - (B) bladder.
    - (C) brain.
    - (D) bone.

18. A method of detecting recurrent ovarian cancer that also may be helpful in early detection of the disease is the use of
     (A) LAK cells.
     (B) open biopsies.
     (C) paracentesis.
     (D) tumor-associated antigen.

19. The treatment of choice for women with a diagnosis of stage I (noninvasive) ovarian cancer is
     (A) intracavitary radiotherapy.
     (B) combination chemotherapy.
     (C) TAH-BSO with omentectomy.
     (D) hormone therapy.

20. Of the following symptoms, the one **most** likely to be experienced by a woman who has vaginal cancer is
     (A) pain with urination.
     (B) bilateral leg pain.
     (C) night sweats.
     (D) changes in libido.

21. Vulvar cancer is **most** commonly detected during
     (A) childbirth.
     (B) urinary catheterization for an unrelated illness or condition.
     (C) routine pelvic examination.
     (D) monthly self-examination.

22. Surgical excision of a stage I vulvar tumor generally includes
     (A) radical vulvectomy only.
     (B) radical vulvectomy and bilateral groin dissection.
     (C) Surgery is not commonly used to treat vulvar cancer.
     (D) individualized surgical treatment.

ANSWER EXPLANATIONS

1. **The answer is (B).**   The term *carcinoma in situ* describes a lesion characterized by full thickness neoplastic change, and there is no evidence of stromal invasion or metastases. **Figure 43-4, text page 1086,** is a schematic representation of the different categories of cervical neoplasia. (1085)

2. **The answer is (D).**   The Pap smear, introduced in 1941, is one of the most effective, accurate, and economical techniques used to detect cervical neoplasia. (1088)

3. **The answer is (D).**   Human papillomaviruses have been implicated in an increased risk for both precancerous cervical lesions and invasive cervical carcinoma. The virus is sexually transmitted and can cause a variety of warty infections. (1084)

4. **The answer is (C).**   Presently, the American Cancer Society recommends that all women who are or have been sexually active or who are 18 years of age or older should have annual Pap smears. After a woman has had three negative annual Pap smears, the test may be performed less frequently at the discretion of the physician. (1089)

5. **The answer is (B).**   The most important diagnostic tool available in vulvar intraepithelial neoplasia is thorough inspection, occasionally with colposcopy and possibly followed by biopsy. A 1% toluidine blue solution can be used to stain suspicious areas, although it has a 20% false-positive rate. (1100)

6. **The answer is (D).**   Twenty-four percent of new cases of cervical cancer and 40% of deaths from cervical cancer occur in women aged 65 or older, making it a significant health problem for elderly women. (1084)

7. **The answer is (D).**   The first symptom of cervical cancer may be a watery vaginal discharge that frequently goes unrecognized. The symptoms that usually prompt the woman to seek medical attention are postco-

ital bleeding, intermenstrual bleeding, or heavy menstrual flow. If the bleeding is chronic, she may complain of symptoms related to anemia. Pelvic pain and regional lymphedema are late symptoms that usually indicate advanced disease. (1088)

8. **The answer is (D).** Many diagnostic tests may be used in the assessment and staging of cervical cancer, among them blood chemistries and CBC, proctosigmoidoscopy, and chest X ray. Other possible tests include cervical biopsy, endocervical curettage, cystoscopy, intravenous pyelography, barium enema, and, in certain cases, lymphangiogram and CT scan of the liver. (1089)

9. **The answer is (C).** Women with later, more advanced forms of cervical cancer are usually treated with high doses of external pelvic radiation, with or without the addition of interstitial parametrial implants. Either radical surgery or radiation therapy are used equally effectively for the earlier stages. (1094)

10. **The answer is (B).** Although in general chemotherapy is not the treatment of choice for women with cervical cancer, because these women often have decreased pelvic vascular perfusion, a limited bone marrow reserve, and poor renal function related to previous treatment with radiation and/or chemotherapy, chemotherapy can effectively treat this disease, especially combination chemotherapy. Of the single agents, the only ones to show significant activity when used alone are cisplatin and 5-FU, and of these two, cisplatin is the one with the greater antineoplastic activity. (1097)

11. **The answer is (A).** The risk factors associated with the development of endometrial cancer are obesity, nulliparity, late menopause, irregular menses, failure to ovulate, infertility, diabetes, hypertension, history of breast or ovarian cancer, adenomatous hyperplasia, and prolonged use of exogenous estrogen therapy. The more of these factors that apply, the greater the risk of developing endometrial cancer. (1067)

12. **The answer is (C).** Endometrial cancer metastasizes primarily to pelvic and para-aortic lymph nodes; less common sites of metastasis include the vagina, peritoneal cavity, omentum, and inguinal lymph nodes. Hematogenous spread occasionally occurs to the lungs, liver, bone, and brain. (1067–1068)

13. **The answer is (B).** The most reliable technique for detecting endometrial cancer, if it is suspected, is an endometrial biopsy. The American Cancer Society even recommends an endometrial sampling for those menopausal women who are at high risk for developing endometrial cancer. A Pap smear is not a reliable method of detecting endometrial cancer, although it too may be performed. (1068)

14. **The answer is (A).** For patients with recurrent endometrial cancer, the synthetic progestational agents (e.g., Megace) have shown some degree of effectiveness. Response appears to be related to tumor grade, the length of disease-free interval, the woman's age, and the presence of areas of squamous metaplasia within the tumor. (1070)

15. **The answer is (D).** Hormonal factors such as nulliparity, infertility, and estrogen therapy have been connected to the development of ovarian cancer, as have marked premenstrual tension, abnormal breast swelling, and dysmenorrhea. A history of breast cancer doubles the risk of ovarian cancer, and a history of colon cancer also somewhat increases risk. (1073)

16. **The answer is (D).** Ovarian cancer is typically asymptomatic in its early stages. As the disease progresses, women may experience vague abdominal discomfort leading to loss of appetite, flatulence, or urinary frequency, but more often than not these symptoms are no more than annoying and not taken seriously by the patient and her physician. By the time a diagnosis of ovarian cancer is made, the cancer has spread beyond the ovary in 75% of cases. (1074)

17. **The answer is (B).** The most common mechanisms for the spread of ovarian cancer are direct extension and serosal seeding. Both of these mechanisms involve neighboring organs such as the bladder and bowel. Hematogenous spread to distant sites (e.g., lungs and bone) also sometimes occurs, but it is less common. (1073)

18. **The answer is (D).** At least two of the tumor-associated antigens specific for ovarian cancer (CA-125 and CA-19-9) have been identified to date, and both seem to correlate relatively closely with disease status. If this method is perfected, then second-look surgery, still commonly used to detect ovarian cancer, may become unnecessary, and early detection, at a point where the disease can still be cured, becomes a possibility. (1077)

19. **The answer is (C).** Total abdominal hysterectomy with bilateral salpingo-oophorectomy (TAH-BSO) and omentectomy is the therapy of choice for the 15%–20% of patients who present with stage I ovarian cancer. At the present time no one adjuvant therapy is being recommended. (1074–1075)

20. **The answer is (A).** The most common presenting symptoms of vaginal cancer are vaginal bleeding, foul-smelling discharge, and dysuria. Urinary symptoms are present because vaginal tumors are in close proximity to the bladder neck and can compress the urethra at an early stage of the disease. (1104)

21. **The answer is (C).** Vulvar cancer's peak occurrence is between 48 and 51 years of age. It is an indolent disease, usually without symptoms in its early stages, and may be detected during routine pelvic examination. (1100)

22. **The answer is (D).** Traditionally, stage I lesions were treated with radical vulvectomy and bilateral groin dissection, but this has been associated with disturbances in sexual function and body image. Recently the trend has moved away from radical surgery to more emphasis on individualized treatment of the patient, taking into account age, location of disease, extent of disease, and psychosocial consequences. (1101–1102)

Head and Neck Malignancies

STUDY OUTLINE

I. **INTRODUCTION**

    1. The challenges presented by the diagnosis of head and neck cancer for the patient are significant since no other tumor site is exposed so completely to society's view.

II. **EPIDEMIOLOGY**

    1. **Approximately 67,000 new cases of head and neck cancer are diagnosed in the United States each year.**
    2. The distribution of primary tumors in the anatomic sites is as follows: **40% oral cavity, 25% larynx, 15% oro/hypopharynx, 7% major salivary glands, and 13% remaining sites.**
    3. The ratio of **male to female incidence is 3:1,** with incidence increasing after the age of 50.
    4. In some locations in the head and neck, pain occurs very late, causing a delay in medical treatment.
        a. Eighty to ninety percent of oral cancers are 2 cm or more in diameter on initial presentation.
        b. More than 60% of cases are diagnosed with advanced disease.

III. **RISK FACTORS**

    1. **Tobacco** remains the **primary risk factor** in the development of head and neck cancer. This includes cigarette and smokeless tobacco use.
    2. The sites at greatest risk for developing cancer from tobacco use are the areas in which **direct contact** with tobacco and tobacco smoke occurs: the **oral cavity, pharynx, larynx, and esophagus.**
    3. The **user group** has changed from men over 50 years of age and older women living primarily in the South to white, male adolescents and young adults in the range of 14–29 years.
    4. It is felt there is a **synergistic effect between alcohol and tobacco,** when consumed in large amounts, in the development of head and neck cancers.
        a. The combination **potentiates carcinogenesis** and creates a significantly higher risk than does either one alone.
    5. Poor oral hygiene and possibly chronic **mechanical irritation** from ill-fitting dentures and plates or sharp, jagged teeth are also predisposing factors in the development of carcinoma of the tongue, the gingiva, and other sites in the oral cavity.
    6. **Nutritional deficiencies** are also seen in patients with head and neck cancer.
        a. **Plummer-Vinson syndrome,** in which an iron deficiency anemia occurs, has been associated with cancers of the tongue, hypopharynx, and esophagus.
    7. See **Table 44-1, text page 1116,** for risk factors in the development of head and neck cancer.

IV. **PRIMARY PREVENTION**

    1. **Avoiding use of tobacco and alcohol** is the key to prevention of head and neck cancer.

V.   **DETECTION**

A. **EARLY DETECTION**

1. Early detection remains the key to successful control of the disease.
2. Five-year disease-free cure rates remain about 30%–40%, regardless of tumor size.
    a. Poor results are due to size of tumor at diagnosis, presence of regional lymph node disease, and distant metastasis.
    b. Often, metastasis to regional lymph nodes has already occurred when the patient first seeks medical care.
3. Head and neck cancers are typically **very aggressive** locally and spread initially to anatomic sites within the head and neck area.

B. **RETINOIDS**

1. **Isotretinoin** has shown some activity in suppressing oral premalignancies and in preventing second primary tumors in patients with squamous cell cancer of the head and neck.
2. Clinical trials are needed to identify the ideal chemopreventive approach to treating oral cancer.

C. **HISTORY AND SYMPTOMS**

1. A thorough review of the patient's medical history should be done, with particular emphasis on **exposure to carcinogens,** as well as a **positive family history of cancer, lifestyle habits,** and **occupation.**
2. Significant **symptoms** include **unilateral nasal obstruction or discharge, persistent ulceration, persistent hoarseness, odynophagia, dysphagia, sore throat,** and **cervical adenopathy.**
3. A thorough assessment should be performed using **inspection and palpation techniques.**
    a. The areas of the **oral cavity** and **oropharynx** are generally considered high-risk areas and should be assessed carefully.
    b. **Regional metastasis in the neck** is the only presenting symptom in more than one-third of patients with head and neck cancers.
    c. An even more thorough exam of the entire head and neck area is next performed under either local or general anesthesia in the operating room.

VI.   **CLASSIFICATION AND STAGING**

1. See **Table 44-2, text page 1118,** for the classification system for head and neck tumors.

VII. **PATHOPHYSIOLOGY**

1. Approximately 95% of all head and neck carcinomas are **squamous cell in origin.**
2. Arising from the **epithelium** that lines the upper aerodigestive tract, the typical mucosal lesion can appear as an ulceration, a roughened or thickened area, a cauliflowerlike lesion, or a combination of all of these.
3. The majority of head and neck tumors **invade locally,** deep into the underlying structures as well as along tissue planes or nerves.
4. See **Figure 44-1, text page 1118,** for lymphatic drainage of the head and neck. Prognosis is strongly influenced by the number of positive nodes, and as tumor spreads to lower nodes in the neck, there is a reduction in the 5-year survival rate.
5. **Lymphatic spread** occurs both locally at the primary site and regionally through lymphatic channels when tumor implantation into the lymph nodes occurs.

VIII. **MULTIDISCIPLINARY MANAGEMENT**

1. **Multimodality therapy** consisting of chemotherapy, surgery, and radiation therapy results in a number of health professionals participating at different intervals in the provision of care.
2. A **multidisciplinary approach** is essential to provide quality care throughout the course of treatment as well as during the rehabilitation period.

IX.   **CARCINOMA OF THE NASAL CAVITY AND PARANASAL SINUSES**

1.   Eighty percent of cancers in the nasal cavity and paranasal sinus area are **squamous cell** in origin. The remainder are adenocarcinomas.
2.   The **maxillary sinus** is the most commonly afflicted site in this area, and most tumors are squamous cell in origin.
3.   Adenocarcinoma is more commonly diagnosed in the **ethmoid sinus,** which accounts for the remainder of tumors in the area.
4.   Most patients are over the age of **40,** and there is a **male predominance** over females of 2:1.
5.   The incidence of nasal cavity carcinoma is increased in persons with occupations in nickel plating, furniture manufacturing, or leather working and in those exposed to chromate compounds, hydrocarbons, nitrosamines, dioxane, mustard gas, isopropyl alcohol, and petroleum.
6.   Chronic sinusitis symptoms may be present, as well as a stuffy nose, sinus headache, dull facial pain, rhinorrhea, epistaxis, cheek hypoesthesia, trismus, and loose teeth, although in the early stages of the disease, the patient may be asymptomatic.
7.   General prognosis is more favorable if the tumor is located anterior and inferior to a plane connecting the medial canthus to the angle of the mandible.

A.   **ANATOMY**

1.   See **Figure 44-2, text page 1120,** for a diagram of the nasal cavity and paranasal sinuses.
2.   Tumor extension in the area of the sphenoid sinus can cause compression of the third, fourth, and sixth **cranial nerves,** resulting in diplopia.
     a.   Pressure on the optic nerve can result in gradual loss of vision.

B.   **TREATMENT**

1.   **Early carcinomas** of the nasal cavity and paranasal sinuses can be effectively treated with either **surgery** or **radiation therapy,** but most tumors are not discovered until they are advanced.
2.   **Maxillectomy** is the treatment of choice for tumors in the maxillary sinus.
     a.   More **extensive disease** with invasion into the floor of the orbit may necessitate combining radical maxillectomy with **orbital exenteration.**
3.   Before surgical excision the maxillofacial prosthodontist will take an impression of the hard and soft palate to create an **obturator,** which is placed following resection and before the patient leaves the operating room.
     a.   The obturator restores oronasal continuity, allows the patient to speak and eat immediately following surgery, and enhances patient comfort by protecting the wound from irritation and debris.
4.   Following surgery, **meticulous wound care** is required in order to avoid drying, crusting, and superficial infection.

C.   **CRANIAL BASE SURGERY**

1.   The craniofacial approach, one of the most challenging areas of head and neck surgery, is used to resect tumors involving the skull base.
2.   Expected outcomes will depend on the surgical approach, the anatomic location of the tumor, and the biologic behavior of the tumor being treated.
     a.   Orbital exenteration may be necessary and will result in loss of **vision.**
     b.   **Temporary facial paralysis** resulting from dissection in the infratemporal fossa commonly occurs.
     c.   **Anesthesia** of the middle or lower face can occur.
     d.   **Loss of smell** will result from transection of olfactory nerves.

D.   **NURSING CONSIDERATIONS**

1.   Patients are monitored very closely in a neurosurgical intensive care unit following surgery.
     a.   Careful monitoring of **fluid balance** must be done because of the effects of extreme fluctuations in blood pressure on cerebral flow, such as inadequate cerebral perfusion and vasoconstriction.
     b.   In addition to careful monitoring of the **neuro status,** another nursing concern is the monitoring and maintenance of the **lumbar spinal drain.**

E. **RADIATION THERAPY**

1. High local recurrence rates of 30%–40% of patients with nasal cavity and paranasal disease, and 60% for patients with maxillary sinus cancer, accentuate the need for early diagnosis and for delivering adequate radiation doses to bulky disease and generous margins of normal tissue.
2. The 5-year survival rate for patients diagnosed early and receiving combined therapy is 40%.

X. **CARCINOMA OF THE NASOPHARYNX**

A. **EPIDEMIOLOGY AND ETIOLOGY**

1. The incidence of nasopharyngeal carcinoma in the United States is only 0.6/100,000 with a **male predominance** of 3:1.
2. The disease strikes men in the 40–44 age group and women between the ages of 60 and 64.
3. Squamous cell carcinomas account for 98% of nasopharynx cancers.
4. Factors postulated to account for the increase in incidence in Eastern populations with the exception of the Japanese include **genetic predisposition, an increased size of the nasopharynx in southern Chinese,** and **environmental relationship to the ingestion of salted fish.**

B. **ANATOMY**

1. See **text page 1122,** columns 1 and 2, for an anatomical description.

C. **SYMPTOMS**

1. Symptoms include **nasal obstruction, epistaxis, hearing impairment, tinnitus,** and **otitis media.**
2. An enlarged node in the neck may be the first indication of nasopharyngeal carcinoma in many patients.
3. Late symptoms include poorly localized headache and facial pain, which can signify advanced disease and bony erosion and pressure on the fifth cranial nerve.
4. Invasion through the base of the skull results in cranial nerve involvement; therefore, cranial nerve abnormalities provide important diagnostic information. See **Table 44-3, text page 1123,** for symptoms of cranial nerve compression from nasopharyngeal carcinoma.

D. **ASSESSMENT**

1. Diagnosis is made by careful examination of the area using a head mirror, tongue depressor, and laryngeal mirror to visualize the area.

E. **TREATMENT**

1. Radiotherapy remains the primary treatment for nasopharyngeal carcinoma; however, surgical treatment following radiation is gaining credibility.
2. Recent retrospective reviews of patients treated with **cisplatin-based combinations** suggest that carcinoma of the nasopharynx should be considered a malignant neoplasm that is distinct from squamous cell cancer of the head and neck and that selected patients with recurrent or metastatic carcinoma of the nasopharynx should receive aggressive combination chemotherapy.
3. The patient with advanced disease often has severe pain and headaches resulting from bony invasion and erosion and may also experience multiple cranial nerve palsies, visual problems, sensory losses, anorexia, severe weight loss, respiratory difficulty secondary to vagal nerve paralysis, and laryngeal edema.

XI. **CARCINOMA OF THE ORAL CAVITY**

A. **PATHOPHYSIOLOGY**

1. If **diagnosed early** when tumor size is small, cure rates for cancer of the oral cavity improve dramatically.
2. Cancers of the oral cavity and oropharynx account for **4%** of all cancers in men and **2%** of all cancers in women.

3. **Positive findings in a patient's history should alert the clinician to the possibility of an oral malignancy:** history of smoking and tobacco use, alcohol abuse, and systemic syphilis.

4. Other potential factors include a **history of poor oral hygiene, poorly fitting dentures** and **dental appliances,** and (particularly among people in India) **the chewing of betel nuts** or the **reverse smoking of cigarettes.**

5. **Alcohol also acts as an irritant to the oral mucosa and, in combination with tobacco, is thought to act synergistically in causing oral cavity cancers.**

6. **Field cancerization** is the development of multiple primary cancers that occur concurrently or subsequently in the same patient.

7. More than 90% of oral cancers are **squamous cell** carcinomas.

B. ANATOMY

1. See **Figure 44-3, text page 1125, and Table 44-4, text page 1124,** for anatomical boundaries of the oral cavity.

2. Squamous cell carcinomas generally **grow** along mucosal surfaces, and in advanced lesions, **infiltration** into deeper structures is seen.

3. As deep invasion occurs, spread may be evident along preformed **pathways of muscle fascia or nerves,** and regional lymph node metastasis frequently occurs.

4. In general, **metastases** occur when a primary lesion has been present for some time, but if the primary tumor is poorly differentiated and aggressive, metastases occur in relatively short periods of time.
   a. Distant metastases occur from cancer cells spreading through the **lymphatic system** and by blood vessel embolization.
   b. When **underlying bone** is affected, the destruction is secondary to tumor invasion.

C. TREATMENT

1. Delays in treatment may occur if the lesion is treated initially as benign.

2. The most common historical complaint may be a **painless lesion** that has existed for some time.
   a. Pain may or may not be present at the primary site and is commonly reported as **referred pain** to the ear or jaw.

3. Treatment options will be determined by the tumor size.
   a. Surgery and radiation alone have comparable cure rates in early-stage lesions.
   b. The **choice** of treatment in early-stage lesions depends on functional and cosmetic results, the patient's general health, and patient preference.
   c. While chemotherapy alone cannot cure oropharyngeal cancer, complete and partial response rates as high as 90% have been demonstrated for **platinum-based combinations.**

D. SURGICAL RESECTION

1. Surgical resection in this area involves a neck dissection in continuity with the tumor and regional metastasis.

2. An **ipsilateral** neck dissection is often done because there is a high frequency of metastasis to ipsilateral nodes.

3. The **guiding principle** of surgical resection is removal of the primary tumor with **adequate margins** that are free from tumor involvement.
   a. Resection of **2 cm** of surrounding normal tissue is usually considered adequate to ensure clear margins.

4. Surgical treatment of stage III and IV lesions often results in a greater degree of tissue resection and thus a greater degree of dysfunction and disfigurement.

5. Patients who have had large surgical resections will have a **tracheostomy** for approximately 7–10 days. An **enteral feeding tube** will be placed, and the patient will be NPO for 10 days to 2 weeks or until all intraoral suture lines are healed.

E. USE OF THE LASER

1. One of the single most important advances in the treatment of head and neck lesions over the past decade has been the increasing use of the laser in **surgical excision of early-stage** oral cavity, pharyngeal, and laryngeal cancers.

a. The CO_2 laser has the advantage of being very precise, and it reduces the possibility of tumor spread by sealing lymphatics as tissue is removed.

2. Laser use has resulted in **reduced patient morbidity, decreased hospital stay,** and an **improved recovery.**

XII. CANCER OF THE HYPOPHARYNX

A. ETIOLOGY

1. The incidence of hypopharyngeal cancer is approximately 8 per 100,000 with the ratio of male to female occurrence 2:1.
2. Specific sites within the hypopharynx that are commonly affected are **the pyriform sinus (70%), the postcricoid area (15%), and the posterolateral wall (15%).**
3. Common etiologic factors that contribute to the development of hypopharyngeal cancer include excessive **smoking** and **alcohol** consumption.
4. Most lesions in the hypopharynx are squamous cell in origin.
5. There is a tendency for submucosal spread, often resulting in what appears to be multiple separate primary tumors.

B. ANATOMY

1. The **three distinct regions** in the hypopharynx are the hypopharynx, the posterior surface of the larynx, and the lower posterior pharyngeal wall.
2. The two recesses on both sides of the larynx are called the **pyriform sinuses.**

C. ASSESSMENT

1. Patients with cancer of the hypopharynx typically present with **odynophagia, referred otalgia,** and **dysphagia.**
   a. **Advanced tumors** of the pyriform sinuses and pharyngeal wall with extension into the larynx may have the associated symptoms of **hoarseness** or **aspiration.**
2. The physical examination includes **visualization** of the pharyngeal wall and pyriform sinus area using a laryngeal mirror and tongue depressor.
3. The pyriform sinuses are best visualized during **phonation.**
4. Diagnostic studies include **CT,** which can help define the extent of the primary tumor boundaries and may demonstrate nonpalpable metastases in the lateral or retropharyngeal cervical lymph nodes.
5. **Direct laryngoscopy** and **biopsy** are performed to confirm a tissue diagnosis.
6. See **text page 1127,** columns 1 and 2, for pertinent findings that may indicate cervical esophageal extension and thereby influence treatment planning.
7. Treatment planning is based on the stage of disease, as outlined in **Table 44-5, text page 1127.**

D. TREATMENT

1. A **combination approach** using surgery, radiation, and chemotherapy is often necessary to control the disease since the majority of patients with hypopharyngeal carcinoma present with **advanced primary tumors.**
   a. Surgery is generally done first, followed by radiation therapy.
2. Because most hypopharyngeal tumors are locally advanced, either partial or total pharyngectomy is required.
   a. It may be necessary to combine this procedure with a partial or total laryngectomy and neck dissection.
3. Approximately 75% of patients with hypopharyngeal cancer present with cervical metastases and require a **radical** or **bilateral neck dissection** to be done along with resection of the primary tumor.
4. The method of reconstruction following laryngo-pharyngectomy depends on the amount of tissue removed from the pharynx and esophageal areas.
   a. If sufficient pharyngeal tissue remains, **direct closure** is the easiest method.
   b. If **primary closure** is performed, great care must be taken to avoid tension on the suture line in order to avoid a postoperative fistula.

c. If a greater amount of tissue is needed to facilitate closure, a **myocutaneous flap** from either the pectoralis major or the latissimus dorsi area can be utilized to close the pharyngeal defect.

E. RADIATION THERAPY

1. The total dose of radiotherapy that is effective in hypopharyngeal tumors is at least 60 Gy.
2. Combining external beam radiation with interstitial radiation is being studied as an adjunct component of therapy.

F. REHABILITATION NEEDS

1. **Swallowing** is often a problem after surgery for hypopharyngeal carcinoma, since the surgical resection may involve the **pharyngeal constrictors,** which assist with control of a food bolus with resultant delivery into the esophagus during swallowing.
2. Patients who have undergone surgical resection will be at increased risk for **fistula** formation, and the **risk is increased** if the patient has had previous radiation therapy.
3. Postoperatively these patients will have a temporary **tracheostomy, enteral feedings,** and **suture line wound care.**
4. **Speech rehabilitation** will depend on the clinical status of the patient.

XIII. CARCINOMA OF THE LARYNX

A. ETIOLOGY

1. **The incidence of laryngeal carcinoma in the United States is 4.2/100,000 with a male to female ratio of 9:1.**
2. **Approximately 80% of laryngeal carcinomas are found in persons over 50 years of age, with the highest incidence occurring in the sixth decade of life.**
3. Over 90% of laryngeal cancers are **squamous cell** in origin, ranging from well-differentiated to undifferentiated tumors, the majority being **moderately well differentiated.**
4. **Tobacco** and **alcohol** use and a history of exposure to ionizing radiation have been implicated as etiologic factors.
5. Cancer of the larynx cannot be considered one disease but rather involves different areas within the larynx, such as the **glottis, supraglottis, and subglottis.**
   a. **Tumors in each region involve distinct signs, symptoms, treatment regimens, and rehabilitation measures.**

B. GLOTTIC CARCINOMA

1. Tumors in this area tend to be **slow-growing, to be well differentiated, and to metastasize late.**
2. Because there are limited lymphatics in the vocal cords, metastasis usually occurs only when the disease **infiltrates muscle** or has spread beyond the limits of the true cord.
3. Important **diagnostic** information includes the mobility of the cords, evidence of fixation of the cord, involvement of the anterior commissure, and involvement of cervical lymphatic vessels.
4. See **Table 44-6, text page 1129,** for classification of glottic cancer.

C. TREATMENT

1. T1 lesions of the membranous cord are treated with equal success by radiotherapy and by conservation surgery.
   a. The **advantage of radiation therapy** in the treatment of early glottic lesions is **preservation** of excellent vocal quality.
2. **Early disease (T1 or T2)**
   a. See **Table 44-7, text page 1129,** for the anatomical limits of hemilaryngectomy surgery.
   b. Following hemilaryngectomy surgery, the individual will have a temporary tracheostomy and receive enteral feedings.
   c. **Vocalization** is accomplished by the adduction of the remaining cord against the scar tissue that eventually takes the place of the resected cord.
   d. Radiotherapy is utilized as an option for cure in early lesions.

3. **Advanced disease (T3 to T4)**
   a. A **total laryngectomy** is reserved for patients who have persistent or recurrent disease after radiotherapy or present with advanced disease.
   b. **Radical neck dissection** is indicated for any patient who presents with obvious metastasis to the lateral neck nodes.
   c. **Preoperative counseling** with a speech therapist is essential to review potential methods of speech rehabilitation.
      (1) **Approaches** that may be used to facilitate communication in the immediate postoperative period range from writing to communication boards to the use of artificial larynges.
      (2) **Electrolarynx, esophageal speech, and esophageal prosthetic voice restoration** are three options for communication on a long-term basis.
   d. It is important for the patient to have choices among different methods of speech rehabilitation at a time when he or she may feel the situation is uncontrollable.
4. **Postoperative care**
   a. In the immediate postoperative period, most patients will have a laryngectomy tube placed.
      (1) The decision to place the tube will depend on the surgical technique used to create the stoma and on the amount of contracture that occurs as healing progresses.
   b. Adequate humidity will be a life-long concern for the laryngectomized patient because the airway is diverted and the patient no longer has the ability to warm, moisten, and filter the air through the nose.
      (1) The patient should be aware of changes in secretions that could signal insufficient humidity, including blood-tinged sputum, an increase in thickness or tenacity of secretions, and increased difficulty mobilizing secretions.
      (2) The goal of patient instruction should be an understanding of the concept of lack of humidity and the subsequent effect on the tracheal secretions.
   c. **Hyposmia occurs to some degree in every laryngectomized patient.**
      (1) The ability to **taste** is closely related to stimulation of olfactory cells and is also reduced.
   d. If the patient has had previous irradiation, the potential for fistula formation is increased, which usually extends the hospital stay.
      (1) In addition, increased scarring in the suture line will contribute to later problems with esophageal strictures and dysphagia.
   e. **Dysphagia** can also occur in the absence of stricture as a result of the uncoordinated contractions of the detached inferior constrictor muscles.
   f. Most laryngectomy patients resume their preoperative lifestyle with only a few limitations.
      (1) Due to the absence of **thoracic fixation** after laryngectomy, the patient is instructed not to lift more than 10 pounds for 4 months after surgery.
      (2) The laryngectomy patient cannot protect the airway during activities such as **swimming** and boating, and these activities should be avoided.
      (3) Special precautions must be taken to avoid getting dust or dirt in the airway when performing activities such as gardening or housework.
      (4) If the patient's occupation depends on communication, the pressure to communicate effectively using an alternative method increases.

D. **SUPRAGLOTTIC CARCINOMA**

1. Supraglottic tumors account for **35% of laryngeal cancers** and are characterized by aggressive growth patterns via both direct extension and lymph node metastasis.
2. Approximately **one-half** of these patients will present with **lymph node involvement,** which occurs because lymphatic channels drain into the jugulodigastric, mid-, and inferior levels of the internal jugular chain.
3. **Clinical manifestations**
   a. Supraglottic cancer is often **advanced** when first detected because there are few early symptoms.
      (1) The patient may complain of **pain** and **poorly defined throat and neck discomfort** that occurs during swallowing.
      (2) Many patients complain of **referred otalgia** in combination with throat pain.
   b. See **Table 44-8, text page 1131,** for the TNM classification system for supraglottic carcinoma.

4. **Assessment**
   a. The diagnosis of supraglottic cancer is usually made through indirect laryngoscopy; direct laryngoscopy is used for obtaining a biopsy specimen.
5. **Treatment**
   a. In some institutions, supraglottic tumors are treated **initially** with radiation therapy.
      (1) This approach remains **controversial** because some clinicians believe that a number of larynges could have been saved with supraglottic laryngectomy as a primary treatment approach.
      (2) If radiation fails, total laryngectomy is usually required as a salvage procedure.
   b. **Postoperative airway obstruction** is common following supraglottic laryngectomy due to edema in the surgical area, and for this reason, patients will have a **temporary tracheostomy tube** placed during surgery.
   c. **Aspiration during swallowing** is one of the major complications following supraglottic laryngectomy.
      (1) The epiglottis, which is a protective mechanism during swallowing, has been removed, and the chances for chronic aspiration have increased. See **Table 44-9, text page 1132,** for the mechanisms of action in the supraglottic swallow.
   d. In some institutions, **cricopharyngeal myotomy** is performed in order to prevent failure of relaxation of the cricopharyngeal sphincter during swallowing.
      (1) **Laryngeal suspension** is another surgical technique that may be performed to decrease aspiration.
   e. A cine-esophogram and videofluoroscopy are usually obtained before the tracheostomy tube is removed to evaluate the patient's ability to swallow without aspirating.
      (1) This exam is often **repeated** at specified intervals to determine the progress of the swallowing therapy.
   f. **Liquids are the most difficult thing for the patient to swallow without aspirating.**
   g. **Tracheal suctioning** is especially important after supraglottic laryngectomy since there is an abundance of secretions caused by **increased edema** in the laryngeal area.

XIV. METHODS OF RECONSTRUCTION

1. The goal of reconstructive procedures in the head and neck is to restore function while **simultaneously** retaining socially acceptable cosmesis.

A. MYOCUTANEOUS FLAP

1. The myocutaneous flap is especially useful when **large** amounts of tissue have been resected and bulk is needed to reconstruct the defect.
2. Flaps consist of **muscle, skin, blood supply,** and in some cases **bone or cartilage.**
3. The muscles most often used to reconstruct defects in the head and neck area include the **pectoralis major, sternocleidomastoid, trapezius,** and **latissimus dorsi.**

B. FREE FLAP

1. The free flap is completely removed from its donor site and placed into the recipient site using microvascular anastomosis.
2. Donor sites that have been used successfully include the **groin** and the **radial forearm.**
3. Some of the major advantages of the free flap: **immediate functional reconstructive replacement of removed tissue is possible, the donor site is not exposed,** and **bulky exposed pedicles are avoided.**

C. DELTOPECTORAL FLAP

1. The deltopectoral flap has the advantage of bringing **well-vascularized tissue** to a previously irradiated surgical bed from an area that has not been treated with radiation.
2. There is no muscle included in the deltopectoral flap, and it maintains its blood supply from its base and consists of skin and the blood supply only.
   a. Disadvantages of this flap include strictures, fistulas, and the fact that several stages are needed.

D. **NURSING CARE OF FLAPS AND GRAFTS**

1. The goal of nursing care of any type of flap is to ensure flap viability.
    a. This is accomplished through frequent and thorough observation and assessment of the flap area.
2. **Skin grafts**
    a. Split-thickness skin grafts are used frequently to reconstruct a primary defect or to protect a major structure.
    b. Skin grafts are composed of **a thin layer of epidermis and a small amount of dermis.**
    c. The skin graft is resected completely from the donor site and sutured into the recipient site.
    d. A **dressing** over the donor site is left in place for 1–2 days after surgery.
        (1) **Re-epithelialization** occurs in the donor site area as the healing process takes place.
    e. The patient will complain of **pain** at the donor site area due to exposure of nerve endings.
3. **Skin flaps**
    a. The viability of any flap depends on adequate vascularization.
    b. The blood supply coming into the flap area must be adequate, and concurrently, the blood flowing out must not be obstructed.
        (1) **Color:** Color is usually the best indicator of adequate blood supply. The color may not match surrounding skin exactly but should be close to the color of the skin at the donor site.
        (2) **Temperature:** The flap should feel warm to the touch.
        (3) **Capillary refill:** The tissue of the flap should blanche with gentle pressure applied to the flap and return to normal color quickly.
    c. Significant changes in any of the above indicators should be reported promptly to the physician. See **Figures 44-6 through 44-10 (Plates 13–17)** for illustration of the sequence of flap failure and repair.
    d. Until flap viability is ensured, care must be taken to avoid any circumferential **pressure** on the flap from dressings, a tracheostomy tube, or neck tapes to secure the tube.
    e. **Surgical drains** placed in the flap area remove any accumulation of blood or fluid from underneath the flap area that could interfere with healing.

XV. **CHEMOTHERAPY**

A. **MODALITIES**

1. **Primary chemotherapy**
    a. There has been an increased interest in the use of induction combination chemotherapy before definitive treatments with surgery or radiation in previously treated patients with stage III or IV disease.
        (1) The rationale for this approach is as follows: Patients will be in **optimal medical condition** and better able to tolerate aggressive chemotherapy; tumor **vascularity** has not been altered by surgery or radiation, so there is adequate drug delivery to tumor tissues; and the **efficacy** of surgery or radiation will be increased by reducing the tumor bulk with chemotherapy.
    b. The regimen that has been most frequently used is a combination of cisplatin at 100 mg/m² followed by 5-day continuous infusion of fluorouracil at 1000 mg/m²/day.
2. **Single-agent chemotherapy**
    a. The overall survival impact of single-agent chemotherapy has been negligible, but it can serve an important role in **palliation** by reducing tumor bulk and promoting comfort in the patient's final days.
3. **Chemotherapy used sequentially with radiation**
    a. In selected situations, chemotherapy has been used **sequentially** with radiation therapy since it is speculated that reducing tumor volume with chemotherapy before administering radiation will increase control of the disease.
    b. The combination of therapies is attractive for advanced-stage head and neck cancer patients, because **functional problems** associated with large surgical resections are avoided.

B. **ORGAN PRESERVATION**

1. Patients who experience **complete response** to induction chemotherapy may be candidates for organ preservation.
2. The objective of organ preservation is to **prevent loss of organ function or severe disfigurement** without compromising survival.

C. **BIOLOGIC RESPONSE MODIFIERS**

1. **Interferon**
   a. Phase I trials have demonstrated some activity in the combination of interferon with 5-FU.
2. **Interleukin-2**
   a. Partial or complete response was noted in four of five patients evaluated in a pilot clinical trial.
3. **Future directions**
   a. Newer biologic agents such as tumor necrosis factor, interleukin-4, and interleukin-6 are beginning to be explored.

D. **CHEMOTHERAPY AS A PRIMARY TREATMENT MODALITY**

1. Randomized trials have indicated that **induction chemotherapy** can **change** the expected pattern of recurrence by decreasing the rate of **metastases.**

XVI. **RADIATION THERAPY**

1. Used as a primary treatment in early lesions, radiation therapy can effect a **cure.**
2. When radiation is combined with surgery for advanced lesions, **control of disease** and decrease of subsequent recurrence are often achieved.
3. The methods of treatment most frequently seen are **external beam, interstitial implantation, and intraoperative therapy.**
4. Head and neck tumors are in the middle range of sensitivity to radiation. They can be controlled with radiation but will require a higher dose than other tumors.

A. **IMPLANT THERAPY (BRACHYTHERAPY)**

1. Implant therapy is the use of radioactive sources placed directly into the tumor with a procedure called **after-loading.**
2. Implants may be used as a **curative therapy** for early-stage lesions in the floor of the mouth and anterior tongue or may be used to boost a tumor that has received prior external beam radiotherapy.

B. **HYPERTHERMIA WITH RADIATION**

1. **Heating** the tumor superficially with ultrasound or microwave increases oxygen in the tumor bed, enhancing the radiation response.

C. **INTRAOPERATIVE RADIATION THERAPY**

1. Intraoperative radiation therapy (IORT) consists of delivery of a **single, large dose of radiation therapy** to either gross disease or a tumor bed after surgical resection and during the operation.

D. **CONCOMITANT RADIATION THERAPY AND CHEMOTHERAPY**

1. The goal of concomitant therapy is to control **regional disease,** thereby decreasing the high incidence of persistent disease.
2. Chemotherapy can be successful at eliminating **systemic micrometastases while concurrently enhancing the activity of radiotherapy in the irradiated field.**

E. **NURSING MANAGEMENT OF PATIENTS UNDERGOING RADIATION THERAPY**

1. Nursing interventions in caring for the patient undergoing radiation therapy are aimed at helping the patient **understand** the goal of therapy, as well as **dealing** with both acute and long-term side effects.
2. Side effects usually experienced by patients receiving radiation therapy to the head and neck area are **mucositis, xerostomia, loss of taste, anorexia, fatigue, and local skin reaction.**
   a. **Mucositis**
      (1) Mucositis is an **inflammatory response** of the oral mucosa to radiation therapy.
      (2) It can occur as early as the first week of treatment, and it generally resolves within 3 weeks after the treatment is completed.
      (3) The oral cavity will appear **reddened** and inflamed, and white patchy areas may be noted on oral exam.
   b. **Xerostomia**
      (1) Xerostomia is a **drying** of the oral mucosa that results from loss of saliva from damage that occurs to the salivary glands subsequent to radiation therapy to the head and neck.
      (2) Salivary changes include a **thicker saliva** by the third week of treatment and are reported to persist for 3 months after treatment is completed in 43% of patients.
   c. **Loss of taste**
      (1) Loss of or alteration in taste occurs when the **taste buds** are included in the radiated field; it is compounded by xerostomia and mucositis.
   d. **Fatigue**
      (1) This is a normal side effect that can occur at any time during the treatment course.
   e. **Skin reactions**
      (1) Wet and/or dry desquamation can occur in the tissues of the radiated site.
      (2) Generally, the patient should be instructed to avoid using harsh creams, lotions, or soaps in the radiated area.

XVII. **MANAGEMENT OF THE ALTERED AIRWAY**

1. If treatment plans include compromise of the upper airway or if the tumor affects the patient's ability to breathe, a **temporary tracheostomy** will be placed.
2. In the postoperative head and neck cancer patient, the massive edema that develops after oropharyngeal procedures necessitates tracheostomy at the time of surgery.

A. **THE TRACHEOSTOMY TUBE**

1. The **type** of tracheostomy tube utilized will depend on the surgical procedure performed and the clinical objectives to be achieved. See **Table 44-10, text page 1139,** for the standard parts of a tracheostomy tube.

B. **TRACHEAL SUCTION**

1. The tracheal suctioning procedure is an important part of postoperative nursing care of the head and neck cancer patient. See **text page 1139,** column 2, for the recommended procedures of tracheal suction.
2. Some points to remember regarding suctioning a tracheostomy: Suction only after a thorough **respiratory assessment** reveals the patient cannot clear the airway effectively; **limit suctioning** to 10 seconds or less; and **hyperoxygenation** and hyperinflation of the lungs are advised both before and after the procedure.

C. **INNER CANNULA CARE**

1. The inner cannula allows for removal and cleaning to maintain patency of the tracheostomy tube.
2. The inner cannula should be removed and cleaned as needed but should be **checked** at least every four hours in the immediate postoperative period.

D. **TRACHEOSTOMY SITE CARE**

1. The tracheostomy site should be treated like any other **surgical wound,** and the nurse must be alert to signs and symptoms that can signal infection, such as erythema or purulent drainage from the site.
2. See **text page 1140,** column 1, for cleaning and tie procedure.

E. **HUMIDITY**

1. The concept of providing adequate **humidity** to the patient with an altered airway is one of the most important points for the patient and family to understand.
2. When breathing through a tracheostomy site, the patient has **lost the functions of the nose** in warming, moistening, and filtering the air.

F. **INSTILLATION OF NORMAL SALINE**

1. If secretions are tenacious and difficult to remove, up to 5 ml of normal saline is instilled directly into the tracheostomy tube to lavage and irritate the trachea and bronchi.

G. **CUFFED TRACHEOSTOMY TUBES**

1. The purpose of a cuff on a tracheostomy tube is to **protect** the airway from aspiration of blood or secretions.
2. A cuff should be used only if indicated and should not be overfilled.
3. Indications for use of a cuff include **chronic aspiration, bleeding in the head and neck area, cardiopulmonary resuscitation, positive pressure respiratory treatments, and emesis.**

H. **LARYNGECTOMY CARE**

1. Care of the altered airway of the laryngectomy patient includes all of the respiratory care mentioned previously.

XVIII. **GENERAL NURSING CONSIDERATIONS**

A. **NUTRITIONAL MANAGEMENT**

1. By virtue of their locations, cancers of the head and neck often impair the patient's ability to take nourishment by mouth.
2. **Enteral therapy**
   a. Patients who undergo surgical resections will have compromised oral intake necessitating placement, at least temporarily, of a feeding tube.
   b. The obstruction in the GI tract is usually seen in the head and neck cancer patient in the **upper area** of the tract, so enteral support must be delivered below the level of the obstruction.
   c. Because there are inherent risks of esophageal perforation and pulmonary intubation with lung puncture, it is recommended that only experienced personnel place the tubes with a stylet.
3. **Oral feeding**
   a. Prior to initiating oral feedings for the postoperative head and neck cancer patient, an assessment of the patient's oral competence is necessary.
   b. The isolation that occurs from an inability to participate in meals and the body image changes associated with an alteration in eating pattern affect the quality of life for many patients.

B. **ORAL CARE**

1. The provision of regular and thorough oral care is **imperative** in the head and neck cancer patient.
   a. **Halitosis** can be a significant problem, but more important, the surgical site of the oral cavity should be kept clean to prevent infection.
2. Oral care should be delivered every 4 hours in the early postoperative period and every 8 hours as wound healing occurs.

C. **SWALLOWING REHABILITATION**

1. The four phases of the normal swallow include the oral preparation phase, the oral phase, the pharyngeal phase, and the esophageal phase. See **Table 44-12, text page 1144,** for the normal sequence of swallowing.

D. **WOUND CARE**

1. The nursing responsibility in wound management lies initially in observation of dressings and the surgical site for any signs of **infection or dehiscence.**
2. A wound that requires **debridement will be treated with wet to dry dressings,** and every 3–4 hours, when the packing is dry, it is gently removed and the necrotic tissue is pulled from the wound.
3. **Wound breakdown**
    a. Wound breakdown with subsequent exposure of the carotid artery is one of the most serious and life-threatening sequelae either of the disease process itself or of surgical therapy. See **Table 44-13, text page 1145,** for carotid precautions equipment.
4. The nursing actions during a carotid hemorrhage focus on maintenance of the airway and control of bleeding.
5. **Carotid hemorrhage in the terminal patient**
    a. The **goal** following a carotid hemorrhage in the terminal patient will not be ligation but providing an atmosphere that minimizes anxiety and ensures death with dignity.

E. **PAIN MANAGEMENT**

1. The type of pain usually experienced by the head and neck cancer patient is described as "throbbing, pounding, and pressurelike."
2. The **goal** is to provide adequate pain relief while simultaneously allowing the patient to function at an optimum level or to die with minimal discomfort.

F. **PSYCHOSOCIAL ISSUES**

1. In addition to coping with a diagnosis of cancer and its subsequent treatment, the head and neck cancer patient must also cope with an **alteration in facial appearance and the possible loss of speech, sight, taste, smell,** and **ability to swallow.**
2. Two parameters must be considered in the adjustment process: **disfigurement** and **dysfunction.**

PRACTICE QUESTIONS

1. The distribution, by sex, of head and neck cancer cases is **best** described by which of the following statements?
    (A) More women than men are diagnosed with head and neck cancer.
    (B) Men are several times more likely to develop head and neck cancer than are women.
    (C) Men and women have similar numbers of head and neck cancers.
    (D) Women have a higher incidence of head and neck cancer than do men.

2. Which of the following is **not** correct in describing the etiology of head and neck cancers?
    (A) Inhalation of certain dusts and chemical exposures are associated with development of nasal carcinomas.
    (B) Viral infection has not been associated with the development of any head and neck cancers.
    (C) Alcohol and tobacco consumption have independent and synergistic effects in head and neck cancer development.
    (D) Poor dentition and poor oral hygiene are risk factors for tongue cancers.

3. Which of the following is of **least** importance in the diagnosis and prognosis of head and neck cancer?
    (A) the lack of lymph node metastasis
    (B) the presence of leukoplakia in a smoker
    (C) the presence of only a small surface lesion
    (D) the lack of pain at diagnosis

4. In working with the patient before the beginning of treatment, the nurse would do all of the following **except**
    (A)   initiate a program of oral hygiene.
    (B)   discuss alternative communication techniques the patient can use postoperatively.
    (C)   reassure the patient with recurrent disease that less intervention is required.
    (D)   assess the patient's nutritional status.

5. The risk of carotid artery rupture after radical neck dissection is associated with all of the following **except**
    (A)   coverage of the artery with a skin flap.
    (B)   infection of the surrounding area.
    (C)   a small trickle of blood from the area.
    (D)   persistent tumor in the area.

6. An example of a postoperative situation requiring immediate nursing intervention is
    (A)   a smooth suture line with no sign of swelling.
    (B)   hematoma formation beneath a skin flap.
    (C)   evidence of cranial nerve damage.
    (D)   clearing of airway secretions by coughing.

7. Skin flaps are used in reconstruction in all of the following ways **except**
    (A)   to prevent wound contracture.
    (B)   to cover a full-thickness surface deficit.
    (C)   to replace mucous production lost by excision.
    (D)   to support other oral structures.

8. Which of the following is the **most** accurate statement reflecting the role of chemotherapy in the treatment of head and neck cancers?
    (A)   Chemotherapy is well-tolerated by patients regardless of previous treatment.
    (B)   Chemotherapy may make a tumor more susceptible to radiation and lead to less extensive surgery.
    (C)   Chemotherapy is not known to have a synergistic impact when administered concurrently with radiation.
    (D)   Chemotherapy has a minor role in the treatment of recurrent or advanced disease.

9. Common symptoms of carcinoma of the nasal cavity and paranasal sinuses include all of the following **except**
    (A)   diplopia.
    (B)   hyperesthesia of the cheek.
    (C)   taste changes.
    (D)   headache pain.

10. Which of the following statements about nasopharyngeal carcinoma is **false?**
    (A)   Radiotherapy is the treatment of choice.
    (B)   It has a high incidence among persons from southern China.
    (C)   Hearing impairment and tinnitus are common symptoms.
    (D)   Distant metastases are relatively rare.

11. Which of the following is an accurate statement about the role of metastases in cancers of the oral cavity?
    (A)   Bone metastasis is a common initial presentation.
    (B)   The presence or absence of metastases does not affect treatment choice.
    (C)   Cervical node masses cannot be palpated.
    (D)   Uncontrolled local disease accounts for most of oral cancer deaths.

12. A patient reports a several-month-long history of hoarseness. The nurse refers the patient for examination of which structure to rule out carcinoma?
    (A)   oropharynx
    (B)   hypopharynx
    (C)   larynx
    (D)   nasopharynx

13. After laryngectomy, heavy lifting is restricted because of the
    (A) lack of thoracic fixation.
    (B) risk of aspiration.
    (C) risk of hiatal hernia.
    (D) reduction in cough effectiveness.

14. Because of the changed configuration of the aerodigestive tract, the person who has undergone a laryngectomy can expect change in all of the following functions **except**
    (A) speaking.
    (B) eating.
    (C) taste.
    (D) smell.

ANSWER EXPLANATIONS

1. **The answer is (B).** Three-quarters of all head and neck cancers are diagnosed in men. (1115)

2. **The answer is (B).** A close relationship has been documented between the Epstein-Barr virus and the development of nasopharyngeal cancer. All other choices contain correct statements about possible head and neck cancer etiologies. (1115–1116)

3. **The answer is (D).** Many head and neck lesions are painless and asymptomatic. Lymph node metastasis is predictable, with the number of involved nodes indicating likely prognosis. Leukoplakia in a tobacco user is considered a precancerous lesion, and actual tumors spread deeply along tissue planes, beyond the anatomic location of the lesion. (1117, 1146)

4. **The answer is (C).** The patient previously treated may be feeling discouraged and depressed at recurrence of second primary tumor after initial treatment. The same assessments need to be made of the previously treated patient as the newly diagnosed patient. (1143–1146)

5. **The answer is (A).** Skin flaps are usually made in order to cover and protect the carotid artery. However, skin flap necrosis leaves the artery unprotected, and infection and persistent tumor raise the risk of rupture. Carotid artery blowout usually is preceded by a small trickle of blood from the area. (1145–1146)

6. **The answer is (B).** Hematoma formation can affect the adherence of skin flaps, resulting in flap necrosis. Excessive bleeding may require return to the operating room for ligation of the bleeding vessel. Choices (A) and (D) are desirable; as to choice (C), cranial nerve damage may have occurred during surgery and cannot be affected by nursing action. (1134, 1145)

7. **The answer is (C).** Skin flaps are used to line the oral cavity, but because they are skin and not mucous membrane, they cannot produce mucus. (1134)

8. **The answer is (B).** Chemotherapy as adjuvant to radiation and surgery improves patient response by medically debulking the tumor and possibly acting synergistically with radiation therapy. (1137)

9. **The answer is (C).** Choices (A), (B), and (D), along with excessive lacrimation and swelling of the cheeks or orbit, are all clinical manifestations of carcinoma of the nasal cavity and paranasal sinus. (1119)

10. **The answer is (D).** On the contrary, nasopharyngeal cancers are a rarity among the head and neck cancers in that they frequently metastasize widely. Bloodborne spread to lung, liver, spine, pelvis, and femur is found. (1122)

11. **The answer is (D).** Eighty percent of oral cancer deaths are due to uncontrolled local disease. Metastasis below the clavicle generally occurs late in the course of the disease. (1124)

12. **The answer is (C).** A two-week history of hoarseness warrants examination of the larynx. Hoarseness is the cardinal symptom of laryngeal cancer. Pain and dysphagia are signs of advanced disease. (1131)

13. **The answer is (A).**   Heavy lifting should be avoided for four months postoperatively and may not be possible in the long term due to lack of thoracic fixation. (1131)

14. **The answer is (B).**   Normal eating remains possible after use of a nasogastric tube for nutrition in the immediate postoperative period. Speech is affected by the excision of the vocal cords—esophageal speech or use of a hand-held artificial larynx is necessary. Hyposomia and decreased taste acuity are also noted post-laryngectomy. (1129–1130)

45   Leukemia

STUDY OUTLINE

I.   INTRODUCTION

    1.   Leukemia is the name given to a group of hematologic malignancies that affect the bone marrow and the lymph tissue.

II.   EPIDEMIOLOGY

    1.   Leukemias account for 3% of all cancers.
    2.   The most common types of leukemias are
        a.   In **adults,** acute myelogenous leukemia (**AML**) and chronic lymphocytic leukemia (**CLL**).
        b.   In **children,** acute lymphocytic leukemia (**ALL**).

III.   ETIOLOGY

    1.   The cause of leukemia is not known. The etiologic factors most commonly considered are **genetic predisposition, radiation, chemicals, drugs,** and **viruses.**

A.   GENETIC FACTORS

    1.   **Familial clustering** is suggested by
        a.   An increased risk among family members of individuals diagnosed with leukemia.
        b.   A 10%–20% incidence among monozygous twins of individuals with leukemia.
    2.   **Chromosome abnormalities** are implicated by an increased incidence among children with Down's syndrome.

B.   RADIATION

    1.   Exposure to **ionizing radiation** is the most conclusively identified etiological factor, with an increased incidence among early radiologists and Japanese survivors of the atomic bomb.

C.   CHEMICALS

    1.   Exposure to **benzene** has been implicated in the development of acute leukemia. Populations at risk include dye users, shoemakers, painters, distillers, and individuals working with explosives.

D.   DRUGS

    1.   Acute myelogenous leukemia (AML) is the most frequent second malignancy following aggressive chemotherapy and is associated with treatment for Hodgkin's disease, multiple myeloma, ovarian cancer, non-Hodgkin's lymphoma, and breast cancer.
    2.   Alkylating agents and etoposide have demonstrated a relationship to the etiology of acute leukemia.
    3.   Characteristics that distinguish treatment-related and de novo (arising without prior chemotherapy or radiation) leukemia are summarized in **Table 45-1, text page 1151.**
    4.   **Chloramphenicol** and **phenylbutazone** are also known to cause acute myelogenous leukemia (AML).

E.   **VIRUSES**

   1.   **Reverse transcriptase** is an enzyme that reverses the transcription of genetic information from DNA to RNA. Reverse transcriptase is present in the virus that causes **feline leukemia** and has been detected in human leukemic blood cells but not in normal blood cells.
   2.   **Human T-cell lymphotrophic virus (HTLV-I)** has been associated with T-cell leukemia in Japan and the Caribbean. **HTLV-II** is probably involved in hairy cell leukemia.

IV.   **CLASSIFICATION**

   1.   **Chronic versus acute**
        a.   In **chronic leukemias** the predominant cell is mature appearing although it does not function normally. The disease has a **gradual onset, prolonged clinical course,** and **relatively longer survival time.**
        b.   In **acute leukemia** the predominant cell is **immature** (i.e., undifferentiated), usually a "blast" cell. The disease has an **abrupt onset, rapid progression,** and **short survival time.** Progress in treatment has significantly lengthened the survival time of children with acute lymphocytic leukemia (ALL).
   2.   **Myelocytic versus lymphocytic**
        a.   **Myelocytic leukemias** develop from abnormalities in maturation and proliferation of the **myeloid cell series.**
             (1)   The myeloid stem cell is **pluripotent.** The immature cells (also called progenitors or precursors) mature in the bone marrow to become **red blood cells, platelets,** and **white blood cells.** See the left side of **Figure 45-1, text page 1152,** for a description of this process.
        b.   **Lymphocytic leukemias** develop from abnormalities in maturation and proliferation of the **lymphocyte series.**
             (1)   The lymphoid stem cell matures to form **plasma cells, T-cells,** and **B-cells.** See the right side of **Figure 45-1, text page 1152,** for a description of this process.
   3.   The French-American-British (FAB) Classification System classifies leukemias according to morphology. See **Table 45-2, text page 1152.**

V.   **PATHOPHYSIOLOGY**

   1.   Manifestations of leukemia are related to
        a.   **Excessive proliferation of immature leukocytes in blood-forming organs** (bone marrow, spleen, and lymph nodes).
        b.   **Crowding of the bone marrow by proliferating leukemic cells,** which results in a decrease in the number of normal leukocytes, erythrocytes, and thrombocytes.
        c.   **Infiltration of various organs** (e.g., lymph nodes, liver, spleen, brain) with proliferating leukocytes.
   2.   **Table 45-3, text pages 1153–1154,** summarizes possible leukemic manifestations, both primary and secondary, although these vary considerably with each type of leukemia.
   3.   **Table 45-4, text page 1154,** summarizes the presenting manifestations, complications, course of disease, and treatment for each type of leukemia. These are discussed in greater detail below.

VI.   **ASSESSMENT OF ACUTE LEUKEMIA**

   1.   **Symptoms** are the result of a large and rapidly growing population of leukemic cells. Factors influencing signs and symptoms include
        a.   **Type of leukemic cell** (myelocytic versus lymphocytic).
        b.   **Degree of leukemic cell burden** (early versus advanced disease).
        c.   **Involvement of organs or systems outside the bone marrow and peripheral circulation.**
        d.   **Depression of normal marrow elements** by the proliferation of leukemic cells.

A.   **PATIENT HISTORY**

   1.   **Acute leukemia has an acute onset.** Usually signs and symptoms have been present for less than 3 months and sometimes for only a few days.

2. **Nonspecific complaints** may include fatigue, malaise, weight loss, and fever.
3. There may be a history of **recurrent infections.** Common sites are skin, gingiva, perianal tissue, lung, and urinary tract. The patient may complain of sore throat and fever with or without symptoms of infection.
4. **Unexplained bleeding** may be present as evidenced by bruising, petechiae, bleeding from gums, heavy menses, or midcycle bleeding.
5. Symptoms of **progressive anemia** may include fatigue, weakness, shortness of breath, palpitations, and anorexia.
6. **Pain** may arise from sources such as the sternum, enlarged lymph nodes, hepatomegaly, and splenomegaly.
7. **Neurologic complaints** attributable to CNS infiltration (especially in ALL) or cerebral hemorrhage include headache, vomiting, visual disturbances, and seizures.
8. Possible **etiologic factors** should be assessed; these may include viral infections, drug exposure, occupational exposure, and family history of genetic abnormalities or cancer.
9. An essential part of the history is the **psychosocial profile,** which encompasses past and present coping strategies, significant others, and the patient's and family's perceptions of the illness.

B. **PHYSICAL EXAMINATION**

1. Vital signs may reveal **fever, tachycardia,** and **tachypnea.**
2. Skin and mucous membranes may demonstrate **pallor** attributable to anemia and **ecchymoses, purpura,** and **petechia** attributable to anemia and decreased platelets.
3. Generalized or localized **adenopathy** may be present as a result of leukemic infiltration or infection.
4. Eye examination may show **retinal capillary hemorrhage** or **papilledema** caused by leukostasis, thrombocytopenia-induced bleeding, and/or increased intracranial pressure.
5. The **oral cavity** should be examined for **gingival bleeding** from thrombocytopenia, **gingival hypertrophy** attributable to leukemic infiltration, and **oral infection** caused by *Candida albicans.*
6. Examination of the lungs and heart may reveal infection or a **cardiac murmur.**
7. Palpation of the abdomen may reveal an **enlarged liver, spleen,** and/or **kidneys.**
8. The only evidence of a **rectal abscess** or a fistula may be perirectal tenderness or swelling.
9. Palpation of **bones and joints** may reveal swelling of joints or pain.

C. **DIAGNOSTIC STUDIES**

1. **Differentiating between AML and ALL is essential because the treatment and prognosis for the two differ markedly.**
2. Ongoing explanations to patient and family are important in order to facilitate cooperation, decrease anxiety, and create an atmosphere of confidence and trust.
3. **Peripheral blood smears**
   a. The white blood count may be low, normal, or high.
   b. Ninety percent of patients have **blast cells** in the peripheral blood.
   c. **Neutropenia** (absolute granulocyte count less than 1000 cells/mm^2) is frequent, and 40% of patients have **thrombocytopenia.**
   d. Blood chemistry studies may reveal hyperuricemia and increased lactic dehydrogenase as well as altered serum and urine muramidase.
4. **Bone marrow biopsy and aspirate**
   a. Bone marrow is usually hypercellular.
   b. **Auer rods** are diagnostic of AML.
5. **Cytogenetic analysis**
   a. Approximately half of patients with de novo acute leukemia exhibit nonrandom chromosome abnormalities, and 40% of adults with leukemia have some cytogenetic translocations.
      (1) Translocations are an adverse feature in ALL, while some translocations in AML indicate a better prognosis.
   b. At the time of diagnosis, cells from the bone marrow or peripheral blood are collected and placed in culture for 24–72 hours.
      (1) After special stains are applied, the cells are examined for abnormalities in number and shape.

(2) These abnormalities are described as translocations, inversions, or loss or gain in chromosome number.

(3) Specific aberrations are related to a favorable or unfavorable outcome.

c. Further information is obtained from immunologic studies.

(1) Monoclonal antibodies reactive to immature cells can identify the predominant cell type and stage of arrested development in the leukemic cell line.

(2) Mixed lymphoid and myeloid surface markers are found in 21% of patients with de novo ALL.

(3) In general, patients with mixed lineage leukemia have a poor response to treatment and should be considered for other investigational therapies.

VII. ACUTE MYELOGENOUS LEUKEMIA

A. CLASSIFICATION

1. **Acute myelogenous leukemia (AML) is the result of an abnormality in the pluripotent myeloid stem cell.**

a. The malignant clone arises in the **myeloid cell lines:** erythrocytes, granulocytes, monocytes, and megakaryocytes. AML is also called **acute nonlymphocytic leukemia (ANLL).** (See **Figure 45-1, text page 1152.**)

b. The rapid accumulation of leukemic cells in the marrow results in "crowding" that both **inhibits the growth of normal blood cells and forces immature blood cells into the peripheral circulation.**

c. Infiltration of organs by myeloblasts causes dysfunction and discomfort.

d. See **Table 45-4, text page 1154,** for a comparison of AML with other leukemias and **Table 45-3, text pages 1153–1154,** for a review of clinical manifestations.

2. The leukemic cells have more abundant cytoplasm, and granulation in the cytoplasm is usually (but not always) present.

a. Auer rods, which are abnormal lysosomal granules, are present and pathognomonic for AML.

3. The type of leukemia is named for the predominant cell.

a. The most common myeloid leukemia is acute myelocytic leukemia (M_1).

b. Acute promyelocytic leukemia (APML, M_3) is associated with an increased risk of disseminated intravascular coagulation.

c. Patients with acute monocytic (M_5) or myelomonocytic (M_4) leukemia often exhibit extramedullary leukemic infiltration with gingival hypertrophy, cutaneous leukemia, and liver, spleen, and lymph enlargement.

d. Erythroleukemia (M_6) has both a chronic and an acute form.

e. Megakaryocytic leukemia (M_7) is quite rare and is less responsive to chemotherapy.

4. By the time an individual is diagnosed with AML, the bone marrow and peripheral blood contain up to 10^{12} leukemic cells.

a. The accumulation within the bone marrow space results in the inhibition and **crowding out** of normal marrow stem cells and the infiltration of other organs by myeloblasts.

B. TREATMENT

1. The goal of antileukemic treatment for AML is the eradication of the leukemic stem cell.

2. Complete remission is defined as the restoration of normal peripheral counts and less than 5% blasts in the bone marrow.

3. The course of therapy is divided into two stages: induction and postremission therapy.

4. **Induction therapy**

a. The cornerstone for remission induction is **cytosine arabinoside (Ara-C),** a cell-cycle-specific agent, for 7 days **plus a non-cycle-specific anthracycline** (e.g., daunorubicin, doxorubicin, mitoxantrone, etc.) for 3 days.

b. The therapy is assessed with a bone marrow biopsy and aspirate on **day 14** (one week after completion of induction therapy), and the induction therapy is repeated if there are residual leukemic cells in the marrow.

c. **Bone marrow recovery** usually takes 14 to 21 days after the completion of chemotherapy.

d. **Response rates** for induction therapy are as follows:

(1) Sixty-five to eighty percent of previously untreated adults achieve a complete remission.

(2) Only 20% remain in complete remission.

5. **Postremission therapy**
   a. **Postremission therapy** is essential to prevent recurrence as a result of undetectable, residual disease. The types of postremission therapy are **consolidation, intensification, maintenance,** and **allogeneic or autologous bone marrow transplant.**
   b. **Consolidation therapy** consists of very high doses of the same drugs used for induction.
      (1) **Toxic effects** are substantial and include extended myelosuppression, cerebellar dysfunction, dermatitis, hepatic dysfunction, and conjunctivitis.
      (2) Two or more courses of consolidation are given.
   c. **Intensification therapy** uses different drugs from those used in induction.
      (1) **Early intensification** begins right after remission is achieved.
      (2) **Late intensification** begins several months later.
   d. **Maintenance therapy** uses lower doses of the same or other drugs at monthly intervals for a **prolonged period of time.** Maintenance therapy is not currently recommended for the treatment of AML.
   e. **Treating relapse after induction or postremission therapy**
      (1) After first relapse, only 30%–60% achieve a second remission with current therapies.
      (2) Patients with early relapses or patients whose leukemia is resistant to therapy should be considered for clinical trials or bone marrow transplantation.
   f. There are several controversies involving the use of **bone marrow transplantation (BMT)** in treating AML.
      (1) The ideal candidate is less than 40 years of age with an HLA-matched donor. However, only 16% of patients with AML are eligible for an allogeneic transplant.
      (2) BMT is associated with significant risks. See **Chapter 18** for an in-depth discussion of BMT.
      (3) The **optimal time** to do BMT is not known.
   g. Options may include a matched unrelated donor obtained through the **National Marrow Donor Program.**
      (1) There are **increased risks** of graft-versus-host disease and lack of engraftment from the histocompatible but unrelated cells.
   h. A **purged autologous** BMT may be performed in a young patient with no HLA match.
   i. In patients **less than 30 years** of age, BMT may offer a higher cure rate than standard treatment.
   j. In patients in the fourth decade, the results of chemotherapy versus BMT vary.
   k. See **Table 45-5, text page 1156,** for prognostic indicators that may be useful in deciding the best course of therapy.
   l. **Multidrug therapy** is a new strategy being offered to patients with risk factors, early relapse, or resistant leukemia to overcome multidrug resistance.
   m. **All-trans retinoic acid** has been used in patients with resistant or recurrent APL, as well as in patients unable to tolerate conventional chemotherapy.

VIII. **ACUTE LYMPHOCYTIC LEUKEMIA**

1. Acute lymphocytic leukemia (ALL) is a malignant disease of the **lymphoid progenitors.**
2. Although the defect does not involve the myeloid cell lines, the secondary effect of the high leukemic cell burden on the bone marrow interferes with normal hematopoietic activity.

A. **CLASSIFICATION**

1. The FAB classification for ALL is based on several cell properties: size ratio of nucleus to cytoplasm; number, size, and shape of nucleoli; and amount and basophilia of the cytoplasm.
2. Another classification system for ALL is based on immune features. Four subtypes are identified by the presence of certain markers on the cell surface.
   a. Common ALL (cALL) is the most frequent and least differentiated ALL.
   b. T-cell markers and T-cell-specific antigens contain another marker, terminal deoxynucleotidyl transferase (TdT).
   c. Other surface and cell immunoglobulins denote the rare B-cell ALL.
   d. About one-fourth are pre-B (formally null) leukemias, which do not have any identifiable surface markers.
3. Lymphoblasts have a propensity for **organ infiltration** and may remain sequestered in sanctuary sites even after remission has been achieved.

        a. Leukemic cells infiltrate into the CNS early in the disease.

        b. Cells can also be harbored in the testes.

        c. Eighty percent of patients have **lymphadenopathy** and/or splenomegaly at the time of diagnosis due to the infiltration of these organs by leukemic cells.

    4. As with AML, long-term survival and cure for individuals with ALL is possible only if a complete remission is achieved, documented by a bone marrow aspirate containing less than 5% lymphoblasts and the disappearance of all peripheral manifestations of the disease.

B. TREATMENT

    1. Unlike AML, chemotherapy regimens for ALL are selectively **toxic to lymphoblasts** and relatively **sparing of normal blood cell precursors.**

        a. **Toxicity associated with treatment is less severe and shorter in duration with greater cell kill.**

    2. Treatment is divided into three phases: **induction, CNS prophylaxis,** and **postremission therapy.**

    3. **Induction therapy**

        a. In **children,** vincristine, prednisone, and L-asparaginase are commonly used and achieve a complete remission in 93% of cases.

        b. In **adults,** vincristine, prednisone, and L-asparaginase plus an anthracycline are utilized, but only 70%–75% achieve complete remission.

        c. Treatment is initiated in the hospital. Once remission is documented, therapy can be completed on an outpatient basis.

    4. **CNS prophylaxis**

        a. **Meningeal leukemia,** present at diagnosis in 2% of patients with ALL, occurs in up to 50% of patients with ALL who do not receive CNS prophylaxis.

        b. The signs and symptoms of meningeal leukemia include headache, blurred vision, nausea, vomiting, and cranial nerve palsies.

        c. **CNS prophylaxis,** involving **cranial radiation** and **intrathecal methotrexate,** should start within a few weeks of the initiation of therapy.

        d. **Side effects of therapy** include somnolence, chemical meningitis, paraparesis, and leukoencephalopathy.

    5. **Postremission therapy**

        a. With prolonged maintenance therapy (duration 2–3 years), cure rates of 40% have been reported. Without maintenance therapy, relapse occurs within 2–3 months.

        b. Maintenance therapy utilizes the same drugs as induction therapy with or without the addition of methotrexate and/or 6-mercaptopurine.

        c. Prognosis is poor if relapse occurs during maintenance therapy.

        d. If relapse occurs after the completion of maintenance therapy, second remission can be achieved in up to 50% of patients with high-dose chemotherapy.

        e. Idarubicin and high-dose cytosine arabinoside have induced second remission in 65% of adults with ALL.

        f. Patients with an unfavorable prognosis should be referred for BMT.

        g. Factors affecting the prognosis in ALL are listed in **Table 45-5, text page 1156.**

IX.   MYELODYSPLASTIC SYNDROMES

    1. **Myelodysplastic syndromes (MDS) are a group of hematologic disorders with an increased risk of transformation to AML.**

    2. Although the etiology is not known, MDS is believed to occur as the result of an **altered stem cell.**

    3. Incidence is greater in men than in women, and 20% of patients diagnosed with MDS are older than 50 years of age.

    4. **Table 45-6, text page 1161,** lists the classifications of MDS, compares the risk of evolution into acute leukemia, and lists the average survival time for each type of MDS.

    5. A bone marrow biopsy and aspirate usually reveal dyshematopoiesis in all cell lineages.

        a. A hypocellular bone marrow with one or more of the lineage defects provides a diagnosis of MDS.

    6. Poor prognostic indicators include **excessive blast cells in the bone marrow, small clusters of immature myeloid precursors, pancytopenia,** and **complex chromosome abnormalities.**

7. Death usually occurs within 2 years from complications related to bone marrow depression or transformation to acute leukemia.
8. Treatment for MDS is as aggressive as the course of the disease.
    a. Supportive therapy includes placement of RBCs or platelets and antibiotics for infection.
    b. Continuous infusion of low-dose cytosine arabinoside is thought to induce differentiation of immature myeloid cells in 25%–35% of patients with MDS.

X. **CHRONIC MYELOGENOUS LEUKEMIA**

1. **Chronic myelogenous leukemia (CML) is a disorder of the myeloid stem cell.**
2. CML is characterized by an increased production of **granulocytes,** especially neutrophils, and **marked splenomegaly.** CML is also called **chronic granulocytic leukemia.**
3. The **Philadelphia chromosome** (Ph[1]) is a diagnostic marker found in 90% of patients with CML. As long as the marker is present, the patient is not cured of the disease.
4. The natural course of CML is divided into a **chronic** and a **terminal** phase.
    a. The **chronic phase,** characterized by an accumulation of **mature granulocytes,** precedes the accelerated phase. Although lymphadenopathy is usually absent, 90% have splenomegaly.
    b. CML usually transforms into a **terminal phase** within 30–40 months. The patient becomes increasingly resistant to treatment.
        (1) Symptoms include **progressive leukocytosis** with increasing myeloid precursors (including blasts), increasing basophils, splenomegaly, weight loss, and weakness. There is increasing resistance to therapy, and cytogenic studies indicate progressive chromosomal abnormalities.
        (2) The accelerated or **blastic** phase of CML resembles AML. **Blast crisis** occurs if the blast cell count rises rapidly, often exceeding 100,000/dL.

A. **ASSESSMENT**

1. Twenty percent of patients with CML may have no symptoms at diagnosis.
2. CML is characterized by a **gradual onset** of symptoms, which are the result of a gradual increase in white blood cells.
3. **Patient history**
    a. Symptoms related to **massive splenomegaly** include left upper quadrant abdominal pain, early satiety, and vague abdominal fullness.
    b. **Nonspecific symptoms** include malaise, fatigue, weight loss, and fever.
    c. The patient may experience **bone and joint pain** related to leukemic infiltration of joints.
    d. Etiologic factors to be assessed are **exposure to ionizing radiation** and **family history of leukemia.**
    e. As with other leukemias, the **psychosocial profile** includes past and present coping strategies, significant others, and the patient's and family's perceptions of the illness.
4. **Physical examination**
    a. **Most patients with chronic myelogenous leukemia (CML) are diagnosed in the chronic phase.**
    b. The individual with anemia appears pale.
    c. Upon EENT exam, **leukemic infiltration** may be evident.
    d. **Splenomegaly** and **hepatomegaly** are common.
    e. In blast crisis, blastic transformation of the leukemic granulocytes has replaced the bone marrow, causing an acute illness with pancytopenia, infection, and hypercatabolism.
5. **Diagnostic studies**
    a. **Peripheral blood count** may reveal
        (1) **Leukocytosis** (>100,000 WBCs/mm³), with a predominance of more mature cells. The white cells are functional but leukemic, which explains the low incidence of infection during the chronic phase.
        (2) Moderate normochromic, normocytic anemia.
        (3) Moderate thrombocytosis.
    b. **Bone marrow biopsy demonstrates hyperplasia,** with an increase in the ratio of white blood cell to red blood cell precursors and normal to increased megakaryocytes (platelet precursors).
        (1) If the abnormal Ph[1] chromosome is found in the granulocytic, erythrocytic, and megakaryocytic series of the marrow, the diagnosis of CML is confirmed.

B. **TREATMENT**

1. **The only chance for cure is with elimination of the Ph¹ chromosome with high-dose therapy followed by allogeneic BMT.**
2. **CML is a chronic disease and is usually suppressed by chemotherapy.**
3. Late in the disease or in blast crisis, high-dose chemotherapy with standard or investigational drugs is used.
4. Recently **interferon** has been found to be useful in early CML.
5. **Chronic phase**
   a. Standard therapy involves **single-agent oral chemotherapy** with **busulfan,** an alkylating agent, or **hydroxyurea.**
   b. Therapy decreases the number of leukemic cells and improves the quality of life, but it does not prevent the inevitable progression to the terminal, refractory stage.
6. **Terminal phase**
   a. The **blastic transformation occurs gradually** and can be detected in the bone marrow 3–4 months before clinical signs are evident.
   b. The length of time from initial evidence of blastic transformation to blast crisis is variable but life expectancy is less than 1 year.
   c. The drugs used to treat the chronic phase are continued until there is clinical evidence of blast crisis.
   d. The intensive chemotherapy used to treat blast crisis in CML is similar to the treatment of AML. If lymphoblastic transformation has occurred, vincristine and prednisone are added.
7. The **prognosis** for patients with CML is
   a. Without treatment: 19 months.
   b. With conventional single-agent chemotherapy: 30–45 months.
   c. If intensive chemotherapy is used during chronic phase: 50–65 months.
8. **Therapies with promise**
   a. **BMT** presently offers the only chance for a cure.
      (1) Only 25% of patients arc eligible.
      (2) Disease-free survivals of 55%–70% at 3 or 5 years have been reported in patients who were transplanted during the chronic phase.
   b. Alpha-interferon, when used alone in patients with early disease, appears to produce a complete hematologic response in 30%–70% of patients.

XI. **CHRONIC LYMPHOCYTIC LEUKEMIA**

1. **Chronic lymphocytic leukemia (CLL) is a disorder affecting the lymphoid cell line.** (Refer to the right side of **Figure 45-1, text page 1152.**)
2. CLL is characterized by an accumulation of **normal, but functionally ineffective, lymphocytes.** As the disease progresses, the abnormal lymphocytes accumulate in marrow, spleen, liver, and lymph nodes.
3. For over 25% of patients, the diagnosis is an incidental finding on routine examination. However, anemia, lymphadenopathy, or infection may be present.
4. Approximately half of patients with CLL have frequent **viral and fungal infections,** while 25% develop an **autoimmune hemolytic anemia.**
5. Three **classification systems** are used: the Rai system, the Binet system, and the International Workshop on Chronic Lymphocytic Leukemias (IWCLL), which combines the Rai and Binet systems. All three classification systems are useful in **projecting survival** for an individual patient. See **Table 45-7, text page 1163,** for a comparison of these three systems.

A. **ASSESSMENT**

1. **Patient history**
   a. **Recurrent infections,** especially of skin and the respiratory tract, are the earliest clinical manifestations of CLL.
   b. Symptoms of more advanced disease include
      (1) Vague complaints of **malaise, anorexia,** and **fatigue.**
      (2) **Lymphadenopathy.**
      (3) **Early satiety** and **abdominal discomfort** related to splenomegaly.

   c. The past medical history may reveal **bleeding tendencies, infectious episodes,** and **auto-immune or immune deficiency disease.**

2. **Physical examination**
   a. In early CLL, the individual appears well and **splenomegaly** may be the only clinical finding.
   b. In advanced CLL, symptoms of **infection** are usually evident, and **lymphadenopathy** occurs in 60% of patients. Nodes are mobile, discrete, and nontender.

3. **Diagnostic studies**
   a. **Peripheral blood examination** may demonstrate **lymphocytosis** with normal or immature lymphocytes. The lymphocyte count is >20,000/mm³ in early disease and may be >100,000/mm³ in advanced disease.
   b. **Protein electrophoresis** shows hypogammaglobulinemia in approximately 50% of patients.
   c. **Bone marrow aspirate** reflects the lymphocytosis seen peripherally, with varying degrees of infiltration.
     (1) The severity of the lymphocytosis reflects the severity of the CLL. In early CLL the marrow has patchy or focal infiltrates of mature-appearing lymphocytes. In advanced CLL, the marrow is "packed" and there are few normal cells.
   d. Pathology on **lymph node biopsy** is similar to well-differentiated lymphocytic lymphoma if the blood count and bone marrow findings are unknown to the pathologist.

B. **TREATMENT**

1. **The treatment for the asymptomatic patient is observation.** Patients may be relatively stable and require no treatment for many years.
2. **The treatment for the symptomatic patient includes**
   a. **Oral alkylating agents** (chlorambucil or cyclophosphamide).
     (1) The response rate is 60%, with complete remission in 10%–20%.
     (2) Prolonged use of alkylating agents is associated with secondary development of AML.
   b. **Corticosteroids** may be used to control leukocytosis and cytopenias mediated by the immune system.
3. Treatments used as **palliative measures** when patients no longer respond to chemotherapy and corticosteroids include
   a. **Splenectomy** to reduce pain and thrombocytopenia.
   b. **Radiation therapy** to treat painful lymphadenopathy or splenomegaly.
4. Treatment of **advanced CLL** (stage III or IV) with anemia or thrombocytopenia involves combination chemotherapy with cyclophosphamide, vincristine, doxorubicin, and prednisone.

XII. **HAIRY CELL LEUKEMIA**

A. **ETIOLOGY**

1. **Hairy cell leukemia (HCL),** an unusual variant of CLL, is named for the hairlike projections of cytoplasm on the circulating mononuclear cells. Clinically, HCL is difficult to distinguish from CLL and malignant lymphoma.
2. Patients present with massive **splenomegaly** but little or no adenopathy, and two-thirds of individuals have **pancytopenia** with symptoms of anemia, bleeding, and infection.

B. **TREATMENT**

1. Historically, patients without cytopenias required no immediate treatment.
2. **Close monitoring** is essential since **infection** is the primary cause of death.
3. **Splenectomy,** which may prolong survival by 15 years, is the treatment of choice for patients with marked pancytopenia, recurrent infections, massive splenomegaly, or rapid disease progression.
4. Complete remissions have been obtained in HCL with 2'-deoxycoformycin and 2-chlorodeoxyadenosine.
5. **Recombinant alpha-interferon** is considered the treatment of choice for those in whom disease progresses either before or after splenectomy.
   a. Alpha-interferon may decrease the need for transfusions, reduce the risk of infection, and improve overall quality of life.

XIII. SUPPORTIVE THERAPY

1. Advances in both antileukemic treatment and supportive therapy, including specialized nursing care, have improved survival and the quality of survival in leukemia. Effective supportive therapy requires an **interdisciplinary** approach.
2. **Nursing** plays a key role in the following areas: **education, physical care, symptom management,** and **psychosocial adaptation.**

A. EDUCATION

1. The teaching plan for all patients includes
   a. **Pertinent information related to the diagnosis.**
   b. **Strategies for self-care in the prevention and treatment of side effects both in the hospital setting and at home.**
   c. **Methods to facilitate coping and adaptation to the illness.**
2. **Patient information** related to diagnosis and treatment includes
   a. Basic physiology of the bone marrow.
   b. Symptoms of leukemia.
   c. Symptom management.
   d. Symptoms to report to the nurse or doctor.
   e. See **Figure 45-4, text page 1165,** for an example of a simplified patient teaching tool. Simplification is essential to facilitate patient learning.
3. **Educational materials** can be obtained from the Leukemia Society, American Cancer Society, and the National Cancer Institute. See the **Yellow Pages: Cancer Nursing Resources** section at the end of the text for addresses and phone numbers.

B. PHYSICAL CARE

1. **Regular and thorough physical examination** is essential in order to detect early signs and symptoms of infection, bleeding, or chemotherapy toxicities.
2. **Early detection** by the nurse in the following areas plays a critical role in assuring that appropriate and potentially life-saving treatment are initiated early.
   a. Subtle changes in vital signs and mentation may indicate **early sepsis.**
   b. Oozing of blood from gums or intravenous site may be the first sign of **disseminated intravascular coagulation (DIC).**
   c. Slight changes in the neurological examination may be the first sign of **cerebellar toxicity from chemotherapy.**
3. Patients with AML are treated with high-dose chemotherapy. The goal of treatment in AML is to achieve complete bone marrow aplasia for several weeks.
4. **The risk of infection is increased and the usual signs and symptoms of infection are reduced or absent.** This is true of all of the leukemias.
   a. Susceptibility to viral and fungal infections is increased because of the decrease in immune globulins.
   b. Fever, inflammation, and pus formation may be absent or muted in a patient with neutropenia.
   c. **Two mechanisms that contribute to infections in patients with lymphocytic leukemias (ALL and CLL) are**
      (1) **Decreased immunocompetence from the decrease in the number of functioning lymphocytes.**
      (2) **Neutropenia from the chemotherapy.**
5. **Management of right atrial catheters (RACs) and vascular access devices (VADs) is an important nursing function.**
   a. A **double- or triple-lumen RAC** is recommended for aggressive induction therapy.
      (1) **Frequent blood drawing** is essential to monitor the patient's response to chemotherapy.
      (2) **Reliable access** for administration of fluids, chemotherapy, antibiotics, total parenteral nutrition, and blood products is essential.
      (3) Double- or triple-lumen catheters are needed to allow **simultaneous administration** of incompatible products and medications.

b. **Single-lumen venous access devices (VADs)** are adequate for patients who
    (1) Require ongoing treatment but less frequent blood drawing.
    (2) Will not require simultaneous infusions of fluids, chemotherapy, blood products, and/or nutritional support.

C. **SYMPTOM MANAGEMENT**

1. **Early detection and prompt treatment of the side effects of leukemic therapy and complications of the disease process are essential.**
2. Knowing which side effects are expected and when they are likely to occur allows the nurse to plan assessment and care appropriately.
3. **Bone marrow depression**
    a. The desired effect of cytotoxic therapy is bone marrow hypoplasia.
    b. The duration of the pancytopenia is variable and depends on the type of therapy and the patient's ability to recover.
    c. Patients with acute leukemia and patients with CML in blast crisis may have severe hypoplasia for weeks at a time.
    d. **Neutropenia**
        (1) Neutrophils are one of the body's first-line defenses against infection.
        (2) Neutrophils (granulocytes) are **particularly sensitive to chemotherapy** because of their short life cycle. Development from precursor to mature granulocyte takes approximately 9–10 days. Mature granulocytes circulate in the peripheral blood for only 6–10 hours.
        (3) Neutropenia is defined as an **absolute neutrophil count lower than 1000/mm³.**
        (4) **Infection is the major complication for patients with leukemia.** The patient with leukemia is at particular risk because
            (a) **Treatment causes a rapid drop in WBCs.**
            (b) **Recovery time is prolonged.**
            (c) Infection develops in approximately 60% of patients with neutropenia.
            (d) **One-third of neutropenic patients have symptoms of infection without documentation of a pathogen.**
        (5) Most infections are due to the organisms that are part of the body's normal flora or are present in the environment.
            (a) The most common sites of infection are the **pharynx, esophagus, anorectal area, sinuses, lungs,** and **skin.**
            (b) *Staphylococcus epidermidis* is the most common Gram-positive organism that causes infection.
            (c) Pneumonia is commonly caused by Gram-negative organisms such as *Pseudomonas aeruginosa, Klebsiella pneumoniae,* and *Escherichia coli.*
            (d) The most serious infections in the neutropenic patient are **fungal infections with *Candida* species or *Aspergillus*, or protozoa such as *Pneumocystis carinii*.** These infections are difficult to treat in the neutropenic and immunocompromised patient, and recovery of the marrow offers the best hope for survival.
        (6) Factors that increase the risk of infection in the leukemic patient include
            (a) **Severity and duration of the neutropenia.** Incidence of infection is 100% if neutrophil count remains lower than 100/mm³ for 3 weeks.
            (b) **Alterations in the mucosa.**
                i. **Chemotherapy** damages the mucosa of the oropharynx and gastrointestinal tract, and neutropenia allows colonization with yeasts or gram-negative bacilli.
                ii. **Perianal infection** occurs in 25% of patients with AML, and the only signs may be induration, erythema, and pain on defecation.
            (c) **Alterations in skin integrity.**
                i. *Staphyloccus epidermidis* is a frequent cause of infection in neutropenic patients.
            (d) **Corticosteroids,** which cause immunosuppression, suppression of inflammatory responses, and protein malnutrition.
        (7) **Empiric antibiotic therapy** is used to treat high-risk patients until an infecting organism is identified.

(8) **Amphotericin B** is used to treat life-threatening fungal infections in myelo-suppressed, immunosuppressed individuals.

    (a) **Side effects** include fever, chills, and rigors; nephrotoxicity; headache; anorexia; vomiting; and anemia.

    (b) **Symptom management** includes interventions to prevent or treat fever, chills, or rigors.

(9) The usual **signs and symptoms of infection may be absent** in the neutropenic patient because there may not be an inflammatory response to infection.

    (a) **Fever is usually the first sign of infection.** Vital signs are monitored every 4 hours.

    (b) **Shortness of breath or cough may be the only evidence of pneumonia** because patients with neutropenia often are unable to produce sputum.

(10) In order to prevent infection in the neutropenic patient, the nurse should

    (a) **Maintain and restore host defenses through rest, sleep, nutrition, and skin integrity.**

    (b) **Decrease invasive procedures.**

        i. If catheterization is necessary, nurses should use the smallest possible lumen and anchor the catheter.

    (c) **Provide meticulous care of intravenous sites or RAC sites and aseptic technique for any invasive procedure.**

    (d) **Take measures to decrease colonization of organisms,** including meticulous hand washing, a private room, restricting visitors, avoiding uncooked fruits and vegetables, removing aerators from faucets, frequently changing water in oxygen humidifiers, and removing live plants or fresh flowers in the room.

(11) **Total reverse isolation for BMT patients.** Total reverse isolation includes

    (a) A sterile laminar air flow room.

    (b) Nonabsorbable antibiotics to sterilize the alimentary tract.

    (c) Frequent cleaning of skin flora with hexachlorophene or an iodine-base soap.

(12) **Granulocyte transfusions** may be indicated for patients with profound neutropenia and documented infections not responding to antibiotics.

(13) **The colony-stimulating factors** G-CSF and GM-CSF seem to reduce myelosuppression and infection.

e. **Erythrocytopenia**

    (1) Patients develop tolerance for the low-grade anemia that develops as a result of intensive chemotherapy.

    (2) Transfusions of red blood cells are only used in the event of symptomatic anemia, sudden blood loss, or severe anemia.

    (3) Multiple transfusions increase the risk of transfusion reactions.

    (4) **Leukocyte-poor red blood cells** may be used to decrease the antibody production against antigens on the leukocytes.

f. **Thrombocytopenia**

    (1) The potential for bleeding occurs with platelet counts $\leq 50,000/mm^3$.

    (2) Spontaneous bleeding may occur with platelet counts $\leq 20,000/mm^3$.

    (3) Patients should be monitored for signs of **bleeding,** including

        (a) Petechiae or ecchymoses on mucous membranes or the skin of dependent limbs.

        (b) Oozing from gums, nose, or intravenous sites.

        (c) Changes in vital signs.

        (d) Headache that may be an early sign of intracranial bleeding.

    (4) **Random donor platelets** are given to keep the platelet count greater than $20,000/mm^3$.

    (5) **Measures to reduce the risk of bleeding include**

        (a) **Avoiding trauma and maintaining skin and mucosa integrity.**

        (b) **Avoiding medications with anticoagulant effects** (e.g., aspirin, ibuprofen, heparin).

        (c) **Taking stool softeners to prevent straining at stool and rectal tears.**

        (d) See **Chapter 25** for a complete discussion of bleeding precautions.

4. **Complications**

  a. Certain complications of the leukemic process or therapy occur with such high frequency that the nursing care plan should anticipate their occurrence.

b. **Leukostasis**
(1) Leukostasis occurs as leukemic blasts accumulate and invade vessel walls, causing rupture and bleeding. **Intracerebral hemorrhage** is the most common and most lethal manifestation of leukostasis.
(2) Patients at increased risk include individuals with **extremely high numbers of circulating blasts** (WBC >50,000/mm³).
(3) Prevention involves **reducing the number of circulating blast cells** through
    (a) High-dose chemotherapy.
    (b) Leukopheresis and cranial irradiation, which may be used to provide immediate reduction.

c. **Disseminated intravascular coagulation**
(1) Patients undergoing **induction therapy** are at increased risk. Although DIC may occur with any acute leukemia, it most frequently is associated with acute promyelocytic leukemia.
(2) Treatment measures include
    (a) **Heparin** to correct the thrombosis.
    (b) **Transfusions of platelets and plasma factors** to prevent bleeding.
    (c) **Correction of the altered coagulation in DIC,** which depends on the successful treatment of the leukemia.
(3) Nursing care of the patient with DIC focuses on
    (a) Prevention of injury.
    (b) Administration of prescribed therapy.
    (c) Monitoring appropriate laboratory studies.

d. **Oral complications** may be the result of the leukemic process or the therapy and include
(1) **Gingival hypertrophy**
    (a) Gingival hypertrophy is caused by infiltration of the gums with leukemic cells.
    (b) Patients at risk are those with acute myelomonocytic leukemia and acute monocytic leukemia.
    (c) Symptoms include swelling, necrosis, and/or superinfection of the gingiva.
    (d) The most effective treatment is therapy for the leukemia.
(2) **Stomatitis**
    (a) Stomatitis is caused by toxicity of chemotherapeutic agents (e.g., anthracyclines or methotrexate) combined with prolonged neutropenia and antibiotic therapy.
    (b) Treatment measures include
        i. **Oral care** with a solution of one quart water with one teaspoon each of salt and sodium bicarbonate.
        ii. **Antifungal mouth rinses.**
        iii. Local or systemic **analgesics** as needed.

e. **Cerebellar toxicity**
(1) Cerebellar toxicity is caused by **high-dose cytosine arabinoside (HDARAC)** in which the ARA-C dose is ≥ 3 gm/m² compared to conventional doses of 100 to 200 mg/m².
    (a) At 3 gm/m², the incidence of cerebellar toxicity is 11%–28%. At 4.5 gm/m², the incidence increases to 67%.
    (b) The incidence of cerebellar toxicity is higher among patients over 50 years of age.
(2) The **symptoms** of cerebellar toxicity are
    (a) Early: ataxia and nystagmus.
    (b) Late: dysarthria and adiadochokinesia (inability to perform alternating movements).
(3) The **treatment** for cerebellar toxicity is to stop HDARAC.
    (a) Symptoms may be irreversible if not detected early.
    (b) A full **neurologic assessment before each dose of HDARAC** is essential. Any changes are reported, and the dose is held until the physician evaluates the patient.

XIV.   PSYCHOSOCIAL SUPPORT

1. **The primary objectives of psychosocial support are**
   a. To facilitate the most effective coping mechanisms for the individual and family.
   b. To enable the patient to live as full and normal a life as possible.

2. Factors to be taken into consideration include the
   a. **Age** of the individual and age-specific developmental tasks and concerns.
   b. Stage and **"curability"** of the leukemia.
   c. **Impact of the therapeutic regimen** on ability to care for oneself and to meet family and/or employment responsibilities.
   d. Impact of the **emotional ups and downs** related to multiple inductions, remissions, and relapses on the patient and family.
   e. Importance of education, reassurance, and consistency of nursing staff members in helping the individual regain a **sense of control** and **hopefulness.**

PRACTICE QUESTIONS

1. Acute myelogenous anemia (AML) is the most frequently reported cancer following treatment with which of the following chemotherapeutic agents?
   (A) alkylating agents (e.g., cyclophosphamide)
   (B) anthracyclines (e.g., daunorubicin)
   (C) vinca alkaloids (e.g., vincristine)
   (D) antimetabolites (e.g., methotrexate)

2. Which of the following statements **best** explains why ongoing monitoring of asymptomatic patients with MDS is important?
   (A) T-cell abnormalities increase the risk of opportunistic infections.
   (B) Compliance with the prescribed treatment will delay or prevent the onset of symptoms.
   (C) All patients with MDS eventually develop life-threatening anemias, thrombocytopenias, and/or neutropenias.
   (D) All patients with MDS eventually develop acute leukemia.

3. The Philadelphia chromosome is only found in which of the following types of leukemias?
   (A) acute lymphocytic leukemia
   (B) acute myelogenous leukemia
   (C) chronic lymphocytic leukemia
   (D) chronic myelogenous leukemia

4. In addition to supportive therapy with transfusions of red blood cells and platelets, patients with hairy cell leukemia may be treated with
   (A) aggressive chemotherapy requiring hospitalization.
   (B) aggressive chemotherapy requiring hospitalization plus CNS prophylaxis.
   (C) low-dose chemotherapy or alpha-interferon as an outpatient; splenectomy may be considered.
   (D) chemotherapy followed by a bone marrow transplant.

5. Acute myelogenous leukemia (AML) occurs **most** frequently in which of the following age groups?
   (A) young children
   (B) teenagers and young adults
   (C) middle-aged adults
   (D) the elderly

6. Acute myelogenous leukemia (AML) and acute lymphocytic leukemia (ALL) have similar symptoms. However, it is essential to differentiate between the two because
   (A) the response rate and survival rate is better in AML than in ALL.
   (B) patients with AML are more susceptible to viral infections.
   (C) bone marrow transplant is the treatment of choice in AML.
   (D) CNS prophylaxis is given routinely in ALL but not in AML.

7. A commonly used induction therapy for acute myelogenous leukemia is
   (A) busulfan and hydroxyurea.
   (B) cytosine arabinoside (ARA-C) and daunorubicin.
   (C) vincristine, prednisone, L-asparaginase, and daunorubicin.
   (D) chlorambucil and cyclophosphamide.

8. A patient has AML and is in a complete remission after two courses of induction therapy. He is beginning postremission therapy in which he will receive very high doses of the same drugs used for induction therapy. This type of postremission therapy is called
    (A) consolidation therapy.
    (B) intensification therapy.
    (C) maintenance therapy.
    (D) CNS prophylaxis.

9. A patient has chronic myelocytic leukemia and is being treated with low-dose busulfan. She complains of left upper quadrant abdominal pain, early satiety, and vague abdominal fullness. These symptoms are **most** likely to be related to
    (A) toxicities of busulfan.
    (B) bowel obstruction.
    (C) splenomegaly.
    (D) hypercalcemia.

10. Busulfan usually is held if the white blood count is less than
    (A) 1000 WBC/mm^3.
    (B) 3000 WBC/mm^3.
    (C) 10,000 WBC/mm^3.
    (D) 20,000 WBC/mm^3.

11. The usual symptoms of infection are absent or muted in the leukemic patient with neutropenia because
    (A) most infections are due to organisms that are part of the body's normal flora.
    (B) the WBCs drop rapidly and recovery time is slow.
    (C) neutrophils are necessary to produce an inflammatory response.
    (D) the immunoglobulins are reduced.

12. Which of the following infections has the **highest** mortality rate in patients undergoing aggressive chemotherapy for acute leukemias?
    (A) viral infections (e.g., herpes simplex).
    (B) fungal infections (e.g., *Candida*).
    (C) Gram-positive organisms (e.g., *Staphylococcus epidermidis*).
    (D) Gram-negative organisms (e.g., *Pseudomonas aeruginosa, Klebsiella pneumoniae*).

13. Nurses should monitor patients with high white blood counts for the complications associated with leukostasis. The most common and most lethal complication of leukostasis is
    (A) intracerebral hemorrhage.
    (B) cerebellar toxicity.
    (C) blast crisis.
    (D) disseminated intravascular coagulation.

14. Patients with acute myelocytic leukemias frequently have gingival hypertrophy with swelling, necrosis, and infection of the gums. All of the following treatments are appropriate. Which one will be **most** effective in relieving the problem?
    (A) oral care with a solution of one quart water with one teaspoon each of salt and sodium bicarbonate
    (B) antifungal mouth rinses
    (C) local or systemic analgesics as needed
    (D) initiating chemotherapy

15. A patient who is receiving high-dose cytosine arabinoside (ARA-C) at 4 gm/m^2 evidences slight difficulty with articulation of words. The patient attributes this to dryness of his mouth and a poor night's sleep. The nurse should
    (A) do an oral examination and offer mouth care; give ARA-C.
    (B) hold ARA-C; do a neurological evaluation.
    (C) hold ARA-C; check renal function tests.
    (D) interview the patient to identify factors contributing to sleeplessness.

ANSWER EXPLANATIONS

1. **The answer is (A).**   Alkylating agents have a demonstrated causative relationship to acute myelocytic leukemia. AML is the most frequently reported second cancer following aggressive chemotherapy for lymphoma, multiple myeloma, ovarian cancer, and breast cancer. These cancers are treated with aggressive chemotherapy regimens containing alkylating agents. (1151)

2. **The answer is (C).**   All patients with MDS will eventually develop life-threatening anemia, thrombocytopenia, and/or neutropenia. Regular evaluation of patients with MDS is important in order to monitor the need for supportive therapy with red blood cells, platelets, or antibiotics. MDS can transform to acute leukemia; however, this does not occur in all patients with MDS. (1161)

3. **The answer is (D).**   The presence of the Philadelphia chromosome is diagnostic of CML. As long as this marker is present, the disease is not cured. (1161)

4. **The answer is (C).**   Hairy cell leukemia is a variant of CLL. Patients without cytopenias require no immediate treatment. Splenectomy is the treatment of choice for patients with marked pancytopenia, recurrent infections, massive splenomegaly, or rapid disease progress. Low-dose chlorambucil and alpha-interferon are also useful in treating hairy cell leukemia. (1164)

5. **The answer is (B).**   AML is typically a disease of teenagers or young adults, with a mean age of 20 years. In contrast, ALL is a disease of young children, with a mean age of 4 years. (1150)

6. **The answer is (D).**   Leukemic infiltration of the central nervous system occurs more frequently in ALL. Relapse occurs in up to 50% of patients who do not receive CNS prophylaxis. Choices (A), (B), and (C) are incorrect because the response rate and survival rate is better in ALL than AML; patients with ALL and patients with AML are equally susceptible to viral infections; and the role for BMT in AML has not yet been established. (1160)

7. **The answer is (B).**   The cornerstone of induction therapy in AML is the cell-cycle-specific antimetabolite cytosine arabinoside, plus an anthracycline such as daunorubicin. Choice (A) includes two drugs used in CML; choice (B) is the induction therapy for ALL; choice (D) includes two drugs used in CLL. (1156–1157)

8. **The answer is (A).**   The purpose of postremission therapies it to eliminate residual microscopic disease. The three types of postremission therapies are consolidation therapy, intensification therapy, and maintenance therapy. Consolidation therapy consists of one or two courses of very high doses of the same drugs used for induction (up to 30 times the induction doses of cytosine arabinoside for AML). Intensification regimens use different drugs in the hope that they will not be cross resistant. Maintenance therapies use lower doses for a prolonged period of time. Maintenance therapy is not currently recommended in the treatment of AML. (1156–1157)

9. **The answer is (C).**   Symptoms of splenomegaly are the result of infiltration of the spleen by leukemic cells. (1162)

10. **The answer is (D).**   Busulfan is taken daily in low doses. Blood counts begin to drop 10–14 days after therapy is begun. To prevent prolonged or severe myelosuppression, treatment is stopped if the WBC is less than 20,000/mm^3. (1162)

11. **The answer is (C).**   The patient with neutropenia is unable to mount an inflammatory response. Fever is usually the first sign of infection. Choices (A), (B), and (D) are all true, but they explain why the neutropenic patient is at greater risk for infection rather than why the usual signs and symptoms of infection are often absent. (1166–1167)

12. **The answer is (B).**   Fungal infections are difficult to treat in the neutropenic and immunocompromised patient, and recovery of the marrow is the best hope for survival. (1166–1167)

13. **The answer is (A).**   Leukostasis occurs as the leukemic blast cells accumulate and invade vessel walls, causing rupture and bleeding. Patients with extremely high numbers of circulating blasts (WBC >50,000/mm^3) are at increased risk for leukostasis. (1168)

14. **The answer is (D).** Gingival hypertrophy is the result of infiltration of the gums by leukemic cells. Chemotherapy will treat the underlying cause. The other measures may reduce infection and add to comfort. (1168)

15. **The answer is (B).** The ARA-C should be held because difficulty in articulating words (dysarthria) is a symptom of cerebellar toxicity. Cytosine arabinoside (ARA-C) can cause cerebellar toxicities that may be irreversible. Patients receiving doses ≥ 3 gm/m^2 are at increased risk. A full neurological examination should be done before each dose, even in the absence of symptoms. (1168)

46 Lung Cancer

STUDY OUTLINE

I. INTRODUCTION

1. **Lung cancer** remains a major health problem in the United States, accounting for more deaths than any other cancer.
2. Advances in therapy have done little to improve long-term survival in lung cancer patients.
3. **Eighty-five percent** of lung cancers could be prevented if people did not smoke.

II. EPIDEMIOLOGY

1. The **incidence** of lung cancer has risen dramatically since the turn of the century.
2. Lung cancer in women began to increase in the late 1960s and is now the leading cause of cancer death in women. In the United States, the mortality rate for women due to lung cancer has increased over 400% since the mid-1950s.
3. Although the lung cancer mortality rates are higher for blacks than for whites, lung cancer incidence rates have been declining for black males since the mid-1980s, and the incidence in black women appears to be leveling off in the younger age groups.
4. Lung cancer is highly virulent and rapidly fatal. In 1992, there were 160,000 new cases and 146,000 deaths.
5. The **five-year survival** is 13% for whites and 11% for blacks.

III. ETIOLOGY

1. Lung cancers occur most commonly following repeated exposures to substances that cause tissue irritation.
2. Exposure to more than one carcinogenic agent has demonstrated **interactive** and **synergistic** effects in the development of lung cancer.

A. TOBACCO SMOKE

1. Epidemiologic studies since the 1950s have proven a **causal link between smoking and lung cancer.** Physiologic changes in smokers reinforce this link.
2. The relative risk of cancer increases with the **number of cigarettes smoked per day** and the **number of years of smoking history.**
3. Individuals who start smoking before age fifteen have a greater risk of lung cancer than those who start after age twenty-five.
4. It is unclear how tobacco smoke causes lung cancer.

B. PASSIVE SMOKING

1. **Passive smoking** is the **involuntary exposure** of nonsmokers to tobacco smoke.
2. Passive smoke is qualitatively similar to the smoke inhaled by the smoker; both are carcinogens.
3. Many fewer lung cancers are attributable to passive than active smoking, but smoke exposure of passive smokers cannot yet be quantified.

C. AIR POLLUTION

1. The three major sources of air pollution are
   a. The sulfur oxide–particulate complex from the combustion of sulfur-containing fuel.

      b.   Photochemical oxidants from motor vehicle emissions.

      c.   Miscellaneous pollutants (e.g., from refineries and factories).

  2. Known carcinogens have been identified in atmospheric pollution, and **lung cancer incidence increases in polluted urban areas.**

  3. It is unclear whether air pollution functions as a promoter or as a carcinogen in the development of lung cancer.

D. OCCUPATIONAL FACTORS

  1. About 12% of lung cancer deaths result from chronic exposure to industrial carcinogens.

  2. See **Table 46-1, text page 1178,** for a list of occupation-related carcinogens, including asbestos and petroleum products.

  3. Smoking compounds the risk of lung cancer in individuals who are chronically exposed to industrial carcinogens.

E. RADON

  1. **Radon** is a naturally occurring radioactive gas found in soil and rocks. It is colorless, tasteless, and odorless.

  2. Radon gas can **migrate** through soils and enter homes through cracks in foundations, drains, or wells.

  3. It has been estimated that radon is responsible for **9000 to 13,000 deaths** from cancer each year.

  4. Home monitoring kits for radon are available. The EPA recommends that steps be taken in homes where the level is greater than 4 pCi/L.

F. VITAMIN A

  1. There is an association between **low vitamin A levels** and lung cancer. Available epidemiologic evidence points to dietary intervention as an encouraging area for further study.

G. CONSTITUTIONAL FACTORS

  1. There is little evidence to suggest a genetic link for lung cancer.

  2. Evidence points to a link between both **chronic obstructive pulmonary disease (COPD)** and **progressive systemic sclerosis (PSS)** and lung cancer.

  3. **Lung scars** from TB or pulmonary inflammatory processes and parenchymal fibrosis can become sites of lung cancers, usually adenocarcinomas.

IV. PREVENTION

A. SMOKING RELATED

  1. Lung cancer, which is both common and lethal, could be controlled by eliminating tobacco use.

  2. In 1990, **25%** of adult Americans smoked cigarettes. Although per capita cigarette consumption has declined in the last 20 years, its use among adolescents and black Americans remains relatively high.

  3. Different types of programs are needed to prevent people from starting to smoke and to help smokers to quit.

      a.   Some steps for reducing the development of smoking behavior in adolescents are listed on **text page 1179.**

  4. Although most smokers want to quit, one of three remains abstinent for one year after attempting to quit smoking.

      a.   The regular use of cigarettes leads to **behavioral** and **pharmacologic dependence** on nicotine, which is a powerful psychoactive and physiologically active drug.

      b.   Success at quitting increases with the number of attempts made.

  5. Nicotine replacement products are available to control symptoms of nicotine withdrawal during smoking cessation.

      a.   Cigarettes with **reduced tar and nicotine** cause less damage to lung tissue than those with more tar and nicotine.

6. Nicotine delivery systems used in combination with counseling sessions can increase smoking cessation rates, at least in the short term (6 months).
7. Government initiatives to control tobacco use can be summarized under the headings of regulatory activities, community education/information, and economic incentives/deterrents.
   a. Examples include **taxation of cigarettes, warning labels, restrictions on advertising,** and **limiting smoking in public places.**

B. **OCCUPATION RELATED**

1. Preventing occupational lung disease depends on **eliminating** or **reducing lung exposure** to toxic substances.
2. The number of cases is relatively small, although occupation-related risk is multiplied if the worker also smokes.
3. **Preventive measures** include
   a. **Premarket testing of new chemical compounds.**
   b. **Use of industrial hygiene techniques.**
   c. **Legal and regulatory approaches and epidemiologic surveillance.**

C. **CHEMOPREVENTION**

1. The National Cancer Institute has undertaken the study of preventive research in nutrition and lung cancer.

V. **EARLY DETECTION**

1. Although lung cancers usually grow for years before clinical presentation, it is rare that they are diagnosed in the occult or localized stage.
2. The only screening tests currently available for diagnosis of asymptomatic lung cancers are **sputum cytologies** and **chest radiographs.**
   a. They are usually used together, but are considered too costly to merit mass screening, even of people in high-risk groups.
   b. Chest radiographs are more accurate in **detecting peripherally located tumors,** and sputum cytologies more often detect **central lung tumors.**
3. Earlier detection seems to lengthen the interval between diagnosis and death without increasing the total life span.
4. Neither serologic testing nor breath analysis has yet proved useful as a screening test to distinguish diagnostic markers for localized lung cancer.

VI. **HISTOGENESIS**

1. Over 90% of all primary lung tumors arise from the **bronchial epithelium.** Normal bronchial epithelium contains both **pseudostratified columnar epithelial cells** and **basal cells,** both with specific functions. (See **Figure 46-3, text page 1182,** for illustration.)
2. Chronic irritation causes the protective **mucus-producing** and **ciliated columnar cells** to be shed at a faster rate than they can be replaced.
   a. **Basal cells** proliferate (basal cell hyperplasia), lose their ability to differentiate, and assume the more primitive appearance of squamous cells and eventually neoplastic cells.
   b. As a tumor grows, tumor cells look less and less like the tissue of origin. Their arrangement in the tissue becomes more chaotic.
   c. Without columnar cell protection, irritants and carcinogens can easily enter lung tissue, exacerbating the destructive cycle.
   d. The developmental period in lung cancer probably depends on the duration and degree of exposure to lung irritants and/or carcinogens.

VII. **HISTOLOGY**

1. The two major histologic classes of bronchogenic cancer are **small-cell lung cancer (SCLC)** and **non-small-cell lung cancer (NSCLC).**
2. All lung tumors probably arise from proliferating **simple pleuropotential reserve cells** rather than from mature epithelial cells.
3. It is not uncommon to find cells of several histologic types in the same tumor.

A. **NON-SMALL-CELL LUNG CANCERS (NSCLC)**

   1. **Squamous cell carcinomas**
      a. **Squamous cell carcinomas** show a strong association with **cigarette smoking:** incidence is directly related to the number of cigarettes smoked.
      b. They comprise about 30% of all lung cancers.
      c. Squamous cells take on several different shapes, and most often arise in the main bronchi or their primary divisions. Their tumors are **slow growing** and tend to remain more localized than other cell types.
      d. Patients with squamous cell tumors have a longer survival period than those with other lung tumors.
   2. **Adenocarcinomas**
      a. **Adenocarcinoma is the most common of the lung cancers.** It is the most frequent type found in women, nonsmokers, and young people.
      b. Adenocarcinoma cells are characteristically found in a **glandular formation** and commonly **produce mucin.** They can develop after **chronic parenchymal irritation, scarring,** or **fibrosis;** the occurrence of adenocarcinoma shows poor correlation with cigarette smoking.
      c. **Hematogenous spread** is common, especially to the brain.
   3. **Large-cell carcinomas**
      a. Lesions that do not fit into the other three categories are called **large-cell carcinomas.** They are histologically **undifferentiated,** and survival is poor.

B. **SMALL-CELL LUNG CANCER (SCLC)**

   1. SCLC is strongly associated with **smoking** and comprises about **25%** of lung cancers.
   2. Malignant cells have large nuclei and little cytoplasm.
   3. Tumors usually arise in the central regions of the lung and metastasize early and widely, features that contribute to a **poor prognosis.**

VIII. **METASTATIC PATTERN**

   1. Patterns of local spread include **invasion through the walls of lung structures** and **along the inside of the bronchial lumens.**
   2. Tumors can cause **bronchial occlusion** by encircling it or by filling it to the point of obstruction. Compression of lung structures is common.
   3. When lymphatic structures are invaded by tumor, the pattern of subsequent spread depends on the tumor cell type and the anatomic location of the tumor.
   4. Metastatic lesions frequently involve the **liver, adrenal glands, bone,** and **brain.**
   5. The widespread pattern of hematogenous metastases in lung cancer is due to the invasion of the pulmonary vascular system and is associated with a poor prognosis.

IX. **PROGRESSION OF DISEASE**

   1. At diagnosis, most tumors have probably progressed through most of their life spans and have metastasized widely.
   2. Though multimodality treatment can prolong survival, the **5-year survival rate is only 11%.**

X. **CLINICAL MANIFESTATIONS**

   1. Presenting symptoms are determined by the location and type of tumor.
   2. **Local symptoms** may include cough, chest pain, hemoptysis, dyspnea, and wheezing.
   3. **Systemic complaints** may include anorexia, weight loss, and fatigue. **Paraneoplastic syndromes,** more common with lung cancer than any other type of cancer, may cause various other systemic complaints.

XI. **CLASSIFICATION AND STAGING**

A. **NON-SMALL-CELL LUNG CANCER**

   1. Staging is based on the **TNM system,** which is defined in **Table 46-2, text page 1186.**
   2. The **stage groupings** of the TNM categories are in **Table 46-3, text page 1186.** They describe levels of **progression of disease.**

3. **The anatomic extent of the disease is the crucial determinant of treatment and ultimate survival** as is depicted in the graphs on **text pages 1186–1187.**

B. SMALL-CELL LUNG CANCER

1. The anatomic extent of disease also is the most important prognostic factor in SCLC.
2. Other factors that have some prognostic significance are **performance status, weight loss,** and **response to therapy.**

XII. DIAGNOSTIC/STAGING TESTS

1. The initial evaluation will include an assessment of the presence, duration, and severity of pulmonary and extrapulmonary symptoms.
2. Initial evaluation of lung cancer also includes a thorough **history of risk factors and symptoms.**
3. A separate diagnostic evaluation is used to examine **tumor sites (T), node status (N), and metastasis status (M).**

A. *T* (TUMOR) SITES

1. A diagnosis of lung cancer is ultimately established by cytologic examination of secretions and/or biopsied tissue.
   a. Centrally located tumors may yield **positive sputum cytologies** and may be accessible for **bronchogenic visualization** and **washing,** brushing, and biopsy.
      (1) Nurses are usually responsible for instructing and assisting in sputum collection and can increase the efficiency of this method of cancer detection by collecting and handling the specimen appropriately.
   b. Cells from peripheral tumors frequently can only be obtained by **needle biopsy.**

B. *N* (NODE) STATUS

1. Seventy percent of all patients with lung cancer have **regional lymph node involvement at diagnosis;** individuals with mediastinal node metastases are usually considered unresectable.
2. Evaluation of the presence and extent of regional lymph node metastases is critical to determining surgical resectability and prognosis.
3. **Thoracic lymph nodes** can be evaluated using **CT scanning.**
4. **Regional nodes** can be sampled using **transbronchial needle aspiration, mediastinoscopy,** and **mediastinotomy.**

C. *M* (METASTASIS) STATUS

1. A **history, physical examination,** and **blood chemistries** are the most useful techniques in evaluating metastatic spread.

XIII. TREATMENT

A. NON-SMALL-CELL LUNG CANCER

1. **Surgery**
   a. **Complete surgical resection** of a lung tumor is generally the only chance for cure, although only 20%–25% of patients have little enough disease at diagnosis to make this possible.
      (1) Occassionally, some patients with localized stage IIIa disease may be considered for surgery, particularly in instances of squamous cell tumors.
   b. **Occult and stage I cancer**
      (1) Localization of the tumor must be achieved before surgery. Traditional **bronchoscopy** or **laser photoirradiation** may be used.
      (2) Surgical procedures include **wedge resection, segmentectomy, lobectomy,** and **pneumonectomy.** All are depicted in **Figure 46-8, text page 1189.**
      (3) **Anatomic location** and **extent of tumor** are critical factors in the selection of a surgical approach.

      (4) Preoperatively, the patient undergoes screening tests to determine probable tolerance to the proposed surgery. The most important test is the **forced expiratory volume in one second (FEV₁)**.

      (5) **Pulmonary toilet** is indicated preoperatively to maximize ventilatory function.

      (6) Twenty to thirty percent of patients will continue to smoke after the diagnosis.

      (7) Postoperative nursing care is outlined in **Table 46-4, text page 1190,** and **Table 46-5, text page 1191.**

  c. **Stage II cancer**

      (1) For non-small-cell tumors, **surgery** is usually the treatment of choice, with cure being the therapeutic goal.

      (2) Although local radiation and systemic chemotherapy have been used both pre- and postoperatively, they have not significantly affected survival rates, although older protocols often tested single agents or agents now known to have only limited activity in lung cancer.

  d. **Stage III**

      (1) Patients in whom the primary tumor and local metastases can be completely resected (stage IIIa) may benefit from surgical resection in combination with radiation and/or chemotherapy.

      (2) Postoperative RT and/or chemotherapy may provide a modest prolongation of life in completely resected patients.

2. **Radiation**

  a. Radiation can be used for cure in certain patients who are not surgical candidates. Most NSCLCs have poor radiosensitivity, however.

  b. It is also used to **sterilize tumors preoperatively** and to **treat regional nodes postoperatively.** However, to date, neither treatment has been shown to affect survival.

  c. **Poor general condition, large tumor size, distant metastases, inadequate pulmonary reserve,** and **malignant pleural effusion** are contraindications to curative XRT.

  d. **Palliative XRT** can improve symptoms by reducing tumor size and impingement on adjacent structures.

  e. **Pneumonitis** and **fibrosis** can occur because of the high doses needed for cure.

  f. **Pharyngitis** and **esophagitis** are common and necessitate a soft diet in many patients.

  g. **Prophylactic brain irradiation** is used in patients at high risk for brain metastasis, especially those with adenocarcinoma.

  h. Brachytherapy may be used as an adjuvant to resectional surgery, as a boost component of initial radiotherapy, or for palliation at the time of recurrent endobronchial disease.

3. **Chemotherapy**

  a. The role of chemotherapy in localized NSCLC is strictly as an adjuvant to radiotherapy or surgery.

  b. Chemotherapy in nonresectable NSCLC has not improved prognosis.

  c. Drug regimens historically have been highly toxic and should be undertaken only in patients with a good performance status.

4. **Chemotherapy combined with radiation therapy**

  a. Because of its demonstrated efficacy against NSCLC as well as its action as a potentiator of radiation therapy, cisplatin is the chemotherapy agent most often selected for combination therapy.

  b. There is evidence from randomized trials that patients with inoperable NSCLC treated with cisplatin and chest irradiation survive longer than patients treated with RT alone.

B. **SMALL-CELL LUNG CANCER**

1. Since SCLC is considered a systemic disease at diagnosis, the mainstay of treatment is **combination chemotherapy with or without radiotherapy.**

2. **Chemotherapy**

  a. Multiple, simultaneously administered chemotherapeutic agents are preferable to single agents in both limited and extensive disease. Drug regimens frequently used against SCLC are listed in **Table 46-7, text page 1193.**

  b. Higher doses produce better responses but more toxicity.

  c. Most responders relapse within a short time, frequently at the initial intrathoracic site.

  d. Tumor drug resistance occurs, necessitating alternating regimens.

     e. Less than 20% of patients survive more than 2 years after diagnosis. Median survival times are on the order of 14 months for limited disease and 7–9 months for extensive disease.

   3. **Radiation therapy**

     a. A reduced frequency of tumor recurrence in the chest and an increased 2-year survival have been reported from combined modality therapy in patients with limited disease.

     b. The value of prophylactic brain irradiation is still unclear, although many patients with SCLC develop brain metastases.

C. SMOKING CESSATION

1. Patients who quit smoking before or at diagnosis have longer survival than those who continue to smoke.
2. Continuing smokers also have a greater risk of developing NSCLC.

D. PHOTOTHERAPY

1. The **YAG laser** is used for **palliation** of symptoms such as airway obstruction.
2. It produces **thermal necrosis** and **shrinkage of the tumor** for easier removal by forceps. Bleeding is a potential complication.

XIV. COMPLICATIONS OF TREATMENT

A. RADIATION THERAPY

1. Effects on pulmonary function include a progressive decline in lung volumes and a decrease in lung compliance and diffusing capacity.
2. **Pulmonary fibrosis, pericarditis,** and **myelitis** are common late effects of chest irradiation.
3. A **"CNS syndrome"** of symptoms, including **memory loss, tremor, slurred speech,** and **somnolence,** has occurred in patients who received prophylactic cranial irradiation.

B. CHEMOTHERAPY

1. The aggressive, multiagent chemotherapy used against lung cancer has caused **preleukemic** and **leukemic** states in patients.
2. Several drugs cause lung injury, especially when chemotherapy is given concurrently with XRT.
3. Risks of pulmonary toxicity for cytotoxic drugs may increase with **cumulative drug dose, age, use of chest radiotherapy,** and **concurrent oxygen therapy.**

XV. SYMPTOM MANAGEMENT

A. COUGH

1. Lung tumor growth can result in dry or productive coughs.

     a. Dry, irritating, nonproductive coughs can be managed with **cough suppressants (e.g., codeine).**

     b. Productive coughs resulting from hypersecretion of mucus require consistent use of **therapeutic coughing** and **deep breathing** to clear secretions. Suction may be necessary.

2. A chronic nonproductive cough in a patient with underlying chronic obstructive lung disease may respond to inhaled bronchodilators.

B. PAIN

1. Chest pain from bronchogenic tumors is usually a **dull ache that is poorly localized.**
2. Pain may increase in intensity and duration with advancing metastatic disease and cancer treatment.
3. If standard cancer therapies fail to relieve or control pain, pharmacologic agents are usually ordered.

C. **DYSPNEA**

1. Dyspnea in a patient with lung cancer is a complex reaction that may involve several physiologic and psychologic processes.
2. Treatment for dyspnea will be dictated by the results of a thorough history of symptoms (including alleviating and exacerbating measures), physical examination, and diagnostic studies.

D. **HEMOPTYSIS**

1. Hemoptysis is caused by **tumor erosion into pulmonary blood vessels.**
2. Persons with mild hemoptysis (less than 50 ml in 24 hours) are usually treated as outpatients using conservative measures.
3. The patient with significant bleeding (200 ml in 24 hours) should be **positioned so that the bleeding lung is dependent** and should be **monitored for increased blood loss, changes in blood pressure and pulse,** and **respiratory distress.**
4. Aggressive measures to control massive bleeding may include angiographic embolization of the bronchial artery source of the bleed or emergency surgery.

E. **WHEEZING**

1. Wheezing is usually caused by a tumor that partially obstructs an airway.
2. **Positioning** may be helpful in alleviating the wheezing.
3. Diffuse wheezing may represent underlying chronic airways obstruction.

XVI. **PSYCHOSOCIAL ISSUES**

A. **QUALITY OF LIFE**

1. The intent of treatment in lung cancer is more often **palliation** than cure.
2. The primary goal of palliative treatment is improving quality of life, a multidimensional construct that includes **physical function, disease- and treatment-related symptoms, psychological functioning,** and **social activity.**
3. Emphasis is placed on assessing the individual's subjective experience.

B. **SOURCES OF DISTRESS**

1. **Social isolation**
   a. Patients with lung cancer usually present with **dyspnea, fatigue,** and **weight loss.** They may isolate themselves socially as a way of coping with these distressing symptoms. If they still smoke, they may want to isolate themselves to protect themselves from criticism.
   b. Patients may need help to balance these coping strategies with the reduced quality of life associated with social isolation.
2. **Limited survival**
   a. Patients with limited prognoses need to be addressed with honesty and hope, in a manner that balances optimism with realism.
   b. Nurses should take cues from the patient when deciding what kind of information and how much information to give.
   c. Patients should have the opportunity to discuss the use of life-saving technologies well before a medical crisis.
   d. Patients and/or family members should be informed of the availability of advance directives such as the Living Will and Durable Power of Attorney for Health Care to document their treatment preferences.
3. **Family disruptions**
   a. Disease progression may be especially rapid in individuals with lung cancer.
   b. Major shifts in family roles and dynamics may occur in a **short time period,** possibly straining family resources and aggravating conflicts predating the cancer diagnosis.
   c. Crises within the family may be controlled by the experienced nurse who **anticipates** problems, **rehearses** approaches and solutions with the family, and initiates early **referrals** to appropriate support systems and personnel.

PRACTICE QUESTIONS

1. What percentage of lung cancers is considered **preventable?**
    (A) 45%
    (B) 50%
    (C) 75%
    (D) 85%

2. Major epidemiologic trends over the last century in lung cancer include a(n)
    (A) overall increased incidence, and a decreased mortality among nonwhites.
    (B) increased incidence, but decreased mortality among women.
    (C) higher mortality rate for blacks than whites, but decreasing incidence for black males.
    (D) mortality that is increasing three times as fast for men as for women.

3. In the course of a physical examination, a steel mill worker asks you about his relative risk of developing lung cancer. The **best** response to his question would be to
    (A) tell him that his risk is increased by his exposure to the fumes from coke ovens.
    (B) ask him about his family history of lung cancer, and explain that multiple factors cause the disease.
    (C) get his demographic information, and ask him about his exposure to tobacco smoke.
    (D) ask him about his diet and his smoking history.

4. Which of the following statements is true?
    (A) Only about one out of three smokers who quit are still not smoking one year after quitting, although an individual's success increases with each attempt made.
    (B) Legislative approaches to preventing lung cancer have included taxation on cigarettes, warning labels, and eliminating smoking in public places.
    (C) Regular use of cigarettes causes behavioral and pharmacologic dependence on tar, a powerfully psychoactive drug.
    (D) More physicians than nurses are active smokers.

5. Early detection of asymptomatic lung cancers is made with the use of such screening technologies as
    (A) carcinoembryonic antigen (CEA) levels, chest radiographs, and sputum cytologies.
    (B) alpha-fetoprotein (AFP) levels and sputum cytologies.
    (C) bronchoscopic exams and chest radiographs.
    (D) chest radiographs and sputum cytologies.

6. Most lung tumors arise in the
    (A) alveolar cells.
    (B) apical lung parenchyma.
    (C) bronchial epithelium.
    (D) alveolar capillaries.

7. The type of lung cancer **most** often found in nonsmokers is
    (A) adenocarcinoma.
    (B) squamous cell carcinoma.
    (C) large-cell carcinoma.
    (D) small-cell lung cancer.

8. Which of the following statements about the metastatic pattern of lung cancer is **false?**
    (A) Local spread includes invasion through the walls of lung structures and along bronchial lumens.
    (B) Metastatic lesions frequently involve the liver, adrenal glands, bowel, bone, and brain.
    (C) Lymphatic and hematogenous spread are common.
    (D) At diagnosis, most tumors have metastasized.

9. The **most** important prognostic factor in non-small-cell lung cancer is
    (A) performance status.
    (B) response to therapy.
    (C) nutritional status and weight loss.
    (D) anatomic extent of disease.

10. Lung cancers are **most** often diagnosed by the use of
    (A) chest radiographs.
    (B) bronchoscopy.
    (C) a microscope.
    (D) chest tomograms.

11. A patient is diagnosed with stage I non-small-cell lung cancer and is to undergo a lobectomy of his disease. He asks you about his preparation for surgery and about whether adjuvant treatment would improve his prognosis. Patient teaching would include all of the following **except**
    (A) describing pulmonary function tests.
    (B) talking to him about the importance of preoperative chest physical therapy.
    (C) telling him that he would probably need some radiation or chemotherapy either pre- or postoperatively.
    (D) telling him that bronchoscopy or photoirradiation would have to be used to localize the tumor.

12. All of the following are contraindications to curative radiation **except**
    (A) the presence of distant metastases.
    (B) a tumor that is larger than 6 cm.
    (C) malignant pleural effusion.
    (D) removal of mediastinal nodes at operation.

13. Which of the following statements about small-cell lung cancer is **false?**
    (A) Surgery is the mainstay of treatment.
    (B) Patients who quit smoking at diagnosis have longer survival times than those who continue.
    (C) Continuing smokers are at greater risk of developing non-small-cell lung cancer.
    (D) The YAG laser can be used to reduce the size of and remove obstructing tumors.

ANSWER EXPLANATIONS

1. **The answer is (D).**   Eighty-five percent of lung cancers could be prevented if people did not smoke. The relative risk of cancer increases with the number of cigarettes smoked per day and the number of years of smoking history. (1177)

2. **The answer is (C).**   Already the source of most male cancer deaths, in 1986 lung cancer became the leading cause of cancer death among women. Although the lung cancer/mortality rates are higher for blacks than for whites, lung cancer incidence has been declining for black males since the mid-1980s, and the incidence in black women appears to be leveling off in the younger age groups. (1176)

3. **The answer is (C).**   By asking him his demographic information, the nurse would be able to assess his exposure to air pollution and possibly his exposure to radon (certain areas have been identified as higher in radon activity than others). Since tobacco has an interactive and synergistic effect on the development of lung cancer when combined with other carcinogens, this would also be a good factor to explore. Genetics and diet have not been shown to have a significant effect on the development of lung cancer. (1178)

4. **The answer is (A).**   The other statements are wrong because legislative approaches have not included **eliminating** smoking in public places, **nicotine** is the addicting substance in smoke, and more nurses smoke than physicians. (1179–1180)

5. **The answer is (D).**   The only screening tests currently available for diagnosing asymptomatic lung cancers are sputum cytologies and chest radiographs. They are usually used together, but are considered too costly to merit mass screening, even of people in high-risk groups. Chest radiographs are more accurate in detecting peripherally located tumors; sputum cytologies more often detect central lung tumors. Most lung cancer patients have elevated carcinoembryonic antigen (CEA) levels, but so do patients with other lung diseases and no cancer. Bronchoscopy is too expensive and invasive to be used as a screening technique. (1181)

6. **The answer is (C).**   Over 90% of all primary lung tumors arise from the bronchial epithelium. In tumorigenesis, the basal cells of the epithelium proliferate, lose their ability to differentiate, and assume the more primitive appearance of squamous cells and eventually neoplastic cells. (1181–1182)

7. **The answer is (A).** Adenocarcinoma is the most common of the lung cancers and the most frequent type found in women, nonsmokers, and young people. Adenocarcinoma cells are characteristically found in a glandular formation and commonly produce mucin. They can develop after chronic parenchymal irritation, scarring, or fibrosis. Hematogenous spread is common, especially to the brain. (1183–1184)

8. **The answer is (B).** Patterns of local spread include invasion through the walls of lung structures and along the inside of the bronchial lumens. Tumors can cause bronchial occlusion by encircling it or by filling it to the point of obstruction. Compression of lung structures is common. Lymphatic and hematogenous spread of tumor cells are common in lung cancers. Metastatic lesions frequently involve the liver, adrenal glands, bone, and brain. Lung cancer does not usually metastasize to the bowel. (1184)

9. **The answer is (D).** The anatomic extent of the disease is the crucial determinant of treatment and ultimate survival, as depicted in the graphs on text pages 1186–1187. The staging of lung cancer is based on the TNM system recommended by the American Joint Committee on Cancer, and describes increasing size or involvement of the primary tumor (T), regional lymph node metastases (N), and the presence or absence of metastases to distant sites (M). (1185)

10. **The answer is (C).** Tumor cells are needed to establish any diagnosis of cancer. Centrally located tumors may yield positive sputum cytologies and may be accessible for bronchogenic visualization and washing, brushing, and biopsy. Cells from peripheral tumors frequently can only be obtained by needle biopsy. (1188)

11. **The answer is (C).** Radiation and chemotherapy, either pre- or postoperatively, have not been shown to affect survival rates in patients with NSCLC. (1188)

12. **The answer is (D).** Poor general condition, large tumor size, distant metastases, inadequate pulmonary reserve, and malignant pleural effusion are contraindications to curative radiation. (1191–1192)

13. **The answer is (A).** Since SCLC is considered a systemic disease at diagnosis, the mainstay of treatment is combination chemotherapy with or without radiotherapy. Higher doses produce better responses but more toxicity. Tumor drug resistance occurs, necessitating alternating regimens. Tumor regression in response to chemotherapy often occurs quickly, but most responders relapse within a short time, frequently at the initial intrathoracic site. Less than 20% of patients survive more than 2 years after diagnosis. (1193)

47 Malignant Lymphomas

STUDY OUTLINE

I. **INTRODUCTION**

1.   The malignant lymphomas constitute a diverse group of neoplasms that arise from the **uncontrolled proliferation of the cellular components of the lymphoreticular system.**
2.   Based on histologic characteristics, the lymphomas are divided into two subgroups—**Hodgkin's disease (HD) and non-Hodgkin's lymphoma (NHL).**
3.   The distinctions between HD and NHL are important because their clinical courses, prognoses, and treatment modalities are substantially different.
4.   The incidence of lymphomas is escalating, particularly NHL, which has now become the **fifth** most common cancer in the United States.

II. **THE IMMUNE SYSTEM AND NEOPLASIA**

1.   See **Figure 47-1, text page 1202,** for the organs of the immune system.
2.   See **Figure 47-2, text page 1203,** for the major lymph node groups.
3.   Lymphomas are mainly a **malignancy of the lymphocyte,** and the process by which a lymphoid neoplasm is generated may be thought of as a series of cellular changes whereby a once normal lymphoid cell becomes refractory to the regulation of its differentiation and proliferation.
4.   Once transformed, the new clone of malignant cells follows the behavior pattern of the stage at which lymphocyte alteration took place.

III. **MATURATION OF THE LYMPHOCYTE**

1.   The origin of the lymphocyte can be traced to a **stem cell** in the bone marrow that has the potential to develop into any of the cells that normally circulate in the blood.
  a.   At each step along the path of differentiation, the cell **loses the capacity to proceed along an alternate route.**
  b.   In the first step, the stem cell matures so that it is either the **precursor of the lymphocyte series** or of **all the other series of the blood,** e.g., erythrocyte.
  c.   The lymphocyte precursor then develops to become one of a number of types of mature lymphocytes.
  d.   An early step in the differentiation of the maturing lymphocyte occurs when the cell is programmed either by the bone marrow to become a B-lymphocyte or by the thymus to become a T-lymphocyte.
  e.   See **Figure 47-3, text page 1203,** for sites of lymphocyte transformation in the lymph node.
  f.   See **Figure 47-4, text page 1204,** for the maturation sequence of the normal lymphocyte.
2.   Eighty percent of lymphomas manifest **B-cell origin,** and most patients present with bone marrow or lymph node involvement.
  a.   B-cell neoplasms tend to follow a more **indolent** course.
3.   Lymphomas derived from T-lymphocytes usually arise in the bone marrow, thymus, lymph nodes, and skin.
  a.   T-cell lymphomas are generally more aggressive and grow more rapidly than B-cell neoplasms.

IV.   **HODGKIN'S DISEASE**

    A.   **HISTORICAL PERSPECTIVE**

        1.   All lymphomas were called HD until around the turn of the century when the giant, multi-nucleated cells in the nodal material of HD patients were characterized by Reed and Sternberg.

        2.   Subsequently, those lymphomas demonstrating the **Reed-Sternberg** cell were classified as HD.

    B.   **EPIDEMIOLOGY**

        1.   HD accounts for approximately 15% of the malignant lymphomas and less than 1% of all cancers.

        2.   In developed countries, the **incidence of HD is bimodal** with a first peak among young adults ages 20–30 years, and a second peak after age 45. This second upslope continues throughout the seventh and eighth decades.

        3.   The **nodular sclerosis** form of the disease predominates in young adults, while **mixed cellularity** is more common in middle age, and **lymphocyte depleted HD** is the predominant histology in the elderly.

    C.   **ETIOLOGY**

        1.   The etiology of HD is unclear.

        2.   Because of clinical manifestations such as fever, chills, and leukocytosis and because of histologic similarity to a granulomatous process, an infectious source has long been a topic of speculation.

            a.   **Epstein-Barr virus** is now recognized as the likely cause of one form of NHL, Burkitt's lymphoma.

            b.   HD in **HIV-infected patients** is a much more aggressive neoplastic process.

        3.   Genetic **and occupational predispositions** for HD may also exist.

    D.   **CELLULAR ABNORMALITIES**

        1.   Patients in all stages of HD exhibit a molecular defect characterized by markedly reduced cellular immunity.

        2.   This deficit is manifested by impaired delayed hypersensitivity skin reactions and reduced T-cell proliferation following antigenic stimulation.

        3.   There is increased **susceptibility to infectious complications** from opportunistic infections.

    E.   **CLINICAL MANIFESTATIONS**

        1.   A typical HD patient presents with a slow, insidious, superficial **lymphadenopathy.**

            a.   **Nodes** of variable size are firm, rubbery, and freely movable.

            b.   Most are located in the cervical and supraclavicular area.

        2.   A second common presentation, **mediastinal adenopathy** is often recognized during routine chest X ray.

        3.   Constitutional symptoms **(B symptoms)** of fever, malaise, night sweats, weight loss, and pruritus appear in about 40% of affected individuals.

        4.   The **spread of HD** is via contiguous nodal groups, and the pattern is quite predictable.

        5.   **Symptoms and prognosis** are related to the location and number of disease sites.

            a.   Local pressure symptoms may arise from enlarged **mediastinal nodes** causing cough, dyspnea, dysphagia, pleural effusions, and in extreme situations, superior vena cava syndrome.

            b.   Left upper quadrant pain results from **splenomegaly.**

            c.   **Extrahepatic bile duct obstruction** can result in jaundice.

            d.   Genitourinary dysfunction, abdominal pain, and ascites can result from **retroperitoneal adenopathy.**

F. **ASSESSMENT**

1. The diagnosis of HD can be established only by biopsy of involved tissue, usually a lymph node.
2. However, there are **many causes of lymphadenopathy,** especially in younger people, including upper respiratory infection, infectious mononucleosis, and allergic reactions.
    a. A careful history and physical examination will determine if an enlarged lymph node should be biopsied.
    b. Older persons with cancer of the head and neck may present with enlarged cervical lymph nodes. A careful search of the mouth, pharynx, and larynx for the presence of a malignancy should be made.
    c. For persistent lymphadenopathy or when etiology is not present, a biopsy is usually indicated.
3. Once the diagnosis is established on the basis of lymph node biopsy, an accurate **histologic typing** and **staging** of the disease is needed to determine the precise prognosis and selection of therapy.

G. **HISTOPATHOLOGY**

1. HD is distinguished from other lymphomas by the presence of the **Reed-Sternberg cell.**
2. See **Table 47-1, text page 1207,** for the frequency and features of four distinct subtypes of HD: **nodular sclerosis, lymphocyte-predominant, mixed cellularity, and lymphocyte-depleted.**
3. Most patients with **nodular sclerosis HD** are asymptomatic at presentation and exhibit stage I or II disease.
    a. Occurs between ages 13 and 34 and is more common in females.
4. The **lymphocyte-predominant (LP)** type is characterized by sheets of mature-appearing small lymphocytes and few Reed-Sternberg cells.
    a. Most patients usually present with localized stage I or II disease.
    b. Peak incidence is during ages 40–50.
    c. **Prognosis** of LP is favorable with B symptoms uncommon.
5. **Mixed cellularity (MC) HD** is intermediate between LP and lymphocyte-depleted (LD) in terms of histology and prognosis.
    a. There is a wide age range that peaks in the 30–40-year-old age group, and it is more common in males.
    b. More than 50% of patients with MC have stage III or IV disease and the majority manifest B symptoms.
6. **LD HD** is the most aggressive of the four types of HD, marked by a paucity of small lymphocytes and an increased number of Reed-Sternberg cells.
    a. Reticular LD-HD patients often present with bone marrow infiltration and peripheral lymphadenopathy while those with diffuse fibrosis are more likely to exhibit lymph node and visceral involvement.
    b. It is more common in elderly males and carries a very poor prognosis.

H. **STAGING**

1. Staging indicates the degree of **systemic progression** and the intensity of treatment that will be required.
2. See **Figure 47-5, text page 1208,** for a schematic representation of the new Ann Arbor-Cotswolds classification system created for both HD and NHL.
3. **Stage I** disease is lymph node involvement in just one area.
4. Involvement of two or more areas confined to one side of the diaphragm constitutes **stage II.**
5. In **stage III,** lymph node groups above and below the diaphragm are affected. The spleen may be involved (stage IIIs), and this often precedes widespread hematogenous dissemination.
6. In HD, stage III is subdivided further into **stage III$_1$,** for disease limited to the upper abdomen, and **stage III$_2$,** for disease involving the lower abdomen.
7. **Stage IV** is marked by diffuse extralymphatic progression that may affect, for example, the liver, bone marrow, lung, and skin.
8. A **subscript E** in stages I, II, and III indicates localized extranodal extension from a nodal mass.

9. Designation of a stage as **either A or B** indicates the absence (A) or presence (B) of unexplained weight loss greater than 10% of body weight in the preceding 6 months and/or fever of greater than 38°C and/or night sweats.
10. **Subscript X** is indicative of bulky disease.
11. The **exploratory laparotomy** is a controversial component of the staging process.
12. Current recommendations advocate that staging laparotomy be used only when surgical findings will either **a) alter the extent of radiation therapy to be administered or b) make chemotherapy rather than radiation therapy the primary treatment modality.**
13. See **Table 47-2, text page 1209,** for staging procedures for HD.

I. TREATMENT

1. The **initial treatment plan** for HD is **crucial** in determining eventual outcome because the overwhelming majority of patients, even those in the most advanced disease stages, are potentially curable if optimal therapy is employed.
2. See **Table 47-3, text page 1210,** for stage-specific therapies for HD.
3. Since nearly one-third of all HD patients die without evidence of lymphoma at autopsy, the prevention of **iatrogenic complications** must be of paramount importance.
4. **Radiation therapy** is curative in most patients with limited disease.
5. For stage IA and IIA disease above the diaphragm, without bulky mediastinal extension, **mantle irradiation** to a total dose of 3500–4400 cGy over a period of 4–6 weeks is advocated.
6. Stage III$_1$A patients having only splenic involvement may be treated with **total or subtotal nodal irradiation.**
7. **Stage IIB disease** may be treated with total or subtotal nodal radiotherapy; otherwise, chemotherapy is indicated.
8. When bulky mediastinal disease is known to be present, **combination radiation and chemotherapy** are unequivocally required.
9. The **combined approach** is usually indicated for patients with adverse prognostic factors such as B symptoms, bulky masses, or disease involving nodes in the lower abdomen.
10. See **Tables 47-4 and 47-5, text page 1211,** for the **MOPP and ABVD regimens,** which have become the benchmarks for combination chemotherapy in HD.
11. The **combined use of MOPP and ABVD,** in three alternating cycles of each, shows evidence of being superior to either regimen alone.
12. The success of aggressive chemotherapy regimens is quite dependent on the dosage and timing of drug administration because even minor **alterations** can have a substantial impact on efficacy.
13. Those who **relapse** following irradiation can be treated with chemotherapy, and, under certain circumstances, additional radiation may be possible.
14. When relapse occurs after chemotherapy, the extent of the disease-free interval is very important.
    a. If relapse takes place **more than 12 months** after initial therapy, the patient can be treated with the same agents and the long-term survival rate remains high.
15. When relapse occurs **less than 12 months** after initial remission, patients are seldom cured with conventional salvage therapies.

V. NON-HODGKIN'S LYMPHOMAS

A. HISTORICAL PERSPECTIVE

1. The non-Hodgkin's lymphomas are a diverse group of neoplasms derived from the different developmental and functional **subdivisions of the lymphoreticular system.**
2. Although these malignancies have many common features, they exhibit a **wide range of immunologic and biologic characteristics.**

B. EPIDEMIOLOGY

1. In the United States, NHL is diagnosed nearly **6 times as often as HD,** and its death rate is 13 times greater.
2. Age-adjusted incidence is somewhat higher in males than in females, and the white population is affected more than the black population.

3. **Age-specific analyses** reveal a preadolescent peak, a late teenage drop, and then a rise with increasing age that persists into the 80s. The average is 50 years of age.

C. ETIOLOGY

1. The heterogeneity of NHL suggests that a variety of factors including **viral infections, genetic abnormalities, and immune disturbances** interact in the pathogenesis.
2. **Epstein-Barr virus (EBV)** is the most likely etiologic agent for one form of NHL, Burkitt's lymphoma (BL).
3. **Environmental factors and exposure to chemicals** in the workplace also are implicated in the pathogenesis of NHL.

D. CELLULAR ABNORMALITIES

1. The molecular pathogenesis of both B- and T-cell origin in NHL reveals several consistent features.
2. Cytogenetic analysis of lymphoma cells has identified other abnormalities as well.
3. At present, the sequence of events that explains the **transformation** of a normal lymphocyte into a lymphomatous cell is unknown.

E. CLINICAL MANIFESTATIONS

1. See **Table 47-6, text page 1213,** for systemic alterations in NHL.
2. The majority of patients present with **advanced disease,** reflected by painless, generalized lymphadenopathy.
3. **Systemic B symptoms** (fever, night sweats, and/or weight loss) are the initial complaint in up to **20%** of cases.
4. **GI involvement** is fairly common at presentation; the most frequent sites of infiltration are the stomach and small intestine.
5. **Pulmonary parenchymal disease** is related most often to lymphatic tumor spread from hilar and mediastinal nodes, and cough, dyspnea, and chest pain are indicative of lung infiltration.
6. Lymphomas can **infiltrate** the skin and liver involvement can occur without signs or symptoms.

F. ASSESSMENT

1. Careful **histologic evaluation** is the most important first step toward initiating proper care of the patient.
2. A careful **history and physical examination** should be precise in evaluating abnormal clinical manifestations and the length of time they have been present.

G. HISTOPATHOLOGY

1. Few areas of pathology have evoked as much controversy and confusion as the **classification** of NHL, and the lack of consistent standardization makes international analysis and comparison extremely difficult.
2. The **Rappaport system** is based on predominant cell type: **well-differentiated lymphocyte; poorly differentiated, histiocytic, undifferentiated, and mixed lymphomas.**
3. The **Lukes and Collins System** proposed an immunological classification system and relates lymphomas to T-cell or B-cell markers.
4. The **Working Formulation** is a translation among the various systems. It distinguishes among low-grade, intermediate-grade, and high-grade types.
5. See **Table 47-7, text page 1215,** for the comparative classifications of NHL.
6. **Low-grade lymphomas**
   a. The low-grade category includes three tumors: **small lymphocytic lymphoma; follicular, predominantly small cleaved cell lymphoma; and follicular mixed (small cleaved and large-cell) lymphoma.**
   b. Usual presenting problems are connected with a painless, progressive, generalized **lymphadenopathy.**
   c. Except for liver and bone marrow involvement, extranodal extension is uncommon.

    d. Most low-grade lymphomas have a **long natural history** that appears to be largely unaffected by treatment.

    e. **Median survival** is 7–9 years.

    f. As the disease **progresses,** patients may complain of increasing fatigue, malaise, low-grade fever, night sweats, and weight loss. Eventually the disease **accelerates** and the majority of indolent lymphomas **convert** from low-grade to intermediate or high-grade malignancies.

7. **Intermediate-grade lymphomas**

    a. There are **four neoplasms** under the intermediate-grade category in the Working Formulation—an uncommon tumor with a follicular architecture and three others with a diffuse pattern.

    b. The **follicular, predominantly large-cell NHL** has a more aggressive clinical course than that of other more indolent subtypes of follicular lymphomas.

    c. These subtypes frequently involve **extranodal progression** to the gastrointestinal tract, skin, and bone.

    d. If left untreated, diffuse NHLs are invariably **fatal** and survival is less than 2 years.

    e. These subtypes are responsive to chemotherapy and a significant chance for cure exists, particularly in patients with localized disease.

8. **High-grade lymphomas**

    a. High-grade lymphomas consist of **three distinct diseases** that are grouped together because of their aggressive clinical behavior and poor prognosis.

    b. The first is the **immunoblast lymphomas.**

        (1) These occur in adults over the age of 50.

        (2) Anemia, B symptoms, and advanced stage are common at **presentation** and cutaneous disease has been reported.

        (3) Poor responses to chemotherapy and survival are characteristic of this group.

    c. **Lymphoblastic lymphoma** is usually a T-cell malignancy that is closely related to T-cell acute lymphocytic leukemia.

        (1) **Adolescents and young adults** are the majority of the cases. Males outnumber females.

        (2) The majority of patients present with a prominent anterior **mediastinal mass** suggestive of thymic origin.

        (3) Unless effectively treated, patients have a **rapidly progressive,** downhill course with dissemination of tumor to the bone marrow, blood, cerebrospinal fluid, and central nervous system.

    d. Within the category of **small, noncleaved cell lymphomas** are two distinct subtypes: Burkitt's lymphoma and non-Burkitt's lymphoma, uncommon in the United States.

    e. **Aggressive lymphomas** exhibit rapid tumor growth and a high mitotic index. Without treatment, survival is less than 18 months.

        (1) Because these neoplasms respond better to chemotherapy than the indolent, low-grade lymphomas, they have a greater potential for **cure,** especially if complete remissions are sustained for at least 2 years.

9. **Mycosis fungoides (cutaneous T-cell lymphoma)**

    a. This is a **rare** disorder and involvement of the skin is a hallmark of this malignancy.

    b. It initially is **indolent** but may evolve into a widely disseminated malignancy.

    c. The disease occurs in **middle age** and is **male predominant.**

H. STAGING

1. Once a histologic diagnosis of NHL has been confirmed by biopsy, a careful, comprehensive **staging work-up** is essential to determine the extent of the disease, the bulk of the tumor mass, and potential complications.

2. **Baseline studies** should include complete history and physical examination with particular emphasis on all lymphoid tissue including liver, spleen, Waldeyer's ring, and lymph nodes.

    a. Also included are complete blood counts, blood chemistries including liver and kidney function tests, erythrocyte sedimentation rate, uric acid, serum immunoglobulin, and bone marrow biopsy.

3. All patients require a **chest X ray** to facilitate detection of hilar adenopathy, mediastinal mass, parenchymal lung infiltration, or pleural/pericardial effusions.

4. **Computed tomography (CT)** of the chest is advised when the X ray is suspicious.

5. Abdominal and pelvic CT should be performed on all individuals.

6. See **Table 47-8, text page 1218,** for staging procedures for NHL.

I. **TREATMENT**

   1. Treatment of NHL is determined by **histology of the tumor, stage of the disease, the physiologic performance of the patient, and extent of the disease.**
   2. See **Table 47-9, text page 1219,** for recommended guidelines for treatment of NHL.
   3. **Indolent lymphomas**
       a. Some physicians advocate a policy of "watchful waiting" until systemic symptoms require intervention.
       b. But evidence is growing that radiation therapy is potentially curative in early-stage disease and intensive combined regimens may be beneficial in some of the advanced stages.
   4. **Aggressive lymphomas**
       a. The recognized treatment of choice for advanced-stage aggressive NHL is **combination chemotherapy.** See **Table 47-10, text page 1220.**

J. **SALVAGE THERAPY**

   1. **Relapsed indolent lymphomas** are rarely resistant to treatment unless they undergo histologic progression.
   2. The outlook for nonresponsive or relapsed aggressive lymphomas is **dismal.**
   3. Patients who **relapse** generally have a reduced bone marrow reserve as a result of primary therapy and tolerate secondary treatment poorly.
   4. With the advent of high-dose therapy followed by ABMT, a substantial number of relapsed patients with aggressive lymphoma are achieving durable second remissions.

VI. **COMPLICATIONS OF TREATMENT**

   1. **Radiotherapy** often causes complications during treatment (acute) or following the completion of treatment (subacute or late).
   2. The most common reactions to **mantle irradiation** are loss of taste, dry mouth, redness of skin, dysphagia, loss of hair at the nape of the neck, nausea, and vomiting.
   3. **Inverted-Y port irradiation** usually results in nausea, vomiting, anorexia, diarrhea, and malaise.
   4. **Total nodal irradiation** leads to all the side effects noted previously and particularly to severe bone marrow depression.
   5. The most frequent side effect of combinations of chemotherapy used in the treatment of HD and NHL is **nausea and vomiting.**
   6. The most serious side effect of all combination regimens is **bone marrow suppression.**

VII. **CONSEQUENCES OF SURVIVAL**

   1. See **Table 47-11, text page 1223,** for a number of long-term complications that may develop in those cured of malignant lymphomas.
   2. Both radiation therapy and chemotherapy promote toxic effects on the **heart and peripheral blood vessels.**
   3. An extension of **injury to the lungs** is common in mantle irradiation, and it may develop as early as 1–3 months after therapy.
   4. Resulting complications of radiotherapy include **pneumothorax, radiation pneumonitis, pulmonary fibrosis, superimposed pulmonary and parenchymal infections, and radiation myelopathy.**
   5. Because both chemotherapy and radiotherapy are immunosuppressive, bacterial as well as other unusual **infections** may occur.
   6. **Herpes zoster** is a complication often seen in individuals with HD and NHL.
   7. Two of the most devastating complications associated with lymphoma treatment are **sterility and second malignancies.**

VIII. **SUPPORTIVE CARE**

   1. Supportive care of the patient with lymphoma begins at diagnosis with
       a. An explanation of the disease.
       b. A description of the steps that will be taken for staging and treatment.

    c.   Generation in the patient of a feeling of confidence in the multidisciplinary team responsible for care.

  2. Individuals must be prepared to cope with the lengthy and highly toxic program of primary treatment.

    a.   Once symptoms have been relieved, the patient may question the need for further therapy with its associated side effects. The nurse must make sure the patient understands that small foci of disease cause no symptoms but may lead to recurrence.

  3. After the primary treatment, there will be a prolonged period during which the patient will be observed for a recurrence.

    a.   The nurse should be sensitive to the patient's fear of recurrence. The individual may perceive every word or facial expression by the treatment team as a potential clue that the cancer has returned.

PRACTICE QUESTIONS

1.   Which of the following statements about lymphomas is correct?
    (A)   Non-Hodgkin's lymphoma (NHL) is distinguished from Hodgkin's disease (HD) primarily on the basis of its different clinical manifestations.
    (B)   Lymphomas are preeminently a malignancy of the lymphocyte.
    (C)   There seems to be a single malignancy for all stages in the developmental sequence from primitive to mature lymphocyte.
    (D)   In general, B-lymphocyte malignancies are more aggressive than T-lymphocyte malignancies.

2.   The incidence curve of HD has two peaks, one during the second and third decades, the second during the sixth and seventh decades. One explanation for this phenomenon is that
    (A)   HD is closely associated with the rise in incidence of AIDS, which primarily affects younger people.
    (B)   the first peak relates to the nodular sclerosing (NS) type of HD, which occurs more often in younger people.
    (C)   one form of HD is genetically based and is programmed to occur during the second and third decades.
    (D)   the second peak represents recurrence of the primary lymphomas that produce the first peak.

A 52-year-old male presents with signs and symptoms of lymphoma. Subsequent assessment and diagnostic tests confirm stage IIB Hodgkin's disease. **Answer questions 3–13 with this diagnosis in mind.**

3.   Mortality in this individual, if it occurs as a result of HD, is **most** likely to result from
    (A)   spinal cord compression.
    (B)   superior vena cava obstruction.
    (C)   failure of the liver or kidneys.
    (D)   infection or hemorrhage.

4.   Which of the following was the **most** likely presenting symptom in this patient?
    (A)   edema in the upper part of the body
    (B)   enlarged cervical lymph nodes
    (C)   a palpable mass in the axillary or inguinal lymph nodes
    (D)   an upper respiratory infection

5.   The diagnosis of either HD or NHL usually is established by
    (A)   cytologic examination of the Reed-Sternberg cells.
    (B)   CT and MRI scans of the nodular tissue.
    (C)   lymph node biopsy.
    (D)   exploratory laparotomy.

6.   Which of the following statements about the staging of this patient's cancer is correct?
    (A)   Stage II malignancy was determined by a positive bone marrow biopsy.
    (B)   Stage II determination is important because it influences what treatment option will be used.
    (C)   Stage II presentation is usually indicative of a more aggressive HD type.
    (D)   HD rarely presents as stage II.

7.   Accurate staging of this patient was **least** likely to include which of the following procedures?
      (A)   a chest radiograph
      (B)   an exploratory laparotomy
      (C)   blood chemistries, including liver and kidney function tests
      (D)   a complete blood count

8.   The prognosis for this patient is **most** closely related to
      (A)   elevated lactic dehydrogenase level.
      (B)   histologic type.
      (C)   abdominal lymph node involvement.
      (D)   stage at presentation.

9.   If careful laparotomy staging has been conducted, the patient is **most** likely to be treated with
      (A)   total or subtotal nodal radiation only.
      (B)   chemotherapy only.
      (C)   total or subtotal nodal radiation combined with chemotherapy.
      (D)   subtotal radiation only.

10.   Which of the following is **least** likely to be a side effect during or following radiation therapy in this patient?
      (A)   dry mouth
      (B)   redness of skin
      (C)   fever
      (D)   nausea and vomiting

11.   Which of the following is the **major** side effect produced by any combination chemotherapy regimen used in the treatment of this patient?
      (A)   nausea and vomiting
      (B)   anorexia and dysphagia
      (C)   permanent aspermia
      (D)   bone marrow suppression

12.   Which of the following statements is true about recurrence of HD in this patient following primary treatment and a complete remission?
      (A)   The complications of secondary treatment for HD are mild compared with those of primary treatment.
      (B)   Cure is rarely possible with HD.
      (C)   HD can be cured with intensive therapy after the first recurrence of the disease.
      (D)   Cure is possible for the patient only if secondary therapy is combined with autologous bone marrow transplantation (ABMT).

13.   Which of the following symptoms should alert the nurse to the possibility of spinal cord compression that may develop in progressive lymphoma?
      (A)   leg weakness or bowel or bladder dysfunction
      (B)   edema of the upper half of the body
      (C)   hypothyroidism with associated lethargy and malaise
      (D)   fever accompanied by a significantly reduced granulocyte count

ANSWER EXPLANATIONS

1.   **The answer is (B).**   Lymphomas are preeminently a malignancy of the lymphocyte. However, there seems to be a separate malignancy for each sequential stage in the developmental sequence from primitive to mature lymphocyte. At each stage of development, the potential exists for the normal maturing lymphocyte to be transformed into a cancer cell. Once transformed, the new clone of malignant cells follows the behavioral pattern of the stage of the lymphocyte at which the transformation occurred. For example, if the function of the maturing cell at the time it is transformed is secretion of an antibody, the tumor cells will continue to secrete that normal protein in abnormal quantities. HD and NHL are distinguished on the basis of the Reed-Sternberg giant cells in NHL. The information in choice (D) is reversed. (1202)

2. **The answer is (B).**   The second peak of the HD incidence curve is similar to that of NHL and is concentrated in the older age group, much like other forms of cancer. The early peak in HD is not understood but is thought to be related to the etiology of the nodular sclerosing (NS) type of HD, the tissue type that is observed commonly in young persons. The text discusses one other hypothesis: that the early peak may represent a disease of viral etiology associated with middle-class families in developed nations. (1205)

3. **The answer is (D).**   The major anatomic characteristic of both HD and NHL is the relentless proliferation of lymphocytes. These proliferating cells invade and compromise the function of various organs, especially bone marrow. Most HD patients exhibit signs of immune deficiency early in the disease. Immunosuppressive therapy makes the patient even more susceptible to infection. Death usually results from infection or hemorrhage due to compromise of bone marrow function. (1201)

4. **The answer is (B).**   Three-fourths of lymphoma patients present with enlargement of cervical lymph nodes, but enlarged axillary or inguinal nodes may be the presenting symptoms. Such nodes are characteristically painless, firm, rubbery in consistency, freely movable, and of variable size. Less common is abdominal HD with malabsorption and autoimmune hemolytic anemia. Weakness, fatigue, and general malaise may be a part of the presenting picture. Poor prognosis is associated with fever, night sweats, or weight loss, which indicate generalized rather than localized disease. Patients with HD also may have pruritis and may complain of pain in enlarged nodes after the ingestion of alcohol. (1206)

5. **The answer is (C).**   The diagnosis of lymphoma can be established only by a biopsy of involved tissue, usually a lymph node. Because there are many causes of lymphadenopathy, however, including upper respiratory infection, infectious mononucleosis, allergic reactions, and, in older people, cancer of the head and neck, a careful history and physical examination must first determine if an enlarged lymph node should be biopsied. For persistent lymphadenopathy or when etiology is not present, a biopsy is usually indicated. (1206)

6. **The answer is (B).**   Determination of the stage of disease in HD is important because it influences which treatment option (radiation therapy or combination therapy) will be used. Radiation is very effective for localized HD and is therefore used in early-stage disease. Chemotherapy is more effective than radiation for late-stage disease, when the number of lymph node groups involved is greater, but it also is as effective as radiation in early-stage disease. NHL, on the other hand, is almost always treated with chemotherapy because it usually presents at an advanced stage. A positive bone marrow biopsy indicates a stage IV tumor. A stage II presentation for HD is more likely to indicate a slow-growing malignancy; it is not at all uncommon. (1208–1209)

7. **The answer is (B).**   All of the other choices, along with a history and physical examination, are standard procedures used in the staging of lymphoma. Others procedures, including a CT scan of the chest and abdomen, a bone marrow biopsy, a percutaneous liver biopsy, a lower limb lymphangiogram (LAG), and an exploratory laparotomy may be done if there is evidence of lymph node involvement below the diaphragm, hepatomegaly or abnormal liver function, extension of the lymphoma to mediastinal lymph nodes, or splenomegaly. Positive results on these tests often mean a stage IV disease. (1206–1207, 1209)

8. **The answer is (D).**   For HD, prognosis is most closely related to stage. Age and the total number of lymph node groups involved (independent of stage) are other prognostic factors. For NHL, prognosis is most closely related to histologic type. The prognosis generally worsens (in the absence of treatment) as one proceeds down the Working Formulation list of types from histologic type A to J. The response to therapy, on the other hand, improves as the aggressiveness of the disease increases. High-grade lymphomas are often cured by intensive chemotherapy; low-grade are not considered curable, although they often demonstrate a long survival without therapy. (1209–1210)

9. **The answer is (A).**   Patients with stage IIB disease may receive total or subtotal nodal radiotherapy if careful laparotomy has been conducted. Otherwise they should receive chemotherapy. Chemotherapy may include either MOPP or ABVD regimens. Either regimen produces complete remission in more than half of the patients who have recurrent disease after treatment with the other regimen. (1210)

10. **The answer is (C).**   Other complications include loss of taste, dysphagia, loss of hair at the nape, anorexia, diarrhea, malaise, and, with total nodal irradiation, severe bone marrow depression. Late reactions may include radiation pneumonitis, transient aspermia in men, and artificial menopause in women who have not had an oophoropexy or shielding of the ovaries. (1222)

11.   **The answer is (D).**   The major side effect produced by all combination regimens is bone marrow suppression, which renders the individual susceptible to infection and hemorrhage. Nausea and vomiting are the most frequent side effects but can be controlled with the use of antiemetics. Transient and sometimes permanent male sterility also may occur, especially if alkylating agents are used in chemotherapy. (1222)

12.   **The answer is (C).**   For the patient with HD, it is possible to obtain a cure with intensive therapy after the first recurrence of disease following a complete remission. Such persons, however, have a reduced bone marrow reserve as a result of primary therapy and tolerate secondary therapy poorly. They need a great deal of psychological support because it rarely escapes their attention that recurrent lymphoma is much more likely to succeed than the initial disease. Cure is rarely possible with NHL. (1211–1212)

13.   **The answer is (A).**   Spinal cord compression is commonly seen in progressive lymphoma and has the potential to cripple the individual with paraplegia. This oncologic emergency develops swiftly, with weakness of the lower extremities, increased tendon reflexes, positive Babinski signs, and the development of a sensory "level" below which sensation is lost. Early diagnosis is critical to prevention of neurologic impairment; patients who have already developed compromised neurologic function usually do not regain function after treatment. The nurse should be sensitive to complaints of leg weakness or bowel or bladder dysfunction, especially if combined with back pain. Precise localization of the compression by myelogram or MRI is essential. Treatment may involve surgery, radiation, or chemotherapy, alone or combined. (1224)

48 Multiple Myeloma

STUDY OUTLINE

I. **INTRODUCTION**

    1. Plasma cell disorders are a group of diseases characterized by the overproduction of **immunoglobulins.**
        a. The malignant cell is the **plasma cell,** which is the functional mature cell that differentiates and develops from the B-lymphocyte.
        b. **Multiple myeloma** is the most common malignant plasma cell disorder.

II. **EPIDEMIOLOGY**

    1. Multiple myeloma represents 1% of all hematologic malignancies in the United States.
    2. There is some evidence that the **incidence** is increasing, which may be due to earlier and improved diagnosis in older, high-risk populations.
    3. The onset is late, with **peak occurrence** between the fifth and seventh decade of life.
    4. Within the United States, multiple myeloma is **more common among blacks** than among whites by 14 to 1.

III. **ETIOLOGY**

    1. A variety of factors have been associated with the development of multiple myeloma, although the **exact** etiology is unknown.
        a. Although a specific chromosomal abnormality has not been detected, frequent **chromosomal abnormalities** have been observed.
        b. Chronic low-level exposure to **radiation** has been associated with a two- to sixfold increase in the incidence, which may develop as late as 20 years after the radiation exposure.
        c. **Chronic antigenic stimulation,** such as recurrent infections and drug allergies, may be part of the medical history in individuals who develop multiple myeloma.

IV. **PATHOPHYSIOLOGY**

    1. The **lymphoid stem cell** resides within the bone marrow and retains the ability to self-replicate or differentiate into either T-lymphocytes or B-lymphocytes.
        a. **T-lymphocytes** regulate the immune response and participate in **cell-mediated immunity.**
        b. **B-lymphocytes,** which are responsible for **humoral immunity,** mature into plasma cells that manufacture and secrete large quantities of immunoglobulins.
    2. In multiple myeloma there is abnormal overproduction of one immunoglobulin called the **M protein;** the M refers to monoclonal antibody, myeloma protein, or malignant protein.
    3. Although an excessive amount of immunoglobulin is being produced, the aberrant M protein is **unable** to effectively produce antibody necessary for maintaining humoral immunity.
        a. Approximately 80%–90% of multiple myeloma patients will show evidence of the aberrant M protein in the serum.

V. **DIAGNOSIS/STAGING**

    1. Once symptoms are present, untreated individuals with multiple myeloma have a **median survival** of 7 months, which can be extended with standard therapy to a median survival of 2–3 years.

2. Individuals may have a long prodromal, indolent, or **asymptomatic period,** but once symptoms occur, systemic therapy becomes necessary.

3. Patients may eventually enter a period where their disease becomes **refractory** or unresponsive to conventional therapy; then experimental therapies are warranted.

4. **Bone pain** is the most frequent symptom at presentation, and the clinical course is complicated by **pathologic fractures, hypercalcemia, spinal cord compression, anemia, thrombocytopenia, recurrent bacterial infections, and renal failure.**

5. Diagnosis is confirmed by **bone marrow biopsy** with histologic confirmation of **increased (greater than 10%) numbers of plasma cells** and the presence of the monoclonal (M) protein in either the serum or the urine.

6. **Osteolytic** "punched-out" lesions may or may not be present at initial diagnosis.

7. See **Table 48-1, text page 1231,** for the diagnostic work-up that is designed to determine the extent of involvement of other organs.

8. Serum B2 microglobulin, platelet count, and the presence of either renal failure and/or infection have been identified as having a role in **predicting prognosis** when diagnosing, staging, and treating myeloma patients.

9. See **Table 48-2, text page 1231,** for the myeloma staging system that integrates clinical and laboratory findings.

VI. **CLINICAL MANIFESTATIONS**

A. **SKELETAL INVOLVEMENT**

1. From 68%–80% of individuals with multiple myeloma present with destructive, painful **osteolytic lesions** at the time of diagnosis.

2. Symptoms associated with osteolytic lesions include hypercalcemia (20%–40% of patients), pathological fractures with acute and chronic pain, decreased mobility, and an inability to fully participate in activities of daily living.

3. Three distinct types of bone lesions are: **(1) a solitary osteolytic lesion, (2) diffuse osteoporosis,** and **(3) multiple discrete osteolytic "punched-out" or "cannon-ball" lesions.**

4. **Bone destruction** is thought to be due to myeloma cell production of **osteoclast-activating factor (OAF),** which has been identified as a class of bone-resorbing factors produced by lymphocytes and monocytes.

5. If untreated, myeloma-induced osteolytic lesions can lead to **compression fractures** of the spine with irreversible neurological sequelae, refractory hypercalcemia compromising renal function, and possibly death.

B. **INFECTION**

1. Fifty to seventy percent of all multiple myeloma patients will die as a result of **bacterial infection,** usually of the **respiratory** or **urinary tract.**

2. Mechanisms identified as being responsible for the immunosuppression and infections associated with multiple myeloma are:
   a. **A deficiency in the normal amount of immunoglobulins.**
   b. **Neutropenia associated with plasma cell replacement in the bone marrow.**
   c. **Qualitative defects in neutrophil and complement system functioning.**
   d. **Decreased physical activity.**

C. **BONE MARROW INVOLVEMENT**

1. **Anemia** is initially caused by **excessive replacement** of erythrocyte precursors with plasma cells in the bone marrow, as well as by **increased red blood cell destruction.**

2. The M protein can coat normal erythrocytes, causing the red cells to line up similar to a roll of coins **(rouleau formation),** which results in capillary sludging with associated hemolysis.

3. **Bleeding** can be caused by:
   a. A decrease in the number of circulating platelets.
   b. The M protein's effect on clotting factors.
   c. Nonspecific coating of platelets with immunoglobulins.

D. **RENAL INSUFFICIENCY**

1. Renal insufficiency is present in **29%** of patients with multiple myeloma; **50%** of these individuals will experience **renal failure** during the course of the disease and its treatment; 15% of this population will die as a result of renal insufficiency.
2. Multiple myeloma can cause intrinsic **renal lesions.**
    a. In **myeloma kidney,** the renal tubules are filled with **damaging, dense casts** surrounded by multinucleated giant cells, which can lead to formation of precipitates in the tubules that can obstruct and rupture the tubular epithelium.
    b. **Interstitial inflammation, fibrosis,** and **tubular degeneration** may occur, resulting finally in renal failure.
    c. The tubular casts contain characteristic light chain immunoglobulins **(Bence Jones proteins),** which may be directly toxic to the renal tubular epithelium regardless of the presence of tubular casts.
    d. Excretion of large amounts of Bence Jones proteins in the face of clinical dehydration with a low urine pH contributes to the risk of **precipitation** of light chain proteins in the renal tubule and possible co-precipitating with calcium, further exacerbating acute renal failure.
    e. **Amyloid deposits** can cause another renal lesion that occurs in approximately 10%–30% of myeloma patients, and they can be found in the tubular basement membrane, renal blood vessels, the interstitium, or glomerulus.
    f. **Amyloidosis** is an adverse prognostic factor and can occur in up to 10% of myeloma patients.

E. **SEQUELAE**

1. Untreated **hypercalcemia** can precipitate renal insufficiency by reducing the glomerular filtration rate, altering renal blood flow, changing the kidney's ability to concentrate urine, and precipitating calcium in the tubules or renal interstitium.
2. Hyperuricemia occurs in multiple myeloma patients as a result of a large tumor burden with an increased rate of cell death.
    a. **Uric acid–induced nephropathy** is caused by precipitation and crystallization of uric acid in the distal tubules.
    b. Elevated uric acid levels will lead to further kidney damage.
3. **Infection is the leading cause of death.** Sepsis associated with **hypotension** or the use or nephrotoxic antibiotics should alert the clinician to closely monitor the individual for renal insufficiency.
4. **Treatment** of renal insufficiency should be directed toward preventing or correcting the predisposing factors and reducing the concentration and/or risk for precipitation of light chain proteins in the renal tubules.

F. **HYPERVISCOSITY SYNDROME**

1. A high concentration of **proteins** that increase serum viscosity and result in vascular sludging causes hyperviscosity syndrome.
2. Initial clinical signs including **blurred vision, irritability, headache, drowsiness,** and **confusion** may indicate neurological impairment.
3. **Plasmapheresis** can be life-saving and is the treatment of choice.

VII. **TREATMENT**

A. **CHEMOTHERAPY**

1. Patients with indolent, asymptomatic multiple myeloma are typically not treated with systemic therapy until clinical symptoms occur.
2. Systemic antineoplastic therapy consisting of **melphalan** and **prednisone** is a first line of therapy. It has a response rate of 30%–60% and a median survival of 24–36 months.
    a. The **intermittent treatment schedule** allows patients to recover from the immunosuppressive effects of the drugs, is associated with fewer acute toxicities, and requires fewer blood counts.

b. Patients are monitored closely for signs of **renal impairment,** and the dose of melphalan may need to be reduced on the basis of the severity of renal toxicity.

3. **VAD (vincristine, doxorubicin, and dexamethasone)** can be safely administered as first-line therapy, with an improved response rate (84%) and improved median survival.

   a. An implantable **intravascular device** enables safe administration of these vesicants and close monitoring of blood counts.

   b. Patients are closely monitored for signs and symptoms of **steroid toxicity,** which are severe dyspepsia, fluid and sodium retention, corticosteroid myopathy, acute pancreatitis, insulin-dependent hyperglycemia, and steroid psychosis. Any of these toxicities mandates at least a 50% reduction of dexamethasone.

   c. Severe **neurologic toxicities** require at least a 50% reduction in the vincristine dose.

   d. **Hepatic toxicity** characterized by a bilirubin greater than 2.0 requires reduction or discontinuation of both doxorubicin and vincristine depending on the severity. If it is greater than 5.0, both doxorubicin and vincristine are discontinued.

4. **Thirty to forty percent** of myeloma patients will **not respond** to first-line therapy, whereas those who initially respond will eventually relapse.

5. The most consistently effective **second-line therapy** resulting in greater than a 70% response rate with a projected survival greater than 1 year is VAD.

B.   INTERFERON

1. Interferon is being used for maintenance therapy in patients who have responded to two courses of induction therapy.

2. The patient is closely monitored for evidence of interferon toxicity: **anorexia, fatigue, hepatic toxicity,** and **neurologic changes.**

C.   RADIATION

1. Radiation has been consistently used in the treatment of multiple myeloma for **palliation of bone lesions** and control of pain.

2. Multiple myeloma is highly **radioresponsive.**

3. **Hemibody irradiation** has been used for refractory myeloma and has been reported to decrease total myeloma cell mass and relieve pain.

4. Toxicities such as **nausea, bone marrow suppression,** and **pneumonitis** may be severe and limit the use of this technique.

5. **Nursing preparation** for hemibody irradiation includes extensive patient and family education and the administration of corticosteroids and antiemetics.

D.   BONE MARROW TRANSPLANTATION

1. **Age restrictions** of donors (syngeneic and allogeneic) may limit the availability of transplant to myeloma patients, and the technical difficulty in **purging** myeloma from the bone marrow limits its usefulness.

2. **Clinical trials** will be required to determine whether this costly and ambitious approach to myeloma will alter the natural history of the disease or affect long-term survival.

E.   TREATMENT-RELATED LEUKEMIA

1. Treatment-related leukemia is thought to result from prolonged exposure to **alkylating agents** and has been reported at a frequency of 20% after 50 months of follow-up.

VIII.   NURSING MANAGEMENT

1. See **Table 48-3, text page 1235,** for an approach to nursing care.

A.   NEUROLOGIC

1. Bone destruction from the myeloma results in osteoporosis and pathologic fractures of long bones and vertebrae that require **aggressive assessment** and **management** of both **acute and chronic pain.**

　　　　2.　Interventions for pain include **assessment, proper positioning of affected limbs, use of supports and braces to prevent additional stress on bones,** and **consultation with physical and occupational therapists.**
　　　　3.　Any change in mental status requires **closer assessment** to determine etiologic factors so the appropriate treatment can be promptly initiated.
　　　　4.　The nurse also plans for **prevention of injury** and **maintaining the patient in a safe environment.**

　B.　**PROTECTIVE MECHANISMS**

　　　　1.　**Infection** is the leading cause of death in patients with multiple myeloma.
　　　　2.　Guidelines for the care of neutropenic patients are principally aimed at the **early recognition** and/or **prevention of infection;** care of the thrombocytopenic patient is directed toward **preventing bleeding.**

　C.　**RESPIRATORY**

　　　　1.　Because the respiratory system is the most frequent site of infection in myeloma patients, nursing care is directed toward **teaching** patients and their families **activities that decrease pooling of pulmonary secretions** and **increase gas exchange.**
　　　　2.　Due to the underlying defect in humoral immunity induced by multiple myeloma, patients should be instructed **not** to receive vaccines with live organisms or be in close contact with others who may have received live organism vaccines that may be shedding organisms.

　D.　**GASTROINTESTINAL**

　　　　1.　Multiple myeloma patients are at risk for **constipation** as a result of decreased physical activity.
　　　　2.　Nursing management includes the assessment of past and present bowel habits, changes in fluid and dietary intake, medication administration, activity changes, and patient and family education.

　E.　**GENITOURINARY**

　　　　1.　Nursing care is directed at **preventing** or quickly **reversing renal insufficiency.**
　　　　2.　Maintaining adequate hydration along with the administration of allopurinol will protect the kidneys from uric acid nephropathy.
　　　　3.　The nurse closely **monitors** the patient for early signs and symptoms of UTI and **educates** patients and families to recognize these symptoms and report them promptly to the physician.

PRACTICE QUESTIONS

1.　Multiple myeloma is a hematologic malignancy characterized by
　　(A)　an abnormal overproduction of plasma cells and an immunoglobulin called the M protein.
　　(B)　excessive production of lymphocytes and monocytes.
　　(C)　profound anemia that is unresponsive to transfusions.
　　(D)　aggressive stem cell proliferation requiring systemic therapy.

2.　The procedure by which blood cell precursors are removed and examined for histologic confirmation of multiple myeloma is
　　(A)　lumbar puncture.
　　(B)　complete blood count.
　　(C)　bone marrow biopsy.
　　(D)　stem cell pheresis.

3.　The **symptom** most frequently presented by patients with multiple myeloma is
　　(A)　anemia.
　　(B)　bone pain.
　　(C)　pathologic fracture.
　　(D)　bacterial infection.

4. Treatment for the patient with indolent, asymptomatic multiple myeloma typically consists of
    (A) systemic, antineoplastic therapy.
    (B) observation.
    (C) intensive therapy followed by stem cell rescue.
    (D) radiation therapy.

5. Which of the following terms applies to the "punched out" bone lesions often identified in patients with multiple myeloma?
    (A) osteoporosis
    (B) osteoclastic
    (C) osteolytic
    (D) osteoblastic

6. A patient with multiple myeloma presents to the ambulatory clinic with a high fever and chills. The nurse's assessment would focus on which two common sites of infection?
    (A) gastrointestinal and urinary tracts
    (B) integumentary and urinary tract
    (C) respiratory tract and integumentary
    (D) respiratory and urinary tracts

7. Because renal insufficiency and renal failure are complications of multiple myeloma either on presentation or during the course of the disease and its treatment, the nurse directs patient and family education at
    (A) increasing fluid intake and following the allopurinal prescription.
    (B) increasing physical activity.
    (C) preventing pathological fractures.
    (D) avoiding a high-sodium diet.

8. A venous access device may be recommended for the multiple myeloma patient who will be receiving VAD (vincristine, doxorubicin, and dexamethasone) both to aid in the close monitoring of blood counts and to
    (A) facilitate high fluid infusion rates.
    (B) enable safe administration of vesicants.
    (C) minimize the number of peripheral sticks from intravenous access.
    (D) promote chemotherapy drug administration in the home setting.

9. Radiation has been consistently used in the treatment of multiple myeloma for **both** palliation of bone lesions and
    (A) control of hypercalcemia.
    (B) stabilization of pathologic fractures.
    (C) control of pain.
    (D) first-line therapy.

10. A patient with multiple myeloma is admitted with confusion, disorientation, an unsteady gait, and a high serum calcium. The staff nurse's **first priority** is to
    (A) assist the patient in sitting comfortably in a chair.
    (B) educate the family about the side effects of hypercalcemia.
    (C) complete the admission history form.
    (D) provide a safe environment and prevent injury.

ANSWER EXPLANATIONS

1. **The answer is (A).**   Multiple myeloma is characterized by the overproduction of immunoglobulins that are produced by plasma cells that are malignant. (1230)

2. **The answer is (C).**   A bone marrow biopsy involves a needle going through the periosteum into the bone marrow and removing blood cells in various stages of development, including the early blood cell precursor stage. A bone marrow biopsy with histologic confirmation of increased number of plasma cells confirms the diagnosis of multiple myeloma. (1231)

3.   **The answer is (B).**   Bone pain is the most frequent symptom at presentation, and the clinical course is complicated by pathologic fractures, hypercalcemia, spinal cord compression, anemia, thrombocytopenia, recurrent bacterial infections, and renal failure. (1231)

4.   **The answer is (B).**   Patients with indolent, asymptomatic multiple myeloma are typically not treated with systemic therapy until clinical symptoms occur. With the onset of symptoms, systemic antineoplastic therapy consisting of melphalan and prednisone is the first line of therapy. Radiation is consistently used for palliation of bone lesions and control of pain. (1233–1234)

5.   **The answer is (C).**   Three distinct types of bone lesions are a solitary osteolytic lesion, diffuse osteoporosis, and multiple discrete osteolytic "punched-out" or "cannon-ball" lesions. Sixty-eight to eighty percent of individuals present with destructive, painful osteolytic lesions at the time of diagnosis. (1232)

6.   **The answer is (D).**   Fifty to seventy percent of all multiple myeloma patients will die as a result of bacterial infection. The two most common sites of infection are the respiratory and urinary tracts. (1232)

7.   **The answer is (A).**   Renal insufficiency is present in 29% of patients with multiple myeloma, and 50% of these individuals will experience renal failure during the course of the disease and its treatment. Patient and family education is directed at increasing fluid intake, allopurinal administration and recognition of the early signs and symptoms of a UTI. (1235)

8.   **The answer is (B).**   An intravascular venous access device enables close monitoring of blood counts and safe administration of doxorubicin, which is a vesicant and can harm tissue if extravasation occurs. (1233)

9.   **The answer is (C).**   Radiation has been consistently used in the treatment of multiple myeloma for palliation of bone lesions and control of pain. It is used to decrease myeloma cell mass thereby relieving pain. (1234)

10.   **The answer is (D).**   Hypercalcemia in patients with multiple myeloma is reflected by clinical signs and symptoms of lethargy, confusion, disorientation, and even stupor. Although admission forms need to be completed and family education is important in understanding what their loved one is experiencing, assuring patient safety and prevention of injury in the disoriented patient is the first priority. (1233)

49   Skin Cancer

STUDY OUTLINE

I.   INTRODUCTION

1. Cancers of the skin consist of **basal cell carcinoma (BCC), squamous cell carcinoma (SCC),** and **malignant melanoma.** Most malignant melanomas are **cutaneous melanoma (CM);** others, which are rare, originate in the eye or viscera.
2. **Nonmelanoma skin cancers** have a higher incidence but a low metastatic potential and mortality rate.
   a. Morbidity is of concern, however, since nonmelanoma cancers often require costly, extensive, and repeated treatments that may result in cosmetic and functional damage.
3. **Malignant melanoma** has a much lower incidence but a mortality rate that is triple that of the nonmelanoma cancers. Increased mortality is directly related to its high potential for metastasis.

II.   EPIDEMIOLOGY

1. **BCC** is the most common form of skin cancer. Both BCC and SCC occur more often in men and have a 5-year survival rate of 95%.
2. **CM** represents only 4% of all skin cancers but accounts for **6700 deaths annually.** It is the most rapidly increasing cancer among white males and fourth most rapidly increasing among white females. Five-year survival rates are 80% for white persons, around 60% for black persons.
3. Skin cancers generally occur in adults between 30 and 60 years of age. Skin cancers of any type are rare in children.

III. ETIOLOGY

1. Multiple etiologic and risk factors are associated with skin cancers.
2. High-risk factors for **CM** include
   a. **A persistent changed or changing mole.**
   b. **The presence of irregular pigmented precursor lesions,** including dysplastic nevi, congenital nevi, and lentigo maligna.
3. High-risk factors for **nonmelanoma cancers** include
   a. **Ultraviolet (UV) radiation,** especially **UV-B** and **UV-A.**
      (1) The incidence of both CM and nonmelanoma cancers is higher in latitudes closer to the equator.
   b. **Skin pigmentation.**
      (1) More deeply pigmented persons, including blacks and persons of Mediterranean descent, have a lower incidence of skin cancer.
      (2) White persons with red hair and fair complexions have higher relative risks.
4. See **Table 49-1, text page 1241,** for a list of other risk factors for cutaneous nonmelanoma and melanoma cancers.

IV.   NONMELANOMA SKIN CANCERS

A.   BASAL CELL CARCINOMA (BCC)

1. **Pathophysiology**
   a. BCC is the **least aggressive** type of skin cancer.

        b. It is an **epithelial tumor** with origins in either the basal layer of the epidermis or in the surrounding dermal structures.

        c. It **grows slowly** by direct extension and has the capacity to cause major local destruction.

        d. **Metastasis is rare** and most often to the regional lymph nodes.

  2. **Assessment**

        a. Types of BCC include **nodular BCC, superficial BCC, pigmented BCC,** and **morphea-like BCC.** See **Chapter 8, Table 8-6, text page 156,** for a review of the clinical characteristics and common sites of occurrence of **nodular** and **superficial** basal cell types.

        b. **Pigmented BCC** is less common and may be nodular or superficial. It occurs most commonly on the head, neck, and face.

           (1) Characteristics include pigmentation of brown, black, or blue and a shiny, pearly, papular border with well-defined margins and telangiectases.

           (2) Biologically, the behavior of pigmented BCC is similar to nodular BCC.

        c. **Morphea-like BCC** is the most rare type. It develops primarily on the head and neck.

           (1) Clinically, it is flat, ivory-colored or colorless, resembles a scar, lacks translucency, and has ill-defined margins.

           (2) It is more aggressive and invasive than nodular BCC.

B. **SQUAMOUS CELL CARCINOMA (SCC)**

  1. **Pathophysiology**

        a. SCC is a tumor that may arise in **any epithelium.**

        b. Cells vary from **well differentiated,** with regular polygonal shapes and round nuclei, to **anaplastic,** with distorted cell and nuclei shapes and more numerous mitoses.

        c. SCC is **more aggressive than BCC,** as it has a faster growth rate, less well-demarcated margins, and a greater metastatic potential.

        d. Metastatic disease is usually first noted in the **regional lymph nodes.**

  2. **Assessment**

        a. See **Chapter 8, Table 8-6, text page 156,** for a review of the clinical characteristics and common sites of occurrence of SCC.

        b. Several preexisting conditions may lead to invasive SCC, including **intraepidermal SCC** (also called **carcinoma in situ**), **keratoacanthomas,** and **epidermodysplasia verruciformis.**

C. **TREATMENT OF NONMELANOMA SKIN CANCERS**

  1. Standard treatment for nonmelanoma skin cancers includes **surgical excision, chemosurgery, curettage and electrodesiccation, radiation,** and **cryotherapy.**

  2. Choice of treatment depends on **tumor type, location, size, growth pattern,** and **whether the tumor is primary or secondary.** No single therapy is applicable to all tumors.

  3. The primary goals of treatment are **cure, preservation of tissue and function, minimal operative risk,** and **optimal cosmetic results.**

  4. The **four** types of **biopsy techniques** used for NMSCs are the **shave** biopsy, **bunch** biopsy, **incisional** biopsy, and **excisional** biopsy.

  5. **Surgical excision**

        a. Surgical excision can be performed for any nonmelanoma skin cancer and may be simple or complex.

        b. Most common is an **elliptical excision,** with suture closure, of a small to moderate lesion that can be performed on an outpatient basis with local anesthesia.

        c. Excision of large carcinomas of the eyelid and lip preserves function and allows reconstruction by **graft** or **flap.**

           (1) A graft or flap is indicated when a lesion is large or located in an area where insufficient tissue for primary closure would result in deformity.

        d. **Advantages** of surgical excision include

           (1) Rapid healing.

           (2) The availability of an entire specimen for histologic examination.

           (3) Favorable cosmetic results.

        e. **Disadvantages** are related to the

           (1) Time-consuming aspect of the procedure.

        (2)   Need for a skilled physician to judge the exact extent of the tumor and the risk of infection.

6. **Mohs' micrographic surgery**
   a. **Mohs' micrographic surgery,** or chemosurgery, involves horizontal shaving and staining of tissue in thin layers, with histologic mapping of all specimen margins. It is the most accurate technique for assessing the actual extent of nonmelanoma skin cancers.
   b. It is most often used for cancers in **high-risk areas** (e.g., the nose) and for **lesions with unclear margins, recurring lesions, aggressive tumors,** and **extensive lesions.**
   c. **Advantages** of Mohs' microsurgery include the
      (1)   Preservation of the maximum amount of tissue for easier reconstruction.
      (2)   Ability to map tumor margins histologically.
      (3)   Fact that the procedure can be performed on an outpatient basis with the use of local anesthetic.
   d. **Disadvantages** are the
      (1)   Requirement of specialized training and equipment.
      (2)   Time-consuming aspects of the procedure.
      (3)   Need for daily wound care postoperatively.
      (4)   Possibility of graft rejection and wound dehiscence.

7. **Curettage and electrodesiccation**
   a. Because of poor margin control, curettage and electrodesiccation is used only for BCE skin cancers that are **small, superficial,** or **recurrent.**
   b. The tumor is destroyed by **scraping out the tumor mass** through curettage and treating the tumor base with a **low-voltage electrode.**
   c. **Advantages** are its rapidity, good cosmetic results, preservation of normal tissue, and the ability to obtain a tissue specimen for histopathologic study.
   d. **Disadvantages** include no margin control, prolonged healing, and the need for a skilled physician to "feel" the tumor tissue.

8. **Radiotherapy**
   a. Radiotherapy is generally recommended only for lesions that are **inoperable,** lesions located in sites such as the **corner of the nose, eyelid, lip, and canthus,** and lesions **between 1 cm and 10 cm in diameter.** Treatment is not recommended for young patients.
   b. **Advantages** are painless treatment, preservation of normal anatomic contours, and the ability to extend treatment into surrounding areas.
   c. **Disadvantages** include lack of histologic tissue for margin control, long treatment periods (3–4 weeks), the risk of radiation-induced malignancy, and the need for clinical facilities with trained radiotherapists.

9. **Cryotherapy**
   a. Cryotherapy involves tumor destruction by the use of **liquid nitrogen** to **freeze and thaw tumor tissue.** It can be used for small to large primary tumors, for certain recurrent lesions, for multiple superficial BCE, and for palliation.
   b. Lesions must have **well-defined margins,** and the procedure is not recommended for areas with cartilage (such as the ear), which can buckle when frozen.
   c. Healing time depends on **tumor location,** with lesions on the back or previously treated sites taking longer than tumors of the face.
   d. **Advantages** include minimal discomfort, performance on an outpatient basis, speed, and good cosmetic results.
   e. **Disadvantages** include the need for wound care, prolonged healing time, possible temporary nerve damage, and bleeding.
   f. Careful follow-up is suggested for 2 years postoperatively to detect secondary tumors, which usually occur within 18 months.

V.   MELANOMA

A.   CUTANEOUS MELANOMA

1. **Pathophysiology**
   a. CM arises from **melanocytes,** cells that specialize in the biosynthesis and transport of melanin.

(1) Melanocytes are found throughout the skin but are most common in the basal layers of the epidermis.

(2) In melanomas, the melanin-synthesizing granule, or **melanosome,** may be abnormal or absent.

b. Three specific **precursor lesions** of CM include **dysplastic nevi (DN), congenital nevi,** and **lentigo maligna.**

c. **Dysplastic nevi (DN)**

(1) Also known as B-K moles and atypical moles, DN may occur in both familial and nonfamilial settings.

    (a) In members of families with **familial** DN, the risk of developing CM approaches **100%.**

    (b) The risk of **nonfamilial DN** in the general population is estimated at **5%–10%;** the upper range of some estimates is 50% or more.

(2) An **early clinical indication** may be the presence of an increased number of histologically normal nevi between the ages of 5 and 8 years, with dysplastic changes occurring after puberty.

(3) DN generally have one or more of the **clinical features of CM:** asymmetry, border irregularity, color variegation, and a diameter greater than 6 mm.

(4) DN appear on the face, trunk, and arms but also may be seen on the buttocks, groin, scalp, and female breast.

(5) **Pigmentation** is irregular with mixtures of tan, brown, and black or red and pink.

(6) A distinctive feature is a **"fried egg" appearance** with a deep pigmented papular area surrounded by an area of lighter pigmentation. The surface is pebbly, and the border is indistinct and irregular.

(7) Individuals with DN or suspected DN should be thoroughly **questioned** about family or personal history of melanoma, atypical pigmented lesions, and prior excisions of any kind.

    (a) The entire skin surface should be examined, including the scalp, axilla, and genitalia, and between the toes and fingers.

d. **Dysplastic nevi** are described in **Chapter 8, Table 8-7, text page 157,** along with accompanying text and guide. Also see **Color Plate 21** for illustration.

(1) The first line of treatment for DN is **excisional biopsy** of the most atypical-looking lesions to document dysplasia and rule out melanoma.

(2) Periodic (3–6-month) skin examinations follow.

(3) New lesions suggestive of melanoma are removed and biopsied.

(4) Individuals with DN are taught to examine the body every 1–2 months.

e. **Congenital nevi** are present at or shortly after birth. They range in size from 1.5–3 cm and cover extensive body surfaces. The lesion surface is irregular and may be raised; borders are fairly regular. Large lesions may contain areas of nodularity. Pigmentation ranges from brown to black.

(1) A careful history and examination is essential to management; dates of appearance and subsequent changes should be noted.

(2) Abnormal-appearing lesions should be biopsied to confirm its histology.

(3) Treatment consists of **surgical excision.** Removal of larger lesions may be disfiguring.

(4) Regular follow-up examinations are essential.

2. **Assessment**

a. Review **study guide Chapter 8, section VIF,** of the outline for a summary of assessment procedures and questions to ask in the patient history.

b. Those patients with melanoma should undergo examinations for metastatic disease. This includes **chest radiography, blood cell count,** and **liver function tests.**

c. Additional tests are performed if clinical findings indicate further metastatic spread. This may include **CT and MRI scans, skin or node biopsy,** and a **bone scan.**

3. **Classification**

a. Melanoma has been classified into several types, including **lentigo maligna (LMM), superficial spreading (SSM), nodular,** and **acral lentiginous.** A comparison of these four major types of cutaneous melanoma is given in **Table 49-3, text page 1246.**

b. Each type of melanoma is characterized by a

(1) **Radial phase,** in which tumor growth is parallel to the skin surface, risk of metastasis is slight, and surgical excision is usually curative, and/or a

  (2) **Vertical growth phase,** marked by focal deep penetration of atypical melanocytes into the dermis and subcutaneous tissue. Penetration occurs rapidly, increasing the risk of metastasis.

 c. **Lentigo maligna melanoma (LMM)** is the least serious type and occurs on body areas that are heavily exposed to **solar radiation.** See **Table 49-3** for characteristics of LMM and **Color plate 22** in Chapter 2 for illustration.

  (1) There is a 25% chance of metastasis in the vertical phase.

 d. **Superficial spreading melanoma (SSM)** accounts for 70% of CM. See **Table 49-3** for characteristics of SSM and **Color plate 23.**

  (1) SSM usually arises in a preexisting nevus.

 e. **Nodular melanoma** constitutes 15%–30% of all CMs. See **Table 49-3** for characteristics of this melanoma and **Color plate 24.**

  (1) Nodular melanoma has **only a vertical phase,** making early diagnosis difficult.

  (2) It is more aggressive than other types of melanomas and has a shorter clinical onset.

 f. **Acral lentiginous** or mucocutaneous melanoma is found in 35%–60% of **dark-skinned persons,** particularly blacks, Asians, and Hispanics and in only 2%–10% of white persons. See **Table 49-3** for characteristics of this melanoma and **Color plate 25** in Chapter 2 for illustration.

  (1) The radial phase may last for years and resembles an early lentigo maligna.

  (2) In the vertical phase, the melanomas are more aggressive and can metastasize.

4. **Staging and prognostic factors**

 a. **Microstaging** is a term used to describe the **level of invasion** of the CM and **maximum tumor thickness.**

 b. The two parameters that are used in assessing the depth of invasion are the

  (1) **Anatomic level of invasion** or the **Clark level.**

  (2) **Thickness of tumor tissue** or the **Breslow level.**

  (3) See **Figure 49-11, text page 1248,** for the corresponding thickness of Clark and Breslow levels.

 c. The **three-stage staging system** for CM is still used, although the American Joint Committee on Cancer's newer **four-stage system** is preferable. See **Tables 49-4** and **49-5, text pages 1248** and **1249,** for a description of these two systems.

 d. As CM **thickness** increases, survival rates decrease. Thus the Breslow level (the system used to assess the depth of invasion of melanoma via the thickness of the tumor) has consistently proved to be a significant prognostic variable in stage I CM.

  (1) Other factors that predict survival are age, sex, and clinical and histologic factors. Younger patients and women have a somewhat better prognosis.

  (2) With equivalent thicknesses, lesions on the hands, feet, and scalp may have a poorer prognosis.

  (3) **Histologic factors** that predict an unfavorable prognosis are the presence of microscopic satellites of tumor, high miotic activity, ulceration, vertical growth phase, and large tumor volume.

  (4) **Stage I** lentigo maligna and superficial-spreading melanomas have better 5-year survival rates (85%–90%) than nodular (about 60%) and acral lentiginous melanomas.

  (5) In **stage II** disease the 5-year survival rates are 36%, but these rates vary according to the clinical status of nodes, the number of nodes involved, and the presence or absence of ulceration in the primary tumor.

  (6) **Stage III** disease is generally incurable secondary to metastases. Median survival is approximately 6 months.

5. **Treatment**

 a. **Surgery**

  (1) **Biopsy** is the initial surgical procedure for suspected CM.

   (a) An **excisional biopsy** that entails removal of few millimeters of normal tissue surrounding the lesion is preferable, since it provides a definitive diagnosis along with microstaging information.

   (b) An **incisional biopsy** can be used for lesions in cosmetically sensitive areas or for large lesions.

(c) Electrocoagulation, curettage, shaving, and burning should never be used to remove a suspicious mole.

(2) **Wide excision** is the standard treatment for stage I CM.

(a) Because risk of recurrence correlates with lesion thickness and not margin size, only a **1 cm** margin of normal skin around the lesion is required for thin melanomas. For thicker lesions a **3–5 cm** margin is left.

(3) **Elective lymph node dissection (ENLD)** has a high degree of morbidity, and use of this procedure is debatable when no clinical evidence of nodal involvement exists.

(4) Standard surgical therapy of clinical stage II disease (clinical, but not histologic, evidence of draining lymph node involvement) includes excision of the primary lesion, along with surgical dissection of the involved nodes.

(a) In cases where the index of suspicion is low for metastatic disease, a palpable node may be biopsied by either the open or the fine-needle approach.

(5) Surgery is also used for **palliation** of disease and symptomatic involvement, especially when a solitary, easily accessible lesion is involved.

b. **Chemotherapy**
(1) Metastatic malignant melanoma is highly resistant to systemic chemotherapeutic agents, indicating the need for further research in this area.

c. **Radiotherapy**
(1) Radiotherapy is most effective when **tumor volume is low** and when a **high dose per fewer fractions** radiation level is used.
(2) Radiation is also used for palliation of neurologic symptoms and bone pain.

d. **Hormonal therapy**
(1) A high incidence of steroid binding in melanoma tissue has led to clinical trials demonstrating some tumor response with several hormonal agents, including tamofixen.

e. **Immunotherapy**
(1) Immunologic intervention by the host may alter the growth pattern of CM. In addition, specific tumor antigen antibodies have been found in melanoma patients.
(2) Immunotherapy is currently being investigated in the context of adjuvant therapy and as treatment for metastatic disease.
(3) Interferon use in CM remains a palliative measure.

f. Melanoma vaccines are under investigation.

B. UVEAL MELANOMA

1. **Uveal melanoma affects the iris, ciliary body, and choroid portions of the eye.** It arises from uveal melanocytes that have a common embryologic origin with melanocytes of the conjuctiva and skin.

2. **Predisposing factors** include ocular melanocytosis (congenital hyperpigmentation), ocular nevi, and neurofibromatosis. Intermittent intense exposure to **UV radiation** may also be an important risk factor.

3. **Choroidal melanoma** is the most common type of uveal melanoma found in adults.
   a. Large lesions left untreated can become invasive, metastasize, and become fatal. Metastasis is to the liver or lung.
   b. Small lesions can be treated surgically or with photocoagulation by laser or xenon arc.
   c. **Radiotherapy** is the most widely used nonenucleation therapy and has the advantage of preserving both life and vision.

VI. PREVENTION

A. PRIMARY PREVENTION

1. See **text pages 1251–1252,** column 1, and **Study Guide Chapter 8, section VIF** of the outline, for a list of preventive measures.

B.   **SECONDARY PREVENTION**

1.   Refer to **Study Guide Chapter 8, section VIF5** of the outline, and **Figure 49-3, text page 1246.**

C.   **TERTIARY PREVENTION**

1.   **Retinoids** (vitamin A and its derivatives) used as biologic treatment agents have shown some effect as chemopreventive agents in persons with BCC and several predisposing conditions of skin cancer.

VII.   **NURSING MANAGEMENT**

1.   Nursing involvement ranges from participation in **prevention and early-detection education** and **screening** of the general population to **posttreatment management** of patients with skin cancer.
2.   Important components of nursing management include **interview, skin assessment, education,** and **posttreatment management.**

A.   **INTERVIEW**

1.   All individuals with skin cancer or those at risk for cancer should be questioned about their knowledge of skin cancers, past medical history, and exposure to risk factors.
2.   A family pedigree ascertains family history of skin cancers.

B.   **SKIN ASSESSMENT**

1.   A thorough skin assessment can initially identify suspicious lesions. Persons with these lesions should then be referred to qualified dermatologists for further review and diagnosis.
2.   Formal skin assessment is performed with the individual seated and in bright, preferably natural light.
3.   The thyroid and regional lymph nodes of the neck should be palpated.
4.   The location and descriptive characteristics of suspicious lesions should be recorded on an **anatomic chart.** Warts, moles, scars, vascularities, and birthmarks should also be documented.

C.   **EDUCATION**

1.   Refer to **Study Guide Chapter 8, section VIF** of the outline.

D.   **POSTTREATMENT MANAGEMENT**

1.   Postoperative nursing management is determined by the **extent of surgical excision.**
2.   Patients who have undergone **skin grafting or flapping** require careful and frequent observation for signs of infection and hemorrhage in both donor and recipient sites.
   a.   The recipient site should be immobilized to prevent separation, and involved limbs should be elevated to minimize edema.
   b.   Minor sloughing of a graft site can be controlled with mineral oil or lanolin.
3.   All patients with a diagnosis of melanoma should be evaluated at regular intervals for recurrence or metastatic disease.
   a.   Intervals should be adjusted according to the risk of metastatic disease.
   b.   Patients must understand the importance of these follow-up visits and inform the physician or nurse of any physical or mental changes that occur.

PRACTICE QUESTIONS

1.   The most common form of skin cancer is
   (A)   basal cell carcinoma (BCC).
   (B)   squamous cell carcinoma (SCC).
   (C)   malignant melanoma.
   (D)   superficial spreading melanoma (SSM).

2. High-risk factors for cutaneous melanoma (CM) include all of the following **except**
   (A) skin pigmentation.
   (B) a persistently changed or changing mole.
   (C) the presence of a precursor lesion such as dysplastic nevi.
   (D) oral contraceptives.

3. One way that basal cell carcinoma (BCC) is distinguished from squamous cell carcinoma (SCC) is by its
   (A) common occurrence on the head and hands.
   (B) lower incidence.
   (C) slower growth rate.
   (D) less well-demarcated margins.

4. Which of the following factors is **least** likely to influence the physician's choice of treatment for nonmelanoma skin cancers?
   (A) the need for a specimen for histologic examination
   (B) the risk of bleeding from surgical excision
   (C) the need for maximum preservation of tissue for favorable cosmetic results
   (D) the size, type, and location of the tumor

5. A graft or flap is most often used in the surgical treatment of a nonmelanoma cancer when
   (A) the lesion is large or located in an area with insufficient tissue for closure.
   (B) risks of bleeding are high and vasculature must be maintained.
   (C) the actual extent of the tumor must be accurately assessed and margins are relatively unclear.
   (D) the lesion is small, superficial, or recurrent.

6. If one were choosing a treatment for a nonmelanoma skin cancer that offered the advantages of minimal discomfort, performance on an outpatient basis, speed, and good cosmetic results, one would be **most** likely to select
   (A) radiotherapy.
   (B) surgical excision.
   (C) chemosurgery.
   (D) cryotherapy.

7. Which of the following statements about dysplastic nevi (DN) is **incorrect?**
   (A) DN may be familial or nonfamilial.
   (B) Most persons affected by DN have about 25–75 abnormal levi.
   (C) DN develop from precursor lesions of CM known as congenital nevi.
   (D) A distinctive feature of DN is a "fried egg" appearance with a deeply pigmented papular area surrounded by an area of lighter pigmentation.

8. Assessment of CM typically would include all of the following measures **except**
   (A) palpation of all accessible lymph nodes.
   (B) a complete visual examination of the cutaneous surface.
   (C) MRI imaging of suspect lesions.
   (D) serum chemistry determinations with liver function tests.

9. The phase of CM tumor growth that is characterized by focal deep penetration of atypical melanocytes into the dermis and subcutaneous tissue is the
   (A) radial phase.
   (B) vertical growth phase.
   (C) nodular phase.
   (D) acral lentiginous phase.

10. Of the following factors related to CM prognosis, the one **most** closely correlated with decreased survival rates in patients with stage I CM is
    (A) anatomic level of tumor invasion.
    (B) tumor location.
    (C) Clark level.
    (D) tumor thickness.

11. The preferred initial surgical procedure for suspected CM is
    (A) excisional biopsy.
    (B) incisional biopsy.
    (C) wide excision.
    (D) curettage and electrodesiccation.

12. The form of skin cancer that affects the iris, ciliary body, and choroid portion of the eye is known as
    (A) malignant angiosarcoma.
    (B) rhabdomyosarcoma.
    (C) uveal melanoma.
    (D) squamous cell melanoma.

13. Which of the following statements about primary prevention of skin cancers is **false?**
    (A) UV radiation is strongest during the mid-part of the day.
    (B) For most people, sunscreen is not required on overcast days.
    (C) Certain medications (e.g., oral contraceptives) can make individuals photosensitive.
    (D) Surfaces such as sand and water can reflect more than one-half of the UV radiation onto the skin.

14. Postoperative nursing management of the patient who has undergone surgery for skin cancer generally is determined by the
    (A) mode of therapy used.
    (B) location of the tumor.
    (C) type of tumor.
    (D) extent of surgical excision.

ANSWER EXPLANATIONS

1. **The answer is (A).** BCC is the most common form of skin cancer in whites and outnumbers SCC by a ratio of 3:1. Nonmelanoma skin cancers, including BCC, have a higher incidence but a lower metastatic potential and mortality rate than malignant melanoma. Malignant melanoma has a much lower incidence but a mortality rate that is triple that of the nonmelanoma cancers. Increased mortality is directly related to its high potential for metastasis. (1239)

2. **The answer is (D).** Multiple etiologic and risk factors are associated with skin cancers. High-risk factors for CM include a persistent changed or changing mole and the presence of irregular pigmented precursor lesions, including dysplastic nevi, congenital nevi, and lentigo maligna. Other possible risk factors for CM include UV radiation, age, hormonal factors, immunosuppression, and a previous history of melanoma. There is no conclusive evidence regarding the use of oral contraceptives and the increased risk of CM. High-risk factors for nonmelanoma cancers include ultraviolet (UV) radiation, especially UV-B and UV-A, and skin pigmentation. (1240–1241)

3. **The answer is (C).** BCC is the least aggressive type of skin cancer and has its origins in either the basal layer of the epidermis or in the surrounding dermal structures. It is most commonly found on the nose, eyelids, cheeks, neck, trunk, and extremities. It grows slowly by direct extension and has the capacity to cause major local destruction. Metastasis is rare and most often to the regional lymph nodes. SCC, on the other hand, may arise in any epithelium. It is most commonly found on the head and hands. It is more aggressive than BCC, as it has a faster growth rate, less well-demarcated margins, and a greater metastatic potential. Metastatic disease is usually first noted in the regional lymph nodes. (1241–1242)

4. **The answer is (B).** Standard treatment for nonmelanoma skin cancers includes surgical excision, chemosurgery, curettage and electrodesiccation, radiation, and cryotherapy. Which of these treatments the physician chooses will depend on several factors, starting with the type of tumor, its location, size, and growth pattern, and whether it is a primary or secondary lesion. The choice also will take into account the primary goals of treatment, including the chances for cure, preservation of tissue and function, minimal operative risk, and optimal cosmetic results. (1243)

5. **The answer is (A).** A graft or flap is indicated when a lesion is large or located in an area where insufficient tissue for primary closure would result in deformity, for example, after excision of large carcino-

mas of the eyelid and lip. Function is preserved in this manner. A skin flap consists of skin and subcutaneous tissue that are transferred from one area of the body to another. A flap contains its own blood supply, whereas a graft is avascular and depends on the blood supply of the recipient site for its survival. (1243)

6. **The answer is (D).** Cryotherapy involves tumor destruction by the use of liquid nitrogen to freeze and thaw tumor tissue. It can be used for small to large primary tumors, for certain recurrent lesions, for multiple superficial BCC, and for palliation, provided lesions have well-defined margins. Its major disadvantages include the need for wound care, prolonged healing time, possible temporary nerve damage, and bleeding. Both surgical excision and chemosurgery, and especially radiotherapy, are fairly lengthy procedures compared with cryotherapy. (1244)

7. **The answer is (C).** DN are precursor lesions of cutaneous melanoma (CM) that develop from normal nevi, usually after puberty. It has been reported that 50% of CM evolve from some form of DN. They may be familial or nonfamilial, with the risk of CM in a family member with DN approaching 100% in melanoma-prone families. DN are often larger than 5 mm and can number from 1–100, with most affected persons having 25–75 abnormal nevi. They appear typically on sun-exposed areas, especially on the back, but also may be seen on the scalp, breasts, and buttocks. Pigmentation is irregular, with mixtures of tan, brown, and black or red and pink. A distinctive feature is a "fried egg" appearance. (1245)

8. **The answer is (C).** Assessment of CM begins with a thorough history and physical examination. The examination includes a visual examination of the cutaneous surface, the questionable lesion(s), and the area surrounding the lesion to determine the presence of satellite lesions or in-transit metastases. All accessible lymph nodes, particularly those in the regional drainage sites, are palpated. Those patients with melanoma should undergo examinations for metastatic disease. This includes chest radiography, blood cell count, and liver function tests. Additional tests are performed if clinical findings indicate further metastatic spread. This may include CT and (rarely) MRI scans, skin or node biopsy for new lesions, and a bone scan for undetermined bone pain. (1245–1246)

9. **The answer is (B).** Melanoma has been classified into several types, including lentigo maligna (LMM), superficial spreading (SSM), nodular, and acral lentiginous. Each type is characterized by a radial phase, in which tumor growth is parallel to the skin surface, risk of metastasis is slight, and surgical excision is usually curative, and/or a vertical growth phase, marked by focal deep penetration of atypical melanocytes into the dermis and subcutaneous tissue. Penetration occurs rapidly, increasing the risk of metastasis. (1246–1247)

10. **The answer is (D).** Microstaging describes the level of invasion of the CM and maximum tumor thickness. The two parameters that are used in assessing the depth of invasion are the anatomic level of invasion or the Clark level and the thickness of tumor tissue or the Breslow level. The prognosis for patients with metastatic disease at the time of diagnosis is poor, with most dying within 5 years. As CM thickness increases, survival rates decrease. Thus, the Breslow level has consistently proved to be a significant prognostic variable in stage I CM. (1247–1248)

11. **The answer is (A).** Biopsy is the initial surgical procedure for suspected CM. Because it provides a definitive diagnosis along with microstaging information, an excisional biopsy that entails removal of a few millimeters of normal tissue surrounding the lesion is preferable. An incisional biopsy can be used for lesions in cosmetically sensitive areas or for large lesions. Electrocoagulation, curettage, shaving, and burning are never used to remove a suspicious mole. (1248–1249)

12. **The answer is (C).** Uveal melanoma derives from melanocytes that have a common embryologic origin with melanocytes of the conjuctiva and skin. Predisposing factors include ocular melanocytosis (congenital hyperpigmentation), ocular nevi, and neurofibromatosis. Intermittent intense exposure to UV radiation may also be an important risk factor. Choroidal melanoma is the most common type of uveal melanoma found in adults. Large lesions left untreated can become invasive, metastasize, and become fatal. Metastasis is to the liver or lung. Small lesions can be treated surgically or with photocoagulation by laser or xenon arc. Radiotherapy is the most widely used nonenucleation therapy and has the advantage of preserving both life and vision. (1251)

13. **The answer is (B).** Sunscreen should also be applied on overcast days because 70%–80% of UV radiation can penetrate cloud cover. (1251–1252)

14.   **The answer is (D).**   Postoperative nursing management is determined by the extent of surgical excision. Patients who have had surgical excision only should be instructed to limit environmental insults to the surgical site and to protect the site against exposure to irritants and mechanical trauma. Patients who have undergone skin grafting or flapping require careful and frequent observation for signs of infection and hemorrhage in both donor and recipient sites. The recipient site should be immobilized to prevent separation, and involved limbs should be elevated to minimize edema. Minor sloughing of a graft site can be controlled with mineral oil or lanolin. In addition, all patients with a diagnosis of melanoma should be evaluated at regular intervals for recurrence or metastatic disease. (1253–1254)

50 Urologic and Male Genital Malignancies

STUDY OUTLINE

I. INTRODUCTION

1. See **Figure 50-1, text page 1260,** for an overview of the sites of genitourinary tumors and metastases in men.
2. See **Figure 50-2, text page 1261,** for an overview of the sites and routes of genitourinary tumors and metastases in women.

II. PROSTATIC CANCER

A. ANATOMY AND PHYSIOLOGY

1. The **prostate** is an organ about the size of a walnut in the adult male located **inferior to the bladder and in front of the rectum.**

B. EPIDEMIOLOGY

1. **Prostate cancer** is the second most common cancer in American men, accounting for approximately **23% of all cancer in men** in the United States and **12% of cancer deaths.**
2. **Black American men** have the highest rate of prostate cancer in the world.
3. The peak incidence is **between 60 and 70 years** of age.

C. ETIOLOGY

1. The three main etiologic agents hypothesized to be related to prostate cancer are **age, sexually transmitted disease,** and **endocrine factors,** such as high levels of serum testosterone.
2. A significant correlation between **family history** and the development of the disease is clearly evident.
3. The possibility that a relationship between **vasectomy** and **prostate cancer** exists is important to investigate in precisely designed research.

D. PATHOPHYSIOLOGY

1. **Cellular characteristics**
   a. Prostatic cancers are almost always **adenocarcinomas arising in the posterior lobe of the organ.**
   b. **Progression of disease**
      (1) Prostatic tumors grow and spread **locally,** usually by way of the **blood vessels and lymphatic system.**
      (2) **Hematogenous spread** typically involves the **lungs, liver, kidneys,** and **bones.**
      (3) Usually slow-growing and indolent, tumors progress slowly and metastasize late. Other cases may be rapidly progressive and fatal.
      (4) Metastases occur to the lungs, liver, kidney, and bone.

E.   **CLINICAL MANIFESTATIONS**

1.   Detection of prostate tumors is often as a result of **routine rectal examination,** since the disease is usually asymptomatic in its early stages.
2.   Presenting symptoms commonly include **weight loss, back pain,** and **prostatism.** Other symptoms include **urinary frequency, nocturia, dysuria, a slow urinary stream,** and **hematuria.**
3.   More than half of patients present with localized disease, 19% with regional involvement, and 23.7% with distant metastases.

F.   **ASSESSMENT**

1.   **Screening**
     a.   Although controversial, screening of asymptomatic males by any means has shown no benefit.
     b.   **Rectal palpation** has been the most important step in detecting prostate cancer, although the positive predictive value of an abnormal rectal examination ranges from 11% to 26%.
     c.   **Transrectal ultrasound** continues to be a controversial screening technique.
2.   **Prostate-specific antigen**
     a.   The most promising **biochemical marker** is **prostate-specific antigen (PSA),** although it may be more useful for monitoring patients with advanced disease.
     b.   It is argued that if the PSA is **combined** with a digital rectal examination and/or transrectal US, it could be part of an effective early detection program.

G.   **DIAGNOSIS**

1.   Every suspected prostatic mass should be biopsied using **transrectal or transperineal needle biopsy.**
2.   **Serial serum prostate-specific antigens** may be the most sensitive marker of localized and metastatic disease.
3.   **Bone scans** have demonstrated metastases in 75% of patients with advanced disease.
4.   **CT scans or MRIs** may help to diagnose pelvic nodal involvement.

H.   **CLASSIFICATION AND STAGING**

1.   **Table 50-1, text page 1267,** provides the **TNM (Tumor/Node/Metastasis)** classification system for prostatic cancer.
2.   A staging work-up to determine the presence of metastases should include a **chest X ray, bone scan,** and **pelvic CT scan.**

I.   **TREATMENT**

1.   **Surgery**
     a.   **Radical prostatectomy** is a common surgical method of choice. A common sequela is **sexual dysfunction** with an impotency rate of up to 90%.
     b.   **Subtotal prostatectomy** is usually performed with a transurethral resectoscope, and almost always causes **retrograde ejaculation.**
2.   **Radiotherapy**
     a.   **External beam radiotherapy**
          (1)   It may be used as either a **curative** or a **palliative** treatment.
          (2)   A curative approach will include **local irradiation of the primary tumor** and **extended field irradiation to encompass first echelon lymphatic drainage.**
          (3)   The dosage is delivered in fractions over a period of about seven weeks.
          (4)   **Side effects** include **proctitis, diarrhea, urinary frequency,** and an **impotency rate of 20%–40%.**
     b.   **Internal radiotherapy**
          (1)   Either **radioactive gold** or **radioactive iodine** is implanted during surgery or using hollow needles inserted at small intervals.
          (2)   Most common **side effects** include **difficulty voiding** and **proctitis.**
          (3)   Sexual function is preserved in 70%–90% of men.

3. **Endocrine manipulation**
   a. About 85% of prostatic cancers are **androgen dependent.**
   b. The primary treatment of advanced prostate cancer is to **decrease the availability of circulating androgens to the tumor by blocking androgen formation or use.**
   c. There are several major methods of endocrine manipulation.
   d. **Surgical castration**
      (1) **Bilateral orchiectiomy** removes the testes, which produce 90%–95% of circulating testosterone, the most powerful androgen.
   e. **Medical castration**
      (1) **Estrogen** is capable of blocking the release of luteinizing hormone (LH) by the pituitary gland. LH stimulates the Leydig cells in the testes to synthesize testosterone. While it is not often used, it is still an option.
   f. **Adrenal suppression**
      (1) **Adrenalectomy** removes the secondary source of androgens, responsible for about 5% of androgen production, either surgically (uncommonly used) or medically through the use of drugs (e.g., aminoglutethemide).
   g. **Pure antiandrogens**
      (1) Administration of **antiandrogen drugs** (e.g., cyproterone acetate, flutamide, megesterol acetate) that interfere with intracellular androgen activity.
      (2) Administration of **gonadotropin releasing hormone** (GnRH) analogs (Lupron, Leuporlide, or Zoladex), which disrupts the release of GnRH, eventually causing the suppression of both LH and testosterone.
   h. **Total androgen ablation**
      (1) **Total androgen ablation,** through a combination of methods, which blocks both adrenal and testicular androgens.
   i. **Evaluation of hormone manipulation**
      (1) Seventy to eighty-five percent of advanced prostatic tumors respond to hormonal manipulation, with a **duration of response from 1–3 years.**

J. **CHEMOTHERAPY**

1. The role of chemotherapy has been limited to **palliation** in men with hormone-resistant tumors.
2. Single agents (e.g., cyclophosphamide, methotrexate) appear to be as effective as combination therapy.

K. **TREATMENT ACCORDING TO STAGE**

1. **Stage A**
   a. The common treatment approach for **stage A disease** (clinically occult cancer) is observation or **prostatectomy** with or without pelvic lymph node dissection.
2. **Stage B**
   a. **Stage B** prostate cancer (palpable tumor in one or more lobes that has not extended through the prostatic capsule) can be treated with either **radical prostatectomy,** with or without node dissection, or **radiotherapy,** with equally curative results. Observation is also an option in elderly men.
3. **Stage C**
   a. Between 40% and 50% of men present with **stage C** prostate cancer, which extends through the prostatic capsule and involves the bladder neck or seminal vesicles.
   b. Therapy may be either one or a combination of treatment methods outlined above.
   c. The choice of therapy depends on the **person's physical condition, extent of cancer spread, degree of tumor differentiation,** and **person's preference.**
4. **Stage D**
   a. **Stage D** disease is the most common presenting clinical stage and involves **metastases,** either confined to the pelvis or distant spread.
   b. There is **no surgical cure.**
   c. Treatment usually involves one or more of the options outlined above, given in combination or sequentially.

L. **RESULTS AND PROGNOSIS**

1. Approximate survival rates after prostatectomy are shown in **Table 50-2, text page 1274.**

M. **NURSING CARE**

1. Nurses should be involved in educating men to have **regular rectal prostatic examinations after the age of 40 years.** Educational efforts should be focused on **high-risk populations** such as black American males.
2. The nursing care of the person undergoing **surgery** for prostate cancer, either radical prostatectomy or transurethral resection, is fully discussed on **text pages 1274–1277,** but includes
   a. Discussion with the patient and family members about such important concerns as **impotence, loss of libido, alternative forms of sexual gratification,** and **urinary control.**
   b. Postoperative care of **three-way indwelling urinary catheters with irrigation.**
   c. **Wound care.**
   d. Instruction regarding methods of regaining **bladder control.**
3. **Nursing care of individuals receiving radiotherapy**
   a. The first step is answering questions and correcting misconceptions regarding what can be a frightening experience.
   b. Nursing care for **external radiotherapy** includes
      (1) Instruction regarding skin care.
      (2) The use of antispasmodics for cystitis and antidiarrheal agents for proctitis.
   c. Nursing care for **internal radiotherapy**
      (1) Must be done quickly and efficiently to minimize nurse exposure, but the patient should not be made to feel abandoned.
      (2) Includes reminding the person he is no longer radioactive after the implants have decayed.
4. Individual agents in **hormonal therapy** have specific side effects that must be monitored and addressed, including **sodium retention, hypercalcemia, nausea, loss of libido,** and **feminization.**
5. **Orchiectomy** can provoke a high degree of anxiety because of its connotation of castration. Discussion of this issue is critical.
6. The nurse should be aware of the major side effects of **chemotherapy** in order to monitor for and teach patients and families about them.

III. **BLADDER CANCER**

A. **EPIDEMIOLOGY**

1. Bladder cancer accounts for **4%–5%** of all cancers in the United States.
2. Most of these cancers occur in **men,** particularly those who are **white** and **over 50 years of age.**

B. **ETIOLOGY**

1. Overwhelming statistical evidence points to **cigarette smoking** as a prime epidemiologic factor, accounting for as much as 50% of bladder cancer in American males.
2. Among **occupational exposure agents, arylamine,** used in the dye industry and as paint pigment, is most strongly related to bladder cancer.
3. Ingestion of other physical agents, such as **coffee, alcohol, saccharin,** and **phenacetin,** is weakly linked to bladder cancer.
4. In areas where the parasite *Schistosoma* is endemic, such as in Egypt and many African countries, the incidence of **squamous cell bladder carcinoma** is much higher.

C. **PATHOPHYSIOLOGY**

1. **Cellular characteristics**
   a. About 90%–95% of bladder tumors in North America occur in **transitional epithelial cells lining the bladder.**
   b. **Grading** of bladder tumors is done to predict the **speed of progression and recurrence,** with well-differentiated (low-grade) tumors having a slower growth rate.

2. **Progression of disease**
   a. The most important growth feature is **the depth of penetration into the bladder wall.**
   b. **Metastasis** takes place through **direct extension out of the muscle of the bladder into the serosa.**
   c. The tumor may involve other adjacent structures such as the **sigmoid colon** or **rectum,** and **hematogenous spread can occur to bones, liver,** and **lungs.**

D. **CLINICAL MANIFESTATIONS**

1. Gross, painless **hematuria** is the most common presenting symptom. Other early symptoms include **dysuria, urinary frequency,** and **urgency.**
2. Symptoms of advanced disease include **pain in the suprapubic region and back** and **urinary hesitancy** if the bladder neck is obstructed.

E. **ASSESSMENT**

1. **Physical examination**
   a. There are no early signs of bladder cancer on physical examination.
2. **Diagnostic studies**
   a. **Exfoliative urinary cytology,** using a total voided specimen, is a simple diagnostic tool.
   b. **Flow cytometry,** a technique used to examine the DNA content of urine cells, is helpful in grading the tumor.
   c. **Excretory urogram** is used before cystoscopy to evaluate a suspected tumor and to show evidence of ureteral or urethral obstruction.
   d. **Cystoscopy** serves to visualize the tumor and provides an opportunity to biopsy it in order to assess the presence of muscle invasion.
   e. The tumor marker **carcinoembryonic antigen (CEA)** is moderately elevated in 50% of late stage bladder cancer.

F. **CLASSIFICATION AND STAGING**

1. **Figure 50-8, text page 1282,** depicts a compilation of the most common staging systems for bladder cancer.
2. Bladder cancer is also often graded from **grade I to grade IV,** with the latter indicating the **least well-differentiated tumor (anaplastic).**

G. **TREATMENT**

1. **Carcinoma in situ**
   a. **Carcinoma in situ** is usually treated either with **electrofulguration and thiotepa** or **radical cystectomy with urinary diversion.**
2. **Superficial, low-grade tumors**
   a. **Superficial, low-grade tumors,** which remain in the epithelium and lamina propria, may be treated with
      (1) Standard treatment of **transurethral resection and fulguration.**
      (2) Intravesical treatment: instillation of **chemotherapy** (thiotepa, mitomycin C, or BCG).
      (3) **Laser therapy.**
3. **Invasive tumors**
   a. **Invasive tumors** have dramatically altered prognoses and are treated aggressively with
      (1) **Definitive radiotherapy:** 7–8 weeks of external radiation to the pelvis and pelvic lymph nodes is usual. Results do not appear to be comparable to cystectomy.
      (2) **Preoperative irradiation,** which is used in an effort to decrease both pelvic recurrence and dissemination during surgery.
      (3) **Radical cystectomy** in men, which includes excision of the bladder with the pericystic fat, the attached peritoneum, and the entire prostate and seminal vesicles (see **Figure 50-10, text page 1285).**
      (4) **Radical cystectomy** in women, which includes removal of the bladder and entire urethra, uterus, ovaries, fallopian tubes, and anterior wall of the vagina (see **Figure 50-11, text page 1285).**

(5) **Urinary diversions** of various types, which are constructed when a cystectomy is performed. Each has advantages, disadvantages, and potential complications.

    (a) Types of diversions are discussed on **text pages 1284–1287.** They include an **ileal conduit, loop stoma, ureterosigmoidostomy,** and **continent ileal reservoir for urinary diversion.**

    (b) A radical cystectomy with urinary diversion can affect many aspects of **sexual function** for both men and women.

    (c) The uses and types of **penile prostheses** are discussed on **text page 1288,** column 1.

    (d) Women may experience sexual dysfunction as a result of perceived losses related to **hysterectomy/oophorectomy, hormonal changes,** or **removal of the anterior wall of the vagina.**

    (e) Both men and women may experience difficulty adjusting to an **external stoma.**

4. **Advanced bladder cancer**

    a. The use of **chemotherapy** early in the course of treatment for high-stage, high-grade bladder cancer may lengthen the disease-free interval and overall survival.

    b. **Intensive combination chemotherapy** that includes **cisplatin** seems to produce a higher complete response rate than single-agent chemotherapy.

    c. The highest response rates documented have been observed with combination regimens that include cisplatin, methotrexate, and vinblastine with or without doxorubicin.

H. RESULTS AND PROGNOSIS

1. **Table 50-9, text page 1289,** shows the approximate 5-year survival rates for bladder cancer in American blacks and whites.

I. NURSING CARE OF INDIVIDUALS WITH BLADDER CANCER

1. **Preoperative nursing care**

    a. Preoperative nursing care involves clear explanations of the procedure and its outcome to the patient and family members, along with emotional support.

    b. Careful **selection of the stoma site** is highly important, involving thorough consideration of

        (1) The **type of urinary diversion** to be performed.

        (2) The patient's **abdominal surface.**

        (3) The patient's **personal habits** pertaining to work and recreation.

    c. A urinary diversion should produce a continuous flow of urine from the time of surgery.

2. **General postoperative care**

    a. Postoperative care will vary **depending on the method of urinary diversion** or bladder substitution.

    b. **Routine postoperative care** is standard as with all patients who have undergone major abdominal surgery.

    c. Continent urinary reservoirs and bladder substitutes produce much mucus and should be **irrigated** regularly in the postoperative period to prevent mucus accumulation.

    d. **Ultrasound** or **intravenous urography** will be performed on a regular basis to check the upper urinary tract for hydronephrosis.

3. **Nursing care following urinary diversion with an ileal conduit**

    a. **Stoma characteristics**

        (1) Protrusion should be about 1/2 to 3/4 inches above the skin surface to allow the urine to drain into the drainage appliance.

        (2) Viability of a stoma is assessed by its **color,** which should be checked regularly in the early postoperative period.

            (a) Normal color is **deep pink to dark red.**

            (b) Sustained color change should be reported.

        (3) **Stoma edema** is normal in the early postoperative period and should resolve in the first 1–2 weeks after surgery.

    b. **Mucus production**

        (1) The intestine normally produces **mucus,** which will be present in all diversions using segments of the bowel, causing the urine to appear cloudy.

    c. **Pouching a urinary stoma**
        (1) Application of a **pouch** to a urinary stoma is described on **text page 1291,** column 2. Applied pouches should remain in place without leakage for 3–5 days.
    d. **Patient teaching for continuing care of a conduit**
        (1) **Patient teaching** for continuing care of a conduit should reinforce the attitude that normal life is possible, include written procedures for stoma care, and provide names and addresses of resource people to contact.
    e. **Follow-up nursing care**
        (1) Periodic **reevaluation of the stoma and function of the conduit** is important to assess for **the need to change the size of the appliance opening, skin integrity and alkaline encrustations around the stoma, stenosis of the stoma, and renal function.**
4. **Nursing care of the individual with a continent ileal reservoir for urinary diversion**
    a. The patient remains in the hospital for 8–10 days postoperatively. See discharge instructions for a Kock pouch with **Medena tube** in **Table 50-12, text page 1293.**
    b. Three weeks after surgery, the individual will be **readmitted.**
        (1) A **radiographic picture** of the pouch will be taken to confirm that there is no extravasation or reflux of urine, and then the Medena tube and ureteral stents will be removed.
        (2) The patient is taught to catheterize the pouch every 2 hours during the day and every 3 hours at night, with gradual decreases in frequency.
5. **Nursing care for a Kock pouch to the urethra**
    a. The male patient who has chosen the continent urinary Kock reservoir to be anastomosed to the urethra following a radical cystectomy is cared for in much the **same way postoperatively as the patient who has had a continent reservoir pouch.**
        (1) The difference is that he has a **#24 French Foley** catheter inserted through the urethra into the reservoir for 3 weeks.
    b. **Table 50-14, text page 1294,** describes discharge instructions for the patients.
6. **Follow-up care**
    a. **Radiological studies** are used to confirm the **integrity of the pouch,** to test the competence of the nipple valves, and to ensure complete emptying of the reservoir.

IV. CANCER OF THE KIDNEY

A. EPIDEMIOLOGY

1. The two major types of kidney cancers are **renal cell cancer,** which occurs in the parenchyma and is the most common form of kidney cancer, and **renal pelvis cancer.** Kidney cancer accounts for only 3% of all cancers in the United States, with 75% of those being **renal cell tumors.**
2. There is a **2:1 male predominance** in kidney cancer.
3. The average age at diagnosis is **55–60 years.**

B. ETIOLOGY

1. **Cigarette smoking**
    a. The only risk factor that has been linked to kidney cancer is **cigarette smoking,** possibly due to the mutagenic chemicals in the urine of smokers.
2. **Occupation**
    a. **Occupational exposure** is associated with only a very small proportion of all renal cancers.
3. **Analgesic use**
    a. Heavy use of certain **analgesics,** including aspirin and acetaminophen, has been shown to increase the risk of cancer of the renal pelvis.

C. PATHOPHYSIOLOGY

1. **Cellular characteristics**
    a. Renal cell carcinoma arises from **tubular epithelial cells** in the kidney parenchyma and are of two broad types.
        (1) **Clear cell tumors.**
        (2) **Granular cell tumors.**
    b. Tumors of the renal pelvis arise from **epithelial tissue anywhere in the renal pelvis.**

2. **Progression of disease**
   a. Somewhere between **30% and 50% of individuals with kidney cancer have metastases at diagnosis.**
   b. Both types of kidney cancers can spread through the venous and lymphatic routes.
   c. Hematogenous spread most often involves the lungs, bones, and liver.

D. **PARANEOPLASIA AND RENAL CELL CARCINOMA**

   1. The term **paraneoplastic syndrome** is used to describe systemic effects of a tumor on the host, through the synthesis by malignant cells of compounds not normally synthesized by cells of that type.
   2. Renal cell carcinomas have an association with paraneoplasia of the endocrine system, through the secretion of hormones such as **parathyroid hormone, erythropoietin,** and **renin.**

E. **CLINICAL MANIFESTATIONS**

   1. **Renal cell carcinoma**
      a. The classic triad of symptoms of renal cell cancer are **hematuria, dull and aching pain,** and a **palpable abdominal mass.**
   2. **Cancer of the renal pelvis**
      a. Most patients with cancer of the renal pelvis present with **hematuria** and **flank pain,** the latter caused by the passage of blood clots through the ureter. Other more generalized symptoms include **fever, weight loss, an elevated erythrocyte sedimentation rate,** and **anemia.**
   3. There are no identified techniques for early detection.

F. **ASSESSMENT**

   1. **Renal cell carcinoma**
      a. **Excretory urograms** and **renal tomography** are considered to be the screening tests of choice for suspected renal mass lesions.
   2. **Cancer of the renal pelvis**
      a. **Excretory urograms, retrograde urogram,** and **urinary cytology** are the most useful techniques for establishing a diagnosis of cancer of the renal pelvis.

G. **CLASSIFICATION AND STAGING**

   1. **Renal cell carcinoma**
      a. **Figure 50-17, text page 1059,** and **Table 50-17, text page 1299,** illustrate two staging systems for renal cell cancer.
   2. **Cancer of the renal pelvis**
      a. The TNM staging system for cancer of the renal pelvis is shown in **Table 50-18, text page 1299.**
   3. **Table 50-19, text page 1302,** shows long-term survival by stage after nephrectomy for renal cell carcinoma.

H. **TREATMENT OF RENAL CELL CARCINOMA**

   1. **Surgery**
      a. Patients with renal cell carcinoma are treated by **radical nephrectomy,** including removal of the lymph nodes in the hilar area.
      b. Various surgical approaches have been used for radical nephrectomy. See **Figure 50-18, text page 1300,** for the boundaries of a left radical nephrectomy.
   2. **Venal cava involvement**
      a. About 5%–9% of persons with renal cell cancer have **tumor thrombus extending into the vena cava,** which is removed in continuity with the tumor to prevent tumor embolization.
   3. **Lymphadenectomy**
      a. Regional lymphadenectomy remains a controversial subject.
      b. Those who favor lymphadenectomy feel that it adds to a more comprehensive and meaningful staging using the TNM system.

    4. **Bilateral tumors or tumors in a solitary kidney**
      a. In bilateral tumors where there is a **larger tumor** in one kidney than in the other, **partial nephrectomy** is performed on the kidney with the smaller tumor, and several weeks later **radical nephrectomy** is carried out on the kidney with the larger tumor.
      b. In cases where there is a tumor in a **solitary** kidney with no evidence of metastasis, partial nephrectomy and radical nephrectomy with subsequent chronic hemodialysis or renal transplantation are treatment alternatives.
    5. **Radiotherapy and chemotherapy**
      a. Renal cell carcinomas and their metastases are usually radioresistant.
      b. Adjuvant chemotherapy has not demonstrated any improvement in survival rates.

I.   **TREATMENT OF ADVANCED RENAL CELL CARCINOMA**

    1. About 30% of persons with renal cell carcinoma present with metastases at diagnosis; this group has a **mean survival rate of 4 months** with only about **10% surviving a year.**
    2. **Palliative nephrectomy** may be justifiable for individuals with disabling symptoms such as local pain and with a life expectancy of greater than 6 months.
    3. **Radiotherapy**
      a. Radiation therapy is an important modality in the **palliation** of patients with metastatic renal cell cancer.
      b. Despite the belief that this is a radio-resistant tumor, effective palliation of metastatic disease to the **bone, brain,** and **lungs** is reported in up to two-thirds of patients.
    4. **Surgery**
      a. **Adjunctive nephrectomy** is done to improve survival, whereas **palliative nephrectomy** is done to relieve symptoms of the primary renal tumor.
    5. **Chemotherapy**
      a. Chemotherapy has little impact on metastatic renal cell carcinoma, although **vinblastine** has shown some success in achieving responses of short duration.
    6. **Hormonal therapy**
      a. The **infrequent responses** to hormonal therapy (rates vary from 2%–15%) have not significantly improved survival.
    7. **Biologic response modifiers**
      a. **Immunotherapy** with **interleukin-2, lymphokine activated killer cells,** and **alpha-interferon** has shown some response in clinical trials with metastatic renal cell cancer. In general, these treatments are complicated, toxic, and expensive.
      b. **Toxicities** include fever, GI bleeding, rash and pruritus, hepatic dysfunction, thrombocytopenia, somnolence, disorientation, and pulmonary edema.

J.   **TREATMENT OF CANCER OF THE RENAL PELVIS**

    1. **Radical nephrectomy,** including the kidney, all perinephric tissue, regional lymph nodes, the ureter, and the periureteral portion of the bladder, is standard treatment for cancer of the renal pelvis.
    2. Radiotherapy has not been proved effective against this tumor, and chemotherapy has been used with only limited results.

K.   **RESULTS AND PROGNOSIS**

    1. Survival rates for patients with renal cell carcinoma are shown in **Table 50-19, text page 1302.**
    2. The overall 5-year survival rates for cancer of the renal pelvis is **40%,** the 5-year survival for persons with differentiated tumors is **60%,** while that for undifferentiated tumors is only **14%.**

L.   **NURSING CARE OF INDIVIDUALS WITH CANCER OF THE KIDNEY**

    1. **Nursing care of individuals undergoing surgery**
      a. The preoperative and postoperative nursing care of the person undergoing a radical nephrectomy is similar to that of the individual undergoing a laparotomy.
      b. It includes **pain relief, prevention of atelectasis and pneumonia, monitoring renal function, watching for paralytic ileus and hemorrhage, wound care, care of any chest tube, and discharge planning.**

2. **Nursing care of individuals receiving chemotherapy**
    a. Although antineoplastic agents have not had a significant effect on kidney cancer, if chemotherapy is used the nurse must be familiar with the agents used and teach potential side effects to the patient and family members.
3. **Nursing care of individuals receiving hormonal therapy**
    a. Progesterone and testosterone agents have been used in hormonal therapy and are generally well tolerated except for mild fluid retention and body weight gain.
4. **Nursing care of individuals receiving biologic response modifiers**
    a. The potential side effects of **biologic response modifiers (BRMs)** used for renal cancer and the nursing care of patients being treated with them are discussed on **text page 1304,** column 1.

V.   **TESTICULAR CANCER**

A.   **EPIDEMIOLOGY**

1. Testicular cancer is an **uncommon cancer,** accounting for only 1%–2% of all cancer in men, although it is the most common solid tumor in men between 29 and 35 years of age.
2. The peak age is **between 20 and 40 years.**
3. There is an association between **higher incidence and higher economic status.**

B.   **ETIOLOGY**

1. Two factors have been associated with an increased incidence of testicular cancer.
    a. Men with **cryptorchidism** (undescended testicle) have a 3-fold to 14-fold risk for testicular cancer.
    b. There is an increased risk of testicular cancer in the male children of women exposed to **exogenous estrogens** (e.g., diethylstilbestrol) during pregnancy.

C.   **PATHOPHYSIOLOGY**

1. **Cellular characteristics**
    a. Cell types are classified in terms of **embryonal tissue.**
    b. A classification system that groups the various histologic types of testicular cancers is found on **text page 1304,** column 2.
    c. The **germinal tumors,** which account for 97% of all testicular cancers, are divided into **seminomas** and **nonseminomas.**
2. **Progression of disease**
    a. Metastases of germinal testicular cancers usually occur either by **direct extension** or through the **lymphatics.**
    b. The tumor may spread by direct extension into the epididymis, spermatic cord, or to the scrotum.
    c. Because of the complicated lymphatic system around the testes, metastasis can occur **while the primary tumor is small.**
    d. Lymphatic spread occurs in a stepwise fashion into the retroperitoneal lymph nodes.
    e. Metastatic spread to the lung, liver, or bone may occur as a late manifestation of disease.

D.   **CLINICAL MANIFESTATIONS**

1. **Painless enlargement of the testicle** is the most common presenting symptom.
2. **Local signs** of testicular cancer include
    a. **A firm, diffuse enlargement.**
    b. **An inability to transilluminate the testis.**
    c. **A lack of pain on palpation.**

E.   **ASSESSMENT**

1. A list of **diagnostic procedures** used for testicular cancer is found on **text page 1065,** column 1.
2. A **high inguinal orchiectomy** with removal of the entire specimen is done for biopsy purposes.
3. **Chest CT scans** are used to detect pulmonary metastases and **abdominal CT scans** are used to determine if retroperitoneal lymph nodes are involved.

4. Two **tumor markers,** alpha-fetoprotein (AFP) and human chorionic gonadotropin (HCG), are useful assessment tools in the following ways:
   a. Detecting whether a germ cell tumor is present.
   b. Determining response to treatment.
   c. Detecting the presence of residual tumor.
   d. Differentiating between seminomas and nonseminomas, thereby aiding in the choice of treatment.

F. CLASSIFICATION AND STAGING

1. Several classification systems are presented in **Table 50-20, text page 1306,** and **Table 50-21, text page 1307.**

G. TREATMENT

1. **Surgery**
   a. A **high radical inguinal orchiectomy** is both a diagnostic tool as well as the first phase of treatment.
   b. Pretreatment **fertility evaluation** should be done for the person who wishes to father a child at a later time. Sperm banking may be possible.
2. **Lymphadenectomy**
   a. **Retroperitoneal lymphadenectomy**
      (1) A **radical retroperitoneal lymphadenectomy** may also be performed as part of the surgical cure. One study reported that over 90% of men who had undergone this procedure had a reduction in or total loss of ejaculatory ability due to damage to nerve supply.
   b. **Modified retroperitoneal lymphadenectomy**
      (1) Modified retroperitoneal lymphadenectomy is a technique that **limits the boundaries of lymph node resection** in those patients determined to be without detectable lymph node metastasis.
      (2) **Advantages** include preservation of ejaculatory ability, fewer complications, and aid in accurate staging of the disease.
3. **Radiotherapy**
   a. **External beam radiotherapy** is directed at lymph node areas in the pelvis and/or chest.
   b. Side effects of radiotherapy are related to the port and dose of irradiation.
4. **Chemotherapy**
   a. The major role of **chemotherapy** in patients with testicular cancer has been in treatment of **disseminated disease,** where it has revolutionized treatment.
   b. Two primary chemotherapy regimens that have been utilized are **PVB** (cisplatin, vinblastine, bleomycin) and **BEP** (bleomycin, VP-16, cisplatin).
   c. Ifosfamide and cisplatin demonstrate a preclinical **synergy.**
   d. The dose-limiting of ifosfamide is hemorrhagic cystitis, which can be managed effectively with mesna.
   e. **Carboplatin,** an analog of cisplatin, is showing promise.
5. **Treatment according to histologic type and stage**
   a. **Seminomas**
      (1) If there is no evidence of metastases and retroperitoneal node involvement is not bulky, **radical orchiectomy followed by radiotherapy** is the primary treatment.
      (2) In case of massive metastases, **preradiation** and **chemotherapy** are commonly used.
   b. **Nonseminomas**
      (1) The most common approach to early-stage nonseminomas is **retroperitoneal lymphadenectomy** and **chemotherapy.**
      (2) Aggressive primary chemotherapy using a **cisplatin-based combination regimen** followed by **lymph node dissection** for any residual disease is generally accepted as standard therapy for late-stage testicular cancer.

H. RESULTS AND PROGNOSIS

1. The advent of tumor markers and sophisticated chemotherapy accounts for the significant improvement in survival of individuals with testicular cancer.

2. Five-year survival rates for **nonseminomas** range from **96%–100%** for early stage disease.
3. Five-year survival rates for **seminomas** range from **98%** in early disease to **71%** for advanced disease.

I. **NURSING CARE OF INDIVIDUALS WITH TESTICULAR CANCER**

1. **Nursing role in early detection**
   a. Nurses should provide information on testicular cancer to young men and instruct them in the important benefits of practicing **testicular self-examination (TSE),** since delay in seeking medical attention accounts for the frequency with which testicular cancer has metastasized by the time it is diagnosed.
2. **Nursing role prior to diagnostic tests and surgery**
   a. Orchiectomy has a tremendous emotional impact on many young men, and the nurse has a responsibility to provide psychological support and teach them the implications of the procedure and subsequent phases of treatment.
3. **Postoperative nursing care**
   a. Perhaps the greatest postoperative complication is **altered body image.**
   b. It is important to assure the man undergoing retroperitoneal lymphadenectomy that his **ability to have an erection and to experience orgasm usually is not permanently impaired by the procedure.**
4. **Nursing care of individuals receiving chemotherapy**
   a. Overall, individuals generally tolerate radiotherapy to the retroperitoneal regions very well. Common side effects include mild nausea and vomiting, diarrhea, myelosuppression, and azoospermia.
   b. The major nursing concern with this type of cancer is to anticipate the **anxiety** these young men will likely experience regarding sexual potency and fertility.
   c. Major side effects of cisplatin are severe nausea and vomiting, ototoxicity, and dose-related nephrotoxicity. See **text page 1311** for further side effects of vinblastine, etopside, and ifosfamide.

PRACTICE QUESTIONS

1. Prostate cancer is the second most common cancer in American men. The highest incidence of prostate cancer is found in
   (A) Asian men.
   (B) black American men.
   (C) Jewish men.
   (D) smokers.

2. Which of the following statements about prostate cancer is true?
   (A) Prostate cancer is usually slow-growing.
   (B) Prostatic tumors are minimally hormone-dependent.
   (C) Screening of asymptomatic males of all ages is effective in early detection of disease.
   (D) Prostate cancer frequently presents with brain metastases.

3. Most cases of prostate cancer are detected
   (A) during self-examination.
   (B) using transrectal ultrasound.
   (C) when abnormally high levels of prostate-specific antigen are found in men age 30–40 years.
   (D) during routine rectal examination.

4. Radical prostatectomy has as a common sequela
   (A) impotence.
   (B) retrograde ejaculation.
   (C) tumor seeding.
   (D) urinary retention.

5. Endocrine manipulation, used to decrease the availability of circulating androgens to prostate tumors, is the primary treatment for advanced prostate cancer. All of the following are methods used to manipulate levels of androgens **except**
   (A) estrogen therapy.
   (B) bilateral orchiectomy.
   (C) radical cystectomy.
   (D) adrenalectomy.

6. Nursing care of the person receiving external radiotherapy for treatment of prostate cancer involves
   (A) care of three-way indwelling urinary catheter with irrigation.
   (B) performing procedures quickly so as to minimize exposure to radiation.
   (C) discussion with the patient and family issues regarding impotence and urinary control.
   (D) instructing the patient in the use of antispasmodics for cystitis.

7. Up to 50% of bladder cancers are thought to be related to
   (A) cigarette smoking.
   (B) alcohol abuse.
   (C) occupational exposure.
   (D) intrauterine exposure to exogenous estrogens.

8. In determining the progression of bladder cancer, the **most** important feature is the
   (A) degree of hematuria present.
   (B) presence of bladder neck obstruction.
   (C) depth of penetration into the bladder wall.
   (D) presence of pain in the suprapubic region.

9. One of the treatments of choice for superficial low-grade bladder cancers is
   (A) radical cystectomy.
   (B) radiation implants.
   (C) laser therapy.
   (D) instillation of single-agent chemotherapy.

10. In women, radical cystectomy includes removal of the
    (A) bladder, urethra, uterus, fallopian tubes, and the anterior wall of the vagina.
    (B) bladder, urethra, and anterior wall of the vagina only.
    (C) bladder and urethra only.
    (D) bladder only.

11. An individual has an ileal conduit placed following cystectomy for advanced bladder cancer. Which of the following would be considered normal?
    (A) a delay of urinary output for 4–5 hours after surgery
    (B) protrusion of the stoma 3 inches above the skin surface
    (C) a stoma dark red in color and slightly edematous
    (D) a small amount of leakage from the appliance

12. If the urine passing from a stoma is cloudy, it may be that
    (A) the patient is dehydrated.
    (B) the stoma was formed from intestinal tissue.
    (C) a leak in the stoma pouch has occurred, allowing air and bacteria to enter a sterile area.
    (D) antispasmodics are indicated.

13. The largest risk group for kidney cancer consists of
    (A) males over the age of 75 years.
    (B) females between the ages of 40 and 50 years.
    (C) females under the age of 30 years.
    (D) males between the ages of 55 and 60 years.

14. In addition to cigarette smoking and occupational exposure, heavy use of which category of drugs has been shown to increase the risk of cancer of the renal pelvis?
    (A) antipsychotics
    (B) non-narcotic analgesics
    (C) narcotics
    (D) hypnotics

15. Standard treatment for renal cell cancer is **most** likely to take the form of
    (A) radiotherapy.
    (B) radical nephrectomy including removal of lymph nodes in the hilar region.
    (C) chemotherapy.
    (D) regional lymphadenectomy.

16. When chemotherapy is used to treat advanced renal cell cancer, it is being used
    (A) in combination with immunotherapy.
    (B) to achieve a response of short duration.
    (C) palliatively, to control symptoms such as pain.
    (D) to shrink tumor burden and allow for effective surgical resection.

17. In determining the survival rate for persons with cancer of the renal pelvis, the **most** important factor seems to be
    (A) the level of tumor differentiation.
    (B) whether or not radiotherapy was used in treatment.
    (C) whether or not the tumor is hormone sensitive.
    (D) the age and physical condition of the patient at diagnosis.

18. One factor that has been associated with an increased incidence of testicular cancer is
    (A) maternal exposure to exogenous estrogens during pregnancy.
    (B) promiscuous sexual behavior.
    (C) narcotic abuse.
    (D) use of anabolic steroids before the age of 20.

19. Metastases are _____ to occur in testicular cancer because _____ .
    (A) likely; both testicular cancer and its metastases are chemotherapy-resistant
    (B) unlikely; most tumors are encapsulated
    (C) likely; the lymphatic network around the testes is complex
    (D) unlikely; it is usually diagnosed early enough to enable swift treatment

20. The **most** common presenting symptom of testicular cancer is
    (A) ureteral obstruction and dysuria.
    (B) painless enlargement of the testicle.
    (C) painful enlargement of the testicle.
    (D) nonproductive cough.

21. CT scans sometimes are used diagnostically in testicular cancer to
    (A) assess distribution of chemotherapeutic agents.
    (B) differentiate between germ cell and non–germ cell tumors.
    (C) determine the extent of lymph node involvement.
    (D) detect liver metastases.

22. A large percentage of men who undergo radical retroperitoneal lymphadenectomy as treatment for testicular cancer experience
    (A) some loss of ejaculatory ability.
    (B) male hormone depletion.
    (C) prolonged pain.
    (D) prolonged bleeding.

23.   A common chemotherapeutic regimen for the treatment of testicular cancer is
      (A)   CMF-cyclophosphamide, methotrexate, 5-FU.
      (B)   PVB-cisplatin, vinblastine, bleomycin.
      (C)   DCP-doxorubicin, cyclophosphamide, cisplatin.
      (D)   MOPP-nitrogen mustard, vincristine, procarbazine, prednisone.

24.   A 5-year survival rate of 98% in early disease is not uncommon in
      (A)   tumors of the renal pelvis.
      (B)   bladder cancer.
      (C)   prostate cancer.
      (D)   germ cell seminomas.

ANSWER EXPLANATIONS

1.   **The answer is (B).**   The highest incidence of prostate cancer in the world is among black Americans. The disease is reportedly less common in African blacks, which indicates that some factor other than genetics is responsible. (1262)

2.   **The answer is (A).**   Most prostatic tumors are slow-growing. Eighty-five percent of prostatic cancers are androgen-dependent, and endocrine manipulation is the mainstay of treatment in advanced prostate cancer. Chemotherapy is felt to be only minimally effective in individuals with hormonally unresponsive tumors. Diagnosis is by rectal examination, but the value of rectal examination in asymptomatic individuals is debatable. Yearly screening rectal examinations are probably unnecessary for men under the age of 50 years. (1264)

3.   **The answer is (D).**   Detection of prostate cancer is most likely to occur during a routine rectal examination. Although measurements of prostate-specific antigen may be useful in monitoring individuals with advanced prostate cancer, its usefulness as a screening tool has yet to be determined. The value of transrectal ultrasound in prostate cancer detection is also questionable. (1264)

4.   **The answer is (A).**   Radical prostatectomy, or the removal of the entire prostate including the prostatic capsule, the seminal vesicles, and a portion of the bladder neck, commonly causes sexual dysfunction, including absence of ejaculation and loss of the ability to achieve an erection. Why impotence occurs, and why 10% of men are still able to achieve an erection after the surgery, is not well understood. (1266–1267)

5.   **The answer is (C).**   Estrogen therapy blocks the release of luteinizing hormone (LH), which stimulates the Leydig cells in the testes to synthesize testosterone. Bilateral orchiectomy is the removal of the testes, which produce 90% of circulating androgens. Adrenalectomy removes the most important secondary source of androgen production, either surgically or through the use of drugs. Cystectomy is not usually indicated in prostate cancer. (1270–1271)

6.   **The answer is (D).**   Cystitis is one the common side effects of external radiotherapy for prostate cancer. Other side effects include proctitis, skin reaction, and radiation syndrome. Cystitis usually occurs during the first 1–3 weeks of treatment, and antispasmodics and analgesics may alleviate some of the symptoms. (1269–1270)

7.   **The answer is (A).**   Recent studies have shown little or no correlation between bladder cancer and alcohol consumption. Similarly, no correlation is felt to exist between bladder cancer and intrauterine estrogen exposure. There are some occupations, among them janitors and cleaners, mechanics, miners, and printers, that place one at higher risk for developing bladder cancer, but by far the strongest correlation is between bladder cancer and cigarette smoking. Since 1956 it has been known that smokers are twice as likely to develop bladder cancer as nonsmokers, with smoking accounting for as much as 50% of all bladder cancer in American men. (1280)

8. **The answer is (C).** Although gross hematuria, bladder neck obstruction, and pain in the suprapubic region can all be clinical manifestations of bladder cancer, the most important indicator of disease progression is the depth of tumor penetration into the bladder wall. (1281)

9. **The answer is (C).** Superficial tumors of the bladder are those that remain in the epithelium and lamina propria. Standard treatment is with transurethral resection (TUR), but because the chance of recurrence is great, adjuvant treatment with combination chemotherapy, hormones, and/or laser beams is not uncommon. Partial cystectomy is indicated for some individuals; radical cystectomy is usually only indicated in high-stage, high-grade tumors. (1283)

10. **The answer is (A).** In women, a radical cystectomy includes the removal of the bladder, urethra, uterus, ovaries, fallopian tubes, and anterior wall of the vagina. In men, the term is synonymous with prostatectomy and includes excision of the bladder with pericystic sac, the attached perineum, the prostate, and seminal vesicles. (1283)

11. **The answer is (C).** A urinary diversion should produce urine from the time of surgery, and flow should be more or less continuous. The stoma should protrude ½–¾ inches above the skin to allow the urine to drain into the aperture of an appliance. Leakage from the appliance is abnormal and could lead to skin breakdown. The stoma itself should be deep pink to dark red in color. (1290)

12. **The answer is (B).** The intestine normally produces mucus, and mucus will almost always be present in diversions using segments of the bowel, causing the urine to appear cloudy. Excessive mucus may clog the urinary appliance outlet, and if this occurs, an appliance with a larger outlet may be used. (1293)

13. **The answer is (D).** The average age of diagnosis in both renal cell cancer and cancer of the renal pelvis is 55–60 years. Both are rare in people under the age of 35 years, but thereafter incidence increases with age. There is a 2:1 male predominance in kidney cancer. (1297–1298)

14. **The answer is (B).** Heavy use of the non-narcotic analgesics aspirin and/or acetaminophen has been shown to increase the risk of cancer of the renal pelvis. Similarly, an association has been made between analgesics and renal cell cancer, but this association has not as yet been substantiated. (1296)

15. **The answer is (B).** The treatment of choice for renal cell cancer is radical nephrectomy, which includes removal of the lymph nodes in the renal hilar area. Regional lymphadenectomy is a controversial procedure, with some experts arguing that the procedure does not improve survival and others feeling that regional lymphadenectomy in combination with radical nephrectomy is potentially curative in some individuals. Renal cell carcinomas and their metastases are usually radioresistant, making radiotherapy an unlikely choice, and adjuvant chemotherapy has not demonstrated much effectiveness against the disease. (1298–1299)

16. **The answer is (B).** Approximately 50% of individuals who develop metastases after radical nephrectomy have an extremely poor prognosis. These individuals, considered to have advanced renal cell carcinoma, may be treated with chemotherapy, which has demonstrated some success in achieving tumor responses, but the response is usually short-lived and the toxicity may be significant. (1301)

17. **The answer is (A).** The overall prognosis for cancer of the renal pelvis is poor, with 5-year survival rates of only approximately 40%. This figure becomes 60% if the carcinoma is well differentiated, and drops to 14% if the carcinoma is undifferentiated. (1302)

18. **The answer is (A).** Two factors have been associated with an increased incidence of testicular cancer: cryptorchidism and maternal exposure to exogenous estrogens during pregnancy, either as birth control agents or as diethylstilbestrol (DES). One researcher has postulated that the abnormal primitive germ cells giving arise to a neoplastic cell line stem from an initial carcinogenic event occurring in utero in response to free estrogen. (1304)

19. **The answer is (C).** Metastases are common with testicular cancer, even while the tumor is quite small, because of the complicated lymphatic network that surrounds the testes. Germ cell tumors, accounting for 97% of all testicular cancers, always spread lymphatically before they spread by direct extension. (1305)

20.   **The answer is (B).**   Painless enlargement of the testicle, often discovered accidentally, is the most common presenting symptom of testicular cancer. Sometimes a sensation described as "heaviness" in the scrotum is what brings attention to the tumor's presence. At other times, trauma, although not an etiological factor, brings to light an already existent condition. (1305)

21.   **The answer is (C).**   Either a CT scan of the abdomen or a lymphangiogram is performed diagnostically in testicular cancer to detect retroperitoneal nodes. These procedures help to assess response to treatment as well as determine the need for retroperitoneal lymphadenectomy. Chest CT may also be performed to detect the presence of pulmonary metastases. (1305–1306)

22.   **The answer is (A).**   Because retroperitoneal lymphadenectomy involves the removal of many of the autonomic nerves necessary for ejaculation and erection, 90% of men who have undergone this procedure have a reduction in or total loss of ejaculate. (1307)

23.   **The answer is (B).**   Patients with testicular cancer have been treated with PVB since 1974. As many as 70% of the individuals treated with this protocol achieve long-term survivor status, with a relapse rate of only 10%. (1309)

24.   **The answer is (D).**   For men with seminomatous testicular cancer that is confined to the testicle (stage A) and treated with radiotherapy, the reported 5-year survival rates are 98%. (1309)

51   Development of Cancer Programs and Services

STUDY OUTLINE

I.   INTRODUCTION

1. The explosion of **technology** in cancer treatment, the **economic constraints** imposed by payers, and the growing **sophistication of consumers** have coalesced to form an unprecedented impetus for integrating cancer care programs.
2. Most consumers are unwilling to accept fragmented care and are seeking **full-service centers** recognized for excellence in cancer care in their communities.

A.   SCOPE OF CANCER PROGRAMS IN THE UNITED STATES

1. The American Hospital Association's (AHA) Division of Ambulatory Care and Health Promotion conducted a **survey** of 1779 hospitals.
   a. Of the hospitals surveyed, 32% had **outpatient oncology services.**
   b. Fifty percent intended to expand oncology programs in the next 2 years.

B.   THE NURSE'S ROLE IN PROGRAM DEVELOPMENT

1. The nurse, as a cancer patient advocate, is in an excellent position to **influence administrators** to provide a full range of services to patients.
2. The nurse chosen for a **development role** generally has well-established relationships with pivotal physicians who can form vital coalitions of health care providers.
3. Every nurse who works in a setting where cancer program development and implementation are in progress can have a positive impact.

C.   MOTIVATIONS FOR DEVELOPING CANCER SERVICES

1. Typical motivations for developing a cancer program can be found in **Table 51-1, text page 1321.** They include
   a. Meeting a community need.
   b. Creating a service niche.
   c. Positively impacting financial success.
   d. Ensuring continuity of care.
   e. Integrating quality, cost containment, and databases.

D.   DEFINING A CANCER PROGRAM

1. The NCI restricts the use of the term **NCI-designated cancer center** to those centers that have been awarded funding through a core grant award and meet eight major criteria.
2. Each Community Clinical Oncology Program (CCOP) is required to enter a certain number of patients annually into clinical treatment and cancer control trials.
   a. Many community cancer programs choose to make their NCI affiliation part of their **marketing strategy.**

3. Many facilities without NCI designation have chosen titles to distinguish themselves in their geographic areas.
   a. In this chapter, the terms **cancer centers** and **cancer programs** are used interchangeably and are defined as hospital-based integrated cancer programs that offer the three major treatment modalities, diagnostic and screening services, in- and outpatient treatment units, and clinical research trial opportunities.

II. PROGRAM DEVELOPMENT

1. It may seem that **bringing together** all the varied components into an integrated cancer center is at worst impossible or at best an arduous task.
2. **Leadership,** the ability to motivate individuals and groups to work for a greater good for the organization and ultimately the patients, is a necessity.
   a. The leadership team that has **experience** in the health care community, knows the **stakeholders,** has the ear of the **top executives,** and can **envision** the future of health care delivery will be successful in planning for a comprehensive program.
   b. The team that can address the need to provide both **quality clinical care** outcomes and **cost-effective care** will succeed in implementing a program and maintaining its viability and growth.

A. STRATEGIC PLANNING

1. The process of developing a strategic plan requires the planners to assess the fundamental variables of **knowing the target, appreciating the organization's mission,** and **taking political factors into consideration.**
2. **Strategic planning** is the process used to determine and evaluate alternatives for an organization to achieve its mission and objectives.
   a. **Planning process—the mission**
      (1) The planning process can be divided into three phases:
          (a) **Clarify values and aspirations.**
          (b) **Analyze information.**
          (c) **Develop a strategy to create the image.**
      (2) The central focus of a strategic plan relies on **shared values.**
      (3) The strategic plan will be based on the few critical phrases of the mission statement.
      (4) The next stage is to identify what service lines will be the cornerstones of future development.
   b. **Planning process—data analysis**
      (1) Identifying who will be involved in the planning process and who will serve as interim and final **decision makers** is imperative.
      (2) One well-utilized framework for data gathering is the SWOT analysis to identify **Strengths, Weaknesses, Opportunities,** and **Threats.** In general, an **internal assessment** results in a list of strengths and weaknesses, while the **external assessment** results in a list of opportunities and threats.
      (3) Internal assessment data for an oncology program include an **evaluation of present services, human resources, current physician strengths and weaknesses,** and **the physical facilities.**
      (4) A careful evaluation must be conducted with the **financial department** regarding present workload, payer mix, cost, charges, and revenue for oncology care.
      (5) An assessment of the **present cancer market** in the service area, demographics, the number of patients, where they are treated, and by whom.
      (6) **Projections** for future workload and revenue are as difficult to develop as they are imperative.
   c. **Planning process—the strategic plan**
      (1) The list of potential plans requires careful prioritization.
      (2) See **text page 1323,** column 2 for an example of a list of major issues.
          (a) For each issue, develop a **philosophical statement** and **long-range goals.**

  (3) The strategic plan is then **presented to the focus groups** who provided initial input, to the hospital administration, to the medical executive committee, and, finally, to the board of trustees for approval.

  (4) To realize the strategic goal, specific programs may be developed. These specific plans are called **business plans.**

  (5) The strategic planning process itself can enable the oncology service to see itself as a **united group** that will work together to implement its plans.

 d. **Planning process—the business plan**

  (1) After a list of potential business plans has been developed from the strategic plan's goals, it is wise to establish a small **working group** to design very specific business plans.

  (2) Most hospitals have **criteria** for the development and approval of new plans.

  (3) A similar but more focused assessment of internal and external environments is required to identify market share.

  (4) Part of a business plan's report should be quality related and part should be financially based.

   (a) **Financial indices** are most easily tracked if a new cost and revenue center is established at the time a new program is established.

   (b) If the new service becomes part of an existing cost center, responsibility for financial indices should be established early.

B. ORGANIZATIONAL STRUCTURES AND OPTIONS

1. External pressures have forced nurses and administrators to view care from the **client's perspective** and not merely from that of the health care provider's perspective or convenience.

 a. This systemwide focus has led to new approaches to managing care.

 b. **Critical pathways** are a method of ensuring timely care and a tool for viewing a total health care experience from emergency room to discharge.

2. Insurers who offer managed care policies are now seeking centers of excellence consisting of inpatient and ambulatory services for their clients.

3. Options for integrating oncology services include

 a. **Product line management (PLM).**

 b. Staff model.

 c. Line model.

4. See **Figures 51-3, 51-4, and 51-5, text pages 1326–1328,** for illustration of three optional structures.

C. MANAGEMENT PERSONNEL

1. The success of an oncology program depends on the ability of leaders to envision the future and to be prepared to meet changing needs quickly.

2. **Administrative director**

 a. **Table 51-3, text page 1328,** lists typical duties of an administrative director such as marketing, education, and program planning.

3. **Medical director**

 a. In general, the medical director of a cancer program is the **liaison** between physicians and administration, overseeing quality, research, education, and new programs.

 b. In facilities where service line management does not include direct reporting relationships of nursing units or other oncology departments, it helps to develop an **executive committee** structure that includes the directors of nursing, radiation therapy, and others.

D. STANDARDS FOR MANAGEMENT

1. Resources for defining quality and program development include

 a. **JCAHO. See Table 51-5, text page 1329.**

 b. The **Association of Community Cancer Centers (ACCC).**

 c. The **Oncology Nursing Society.**

 d. The **American College of Surgeons' Commission on Cancer.**

III.   **COMPONENTS OF A CANCER PROGRAM**

    1.   See **Table 51-6, text pages 1330–1331,** for some of the hundreds of components program designers may consider.

A. **INPATIENT ONCOLOGY UNITS**

    1.   In a recent survey of 398 cancer programs, **39% had dedicated medical oncology units** and **33% combined medical and surgical oncology units.**

    2.   If the average **daily census** of oncology patients approaches 20, the argument to establish a dedicated nursing unit is strong.
        a.   By centralizing patients, nursing and support staff who prefer to care for cancer patients can be recruited.
        b.   Daily experience with oncologic nursing problems increases the potential for expert nursing assessment and intervention.

    3.   In designing an oncology inpatient unit, Goldsmith's prediction that **inpatient hospital use will decline** by 20%–30% over the next 10 years should be taken into account.

    4.   Creating an **ICU** within an oncology unit or transforming an ICU into an oncology ICU is widely debated.

    5.   The decision to develop a **bone marrow transplant** program is major in terms of volume, expertise, equipment, and facilities.

B. **AMBULATORY CLINICS**

    1.   Oncology care, like health care in general, is **shifting** to the outpatient arena due to technological changes, cost constraints, and quality issues.

    2.   The strategic decision to develop or expand outpatient oncology services hinges heavily on the needs of the practicing **physicians.**
        a.   **Physician payment** has caused many physicians to attempt to capture a larger share of ambulatory care within their offices.

    3.   See **Table 51-6, text pages 1330–1331,** for the scope of ambulatory services for cancer care.

    4.   Ambulatory settings should be physically situated so they are easily accessible to cancer patients.

    5.   The challenges of ambulatory care also include the future of **reimbursement** and our ability to prepare patients and families for self-care.

    6.   See **Chapter 54** for an exploration of a variety of ambulatory settings, including
        a.   The **24-hour clinic,** where patients can receive routine treatment or seek urgent care at a time most convenient to them, is gaining popularity.
        b.   The **day hospital clinic** offers similar services during expanded hours, but **not** 24 hours a day.
        c.   Some centers have patient volume that supports the development of **site-specific, symptom management,** and/or **pain management clinics** that may be nurse-managed with physician back-up or physician-run.
        d.   Outpatient rehabilitation services are available in most hospitals, but few have developed oncology-specific **outpatient rehabilitation centers** to provide exercise classes, support groups, and nutritional counseling in addition to physical, occupational, and vocational therapies.

    7.   Breast health centers have developed in many centers as a way to provide "one-stop shopping" for patients and clients.

C. **RADIATION THERAPY**

    1.   More than the other treatment modalities, radiation therapy requires a major commitment in terms of **equipment** and **facilities.**

    2.   The capital investment can prove profitable if a need for services exists.
        a.   A rule of thumb widely circulated purports that a volume of 20–25 patients per day will result in at least a break-even business venture.

    3.   **Staffing** a radiation department has become more problematic over the last few years since there are shortages of radiation technologists, physicists, and dosimetrists.

    4.   Many programs include department-based computerized tomography machines to aid in treatment planning and high-dose afterloading brachytherapy (HDR) equipment.

D. **SURGERY**

    1. Nearly every cancer patient will undergo surgery during the course of the disease.
        a. Future improvements in surgical success will relate more to the technical ability of the surgeon to locate and remove tumor growth than to equipment or technology breakthroughs.
    2. The cancer program administrator wishing to enhance surgical treatment looks to recruiting and retaining skilled **specialists.**
        a. In a study by Munoz et al. of 2627 elective surgical oncologic admissions, low-volume surgeons utilized greater hospital resources and had a greater patient mortality than did high-volume surgeons.
        b. The development of surgical expertise is part of the overall strategic plan.
        c. Goldsmith estimates that by the year 2002, ambulatory surgery will account for 85% of all surgery.

E. **DIAGNOSTICS**

    1. Predictions are that the revolution in health care during the next 15 years will originate in the clinical **laboratory** and the **pharmacy.**
        a. All health care managers should, however, be prepared to rethink health care in terms of predictive tools, genetic counseling, and risk reduction classes in lieu of the present acute care model.
    2. **Basics** for a cancer program include **excellent pathologists, timely turnaround for routine blood work,** and **cytology on minute products** (e.g., fine-needle aspirates).
        a. Reimbursement for these and other procedures is changing rapidly.
    3. With the exception of radiation therapy, imaging technology is the most **expensive** equipment-related component of oncology care.

F. **PHYSICIANS**

    1. It is imperative for a hospital wishing to excel in cancer care to have a cadre of oncology physicians who are board-certified clinical experts with good interpersonal relations skills involved in priority setting and program development.
    2. **Consumers** are accepting more responsibility for decisions regarding their care and frequently have an impact upon which facility and physician will be involved in their care.
    3. The recruitment of oncology surgeons must be weighed against the **potential** of negatively impacting a group of general surgeons, particularly in a smaller community or facility.

G. **AMERICAN COLLEGE OF SURGEONS ACCREDITATION**

    1. More than 70% of patients newly diagnosed with cancer receive their initial care at an institution that is accredited by the **American College of Surgeons' (ACOS) Commission on Cancer;** 1200 hospitals are accredited nationally.
        a. See **text page 1334,** column 1, for ACOS requirements.
    2. Building a cancer program around ACOS accreditation criteria will urge employed staff and physicians to **interact** for the good of the overall program.
    3. The **tumor registry** is a cornerstone of the broad oncology database necessary for an integrated cancer program.
        a. Because the registry is entirely overhead expense, it requires administrative support and frequently does not receive the attention it deserves for staffing and computerization.

H. **SUPPORT SERVICES**

    1. The decision to include specific services and the staffing required for each is dependent on the volume of patients served and the mission of the organization, but there are some basic services that are necessary.
        a. Ideally, support services are provided by team members who have special education in oncology and devote **100%** of their time to oncology, but that is not always practical for a small program.

b. The reasons for developing a designated oncology nursing unit apply to each team member as well: **Experience leads to expertise, continuing education is focused, team collaboration is enhanced,** and **improved-quality patient care results.**

2. A **patient education department** is in the best position to manage a resource center where patients and others can seek information on an as-needed basis.

3. **Support groups** and **wellness groups** are other services that can be offered regardless of size or complexity of the cancer program.

    a. Support programs for **cancer survivors** help clients become maximally functional again.

4. The list of **additional support services** to benefit patients and distinguish a program is limited only by imagination.

I. HOME CARE AND HOSPICE SERVICES

1. As cancer treatment has advanced and cost containment has become an everyday fact of life, the need for **home care** and **hospice services** has exploded.

2. The question for the hospital-based cancer team is not whether home care and hospice programs are required but whether the **hospital** chooses to provide the service itself.

    a. The **strategic plan** should spell out this choice based on patient need, existing programs, and existing resources.

3. The advantages to developing in-house programs are **continuity of care** and a **broad philosophical base in holistic care.**

J. REHABILITATION SERVICES

1. An oncology program or cancer center can develop a team of **oncology-focused rehabilitation specialists.**

2. **Chapter 53** contains a thorough review of cancer rehabilitation.

K. RESEARCH

1. The **purpose** of cancer research is to improve the survival and quality of life of cancer patients by providing care and documenting it so that others will benefit from our experience.

2. Many agree that until we can consistently cure cancer we must conduct **prospective** randomized clinical trials of treatment options to determine efficacy.

3. The humanitarian reason for participating in clinical trials is obvious but Borzo identifies additional advantages:

    a. **Increased patient referral.**

    b. **Marketing opportunities.**

    c. **Early access to advanced treatment.**

    d. **Facilitation of staff recruitment and retention.**

    e. **Program prestige.**

4. Clinical research can be conducted through **cooperative groups,** the Community Clinical Oncology Program, pharmaceutical companies, and other agencies such as the American Cancer Society (ACS).

5. A **community hospital** that provides the opportunity for patients to be entered into clinical trials must be prepared to develop an infrastructure to oversee the process.

6. Small facilities and programs can accommodate cooperative clinical trials if they commit to providing the diagnostic imaging and laboratory procedures necessary and the personnel to manage the protocols and data.

L. ONCOLOGY DATABASE

1. Many software packages exist for capturing data to meet **strategic requirements.**

2. **Insurers' requirements,** particularly those of prospective payment insurers, have resulted in the proliferation of **financial software packages** that generally report patient charges by admission.

3. Clinical trial reporting requirements focus on the process and outcome of a particular treatment.

4. Developing the linkages between data sets can require expensive programming time and frequently does not match organizationwide data processing priorities.

M. **PROFESSIONAL EDUCATION**

1. Providing professional education programs can meet a variety of goals for a hospital-based cancer center.
    a. Such education **increases** the skills and knowledge of the program's physicians and staff and optimally leads to a better quality of day-to-day care.
2. The oncology team can develop a **menu of basic classes,** such as radiology, financial counseling, and housekeeping, to be offered to departments who care for cancer patients.
3. **Regional conferences** or outreach education programs establish the center as a referral center for a geographic area.

N. **COMMUNITY EDUCATION**

1. The purposes of health education are to provide the public with **health information** and to inspire them to **adopt** new health practices.
2. **Community education** strategies are wide-ranging and should be linked to the target population and goals.
3. **Families** of cancer patients are another population that is eager for health promotion and cancer prevention information.
4. **Mass media** offer a different level of community education.
    a. The disadvantage to the use of mass media is the lack of a target audience and the lack of control over the timing of message delivery.
5. The degree to which public education can be emphasized is dependent on the program goals and resources.

O. **SCREENING PROGRAMS**

1. Screening programs offer an added benefit because they actually **engage** clients in a positive behavior that results in new knowledge about their health.
2. A broad scope of programs exists for developing cancer programs.
    a. Many local units of the ACS assist in screening programs at many facilities by offering group advertising and aggregate results.
3. The facility choosing to participate in mass screenings should carefully evaluate the medical evidence supporting the efficacy of screening, their ability to follow up with individuals regarding results, and their moral obligation to provide continuing care if disease is detected.
4. Mobile vans equipped to provide cancer screening can now provide this service at work sites, shopping centers, and health fairs.

IV. **MAINTAINING PROGRAM PROMINENCE**

A. **ONGOING EVALUATION AND REPRIORITIZATION**

1. The director(s) is responsible for establishing **monitoring criteria** and ensuring that data are collected.
    a. A small executive team periodically (usually quarterly) analyzes the results of the data and revises the course of action as necessary.
2. **Quality evaluation**
    a. Integrated cancer programs have an excellent opportunity to be the leaders in their facilities to establish system-oriented quality improvement.
        (1) The active involvement of **physicians** is integral to successful quality improvement, and the cancer team's medical director can play a major role.
    b. It is ideal to have **one** quality manager responsible for assisting the oncology team and its components to develop and monitor their quality improvement strategies.
    c. The quality of programs is **judged** differently by different audiences.
        (1) The organized oncology program also has the opportunity to conduct **patient satisfaction** surveys that relate to the entire system that has an impact on the patient, not just one department or service.
    d. The results of the cancer program's evaluation should be reported not only to the oncology team but **also** to the cancer committee and general hospital administration.

3. **Financial evaluation**
    a. The cancer program's strategic plan sets overall goals for **volume** and **income growth.**
        (1) Individual departments and services will have similar growth projections or goals.
        (2) One method for ensuring support for nonreimbursable services is to ensure that aggregated oncology revenue and expenses are **reported.**
    b. Outpatient data, especially comparable outpatient data, are much more **difficult** to determine in most facilities.
    c. An integrated information system should be able to identify that a patient having an outpatient procedure is part of the cancer service line.
        (1) Only by **combining** inpatient and outpatient data for an individual patient can actual resource consumption be measured and the actual profitability of the service line be judged.
    d. Each cancer center will choose the data most important to its particular program. See **Figure 51-6, text page 1340,** for a sample annual tracking form.
    e. A grand **total** for all oncology care revenue in excess of cost is probably the critical figure that will allow for future program development or will necessitate that the program determine what services are to be eliminated.
    f. **Plotting volume growth** and **income** for oncology services can be enlightening. See **Figure 51-7, text page 1341,** for an example in which, in a hypothetical hospital, support group volume is growing but contributes negatively to the overall income, while surgical oncology admissions are growing slightly in volume and are profitable.
        (1) A high-growth, low-income service may cause the oncology management to **rethink their commitment** to research, **identify new funding sources, concentrate on cost-cutting measures,** or **consider an increase in prices for other services to support research.**
4. **Shifts in reimbursement**
    a. **Changes** in payer mix and revenue from specific payers can have a significant impact on a program's strategy.
        (1) The prudent oncology manager is well versed in upcoming legislation and **local market shifts** so quick action can be taken.
    b. A cancer program's database, again, can assist it in preparing to negotiate with managed and contracted care.
5. **Demographic shifts**
    a. In addition to focusing the annual review of the strategic plan on internal strengths and weaknesses, it is also wise to evaluate shifts in the **service area's demographics.**
6. **Changes in technology**
    a. The more dynamic the oncology program team is, the more innovations they will be eager to implement.
        (1) Most programs are not in a position of unlimited resources, either human or financial, and must make difficult and careful choices.
    b. **Table 51-7, text page 1341,** describes a process of **evaluating new technology** that has five basic steps:
        (1) Determining decision makers.
        (2) Oncology team evaluation.
        (3) Oncology team recommendations.
        (4) Business planning.
        (5) Organizational approval.
    c. It is advantageous to **build consensus** among the oncology stakeholders before organizational approval is sought.
    d. Before the financial analysis is undertaken, the oncology leadership should have evaluated its scientific merit, fit with the strategic plan, resources required, and relative benefit.

B. **PHYSICAL FACILITIES**

1. Perhaps the **biggest undertaking** for any oncology program is the development of new facilities or the renovation of existing facilities.
    a. The decision to develop or renovate is based on the need for new space to meet **projected volume of patients, new technology being introduced,** or the **need to consolidate present services in contiguous space.**

2. **Small work groups** are established to work with the architects to perform functional analysis and help design the structure.
3. A **matrix** is frequently used to determine how closely adjacent new departments must be to each other and to existing departments within the facility.
4. It is important to not become so mired in space details that systems planning is neglected.

C. **MARKETING**

1. Developing a **marketing strategy** and planning specific activities are increasingly important in this time of escalating health care competition.
2. Gilden points out that "cancer care marketing requires scrupulous sensitivity to even implied promise of the one real sought-after benefit from cancer care—cure for the disease."
3. Developing the marketing plan is a four-step process:
   a. **Conduct an internal and external assessment annually.**
   b. **Define the products and marketing objectives.**
   c. **Identify target audiences.**
   d. **Plan specific activities to implement strategy.**
4. Most facilities have some kind of marketing or community relations department staffed by professionals who can guide clinicians in developing and implementing plans.
5. **Table 51-9, text page 1343,** lists examples of marketing activities for specific target audiences.

D. **SATELLITES AND MANAGEMENT CONTRACTS**

1. Depending on size and sophistication, a cancer program may look for a large center with which to **affiliate** or may develop a network of smaller referring facilities.
   a. Affiliations positively impact the image of a smaller facility.
   b. Affiliations make new research protocols or treatment plans available.
   c. Affiliations allow attendance at educational programs.
   d. Affiliations provide consultation at a reduced rate.
   e. Affiliations create confidence that patients referred for specialized treatment will be returned to the referring physician.
2. Due to physical constraints or shifting demographics, opening **satellite treatment facilities** may meet a program's strategic goals.
3. Another option for expansion is to **offer management services** to smaller community hospitals.
4. The decision to expand should be based on sound strategic and financial **planning.**

PRACTICE QUESTIONS

1. Fifty percent of hospitals surveyed by the American Hospital Association plan to expand their oncology programs. The **most** likely reason for expansion is
   (A) governmental mandates.
   (B) increased reimbursement for outpatient procedures.
   (C) the unwillingness of consumers to travel long distances for care.
   (D) a desire to distinguish a hospital's services from competitors.

2. Because oncology is not considered one of the highest-ranking service lines from a financial perspective, which of the following is the **most** likely reason for oncology program expansion?
   (A) Expansion into outpatient cancer services helps maintain market share as care shifts to the ambulatory setting.
   (B) It helps the hospital provide quality care.
   (C) It assists in retaining primary care physicians.
   (D) Prospective payment systems require full-care facilities.

3. The ultimate objective of strategic planning is to
   (A) develop a clear picture of the hospital's mission.
   (B) determine and evaluate alternatives for an organization.
   (C) cultivate collegiality among physician groups.
   (D) analyze the productivity and outcomes of the previous year.

4. The **most** important benefit of product line management or service line management is that
    (A) outcome indicators are established for tracking the patient's outcome through the spectrum of health care interventions.
    (B) critical pathways are in place for reimbursement purposes.
    (C) a team of administrators or the executive committee is responsible for the day-to-day management of the hospital.
    (D) one individual is responsible for developing, maintaining, and ensuring the quality and financial viability of a group of patients.

5. Centralizing patients onto an oncology floor results in the ability to recruit nursing and support staff who prefer to care for patients with cancer. An additional benefit of a consistent nursing staff is
    (A) decreased overtime needs.
    (B) decreased turnover rate.
    (C) increased potential for expert nursing assessment and intervention.
    (D) decreased overall expenses.

6. In a cancer program, the treatment modality requiring the **largest** commitment in terms of equipment and facilities is
    (A) radiation therapy.
    (B) simulation.
    (C) inpatient surgery.
    (D) outpatient surgery.

7. Which of the following educational formats has the **least** control over the target audience?
    (A) public service announcement
    (B) regional conference
    (C) support group
    (D) educational resource center

ANSWER EXPLANATIONS

1. **The answer is (D).**   Most consumers are unwilling to accept fragmented care that causes them to traverse the country or even their communities to access the complex services they require. Consumers are seeking full-service centers recognized for excellence in cancer care in their communities. But health care facilities are now faced with declining bottom lines from prospective payment systems and a desire to capture the ever-increasing ambulatory-based care market. Oncology physicians want major cancer treatment facilities to be available where they practice as well. In addition, today's emphasis has shifted to development of well-integrated, full-service, highly technical cancer care programs of high quality that distinguish one hospital's services from its competitors. (1320–1321)

2. **The answer is (A).**   The utilization of outpatient services for cancer care is high. Even if oncology inpatient care is at the break-even level, expansion of outpatient cancer care services will help maintain market share as care shifts to the ambulatory setting. Also, the hospital that can provide a broad range of services and a solid base of referring primary care physicians will have less difficulty recruiting oncology specialists. (1321)

3. **The answer is (B).**   Strategic planning is the process used to determine and evaluate alternatives for an organization to achieve its mission and objectives. A clear picture of the hospital's mission needs to be understood prior to developing the plan in order to prioritize major initiatives set out in the plan and for future decision making. The process includes data analysis and financial analysis of present services in order to determine assets and drains on the hospital. A positive outcome of the process is an opportunity for groups from divergent oncology departments to become a multidisciplinary team and to see itself as a united group. (1322–1324)

4. **The answer is (D).**   One sweeping definition of PLM or SLM states that one single administrator is responsible for strategy formation, coordination of resources, monitoring of production and marketing, budgeting, and measuring results for each product line within the hospital. It requires that one individual be responsible for developing, maintaining, and ensuring the quality and financial viability of a group of patients. Critical pathways and outcome indicators assist in tracking patients' courses through the hospital system, which facilitates reimbursement and means of evaluation for continuous quality improvement. (1325–1326)

5. **The answer is (C).**   A dedicated unit enables cancer team members to interact with each other continuously; therefore, they can appreciate the skills of each team member and use them appropriately. Daily experience with oncologic nursing problems increases the potential for expert nursing assessment and intervention. (1329)

6. **The answer is (A).**   External beam radiation requires a minimum of 4000 square feet of partially lead-shielded space. Equipment, including a linear accelerator, simulator, and computerized treatment planning systems, can cost $1.0–$1.5 million. (1332)

7. **The answer is (A).**   The disadvantage to the use of mass media is the lack of a target audience and the lack of control over the timing of message delivery. The other educational formats are structured so that specific information is relayed to specific audiences. Learners choose to attend and/or participate because they have reviewed what information will be presented and who would benefit from the information and format. (1335, 1337–1338)

52   Continuity of Care

STUDY OUTLINE

I. INTRODUCTION

1. This chapter discusses the concept of continuity of care, care setting alternatives and issues, selecting and recommending settings, and the transition from hospital to the community.

II. CONTINUITY OF CARE—AN OVERVIEW

A. DEFINITION

1. Continuity of care implies a **standard of care in which there is planned coordination of care that results in improved outcomes for the patient, irrespective of care setting or provider.** It is distinct from **discharge planning,** the process of preparing the patient for transfer from one system and entry into the next phase of care.
2. Several social and health care factors have stimulated increased emphasis on the concept of continuity of care, including
   a. The **implementation of DRGs,** resulting in restricted use of acute care settings and reliance on alternative care systems.
   b. **Shortened hospital stays, combined with complex "high-tech" care,** resulting in patients and their families assuming a greater share of care responsibility at home.
   c. The **evolution of cancer care delivered in multiple health care settings** (e.g., diagnostic clinics, ambulatory care centers, hospices, home care), resulting in patient care that is less linear and more a trajectory with multiple transitions between systems.
3. Studies have documented benefits of continuity of care that include
   a. Decreased hospital stays.
   b. Fewer hospital admissions.
   c. Increased patient satisfaction.
4. **Figure 52-1, text page 1348,** presents a model of continuity of care that illustrates the continuing needs of the patient during the care experience.

B. PRINCIPLES UNDERLYING EFFECTIVE CONTINUITY OF CARE

1. See **Table 52-1, text page 1348,** for a list of major characteristics of continuity of care. This table can be used as a checklist by nurse managers or clinicians to evaluate their own settings.
2. The standards used in continuity of care emphasize an interdisciplinary approach and identify patient needs to include such issues as **comfort, coping, mobility,** and **elimination.**

C. SPECIFIC CONCERNS RELATED TO THE PERSON WITH CANCER

1. **The complex physical and psychologic needs of the cancer patient, along with the wide range of types of therapies and health care providers, make continuity of care an essential element in achieving quality of care.**
2. Elderly cancer patients have special needs for continuity of care. Coupled with the burdens of a cancer diagnosis are the factors associated with aging, including **decreased social supports, diminished financial resources,** and **multiple medical problems.**
3. The oncology nursing profession must evaluate current systems and devise strategies for enhancing continuity of care. This is best accomplished through

    a.   Careful evaluation of the specific settings used by cancer patients.

    b.   Planning of the transition from the acute care hospital to these settings.

III. **CARE SETTING ALTERNATIVES AND ISSUES: FROM HOSPITAL TO COMMUNITY**

  A. **HOSPITAL TO HOSPITAL**

    1. **Written care instructions** are essential between hospital settings but are particularly important when the patient will continue to receive acute care and complex treatments.

    2. **Verbal communication among nurses** is an effective avenue for exchanging information about the patient.

  B. **NURSING HOME OR SKILLED NURSING FACILITY**

    1. **Nursing homes** care for a dynamic population of patients constantly in transition between settings, including home, hospitals, and other long-term care institutions.

    2. Limitations to continuity of care in these settings include

      a. **Reliance on a predominantly nonprofessional staff of nursing assistants and medication aids.**

        (1) Certain patients, especially those requiring aggressive management of pain or continuous parenteral infusions, may receive inadequate care.

        (2) Oncology nurses from the acute care hospital can help by offering education programs related to cancer care.

      b. Inadequate documentation in the medical record.

        (1) Patients in this setting are often unable to provide this information because of communication deficits, dementia, or poor memory.

        (2) Adverse drug reactions and inappropriate prescriptions have been associated with inaccurate diagnosis and poor medical records.

    3. Knowledge of those nursing homes in the community that provide excellent care is valuable.

    4. In addition to the basic nursing plan, other specific information may be needed on transfer to a nursing home, including **mental status information, last medication administration, functional status, specific nutritional needs,** and **skin condition.**

  C. **HOSPICE**

    1. Two important issues that relate to the transition from acute care to the **hospice setting** are

      a. **The psychologic impact on the patient and family.**

        (1) Patients and families may be facing the reality of terminal illness for the first time.

      b. **The need for continuous symptom control.**

        (1) The burden of providing symptom control shifts to the family.

  D. **AMBULATORY CARE**

    1. The major issues in continuity of care in the **ambulatory care setting** are

      a. **Teaching patients and families self-care measures.**

      b. **Preparing patients to detect an adverse reaction early enough to avoid serious sequelae or hospitalization.**

    2. Patients who receive adequate education are more capable of self-care activities.

  E. **HOME CARE**

    1. The major issues in continuity of care in the **home setting** are

      a. **Management of cancer pain and other symptoms.**

        (1) Families member tend to undermedicate because of their fears of drug addiction and respiratory depression and their general misunderstanding of pain relief.

        (2) Some home care agencies are not skilled in the special needs of cancer patients.

      b. **The effects of home care on the physical and psychologic health of surviving family members.**

        (1) Home health care is often immensely burdensome on family members.

c. Research suggests that while family members want to care for the dying patient at home, the experience may have deleterious effects on the physical and psychological health of surviving family members.

d. The family caregiving experience can be supported and patient and family quality of life enhanced through **accurate assessment of the family** prior to implementing home care, **management of symptoms,** assessment of **psychological needs** and moods, provision of **continuity of care,** and **appropriate use of technology** in the home care setting.

e. **The increase in "high-tech" home care of oncology patients,** including such procedures as tube feedings, epidural catheters, intravenous transfusions, or blood transfusions.

   (1) Family members must learn special skills to provide care when the patient goes home.

F.   REHABILITATION FACILITY

1. Both **skilled nursing facilities** and **rehabilitation settings** are designed as interim care facilities to help in the patient's transition from acute care to home or alternate care. Patients need time and skills to adjust to the deficits or changes they have incurred.

2. Rehabilitation includes both the traditional areas of **physical rehabilitation and mobility** and **psychological and social recovery** (e.g., return to work, recovery from mastectomy). In the transition to the rehabilitation setting, it is important to communicate information regarding the patient's psychological status and social concerns.

G.   THE PATIENT WITH NO FOLLOW-UP CARE

1. The majority of cancer patients are discharged from hospital settings to **self-care or family care only.** Financial constraints, geographic location, and resource limitations are the primary barriers to continuing services.

2. One way of facilitating the transition for these patients is to designate a **primary care provider** at home. This person is targeted to receive instructions.

3. Families also should be advised on how to obtain services at a later time if required.

4. The nursing staff can help the family address the responsibilities for assuming care at home.
   a. Procedures such as dressing changes and tube feedings should be demonstrated during the patient's hospitalization.
   b. Family responsibilities should be assumed gradually.
   c. The first 24 hours after discharge can be planned in great detail.
   d. Family "care plans" and a "cardex" can be used. (See **Figure 52-2, text page 1352,** for illustration.)
   e. Volunteer groups may be able to offer some relief or assistance.

IV.   SELECTING AND RECOMMENDING SETTINGS

A.   ASSESSMENT OF PATIENT AND FAMILY NEEDS

1. Continuity of care must be based on a comprehensive nursing assessment **specific to the needs of the cancer patient.**

2. Assessment of need includes
   a. Identifying who is "family" to the patient.
   b. Evaluating the normal family routine, normal roles in the family, and the health status of family members. The various strengths of different family members should form the basis of their interventions.
   c. Balancing patient and family needs.

B.   COLLABORATIVE PLANNING AND ROLES OF THE HEALTH CARE TEAM

1. Patients benefit from **clear communication between health care providers** and from **consistent goals of care.** Care should be based on collaborative, multidisciplinary planning; conflicts and "territorial struggles" among providers should be avoided.

2. **Discharge-planning teams** exist in most acute care settings. They include
   a. **Formal teams** who develop coordinated plans of care through conferences.
   b. **Discharge planners** functioning as consultants to staff.
   c. **Staff nurses** or **social workers** who assume discharge-planning functions within their normal roles.
3. The nurse, as the primary provider of inpatient care of the patient, has the **central role in the discharge-planning team.** The nurse may be an advanced practitioner, a clinical specialist, or the staff nurse. Nurses and social workers collaborate to provide a comprehensive approach to discharge planning.
4. Written documentation is essential as discharge plans are made. Other forms of verbal and written communications are vital to the process.
5. **Case management** is a care-delivery system with increasing value to continuity of care.
   a. It involves a primary nurse/case manager who uses a systematic plan to organize, direct, revise, and evaluate care.
   b. It emphasizes the need for interdisciplinary collaboration while maintaining the central role of the nurse as case manager.
   c. It uses specific outcome criteria and predicted time frames to monitor the patient's hospital stay and discharges. Critical paths are used to map out the patient's expected progress.

C. EVALUATION OF ALTERNATIVES

1. The evaluation and selection of **alternative care arrangements** require individual attention to the needs and goals of the patient.
2. Two important considerations in this selection process are
   a. **Cost** and the **patient's financial resources,** including **insurance coverage and benefits.**
   b. **Quantity and quality of care** provided by alternative care settings or agencies.

D. CHOICES

1. After alternatives are assessed and evaluated, a choice can be made and specific arrangements can begin. However, patients should be reminded that choices may be flexible and that alterations can be made at any time.
2. The nurse should encourage the patient and family to be assertive consumers in their choices of care, e.g.,
   a. Does a nursing home have experience in providing care to cancer patients?
   b. What is a hospice's extent or limit of emergency on-call services?

E. ASSESSMENT OF THE CARE SETTING

1. The nurse determines how the patient's needs were met before the current hospitalization in order to evaluate future plans.
   a. A visit to the patient's hospital and home may be valuable in assessing past and existing needs.
   b. The patient can be asked to describe the environment and routines that existed before the present hospitalization.
2. If the patient is not going home, the family should be encouraged to visit the alternative care setting in advance of discharge.
3. If the patient is going to a hospice, a visit by the hospice nurse may allay the patient's and family's anxieties.
4. Some patients may be best served through a short stay in a skilled nursing facility.

V. TRANSITION

A. COORDINATION

1. The stress of transition may be greatly reduced by active involvement of the staff nurse.
2. Discharge instructions are better given over a period of time rather than on the day of discharge, when anxiety levels are highest.
3. The **case management** delivery method facilitates the exchange of information between inpatient and outpatient services.

4. The case management model stresses **the patient and family as the primary focus.**
5. Case management **promotes a cooperative relationship among the patient and family, nurse case manager, physician, and other members of the interdisciplinary team.**

B. COMMUNICATION PROCESS AND TOOLS

1. Providing **continuity of care** requires complex interactions between the patient, family, and health care team.
2. In order to achieve continuity of care, there is a strong need for **shared information.**
3. Several continuing care models identify the need for a specific professional manager.
4. Final decisions regarding care should rest with the patient after open interaction and sharing of information with the family and all members of the health care team.
5. One new communication strategy that has been developed is a statewide telecommunication system entitled **CHILD (Continued Help in Lending Direction).** This system facilitates communication among nurses at a tertiary referral center and a community hospital and has resulted in improved patient outcomes, increased patient satisfaction, and continuity of care.
6. Other tools have been developed to help in the transition from the hospital to the community setting. See **Figure 52-3, text page 1356–1357,** for a description of one of these tools.

C. ACCEPTANCE AND ADJUSTMENT

1. Gradual transition from the acute care setting to the community is best accomplished through **transfer to a day hospital, respite care,** or **gradual assumption of care by the family during hospitalization.**
2. However, hospitals can play a role in coordinating continuity of care after the patient has been discharged. For example, the Memorial Sloan-Kettering Cancer Center's Supportive Care Program emphasizes the central role of nursing in the extension of the acute care setting to the community.

VI. EVALUATION AND FOLLOW-UP

1. Further research is needed to determine the quality of transitions of cancer patients among the various settings and to evaluate such settings according to standards of care.

PRACTICE QUESTIONS

1. Each of the following is an important element in the definition of continuity of care **except**
   (A) planned coordination of care.
   (B) improved outcomes for the patient.
   (C) improved outcomes regardless of care setting or provider.
   (D) preparation for patient transfer.

2. One factor that has stimulated an increased emphasis on the concept of continuity of care is
   (A) the trend toward fewer health care settings.
   (B) the implementation of DRGs.
   (C) longer hospital stays coupled with diminished technical resources.
   (D) the assumption of greater nursing responsibility by acute care hospitals.

3. Probably the **most** important part of the oncology nursing profession's strategy for enhancing continuity of care is
   (A) planning the transition from the acute care hospital to alternative care settings.
   (B) advising patients on the complex issues related to choice of treatment.
   (C) working with hospices, ambulatory care settings, and other providers in staffing care facilities.
   (D) developing procedures for providing financial support to patients in need of help.

4. One of the major limitations to continuity of care in the nursing home setting is
   (A) inadequate documentation in medical records.
   (B) undermedication of patients because of a general misunderstanding of pain relief.
   (C) an overemphasis on the patient's psychological and social needs.
   (D) the lack of opportunity for intervention by family members.

5. Several issues relate to the quality of care a cancer patient receives in the home setting, including the family's management of symptoms and the effects of home care on the psychological health of surviving family members. A third issue that affects many families providing oncologic care is the
    (A) psychological impact of home care on home care agencies.
    (B) increase in "high-tech" home care procedures such as tube feedings.
    (C) physical health status of family members.
    (D) lack of communication between the family and the primary health care provider.

6. The majority of cancer patients are discharged from hospital settings to
    (A) hospices.
    (B) nursing homes.
    (C) self-care or family care.
    (D) rehabilitation facilities.

7. The central role in the discharge-planning teams that exist in most acute care hospitals is held by the
    (A) discharge planner.
    (B) social worker.
    (C) nurse.
    (D) physician.

8. Along with the quantity and quality of care provided by alternative care settings, the other important factor that influences the selection of a care setting for the cancer patient is
    (A) its proximity to the acute care hospital.
    (B) its cost and the patient's financial resources.
    (C) the professional training of its medical staff.
    (D) its policies relating to the multidisciplinary, team approach.

9. One step the nurse can take to determine how the cancer patient's needs were met before the current hospitalization in order to evaluate future plans is to
    (A) visit the hospice nurse if the patient is being released to a hospice.
    (B) encourage the patient's family to visit the alternative care setting in advance of the patient's discharge from the hospital.
    (C) encourage the patient to spend a brief period in a skilled nursing facility.
    (D) ask the patient to describe the environment and routines that existed prior to hospitalization.

10. A common nursing strategy for assuring the cancer patient's smooth transition from the acute care setting to the community is
    (A) involving members of the community in the discharge-planning process.
    (B) avoiding doctrinaire approaches to alternative care such as the case management approach.
    (C) providing insurers and appropriate agencies with the patient's complete medical records.
    (D) allowing the family to assume gradual care of the patient during hospitalization.

ANSWER EXPLANATIONS

1. **The answer is (D).**   Continuity of care implies a standard of care in which there is planned coordination of care that results in improved outcomes for the patient, irrespective of care setting or provider. It is distinct from discharge planning, the process of preparing the patient for transfer from one system and entry into the next phase of care. (1347)

2. **The answer is (B).**   Among the social and health care factors that have stimulated increased emphasis on the concept of continuity of care are the implementation of DRGs, resulting in restricted use of acute care settings and reliance on alternative care systems; shortened hospital stays, combined with complex "high-tech" care, resulting in patients and their families assuming a greater share of nursing responsibilities; and the evolution of cancer care delivered on multiple health care settings (e.g., diagnostic clinics, ambulatory care centers, home care), resulting in patient care that is less linear and more a trajectory with multiple transitions between systems. (1347)

3. **The answer is (A).**   Continuity of care is an essential element in achieving quality of care. The oncology nursing profession can help address the issue of continuity of care by evaluating current systems and de-

vising strategies for enhancing the concept. This is best accomplished through careful evaluation of the specific settings used by cancer patients and planning of the transition from the acute care hospital to these settings. (1349)

4. **The answer is (A).** Nursing homes care for a dynamic population of patients constantly in transition between settings, including home, hospitals, and other long-term care institutions. One of the primary limitations to continuity of care in these settings is reliance on a predominantly nonprofessional staff of nursing assistants and medication aids, which may result in certain patients, especially those requiring aggressive management of pain or continuous parenteral infusions, receiving inadequate care. Another is inadequate documentation in the medical records of transferred patients. Frequently, patients arrive from the hospital with little or no medical history and are unable to provide this information because of communication deficits, dementia, or poor memory. (1349)

5. **The answer is (B).** The increase in "high-tech" home care of oncology patients, including such procedures as tube feedings, epidural catheters, intravenous transfusions, or blood transfusions, requires family members to learn special skills to provide care when the patient goes home. Instructions given to families in the final hours before discharge are easily forgotten and can result in compromised care for the patient. (1351)

6. **The answer is (C).** Because of financial constraints, geographic location, and resource limitations, the majority of cancer patients are discharged from hospital settings to self-care or family care only. The nursing staff then must help the patient and family address the responsibilities for assuming care at home. Procedures such as dressing changes and tube feedings can be demonstrated during the patient's hospitalization. The first 24 hours after discharge can be planned in great detail, and family "care plans" and a "cardex" can be used. (1352)

7. **The answer is (C).** Discharge-planning teams generally consist of formal teams who develop coordinated plans of care through conferences, discharge planners functioning as consultants to staff, and staff nurses or social workers who assume discharge-planning functions within their normal roles. The nurse, as the primary provider of inpatient care of the patient, has the central role in the discharge-planning team. Nurses and social workers collaborate to provide a comprehensive approach to discharge planning. (1353)

8. **The answer is (B).** The evaluation and selection of alternative care arrangements requires individual attention to the needs and goals of the patient. Two important considerations in this selection process are cost and the patient's financial resources, including insurance coverage and benefits, and the quantity and quality of care provided by alternative care settings or agencies. (1353)

9. **The answer is (D).** Continuity of care requires integration of the patient's past, present, and future in the planning and provision of care. The nurse must remember that some of the patient's needs could have existed before admission to a health care facility. One way to determine how the patient's needs were met before the current hospitalization is a visit to the patient's hospital and home. Another is to ask the patient to describe the environment and routines that existed before the present hospitalization. (1354)

10. **The answer is (D).** Gradual transition from the acute care setting to the community is best accomplished through transfer to a day hospital, respite care, or gradual assumption of care by the family during hospitalization. However, hospitals can play a role in coordinating continuity of care after the patient has been discharged. (1355)

53 Rehabilitation of the Person with Cancer

STUDY OUTLINE

I. INTRODUCTION

1. **Rehabilitation** refers to "the process by which individuals, within their environments, are assisted to achieve optimal functioning within the limits imposed by cancer."
2. The basic principles of cancer rehabilitation include **using an interdisciplinary team approach, emphasis on maximizing strengths, focus on practical day-to-day issues, facilitation of coping with loss, family care,** and **focus on prevention in areas of high risk for complications.**

II. REHABILITATION GOALS

1. The **overall goal** of rehabilitation is to help the individual reach an optimal level of independence while preventing disabilities that might limit the individual's potential.
2. Four categories for rehabilitation goals were defined originally by Dietz:
   a. **Preventive:** To prevent or reduce the impact of expected disabilities.
   b. **Restorative:** To return the individual to optimal functional status with expected complete medical recovery.
   c. **Supportive:** To maximize function and prevent secondary disabilities while the disease persists and the possibility of progressive disability exists.
   d. **Palliative:** To assist the dying person and his or her family in maximizing their independence, while providing comfort.
3. Over the course of a person's cancer history, these goals are **continually assessed, defined, reached, and modified.**
4. Goals are a **balance** between having a hopeful vision of tomorrow and being realistic about current limitations.

III. REHABILITATION NEEDS

1. Rehabilitation needs are related to the **type of cancer site** and **stage of disease, type of treatment** and **side effects experienced, length of illness, coping skills, family and other medical history, social issues,** and the individual's response.
   a. **Severity** or **duration** of disease is **most related** to the cancer patient's rehabilitation needs.
2. **Health care professionals** can help to identify unmet patient needs and enhance the individual's ability to adjust to cancer and comply with the treatment plan.
3. Some problems are more **chronic** or long term than others.
   a. Fatigue, anorexia, and weakness may be associated with recovery from surgery and be of short duration, while at other times these symptoms are associated with metastatic or advancing disease and are of longer duration.
4. A **multidisciplinary cancer rehabilitation team or service** may be the most prepared with the resources and skills to deal with the challenges of addressing the changing and varying rehabilitation needs of patients.
5. Rehabilitation needs fall into **categories** that include physiological, functional, emotional, spiritual, and social. See **Table 53-1, text page 1362.**

A. **PHYSIOLOGICAL NEEDS**

1. Many physiologic needs of individuals with cancer related to alterations in mobility are best addressed with preventive measures. These needs include those related to skin and wound care and to fatigue.

B. **FUNCTIONAL NEEDS**

1. This category includes the problems related to **day-to-day practical issues** of living that may be temporary or permanent, such as mobility and swallowing.
2. Functional needs of the cancer patient are often **unrecognized** or not appreciated by acute care providers.
3. For the patient, physical dependence can be a constant **reminder** of life-threatening illness.
4. Functional rehabilitation needs can arise at any time during the course of a person's cancer experience, even for long-term cancer survivors.

C. **EMOTIONAL NEEDS**

1. Major emotional needs include **hope, honesty, information, emotional expression,** and **discussion of issues related to death.**
    a. These emotional issues may be **affected** by the patient's prognosis or change in status as well as functional and physical limitations.
    b. **Psychological needs** may be in response to a new event or may be related to coping with the chronic uncertainty about the future.
    c. **Family members** may each be coping with different fears and concerns, such as the stress of family role changes.

D. **SPIRITUAL NEEDS**

1. Patients with cancer will frequently reexamine their priorities and their beliefs and values throughout their experience with cancer.
2. **Assessing** spiritual needs can be done as an extension of a psychosocial assessment, as beliefs, values, and faith can be the foundation for coping.

E. **SOCIAL NEEDS**

1. Like other chronic illnesses, cancer can have an impact on **family, friends,** and **coworkers.**
2. Many cancer patients fear **withdrawal** of their family, friends, and colleagues. This is often **enhanced** if there are any noticeable physical changes as a result of the cancer.
3. Early in the rehabilitation process, **social assessment** is important to understanding the extent and depth of the person's social and support network and resources.
4. Northouse and Sivcun found that a **partner's distress** is equally as intense as that of the one experiencing the cancer.
5. **Separate support groups** for family members or caregivers may help them openly acknowledge their own needs.
6. Social needs may have an impact on the individual's ability to **continue treatment.**
    a. Transportation, financial, and work-related problems must be assessed early so appropriate referrals can be made and resources utilized.

IV. **NURSING ASSESSMENT OF REHABILITATIVE NEEDS**

1. Careful assessment of the patient's needs is critical since each individual has unique needs and may not require all the resources of a cancer rehabilitation team.
2. Rehabilitation assessment should begin at the **onset** of a cancer diagnosis and be repeated regularly and when changes in status occur.
3. The initial assessment may be global, followed by a more detailed evaluation by the appropriate health care discipline.

A. **ASSESSMENT TOOLS**

1. Most cancer rehabilitation services use some type of **instrument**—an informal inventory of needs, a survey, or a specially designed self-assessment tool—as a systematic way to gather information and identify the need for assistance.
2. When evaluating the effectiveness of an assessment tool, consider **whether the patient can understand the questions, the restrictiveness of the form, the patient's state of health (influencing one's ability to complete the tool)**, and **the patient's willingness to acknowledge** and **confront his or her needs openly.**
3. An **inventory of needs** can be used by the assessor as a checklist so that actual or potential problems frequently experienced are not overlooked.
4. A **self-assessment tool** is designed to be completed by the patient on each visit to the clinic, and once completed, the tool is followed up by an interview with an oncology nurse.
5. The **Karnofsky Performance Status** is limited for identifying rehabilitation needs; however, it can indicate to the assessor the need for a more detailed clinical evaluation by the rehabilitation team.

B. **ASSESSMENT PROCESS**

1. The use of an assessment tool is optimally **followed by observation** or a more detailed assessment of particular problems.
2. Depending on the **severity** of the problem and the degree to which the person wants the problem addressed, other team members are involved.
3. An **open, accepting style** of assessment allows feelings such as anger, frustration, or guilt to be aired and then dealt with productively.
4. As needs are identified, a more **detailed evaluation** and development of a treatment plan are initiated by the appropriate rehabilitation team member. See **Table 53-2, text page 1365,** for a sample rehabilitation plan.

V. **REHABILITATION RESOURCES**

A. **ORGANIZATION OF CARE**

1. The design of a cancer rehabilitation service includes **basic elements** such as a comprehensive approach to addressing needs and an interdisciplinary team knowledgeable about cancer, family care, and coordinated services integrated into the acute care of the cancer patient.
2. The tumor registry can help to **identify** the largest cancer populations being served and therefore potential referrals for rehabilitation services.
3. The most successful cancer rehabilitation programs have a broad base of support and **interdepartmental teamwork** in the assessment and planning of a program or service.
4. The delivery of cancer rehabilitation services is dependent on the coordinating structure, but there are various organizational models, ranging from informal to formal structures.
5. See **Table 53-3, text page 1366,** for organizational options for a rehabilitation service.

B. **CANCER REHABILITATION TEAM**

1. The cancer rehabilitation team is a **cohesive group** of interdisciplinary members who apply their professional expertise to the benefit of individuals with cancer.
2. Although each team member has his or her own professional knowledge base, together the team develops a **common knowledge base** that includes cancer pathophysiology, cancer treatments and their side effects, emotional responses to cancer, coping styles, family dynamics, and symptom control.
3. A team's **effectiveness** is related to its capabilities to do the work and its ability to manage itself as an interdependent group of people.
4. Four **barriers** to team effectiveness are goal conflicts, organizational structure, interprofessional conflicts, and lack of communication.
5. Several critical areas for **effective team communication** are assessment, rehabilitation plan and referrals, further assessment, progress notes, interdisciplinary conferences, and discharge plans.
6. **Informal communication** becomes important as changes occur in day-to-day patient care.
7. A **designated leader,** whether formal or informal, is needed to monitor the team's needs and facilitate its effectiveness.

C. **COORDINATION OF CARE**

1. Following the assessment and development of a plan, a coordinator involves and updates the necessary team members. See **Figure 53-1, text page 1368,** for a coordinator model of cancer rehabilitation service.
2. In partnership with the acute care oncology nurse, the coordinator is central to the interdisciplinary conference, which is usually held weekly.

D. **OUTPATIENT NEEDS AND CONTINUITY OF CARE**

1. With hospitalization periods shortening, there is an **increasing need** for pre- and posthospital rehabilitation.
2. If rehabilitation is to be involved early in the cancer care, outpatient rehabilitation is required.
3. Access to rehabilitation services **prior** to hospitalization allows the individual to become familiar with the team and the resources that can help through this time of change and uncertainty.
    a. The team's subsequent involvement during the hospitalization period becomes one of continuation rather than introduction of a new service.
    b. The individual and health care team can proceed through this period of cancer care with a foundation based on familiarity and clarity in goals for the rehabilitation process.
    c. The rehabilitation team can enhance **continuity of care** by coordinating and providing services in most care settings.
4. Cancer rehabilitation services can complement outpatient chemotherapy clinics and radiation oncology centers.

E. **EDUCATION AND SUPPORT GROUPS**

1. An advantage of education and support groups is that the **individual can choose** to participate to the degree desired.
2. When the acute care team and the rehabilitation staff facilitate and teach these sessions together, individuals become **familiar** with not only the acute and chronic issues but with the resources that can help as well.

F. **EXERCISE GROUPS**

1. Modified exercise classes accentuate the value of **physical activity** and **support combined.**
2. An exercise program focuses on the physiologic and psychosocial issues of living through energy conservation, energy utilization, and restoration strategies.

G. **SURVIVOR NEEDS**

1. In the outpatient setting, patients and families discuss the **transitional issues of reintegration** from an illness to wellness orientation such as **workplace concerns, sexuality and intimacy, issues related to body image and self-esteem,** and a **reexamination of one's values and beliefs.**
2. Outpatient rehabilitation services, particularly support groups and counseling services, can continue to **facilitate emotional independence.**
3. Workplace issues include both emotional and functional factors.
    a. Of persons with cancer, **80% will return to work,** and **25% will have problems in the workplace.**
    b. Issues may be **difficulties peers and supervisors have; withdrawal; facing questions one would rather not discuss;** or **fatigue, which impairs ability to work a full shift or presents specific functional limitations.**

PRACTICE QUESTIONS

1. The overall goal of rehabilitation for the person with cancer is to
    (A) return to baseline performance prior to the cancer.
    (B) anticipate and prepare physically for future debilitating effects of cancer.
    (C) achieve optimal functioning within the limits of cancer.
    (D) maintain an active, busy life.

2.   Which of the following factors have been found to be **most closely** related to rehabilitation needs of the cancer patient?
     (A)   medical and family history
     (B)   type of treatment and side effects experienced
     (C)   cancer site and stage of disease
     (D)   severity or duration of disease

3.   Physiologic distress can be minimized by teaching the patient
     (A)   preventive and self-care measures.
     (B)   the location of social support systems.
     (C)   how to access counseling services.
     (D)   strength and endurance exercises.

4.   Which of the following patient indicators observed by the rehabilitation nurse during an assessment suggests that the techniques used may **not** be effective in obtaining all the information?
     (A)   The patient has just completed a card game with his brother and reports feeling energized.
     (B)   The patient asks questions and completes full thoughts in response to the questions.
     (C)   The patient insists that he has no rehabilitation needs.
     (D)   The patient shares his pride in successfully being a trial lawyer for 30 years.

5.   The effectiveness of rehabilitation teams can be impaired by four barriers: goal conflicts, organizational structure, interprofessional conflicts, and
     (A)   lack of nursing leadership.
     (B)   lack of communication.
     (C)   lack of sufficient reimbursement.
     (D)   lack of 100% time commitments.

6.   The success of a rehabilitation team is related to its ability to work together and manage itself as a(n)
     (A)   co-dependent group of people.
     (B)   independent group of people
     (C)   interdependent group of people.
     (D)   consistent group of people.

7.   The person responsible for providing updated information to the rehabilitation team members is vital to an effective cohesive cancer rehabilitation program. This is the
     (A)   coordinator.
     (B)   medical director.
     (C)   discharge planner.
     (D)   patient.

ANSWER EXPLANATIONS

1.   **The answer is (C).**   Rehabilitation refers to the process by which individuals, within their environments, are assisted to achieve optimal functioning within the limits imposed by cancer. The goals are to improve the quality of life for those experiencing cancer and to help the individual regain "wholeness." (1361)

2.   **The answer is (D).**   Severity or duration of disease is the factor most closely related to the cancer patient's rehabilitation needs. The physical needs frequently occurring with a variety of cancers included general weakness, limited activities of daily living, and issues related to limited mobility. (1361)

3.   **The answer is (A).**   Physiological needs relate to skin care, bowel and bladder dysfunction, ostomy and wound care, fatigue, symptom control, lymphedema, nutrition, cognitive skills, and sleep. Teaching patients how to prevent problems with these areas and what the patients can do for themselves minimizes the distress they experience. Choices (B) and (C) would be more in response to rehabilitation needs falling into the emotional, social, and/or spiritual categories. Strength and endurance exercises may be more appropriate for rehabilitation needs falling into the functional category. (1362)

4.   **The answer is (C).**   When evaluating the effectiveness of an assessment tool, points to consider are whether the person can understand the questions, the restrictiveness of the form, the person's state of health that

could influence one's ability to complete the form, and the person's willingness to acknowledge and confront his or her needs openly. Choices (B) and (D) suggest that the patient understands the questions, and choice (A) suggests that he or she is not fatigued, compromised physically, or unable to answer the questions. The fact that the patient insists he or she has no needs might suggest that there is a lack of willingness to acknowledge and confront those needs. (1364)

5. **The answer is (B).** Poor communication, the most common barrier to the team's efficiency, is frequently an issue of accessibility of one team member to another. Strategies for prevention of communication problems include defining clinical communication methods such as documentation, team log books, scheduling boards, and care plans. (1367)

6. **The answer is (C).** A team's effectiveness is related to its capabilities to do the work and its ability to manage itself as an interdependent group of people. The team needs to come together and work together to solve problems and meet patient needs. Therefore, independent practice would lead to redundancy of interventions as well as interventions and care needs going unaddressed. Co-dependence would be an unhealthy way of relating to each other and it could interfere in meeting patient needs because the individual's own needs would most likely come first. Although consistency is helpful in solidifying team relationships, the respect and behaviors that are in accordance with interdependence and interprofessionalism are the priority. (1367)

7. **The answer is (A).** Coordination of care is vital to a rehabilitation program because each patient situation requires a unique subset of team members. Coordination of care includes ongoing monitoring with input from the primary nurse as to the status of each problem area and the identification of new areas of need. Any changes in medical status, caregiver issues, and discharge planning are important communications for team members so that their interventions can be relevant and timely. This requires the coordinator to have frequent communication with the acute care team and the family, who along with the rehabilitation team depend on the coordinator for information relevant to the rehabilitation status, assessment of the individual and family's ability to function independently, and availability of community resources. (1367–1368)

54   Ambulatory Care

STUDY OUTLINE

I.   AMBULATORY CARE OVERVIEW

1. Ambulatory care is **synonymous** with **outpatient care** and includes services such as diagnostic testing; screening and detection; treatment modalities such as chemotherapy, biotherapy, radiation therapy, and minor surgical procedures; as well as psychosocial intervention.
2. **Advances** in cancer treatment and technology and the influences of economics and **quality-of-life issues** have promoted ambulatory services as a method for providing cancer patient and family care.
3. Already **80%–90%** of all cancer care is delivered in outpatient settings such as physicians' offices, freestanding oncology centers, and hospital outpatient departments.

A.   AMBULATORY CARE SETTINGS

1. A wide **variety of ambulatory care settings** available are community cancer centers, freestanding cancer centers, 24-hour clinics, chemotherapy and blood therapy infusion centers, day hospital clinics, physicians' offices, outreach and network programs, and other specialty centers that focus on screening, rehabilitation, and symptom management.
2. The **distinction** between models or types of cancer centers and ambulatory settings is not always clear, but it usually reflects purpose, organizational structure, or source of funding.
3. **Freestanding centers**
   a. A freestanding cancer center (FSCC) may be a facility **separate from an existing medical care delivery building** such as a hospital, or it may be **contiguous with** or within a hospital facility.
   b. An FSCC may be a **joint venture** between hospitals or a hospital(s) and a group of community oncologists or it may be physician-owned and -operated.
   c. The movement toward FSCCs resulted from the **shift** in medical care delivery from inpatient to outpatient settings and from patient demand for sophisticated therapies in the local community.
   d. FSCCs are usually based within the community, do not incorporate training of oncologists, and are not involved with on-site basic research.
   e. **Affiliation** of community programs with university-based cancer centers is emerging.
4. **Twenty-four-hour clinics**
   a. The **need** for ambulatory services on a continuous basis has precipitated the development of a number of 24-hour services across the country.
   b. **Two categories** of service are typical: urgent oncology care and traditional infusion therapies given during expanded hours.
   c. Such settings are specifically designed to deal with **side effect management** and **unpredictable changes** in the patient's condition following therapy.
5. **Day hospitals**
   a. The day hospital provides a system of **partial hospitalization.** Individualized care, treatments, and diagnostic tests are provided for extended periods.
6. **Outreach and satellite centers**
   a. Since patients often want to remain in their own communities to receive cancer treatment, linkages between tertiary and rural hospitals are being developed.
7. **Physician office practices**
   a. Physician office practices continue to expand the scope of services provided, i.e., lab, nutrition, counseling, education, and support groups.

8. **Other ambulatory centers (screening, rehabilitation)**
    a. The basic focus of these newly developing screening programs is directed at low-cost cancer detection services.
        (1) Among the factors contributing to a successful screening center are **convenience** and **visibility, adequate volume to keep the cost affordable,** and an **approach directed at screening programs outside the usual programs.**
    b. Cancer rehabilitation services, symptom control clinics, pain management centers, and cancer psychosocial clinics are also offered through a variety of settings.
    c. Another recent trend is the development of **site-specific cancer centers,** such as breast clinics or centers. See **Table 54-1, text page 1374,** for operational and programmatic components.
        (1) Services not generally available in the community can be offered in these site-specific centers and can include risk assessment, screening for the disadvantaged and minorities, and educational programs for both professionals and the public.
    d. Specialized programs for all major cancers may soon be developed, most likely in larger institutions due to the cost of setting up the programs and the need for large populations of patients.

B. **PLANNING ISSUES**

1. Consideration should be given to **space, staffing, equipment needs, management support,** and **how the services will be delivered.**
2. A functional development **plan** including the elements of **present services, physician referral patterns, the patient population, financial** and **human resources, as well as local reimbursement policies should be written using information elicited from both external and internal surveys.**
3. Increased competition has changed the focus of ambulatory care to be more responsive to the patient's and family's requests.

II. **THE ROLE OF THE NURSE IN AMBULATORY CARE**

1. Three elements make the role of the ambulatory care nurse unique:
    a. The **scope of practice.**
    b. The **use of the telephone in delivery of care.**
    c. The nurse's **role in continuity of care.**

A. **AMBULATORY CARE STANDARDS**

1. Standards that have applicability to the ambulatory oncology nurse have been developed by
    a. The American Academy of Ambulatory Nursing Administration.
    b. The American Nurses' Association.
    c. The Oncology Nursing Society.

B. **AMBULATORY CARE RESPONSIBILITIES**

1. See **Table 54-2, text page 1376,** for responsibilities of the nurse in the ambulatory care setting as researched by Verran and adapted by Tighe.
2. Oncology nurses reported most frequent involvement in **health care maintenance activities, followed by counseling** and **communication.**
3. Continued research is needed to develop a **consistent vocabulary** to describe the practice of ambulatory nursing and to develop a consensus about the role of the nurse.

C. **OFFICE-BASED NURSING**

1. Choosing the office for oncology care may be a result of **increasing health care costs, consumer demand,** and the **chronicity of the disease.**
2. The office-based oncology nurse must possess sharp **assessment skills** in order to handle the large patient population in which patient care is intermittent and brief.
3. See **Table 54-3, text page 1377,** for a summary task profile of office-based oncology nurses.

4. **Triaging phone calls** appropriately and efficiently is a major role of the office-based nurse.
   a. Phone calls may relate to **symptom complaints, clarification of information, prescription refills, crisis management, reporting and interpreting lab tests, referrals to community resources, assistance with reimbursement,** and **counseling.**
   b. Phone calls may also be made for follow-up purposes and provide an opportunity to reinforce symptom management and preventive actions.
   c. **Documentation** of phone calls and interventions must be done as a minimum standard of care. See **Figures 54-1 and 54-2, text page 1379,** for examples of two different forms that can be used for this purpose.
   d. Communication among all care providers of each phase of the patient's care is critical and facilitates the exchange of information.
      (1) **Figure 54-3, text page 1380,** provides an example of an interagency referral form that can be used to promote continuity.

D. **RADIATION ONCOLOGY PRACTICE NURSING**

1. Hilderley has described the role of the clinical nurse specialist in a radiation oncology private practice as having the characteristics of **"mutual trust, understanding, open communication, flexibility, common goals, competence, independence as well as interdependence,** and a **strong desire to make it work."**
2. In a survey of radiation-therapy-based oncology nurses, results showed that nurses principally **performed patient assessments, patient teaching,** and **care of catheters, ports,** and **pumps.**
3. See **Chapter 13** for a discussion of the role of the nurse and management of care in radiotherapy.

III. **NURSING ISSUES**

A. **MODELS OF NURSING CARE DELIVERY**

1. The evolution of the role of the ambulatory nurse and the complexity of care requirements have resulted in several models, including **primary nursing, multidisciplinary teams,** and **collaborative practice.**
2. **Primary nursing** is designed to improve the quality of nursing care; recognize the patient and family as the unit of care, with the care designed accordingly; improve coordination of care among specialties; and ensure continuity of care between settings.
   a. The **reality** of high patient to low staff ratios in a complex and sophisticated environment makes the primary nursing model even more of a challenge today.
   b. **Selection** of the primary nursing model will depend on the philosophy and resources of the particular setting.
   c. Creativity in adapting the model to a particular setting is encouraged.
3. The **multidisciplinary team model** emphasizes the important element of **teamwork** necessary to address patient and family needs in the ambulatory setting.
4. The **collaborative nurse-physician model** has been implemented in all types of ambulatory settings. This model has five components: primary nursing, increased clinical decision making by the nurse, a collaborative practice committee of nurses and physicians, joint record review, and an integrated medical record.
   a. This model allows nurses to manage resources so that triage occurs appropriately and there are designated appointment systems, easy access, and long-term follow-up.

B. **PATIENT CLASSIFICATION AND PRODUCTIVITY**

1. Patient classification systems are used extensively in the **inpatient setting** and can be useful in the ambulatory area, with some adaptation.
2. Developing a system for ambulatory care is complex due to the many variables affecting the nursing role as well as the variety of facilities and types of clinics.
3. **Workload** is generally influenced by **patient characteristics, nursing role characteristics,** and the actual **number of patients who require care.**
4. **Workload analysis** can be used to develop the **staffing plan** by classifying workload variables so they can be assigned a numerical value that is then converted into hours of staff time.
5. Two types of patient classification instruments are **factor** and **prototype.**

    a. **Factor classification** requires the nurse to rate the patient on the basis of specific characteristics such as independence in activities of daily living, medications, treatments, and psychological needs.

    b. **Prototype instruments** require an evaluation of the overall status of the patient and placement into a defined category, and the resulting score is then computed to reflect the amount of nursing time and effort required.

6. When considering a classification system, it is important to account for time spent in **indirect care** and in **telephone activity.**

7. In the outpatient setting, classification systems are typically used for **retrospective trending of patient characteristics, justification of resources, use of monitored trends for program planning, nursing workload analysis, patient care charges, validation of nursing care provided,** and **quality assurance.**

8. Effectively utilizing resources can result in improved profitability. Five **techniques to improve productivity** are improving scheduling, staffing only for current workload, improving functional design of facilities, ensuring employee motivation, and increasing patient volume.

9. The ideal ambulatory care classification system has yet to be developed, and its importance will not be fully realized until a prospective payment system for outpatient visits is implemented.

10. **Three motives** for redesigning the reimbursement system for ambulatory care are the need for a rational system that is consistent, cost containment, and the need to shift the focus of patient care to a primary ambulatory setting and away from excessive use of hospitals and costly subspecialty services.

C. QUALITY ASSURANCE/IMPROVEMENT

1. The **goal** of a quality assurance/improvement program is to ensure that care is provided according to established standards and procedures.

2. It is essential to identify major aspects of care and **critical indicators** to monitor and evaluate.

3. **AmbuQual,** a computer-supported ambulatory quality assurance system, is based on ten parameters that define quality health care in diverse ambulatory settings.

4. With an emphasis on "total quality management" or "continuous quality improvement" interest has been renewed in identifying problems/deficiencies from a **systems approach.**

5. Another approach to quality improvement may be the development of indicators **standard to all oncology settings,** with reports given to the hospital or clinic cancer committee.

6. See **Table 54-4, text page 1383,** for a list of ten items with the highest and lowest ratings of patient satisfaction with care.

D. OCCUPATIONAL HAZARDS

1. Oncology nurses working in ambulatory settings are involved with specific occupational hazards such as the safe handling of **antineoplastic agents, radioactive materials,** and **blood** and **body fluids.**

    a. Guidelines for protection in handling antineoplastic agents were issued by the Occupational Safety and Health Administration (OSHA) in 1986.

    b. The subject remains controversial, and wide variations in practice exist.

2. It is highly desirable to implement a facility-wide chemotherapy and radiotherapy **task force** to establish standards, protocols, and procedures; recommend protective equipment purchases; and evaluate compliance with the accepted standards.

3. The exposure of staff to patients' blood and body fluids is common in all oncology settings, and strict adherence to the guidelines is essential for protection of both staff and patients.

E. CONTINUITY OF CARE

1. The oncology nurse in the ambulatory setting is the person who frequently maintains continuity of care with the patient and family.

2. Continuity of care involves the **multifaceted processes** requiring mutual patient, family, and professional planning as well as the advocacy, coordination, and implementation necessary to achieve an optimal outcome.

3. See **Table 54-4, text page 1384,** for key components of continuity of care planning and implementation, such as
   a. Uniform access.
   b. Comprehensive medical and psychosocial planning.
   c. Responsiveness to patient/family needs.
   d. Availability of resources and services.
   e. Coordination of medical and psychosocial care.
   f. Monitoring and accountability.
4. Issues that have an impact on continuity of care include **economic forces, health care provider concerns, patient interests, family involvement,** and **demographic factors.**
5. Several models of providing continuity of care are described on **text pages 1384–1385.**
6. The technical capability of the **computer** to integrate information from multiple sources, store, and then later transmit the data to another location is especially advantageous for care of patients with cancer and is an ideal way to enhance continuity.
7. **Multidisciplinary care conferences** increase communication and knowledge among departments providing oncology services.
   a. The **goals** of multidisciplinary conferences are to provide a forum for education and communication among those involved in the care of the patient and to develop and evaluate individualized multidisciplinary care plans for oncology patients.
8. Another important aspect of continuity of care involves defining **who** the patient should call if a question or concern comes up after traditional working hours.
9. Another method for ensuring improved continuity of care is the daily morning conference to discuss new patients coming on a given day, problems that have arisen, or general issues.

IV. **NURSING CARE DELIVERY**

A. **ADMISSION AND ASSESSMENT**

1. The patient's first visit to the ambulatory setting provides an opportunity to establish what may be a **long-term** relationship.
2. The first visit is a time that can be utilized to give important details of parking facilities, how to find the department, the routine at the time of the visit, and how long to plan to be there.
3. Knowing as much as possible about the patient **prior** to the first visit is ideal.
   a. Obtaining **reports** and **old charts** is helpful.
   b. Most ambulatory settings require that the patient complete the **routine admission procedure,** at least on the first visit.
4. Many excellent **assessment forms** exist, and most ambulatory settings have developed one specific to their setting.
5. A thorough explanation of **future visits** is reviewed with the patient and family.

B. **PATIENT EDUCATION**

1. Patient education is a key component of the nurse's role in the ambulatory setting.
   a. Challenges involve determining the appropriate **time** to teach and having specific materials available.
2. Nurses in the ambulatory setting are fortunate that there is a great deal of **printed material** available related to cancer, cancer treatment, and management of side effects.
3. Nurses should be involved with the planning, development, and testing of educational materials.
4. The readability of cancer patient education materials has recently been addressed in the literature, and a discrepancy exists between the reading level of the average adult and the reading level of many printed materials.
   a. Because low-income, low-education subgroups are at high risk for cancer, much of the available literature may be of limited value.
   b. Suggestions for **improving readability** include determining the medical terms that need definition and substituting simpler terms whenever possible.
5. More intensive **one-on-one discussions** or use of picture cards, flipcharts, and videos rather than the written material may help in the education process.
6. A **lack** of interest in the material, lack of reading speed, expressions of frustration, inability to answer questions about the material, or the desire to let another person read the text may all be cues to the patient's inability to read at the needed level.

7. Reading ability will **not** necessarily predict how well a patient understands what he or she has read.
8. Nurses can provide important information to families through
   a. Serving as a **guide** through vocabulary and procedures common to the cancer setting.
   b. **Treating family members as part of the treatment team.**
   c. Offering **assurance that the patient is being well cared for.**
      (1) Strategies for meeting the information needs of families are described in **Table 54-7, text page 1387.**
9. Patient teaching in the ambulatory setting has **changed** to incorporate an increased emphasis on **prevention** and **management of problems** as well as therapeutic goals.
10. Factors affecting patient education include the **patient variables** of acuity; psychosocial issues and resources; and the **institutional variables** of time, money, and environment.
11. The **level of illness** of patients often presents a learning barrier.
    a. Education can only be accomplished after the patient has achieved **symptom relief.**
    b. **Psychosocial issues** may either help or hinder the patient's ability to learn about the disease, treatment, and self-care.
12. Promoting effective patient education includes **active involvement** by the nurse in planning and presenting material and evaluating learning.
13. **Newsletters** can be valuable for patient education.
14. Group teaching and classes provide opportunities for patients to interact with each other and to share common experiences.
15. **Table 54-8, text pages 1388–1389,** is an example of an ambulatory continuous infusion chemotherapy teaching plan that delineates teaching activities as well as expected patient/family outcomes.
16. Another approach is the development of a **"learning center"** or lab-like environment for learning, practicing, and demonstrating skills necessary for self-care.

C. TELEPHONE TRIAGE/COUNSELING

1. The **amount of time** spent on the telephone is a unique feature of ambulatory nursing practice.
2. Telephone activities include **assessing patients' responses to the treatment given, providing information about prevention of side effects and symptoms,** and **evaluating patient outcomes.**
3. A high potential for **liability** exists when medical advice is given over the telephone to patients and families.
   a. It is important to maintain a **record of phone calls** with specific data about the purpose, duration, and outcome of each call.
4. Even though there are some differences among the duties of ambulatory oncology nurses in different settings, the primary telephone activities of all groups include symptom management, follow-up, physician contact to discuss patient care issues, and provide education.
5. Providing patients with instructions and a way to reach someone after routine hours is critical and can be accomplished in a variety of ways.
6. **Follow-up phone calls** after treatment has been completed are a routine practice in many settings.
   a. This provides an excellent opportunity for patient **assessment** and **further self-care instructions.**
   b. Patients receiving chemotherapy through an ambulatory infusion pump should be given precise instructions about how to handle a problem after routine office hours.
7. See **Figure 54-4, text page 1393,** for an example of a form that can be used in interagency referral communication.

D. DOCUMENTATION

1. Documentation is a major challenge facing nurses in ambulatory settings because greater complexity of care and higher patient-nurse ratios **demand** accurate, concise, clear, and objective documentation.
2. Documentation includes the **nursing process, fulfills legal requirements, describes the nursing care delivered,** and **reflects the quality of nursing care.**

3. Flow sheets have been developed to fulfill a number of patient care needs.
   a. Specific to the oncology settings are **flow sheets to record side effects, laboratory data, chemotherapy administration information,** and **patient teaching.**
      (1) **Figure 54-5, text pages 1394–1395,** is an example of a flow sheet specific to therapy side effects.
4. Another approach to documentation is a **patient self-assessment tool.** See **Figures 54-6 and 54-7, text pages 1396 and 1397.**
5. Use of **point-of-care computer terminals** has the potential for simplifying documentation issues by enabling the nurse to immediately enter data into the computer, thus decreasing documentation time and improving accuracy.
6. A frequent **omission** in ambulatory care is the nurse's documentation of **behavioral expectations** for patients providing their own care.
7. For assessing quality of care, complying with regulations, and a multitude of other reasons, documentation will remain a **significant challenge** to the oncology nurse in the ambulatory setting.

V. **PATIENT-RELATED ISSUES**

A. **SELF-CARE**

1. **Transition** of patient care from the hospital to ambulatory and home settings has resulted in a shift in responsibility to family members caring for patients receiving treatment.
2. Self-care is **defined** as how individuals care for themselves or alter conditions or objects in their environment in the interest of their own lives, health, or well-being.
   a. Applying this definition to oncology, the actions **initiated** by patients and families to prevent, detect, and manage side effects of radiation and chemotherapy can be defined as self-care.
3. **Diary entries** can form the basis for evaluating the effectiveness of self-care activities and adjusting as necessary for future treatments.
4. Self-care is an important behavior for **cancer survivors** also, since they need to be motivated to take an active role in their own health care, thus lessening their feeling of hopelessness.
5. For optimal self-care behavior, patients and families need to be adequately **taught about the specific treatment modality** and **side effect management.**
6. **Encouraging** and **supporting self-care** is a critical component of the nurse's role in the ambulatory oncology setting.

B. **ETHICAL ISSUES**

1. Ethical issues encountered in ambulatory care are **similar** to those that arise in other settings, i.e., informed decisions, quality of care, and research issues.

C. **ECONOMIC ISSUES**

1. Access to health care has become a major concern for many Americans.
2. **Poverty** has been shown to **correlate** with poor prognosis for all types of cancers.
3. **Refusal by insurers** to pay for research treatments tends to limit participation in studies.

PRACTICE QUESTIONS

1. Ambulatory oncology services have increased over the past 10 years for all of the following reasons **except**
   (A) economic pressures.
   (B) developments in cancer treatment.
   (C) innovation in cancer technology.
   (D) decreased patient acuity.

2. Which of the following components is **not** a component of the collaborative nurse-physician model?
   (A) primary nursing
   (B) joint record review
   (C) integrated medical record
   (D) nurse reports to the physician

3. What are the **three** factors that generally influence workload?
   (A) patient characteristics, nursing role characteristics, volume of patients
   (B) patient volume, physician characteristics, nursing role characteristics
   (C) patient characteristics, physician characteristics, number of indirect care activities
   (D) nursing role characteristics, number of indirect care activities, patient volume

4. The role of the oncology nurse in the office practice includes numerous activities and tasks. Which of the following activities is considered an **indirect** nursing action?
   (A) receiving phone calls from patients
   (B) providing psychological support
   (C) teaching chemotherapy side effects
   (D) accessing a venous access device

5. An important aspect for ensuring continuity of care for an ambulatory patient is knowing
   (A) what side effects to expect in the 48 hours after treatment.
   (B) whom the patient should call if concerns arise after working hours.
   (C) what home care coverage will be reimbursed.
   (D) what the long-range treatment plan is.

6. The ambulatory nurse about to provide an immigrant couple with patient education regarding lymphoma decides to utilize a video and a flipchart rather than cancer society booklets because
   (A) the nurse is concerned about the couple's not being able to afford the booklets.
   (B) the nurse is concerned that the reading level of the booklets might be too high.
   (C) videos contain more information than the booklets.
   (D) the prime time for learning is in the ambulatory department.

7. Which of the following are **not** telephone activities often engaged in by the ambulatory nurse?
   (A) coordinating follow-up tests, clinic visits, and transportation
   (B) communicating changes in the care plan
   (C) recording messages for the patient's physician
   (D) providing information about the prevention of side effects and symptoms

8. Successful nursing documentation can best be achieved by all of the following **except**
   (A) the point-of-care computer terminal.
   (B) the therapy side-effect flowchart.
   (C) the patient diary.
   (D) the nursing diagnosis flow sheet.

9. Applying the definition of self-care to oncology, an example of self-care actions initiated by patients would be
   (A) to keep a diary of their side effects and the efficacy of their efforts to control the side effects.
   (B) to entrust their loved one with the care of their venous access device.
   (C) to trust that their care providers would provide total care.
   (D) to have their significant other review the patient education material for them.

ANSWER EXPLANATIONS

1. **The answer is (D).** Advances in cancer treatment and technology, the influences of economics, and quality-of-life issues have promoted ambulatory services as a method for providing cancer patient and family care. With shortened hospitalizations driven by reimbursement changes, patients are being discharged quicker and sicker; therefore, the patient acuity is actually higher. (1372)

2. **The answer is (D).** The nurse does not necessarily report to the physician. Rather, the model has five components: primary nursing, increased clinical decision making by the nurse, a collaborative practice committee of nurses and physicians, joint record review, and an integrated medical record. (1381)

3. **The answer is (A).** Workload is generally influenced by patient characteristics, nursing role characteristics, and the actual number of patients who require care. Workload analysis can be used to develop the staffing plan by classifying workload variables so they can be assigned a numerical value that is then converted into hours of staff time. (1381)

4.   **The answer is (A).**   Telephone triage and counseling are unique and major aspects of the ambulatory and office-based nurse's role. Telephone activity is considered an indirect nursing care activity in the context of a nurse's workload and/or a patient classification system. (1377, 1382)

5.   **The answer is (B).**   The patient and family must clearly understand who should be called and when to call. An important aspect of continuity of care involves defining whom the patient should call if a question or concern arises after traditional working hours. (1385)

6.   **The answer is (B).**   There is a discrepancy between the reading level of the average adult and the reading level of many printed materials. Using the SMOG formula, the reading level of the American Cancer Society's booklets ranges from grade 5.8 to grade 15.6, with a mean reading level of 11.9, whereas the reading level of most Americans is closer to grades 8–10. It is important to assess the patient's reading level using informal cues and to make sure the readability of the provided information is appropriate. More intensive one-on-one discussions or use of picture cards, flipcharts, and videos rather than the written material may help in the education process. (1386)

7.   **The answer is (C).**   The amount of time spent on the telephone is a unique feature of ambulatory nursing practice. Although there may be some coordination activities involved in the nurse's role, these activities are not the major aspects. Telephone activities include assessing patients' response to the treatment given, providing information about prevention of side effects and symptoms, and evaluating patient outcomes. Patient care–oriented calls can have multiple purposes: communication of changes in the care plan, reassurance of the patient and family about side effects, instructions to lessen the severity of the side effect, and assessment of supportive services. (1388)

8.   **The answer is (C).**   A patient diary can be helpful in identifying side effects and responses to treatments and interventions, but it does not replace the need for documentation. Flow sheets can be specific to therapy side effects as well as patient care needs. They can decrease documentation time and improve consistency of charting details. Point-of-care computer terminals enable the nurse to enter data into the computer immediately, thus decreasing documentation time and improving accuracy. (1398)

9.   **The answer is (A).**   Maintaining a diary with recorded side effects, severity of each, and the recorded efficacy of self-care activities is an example of self-care actions. Any action initiated by the patient and family to prevent, detect, and manage side effects of radiation or chemotherapy can be defined as self-care. (1398)

55   Home Care

STUDY OUTLINE

I.   OVERVIEW OF HOME HEALTH CARE

1. Home health care is one of the most **rapidly growing** and changing fields in health care.
    a. In 1986, 1.6 million persons received an average of 24 home visits.
    b. From 1974 to 1986, Medicare program expenditures increased at an average annual rate of 23.6%.
    c. The number of home health agencies increased from 2250 in 1975 to approximately 5700 in 1990.
2. Factors influencing the consumption of health care services include the **increase in our elderly population and their increased life span, changes in family structure, and the increase in women working outside the home. The mobility of our society has decreased the support from family members who traditionally have provided the care needed to enable the elderly to remain in their homes.**
    a. Use of home health care services was significantly affected by the enactment in 1982 of the **prospective payment system (PPS)** for hospital care.
3. As defined by insurance eligibility guidelines, care at home can be **preventive, diagnostic, therapeutic, rehabilitative,** or **long-term maintenance care.**
4. Home health care is an **extension** of the medical care system in which a physician oversees the care, and the nurse is a primary provider and care manager through collaboration with the patient's physician.

A.   HOME CARE SERVICES

1. The goals of home health care are to **promote, maintain,** or **restore health; to minimize the effects of illness and disability;** or **to allow for a peaceful death.**
2. The services provided depend on the needs of the individual and the family.
3. **Nursing**
    a. Federal legislation has reinforced the position of nursing in home health care by **requiring that nursing services be available** in all home health agencies certified to receive Medicare or Medicaid funds.
    b. Home care nursing **responsibilities** include assessment, direct physical care, evaluation of patient progress, patient and family teaching, supervision and coordination of patient care, and provision of psychosocial support.
    c. Home health care nursing **differs** from private duty nursing in that care is provided on an intermittent basis rather than daily or for extended time periods.
4. **Homemaker-home health aide**
    a. The **homemaker-home health aide** is responsible for assisting with personal hygiene and homemaking tasks.
    b. The aide must have successfully completed a **home health aide certification course** and is **supervised by the home care nurse.**
    c. Aides do **feeding, bathing,** and **grooming** and may also do **marketing, laundry,** and **light housekeeping.**
5. **Physical therapy**
    a. **Physical therapists** provide **maintenance, preventative,** and **restorative treatment** for individuals at home to promote patient functioning to the optimal level.
    b. **Physical therapy** emphasizes **restorative function** in the home care setting, because Medicare restricts reimbursement to restorative work.

6. **Occupational therapy**
   a. **Occupational therapists** assist individuals to achieve their highest functional level and to be as self-reliant as possible.
   b. **Occupational therapy** helps the individual to develop and maintain the ability to perform **those tasks essential to daily living.**
   c. Occupational therapists use adaptive equipment, prostheses, and splints.
7. **Speech and language pathology**
   a. **Speech pathologists** provide therapy to individuals with communication problems of speech, language, or hearing and those with swallowing disorders.
8. **Social work**
   a. **Social workers** work as referral agents, counselors, and patient advocates.
9. **Nutrition services**
   a. **Nutrition services** consist of diet counseling, staff consultation, and education.
   b. Direct patient counseling is often not covered by third-party payers.
10. **Additional care services**
    a. A diverse assortment of services for the patient in the home are provided by physicians, dentists, chiropodists, respiratory therapists, vocational rehabilitation personnel, barbers, hairdressers, in-home companions, and homemaker/chore workers.

B. **TYPES OF HOME CARE AGENCIES**

1. Selection of the most appropriate type of home care agencies is based primarily on
   a. Patient/family needs.
   b. Financial arrangement or health care insurance.
   c. Family and community support.
   d. Type of home care services available in the patient's community.
2. Three classifications of agencies provide home care:
   a. Official public health agencies.
   b. Medicare-certified home health agencies.
   c. Private duty agencies.
3. **Official public health agencies**
   a. **Official public health agencies** are either city, county, or multicounty agencies. They are usually prevention-oriented, and nurses visit on a weekly or biweekly basis.
   b. A number of official public health departments have expanded the scope of their services and have developed Medicare-certified home health agencies.
4. **Medicare-certified home health agencies**
   a. **Medicare-certified home health agencies** are operated within the guidelines of the HFCA so that they can be reimbursed by Medicare and Medicaid.
   b. Private insurers usually require Medicare certification for their reimbursement as well.
5. **Private duty agencies**
   a. Private duty agencies provide nursing care in the home by registered nurses, licensed practical nurses, home health aides, or companions for specific periods of time.
   b. Services may be contracted and paid for by the patient or family or arranged through a case manager from the patient's health insurance company.
6. **Other agencies**
   a. As home care agencies have become more comprehensive in scope, other agencies have emerged, such as **durable medical equipment (DME)** companies and infusion therapy agencies.
   b. DME companies provide medical equipment and supplies, including respiratory equipment, ostomy appliances, and parenteral feedings and supplies.
   c. **Infusion therapy agencies** provide parenteral medications, total parenteral nutritional feedings, parenteral solutions, infusion devices, and equipment necessary for provision of infusion therapy at home.

C. **CONTINUITY OF CARE**

1. The processes most frequently used to ensure a comprehensive multidisciplinary approach to patient care are case management and discharge planning.
2. **Case management**
   a. Case management is a multidisciplinary approach identifying patient needs and coordinating the appropriate use of services and the health care system.

3. **Discharge planning**
    a. Discharge planning is an **interdisciplinary** approach that centers on the family or significant other to facilitate the transition of the patient from one level of care to another.
    b. A continuing care program begins with a **comprehensive assessment** of patient needs and the patient's and family's ability to comply with the treatment plans and cope with the disease.
    c. The majority of individuals diagnosed with cancer whose situations are appropriate for home care have **advanced disease** that is metastatic and incurable but not imminently terminal.
    d. The potential for success in home care is increased if the types of home health services necessary to assist with the supervision and management of the patient are available.
        (1) The degree of **informal support** available also affects the family's ability to manage home care, referring to support systems such as friends, neighbors, and church groups.
        (2) Continuity of care can be enhanced through the appropriate use of community resources.
    e. The continuing care plan developed by the discharge planner or case manager in the acute care setting includes goals based on essential assessment data and interventions that address the patient's overall care needs.
    f. To promote continuity of care, it is essential to have **effective communication** between the referring professionals and the community service agency staff who are caring for the patient during the next phase of care.
    g. **Shortened hospital stays** have resulted in the early discharge of cancer patients with highly complex treatment plans that must be managed in the home by families.

D. **UNIQUE CHARACTERISTICS OF THE HOME**

    1. The home presents the nurse with **conditions** unlike those encountered in other health care settings.
    2. In the home, the patient and family determine when and how the patient's plan of care will be implemented.
    3. The overall goal of home care is to have the **patient and family assume responsibility for the care** of the patient. When an individual or family member states how things will be done, it reflects a desire to maintain independence.
    4. It is critical that the home health care nurse **evaluate** the physical and financial conditions to support the care required by the patient at home.

II. **ROLE OF THE NURSE IN HOME HEALTH**

    1. The advances in treatment of disease and changes in reimbursement of health care services have shifted the focus of home care nursing in the 1990s to one that emphasizes care of the acutely ill patient in the home.

A. **THE PATIENT AND FAMILY AS THE UNIT OF CARE**

    1. For home health nursing care to be successful, the nurse assesses the family's structure and processes, develops a plan of care that is congruent with the family's values and lifestyle, and includes the patient and family in the decision-making process.
    2. Three types of family units identified are **supportive, ambivalent,** and **hostile.**
        a. The way a family functioned in the past is generally the way it will confront the current crisis of cancer.
        b. Family behavior can be described in terms of **cohesion, adaptability,** and **communication.**
            (1) Cohesion is the emotional bonding of family members.
            (2) Adaptability is the ability to change structures, roles, and relationships.
            (3) Family communication is a facilitator; it can enhance or restrict movement on the cohesion and adaptability dimensions.
    3. **Family assessment**
        a. Assessment of family organizations begins with obtaining a **history of family functioning, ages, geographic location, socioeconomic status, cultural and ethnic background, roles, relationship to patient, developmental level, major stressors, alliances,** and **frictions.**

b. In addition to the previous criteria, the assessment includes **patterns of authority, level of family development, values, behavior, coping ability, health and functional status, stressors, support systems,** and **knowledge of the illness and health practices.**

c. See **text page 1408** for questions that should be addressed during assessment of the family.

4. **Demands on caregivers**

a. Most caregivers report that the patient's daily physical needs are being met by immediate relatives and close friends.

b. The problem most often identified was a **lack of knowledge in management of the patient's physical symptoms, such as pain,** and **nutritional** and **elimination problems.**

c. Caregivers have reported a decrease in their abilities to cope when changes occur in the patient's health status.

   (1) See **Table 55-1, text page 1409,** for home care situations that have been identified as evoking the greatest stress for families and caregivers.

d. The nursing intervention most often cited by patients and caregivers as the most helpful is for the nurse to give excellent, knowledgeable, skilled, and personalized nursing care to the patient.

   (1) See **Table 55-2, text page 1409,** for other helpful nursing interventions.

B. **IMPLEMENTATION OF THE NURSING PROCESS**

1. **Assessment**

a. The assessment of health problems in the home setting includes the patient's **actual** and **potential health problems** as well as relevant characteristics of the family and the environment.

   (1) See **Table 55-3, text page 1410,** for assessment parameters at the time of admission.

2. **Planning**

a. The problem areas of comfort, nutrition, protective mechanisms, mobility, elimination, sexuality, ventilation, and circulation provide the framework for assessment and planning.

   (1) See **Table 55-4, text page 1411,** for a detailed tool to anticipate requirements.

3. **Nursing interventions**

a. Nursing functions and activities in home health assist the patient and family by providing direct care and treatment, supervision of patient care, health and disease management, teaching, counseling, and coordination of health care services.

   (1) See **Table 55-5, text page 1412,** for detailed interventions.

4. **Evaluation**

a. **Outcome measures** can be used to assess the quality of nursing care in specific areas based on predictable results.

   (1) Outcome measures are influenced by the multifactorial aspects of a patient's care environment and the natural history of the disease, which are beyond the nurse's control.

C. **COORDINATION OF SERVICES**

1. **Coordination** and **collaboration skills** are essential to promote continuity of care from the acute care setting, coordination of services in the home setting, and achievement of rehabilitation goals.

2. Care coordination and collaborative activities of the home health nurse often expand to become **case management,** especially when the patient has advanced metastatic disease or severe functional limitations.

D. **DOCUMENTING NURSING CARE**

1. **Legal responsibilities** of the home health oncology nurse include knowledge of and compliance with the nursing role as defined in the state Nurse Practice Act, the regulations that govern home health, and the standards of nursing practice for the nurse's community.

2. The best evidence that the nurse has **complied** with these regulations and standards is the documentation of patient care.

a. Documentation must be complete, clear, accurate, objective, and timely to fulfill federal and state certification requirements and Medicare and third-party reimbursement requirements.

b. **Inadequate documentation implies inadequate nursing care** and negatively affects the agency's fulfillment of state licensure and certification requirements, delays or prohibits third-party reimbursement, places the agency at risk of a legal suit, and reflects a negative image of the agency and the quality of care provided.

c. The legal criterion for timeliness is the recording of an event at the time the care is given.

E. **REHABILITATION NURSING**

1. The **underlying concepts** of rehabilitation focus on interdisciplinary collaboration, comprehensive services, self-care, maximum function, prevention, family and cultural values, and the patient and family as a unity of care in the community.

2. When patients and families become co-partners with the rehabilitation team, they **contract mutually agreeable goals,** foster empowerment, educate for self-care, and enhance positive behaviors.

3. **Education** is the key to enhancing patient independence and promoting self-care.

4. The greatest needs of patients with cancer and their caregivers have been found to be primarily **psychological** and **informational.**

5. The debilitating sequelae of cancer and treatment often necessitate the use of adaptive equipment to maintain the optimal level of independence and meaningful activity.

6. Encouraging the patient and family to develop networks and supports in the community fosters independence and facilitates patient discharge from the home health agency.

7. To **prevent fragmentation of care,** referrals to appropriate agencies are carefully timed so they can begin their services when the patient is discharged from home health care.

8. As the disease advances and ability to maintain activities for independent functioning wanes, it is important to recognize that cancer patients are likely to need services such as personal care, meal preparation, shopping, housekeeping, and transportation.

F. **ROLE OF THE ONCOLOGY CLINICAL NURSE SPECIALIST (OCNS)**

1. **Practitioner role**
   a. **Direct care** activities provided by the OCNS in home health care include advanced services and skills not usually available from the general nursing staff.
   b. **Restructuring** the OCNS's role to include sharing complex cases with staff nurses provides the opportunity for the OCNS to increase the knowledge of agency staff in new complex skills, fosters patient and family confidence when the OCNS is not available, and increases the availability of the OCNS to additional patients.

2. **Educator role**
   a. Educational activities for both **individual** and **group** instruction of staff and families are usually included in the OCNS role.

3. **Consultant role**
   a. Consultation may include assisting staff with managing difficult cases or providing information to improve their skills, knowledge, self-assurance, or objectivity.
   b. The OCNS may develop or revise agency programs or assist with counseling staff.

4. **Researcher role**
   a. Research activity for the OCNS varies from the basics of interpreting, evaluating, and communicating research findings to caregivers to the advanced level of research collaboration and actively generating or replicating research projects.

5. **Evaluation of the OCNS role in home health**
   a. Evaluation of the OCNS role is **limited.**
   b. The OCNS has produced revenues through home visits, participated in revisions of policies, procedures, and charting forms; developed and conducted nursing process audits; served as home health liaisons to community health care organizations; and participated in professional oncology nursing activities in the community.

III. **ECONOMIC ISSUES**

A. **FINANCING HOME HEALTH CARE**

1. Knowledge of the services, equipment, and supplies covered by the individual's insurance is essential.

2. Home health services available to **Medicare recipients** include nursing, physical therapy, speech therapy, occupational therapy, home health aid, and social work services.
3. **Medicare eligibility requirements** state that the beneficiary must be homebound and require skilled nursing, physical therapy, or speech and language pathology services ordered by a physician.
4. Services must be provided on a **part-time, intermittent basis.**
   a. **Intermittent** is currently defined as services required at least every 60 days and daily visits limited to 21 consecutive days or having a predictable and finite end if daily visits extend beyond 21 days.
5. **Medicare reimburses** at the lower end of a reasonable cost or agency charge, up to a limit that is set annually by the U.S. Health Care Financing Administration (HCFA).
6. **Medicaid funding** for home health services is a joint federal-state assistance program for the poor of all ages.
   a. Federal regulations require states to provide a minimum range of home health services, including part-time nursing care, home health aides, medical supplies, and equipment.
   b. **States** receive matching funds for their expenditures and are allowed extensive flexibility in determining eligibility, services, and reimbursement.
7. **Private insurance carriers** vary significantly in their coverage for home health services and should be contacted prior to admission to determine the patient's specific coverage.

B. DOCUMENTING FOR REIMBURSEMENT

1. Accurate and comprehensive nursing documentation, although time-consuming and requiring thoughtful deliberation, is essential for procuring reimbursement.

C. HOME CARE FOR THE SOCIALLY DISADVANTAGED

1. Since home health reimbursement by payers is computed on the cost per visit, most home health agencies have **limited funds** available for services to persons without home health insurance.
2. The Medicare home health benefit does **not** cover long-term or chronic care.
3. When a patient has a limited income, the oncology home care staff are faced with the problem of locating a community service agency that provides follow-up monitoring and support services for personal care or homemaking without cost.
4. **States have been slow to expand home care services** because soaring costs have strained the state Medicaid budget.
5. In 1989, the HCFA **expanded reimbursable home health services** to include assessment, monitoring, teaching, and revisions of the plan of care for persons whose condition has stabilized but who are at risk for complications or require frequent unskilled care from caregivers.
   a. Implementation of this benefit has been **limited.**
   b. Agencies must interpret its "management and evaluation" terms, identify categories for patient selection, determine appropriate criteria to be included in documentation, and evaluate the extent of Medicare reimbursement.

IV. ETHICAL CONCERNS

1. Personal lifestyle, financial means, possessions, routines, and family structures may not be conducive to the provision of health care in the home.
2. Ethical concerns of home health providers are **primarily**
   a. Maintaining agency solvency while not denying care to indigent patients.
   b. Responding to conflicts between patients and families.
   c. Providing care to abused or neglected patients.
   d. Candidly addressing decisions about treatment with the terminally ill.
3. Home health nurses are usually familiar with the ethical principles of **advocacy for patient autonomy** and the **patient's right of self-determination** to refuse treatment when incapacitated.

A. MORAL VALUES

1. The values of the patient, family, and caregiver are not usually known when a patient is admitted to home care, nor are they easily assessed during the initial visit.

2. **Ongoing assessment** of the values of the patient, family, and caregivers is essential to identify potential ethical conflicts and plan for nursing care that is comparable with their needs and values.

B. **ETHICAL PRINCIPLES**

1. The six principles of autonomy, beneficence, justice, veracity, confidentiality, and fidelity identified by the ANA Code for Nurses should be used by the nurse as guides to action.
    a. **Autonomy.** Conflicts arise in the home setting if a patient's decisions are detrimental to his or her health.
    b. **Beneficence.** A conflict may occur for the home care nurse when the patient lives in an apartment or neighborhood that is a risk to the personal safety of the nurse or when threats or attempts to do bodily harm may necessitate closing or not opening a case to a home care service.
    c. **Justice.** The principle of justice guides the nurse to treat all persons equally and to give individuals what is owed to them by another person or society.
    d. **Veracity.** Conflicts may arise when the family or caregivers insist that the patient not be given specific information because it may distress the patient.
    e. **Confidentiality** requires the nurse to respect and hold confidential all information shared by the patient.
    f. **Fidelity** requires the nurse to be faithful to his or her commitments and profession.

C. **ETHICAL DECISION MAKING**

1. When conflict occurs, the nurse uses a **decision-making process** to assess the problem and potential courses of action and to consider what is right or good on the basis of the ethical principles and values of the persons involved.
    a. See **Table 55-6, text page 1418,** for the process of ethical decision making.

V. **INFUSION THERAPY IN THE HOME**

1. Infusion therapy is one of the most rapidly growing segments of home care.
2. The growth of home infusion therapy has been stimulated by **cost-containment pressure from third-party payers, the increase in the aging population,** and **advances in technology that have increased the safety, effectiveness, and availability of home infusion therapies.**
3. Advanced technology has produced an array of **long-term central venous access devices** and **infusion pumps that simplify parenteral administration of drugs in the home** and have less risk for complications.
4. The **peripherally inserted central catheter (PICC)** is used frequently in the home because it can be inserted by a nurse who is certified in the procedure.
5. Home health management of the cancer patient receiving infusion therapy that incorporates sophisticated infusion pumps and VADs focuses on caring for the patient and family rather than on management of the equipment.
6. Communication between the infusion therapy personnel and the home health nurse for coordination of services and delineation of responsibilities will also decrease patient and family confusion and anxiety. Examples include a **joint visit** by the home health and infusion therapy nurses at the patient's home when home infusion therapy is initiated and an infusion therapy/home care record.

A. **CHEMOTHERAPY ADMINISTRATION**

1. The demand for more cost-effective methods of treating cancer patients has stimulated the development of comprehensive services, including administration of chemotherapy.
2. **Criteria for patient selection**
    a. See **text page 1419** for specific criteria that must be met for chemotherapy administration in the home.
    b. Insurance **reimbursement** for antineoplastic drugs, equipment, supplies, and nursing services varies and should be reviewed prior to referring a patient for home chemotherapy.
3. **Policies for chemotherapy administration**
    a. See **text page 1419** for specific policies and procedures of home health agencies that offer

chemotherapy. Such policies address patient eligibility, approved drugs, laboratory parameters, administration procedures, criteria for withholding chemotherapy, and educational requirements for the nurses involved.

    b. Some agencies **limit** approved antineoplastic agents given at home to nonvesicant and noncaustic drugs.

    c. An agency must determine whether the nurses will perform **venipunctures** if a VAD is not in use.

    d. Specific **hematologic parameters** must be designated for white blood cell and platelet levels at which chemotherapy will or will not be administered.

4. **Staff education**

    a. Nurses eligible to administer chemotherapy at home must understand the purpose, action, and side effects of the drugs.

    b. They must also know how to prepare and dispose of the drugs and operate the equipment involved.

5. **Safety considerations**

    a. **Potential risks** to persons who come into contact with chemotherapy drugs and associated safety measures should be discussed with the patient and family prior to the initial home chemotherapy treatment.

    b. Safety considerations include transport of drugs, preparation of drugs, spills, patient care, and disposal.

        (1) **Transport of drugs:** The drugs should be labeled as cytotoxic, securely capped or sealed, and packaged in an impervious packing material for transport.

        (2) **Preparation of drugs:** An area of the patient's home that is apart from frequent family activity and food preparation should be selected to prepare drugs.

            (a) A closable, puncture-resistant, shatter-resistant container is necessary for the disposal of contaminated sharp or breakable materials.

            (b) While administering antineoplastic drugs, observe universal precautions for preventing transmission of HIV, hepatitis B virus, and other blood-borne pathogens.

        (3) **Spills:** Liquids and solids are wiped up with absorbent pads or gauze, and the area is cleaned three times with detergent solution and rinsed with clean water. Protective equipment is needed for cleanup and disposal.

        (4) **Patient care:** Blood, emesis, and excreta from patients who have received antineoplastic agents within 48 hours may be contaminated, and precautions must be taken.

        (5) **Disposal:** When administration is completed, all items that have been in contact with the drug are wrapped in an absorbent pad and placed into the plastic bag labeled "Biologic Hazard."

6. **Patient and family responsibilities**

    a. **Written information** about potential side effects is provided along with the descriptions of symptoms that need to be reported immediately to the physician or nurse.

    b. Nontraditional methods of chemotherapy administration, such as **continuous infusion** and **regional infusion** of antineoplastic drugs, are being used more frequently today since these methods can increase exposure of tumor cells to higher total dose of drug, theoretically increasing tumor cell kill.

    c. **Reimbursement** for chemotherapy administration in the home varies according to the reimbursement policies of the third-party payers.

B. **HOME PARENTERAL NUTRITION**

1. The administration of parenteral nutrition at home is a rapidly growing option for cost-effective and beneficial therapy for the malnourished patient with cancer.

2. **Criteria for patient selection**

    a. See **text page 1422,** column 2, for certain criteria that are recommended for acceptance of a patient into a home parenteral nutrition (HPN) program.

    b. The patient and family must assume **primary responsibility** for the administration of HPN.

    c. The patient's **medical insurance** must be reviewed by the discharge planner or home infusion company to determine HPN coverage.

3. **Initial home assessment**

    a. The initial visit by the home care nurse should occur soon after the patient's arrival at home and should coincide with the arrival of the supplies, equipment, medication, and home infusion therapy company personnel.

    (1)   It is essential that agencies administering HPN provide **24-hour service.**

  b. The initial assessment **includes** the type and status of the venous access device, the patient's and family's knowledge of the management of HPN, and evaluation of the home environment for safety and cleanliness factors required for HPN.

  c. Most acute care facilities have developed complete teaching programs.

  d. Adequate **refrigeration** must be available in the home to store the 2- to 4-week supply of solutions. Most infusion companies will provide a small refrigerator if needed.

  4. **Nursing management**

    a. The role of the nurse encompasses ongoing assessment and evaluation of the patient's status, direct patient care, supervision of the patient/family management of HPN, and **patient/family education.**

    b. HPN is often administered over 10–16 hours, including the patient's sleeping time.

    c. A **flow sheet** for documenting monitoring tasks is necessary, and the facts that must be recorded can be found on **text page 1423,** column 2.

C. INTRAVENOUS ANTIBIOTIC THERAPY

1. Antibiotic therapy is the most commonly used IV therapy at home.

2. Home parenteral antibiotic therapy (HPAT) is a preferred method for delivering a course of therapy for many infectious diseases because of the **significant cost savings** as compared with hospitalization costs.

3. **Criteria for patient selection**

  a. See **text pages 1423–1424** for criteria for patient selection for HPAT.

4. **Nursing management**

  a. Infusion therapy agencies with pharmacies will prepare and deliver the antibiotics and the supplies on schedule.

  b. During the active treatment phase, nursing visits may vary in frequency from three times a day to once a week.

    (1)   On each visit, the nurse monitors **vital signs, laboratory tests, equipment operation, supplies, adverse drug effects,** and **signs/symptoms of complications.**

  c. In the cases where the **infusion rate** is a critical factor in administration, it is preferable to use a mechanized infusion pump.

  d. Factors such as dosing interval and adverse effects profile are important in selecting a drug.

  e. Consideration must be given to the **stability** of the medication and type of storage required.

  f. **Patient education** is the key to safe administration of antibiotics in the home.

  g. **Reimbursement** for HPAT varies according to the reimbursement policies of the individual third-party payer.

  h. A **quality assurance instrument** for at-home IV antibiotic care has been developed that identifies outcome criteria in six areas: infusion-related complications, drug-related complications, home care management, psychosocial response of patient/caregiver, cost, and recovery.

D. PAIN MANAGEMENT

1. Six principles of pain management in the home setting can be reviewed on **text page 1425,** column 1.

2. The **oral route** for analgesic administration is preferable for long-term cancer pain management for a number of reasons: comfort, ease of administration, increased compliance, no restriction of movement, and no equipment requirement.

3. **Morphine** is the prototype agent for cancer pain and is often the analgesic of choice, since it is easy to use, safe, versatile, effective, and well tolerated.

4. **Intermittent** or **continuous infusion pain therapy** is being utilized in the home setting by a variety of routes: subcutaneous, intravenous, epidural, and subarachnoid.

  a. The epidural or subarachnoid route is indicated for pain that is **refractory to analgesics** administered by conventional means and for analgesics that have produced severe, intolerable side effects that cannot be modified by alterations in drug therapy.

5. Patients and families are taught preparation and administration procedures, dressing change procedures, and emergency administration of naloxone for severe respiratory depression.

6. **Patient-controlled analgesia (PCA)** provides the ability to self-administer medication and manage pain.
    a. This produces a sense of control for patients that seems to decrease feelings of powerlessness and vulnerability.
    b. Small, portable, computerized PCA pumps are available for home use.
7. Difficulty in **obtaining** narcotics for home use must be considered. Community pharmacies do not routinely stock potent narcotics and may need 1 or 2 weeks to obtain the drugs.
8. Measures other than narcotic analgesics to decrease pain may be more effective in the comfort of the patient's home. These methods include behavioral strategies and relaxation techniques.
9. Assessment of pain is **ongoing.** A change in the location, severity, or type of pain may indicate an acute problem that requires other interventions.
10. Patients and caregivers often **negatively influence** the treatment of pain as a result of their fears about potent narcotics.
    a. They may increase the dose interval, withhold doses, or refuse certain medications or certain routes as they attempt to prevent dependence, addiction, somnolence, or sedation.

VI.   DISCHARGE FROM HOME HEALTH CARE

1. It is **rarely** the case that individuals receive care for longer than necessary, since the overall goal of home health care is to facilitate the patient's and family's independence in managing daily life within the constraints imposed by the malignant disease. See **Table 55-9, text page 1427,** for components of a discharge plan.
2. Guidelines for reimbursable services are specific, and services are monitored so that home health services are discontinued or modified when the **level of care** required by the person changes.
3. The obvious reason for discontinuing home health services is that the patient and family have **achieved the identified outcomes** developed by the nurse, patient, and family.
4. Patients will be discharged from home health care when an exacerbation of the disease process produces symptoms that require management in an inpatient setting or when service needs change.
5. An **area of concern** in patient discharge from home health care occurs when the patient and family desire to continue services but the nurse must discharge the patient because his or her physical status has changed and no longer meets the requirements for reimbursable home health care.
6. When one is **evaluating** the discharge process, important points to consider and document are the patient's status on discharge, evidence of planning for discharge, and timeliness of the decision to discharge.

VII.   QUALITY ASSESSMENT IN HOME CARE

1. Quality assessment as an **evaluation strategy** is essential in home health care in light of recently enacted federal regulations; the increased risks associated with expanded, highly technological services; and a growing industry's need to quantify credibility.
2. A quality assessment program begins with identification and adoption of standards for home health care.
3. Quality is evaluated by the level of achievement of each identified standard of care.
4. Health care providers, recipients, payers, and the general public are attempting to design new models to define quality and effective systems to assess, monitor, and improve the care provided to patients.
    a. A sample of quality indicators appears in **Table 55-10, text page 1427.**

PRACTICE QUESTIONS

1. The potential for success in home care is **increased** by the
    (A) support received by friends and family.
    (B) degree of complexity of care.
    (C) age of the patient.
    (D) need for colostomy.

2. Homebound is defined as
    (A) being able to leave one's home only with great difficulty.
    (B) being confined to a wheelchair.
    (C) requiring home care for over 35 hours per week.
    (D) requiring intermittent care.

3. The family assessment in home care is **least** likely to include which of the following questions?
    (A) What is the pattern of authority at home?
    (B) What is the functionality of the caregiver?
    (C) How many fire exits are available?
    (D) What other support systems are there?

4. In the nurse's planning of home care, which of the following measures is **most** important?
    (A) Schedule extra visits during the working stage.
    (B) Avoid upsetting the family by discussing possible emergency situations.
    (C) Wait until discharge to order materials and supplies.
    (D) Be realistic about expected outcomes.

5. One of the nurse's roles in home parenteral nutrition (HPN) is to
    (A) keep records of times of infusion, intake, and output.
    (B) deliver supplies, equipment, and medicines to the patient.
    (C) evaluate the patient, the home environment, and the family's ability to manage HPN.
    (D) perform all infusion regimens at home.

6. Accurate and timely documentation is crucial to the solvency of a home care agency since it is required for
    (A) reimbursement.
    (B) continued referrals.
    (C) medical consultations.
    (D) access to hospital records.

7. Upon conducting a family assessment, the home health care nurse identifies conflict among the family members caring for the patient. Upon inquiry, the nurse learns that the conflict is "not new" and has existed "for years." Utilizing this information, the home health care nurse establishes a plan of care that
    (A) attempts to change the behavior among the family members since the patient is upset by the conflict.
    (B) involves having psychological services counsel the "conflicting members."
    (C) schedules family meetings about how the conflict is affecting the patient and what can be done to resolve it.
    (D) is sensitive to the feelings of the members in conflict but does not attempt to treat the causes of the conflict.

8. Which of the following activities would most likely **not** be found in the oncology clinical nurse specialist's job description in the home health care setting?
    (A) Revise nursing practice standards according to research findings.
    (B) Maintain a caseload of all the complex patients.
    (C) Present weekly patient care conferences.
    (D) Conduct nursing audits as needed.

9. A **major advantage** of the peripherally inserted central catheter (PICC), in addition to long-term life span, is that
    (A) it does not require frequent flushing due to the one-way valve.
    (B) dressing changes are simpler and more cost-effective.
    (C) it can be inserted by a certified home health nurse.
    (D) it has a separate designated port for blood withdrawal.

10. The overall goal of home care is
    (A) to provide complete and holistic care for the patient.
    (B) to assist the patient in a peaceful death with dignity.
    (C) to provide palliative care.
    (D) for patients and families to assume responsibility for the care.

11.   Guidelines for the handling of antineoplastic agents in the home are in accordance with those established by:
      (A)   the Food and Drug Administration.
      (B)   the Occupational Safety and Health Administration.
      (C)   the American Nurse's Association.
      (D)   the Health Care Financing Administration.

12.   Which of the following activities or facts is the home health care nurse most likely **not** to teach the patient and/or family in order to ensure safe antibiotic administration in the home?
      (A)   at what temperature to store the medication
      (B)   what signs/symptoms of drug side effects to report
      (C)   how to withdraw heparin from a vial
      (D)   how to prepare and mix the antibiotic

13.   Upon a return visit to a man with metastatic prostate cancer to the ribs, the home health nurse notes that he is in pain and has not been receiving the morphine at the increased frequency prescribed 48 hours earlier. The wife is visibly upset at his discomfort yet is confused by his increased lethargy when the drug interval was first changed. She does not understand why he is not reporting relief when she knows that he has been sleeping more. The nurse's interventions at this point would be directed at
      (A)   explaining to the wife that increasing the frequency of the drug is what probably gave him some pain relief and his sleep was a sign that he was comfortable.
      (B)   empathizing with the wife over her concerns that the decreased drug interval was a sign that her husband was becoming addicted.
      (C)   congratulating the wife for being astute enough to recognize that the drug was building up in his system.
      (D)   changing the pain regimen to include a different narcotic.

ANSWER EXPLANATIONS

1.   **The answer is (A).**   It is important to the family and the caregiver to be able to draw on other people and institutions for support at this time. Success in home care requires that the services needed be available, but the degree of informal support from family, friends, neighbors, church groups, and the like is critical. (1406)

2.   **The answer is (A).**   The homebound status is necessary for insurance and Medicare coverage, and it has to be established and documented by the health care nurse. Homebound means that leaving the home requires considerable effort. (1415)

3.   **The answer is (C).**   A detailed family assessment is important, particularly with regard to the status of the caregiver. Families are categorized as supportive, ambivalent, or hostile, and they generally continue to act in this crisis as they reacted to other crises in the past. (1407)

4.   **The answer is (D).**   Evaluation of care is based on patient outcomes. Expected outcomes should be realistic and achievable so that the patient, caregiver(s), and health care providers are able to provide good care and to feel a sense of satisfaction and accomplishment. The family should know what is realistic and achievable from the start. Choice (B) would be especially damaging—families are better off if they know how to deal with emergencies. (1410)

5.   **The answer is (C).**   Home care assessment for HPN begins with a visit coincidental with the arrival of equipment. The nurse should review orders for HPN with the supplying agency. The assessment should include the type and status of the venous access device, the patient and family's knowledge of the management of HPN, and an evaluation of the home for safety factors. Adequate refrigeration should be available in the home for a 2–3-week supply of solutions. An electric infusion pump with a battery backup is normally part of the equipment. Choices (A) and eventually (D) are handled by the family; (B) is done by the home infusion therapy company personnel. (1423)

6.   **The answer is (A).**   Accurate descriptive documentation of home health nursing care is vital to reimbursement and continuation of home health services. Articles have been published describing methods of documentation to ensure successful reimbursement. It has been postulated that the rise in health care expenditures, including those for home health care, has led the government and fiscal intermediaries to

enact regulations requiring specific documentation and has increased focused review in an effort to decrease costs by denial of payment for services designated by the reviewer as "noncovered." (1416)

7.   **The answer is (D).**   Family units can be identified as supportive, hostile, or ambivalent with behavior described in terms of cohesion, adaptability, and communication. When crisis occurs or families are faced with the serious and difficult implications of cancer and its treatment, their behavior does not change and in some cases can intensify. Therefore, if a family was dysfunctional, hostile, or in conflict, it is very likely that the behavior will continue. The home health care nurse's primary concern is to support and care for the patient. The chances are high that the home health care nurse would be unable to change the behavior of the family members in conflict. (1407–1408)

8.   **The answer is (B).**   Although the OCNS is particularly adept in management of complex physical and psychological care requirements, staff nurses may feel frustrated by the loss of challenging cases, the lack of freedom to select cases, and the absence of recognition for services they have provided in the past. Instead, complex cases could be used as teaching examples for the OCNS and the staff nurses. In addition, having the OCNS available for consultation on complex cases helps the staff nurses deliver quality care and fosters collegiality. (1414)

9.   **The answer is (C).**   The PICC catheter does require daily flushing and central line dressing changes as frequently as every 3–7 days. Although some PICC catheters have more than one lumen, any lumen can be used for blood withdrawal. The major advantage is that the catheter can be placed by specially trained nurses in the home without the patient's needing to go to the hospital or doctor's office. (1418–1419)

10.   **The answer is (D).**   Although care does consist of holistic and direct physical care, the ultimate goal is to enable the family and/or patient to provide the care. Choices (B) and (C) apply more to hospice care and not necessarily to home care. The patient and family are encouraged to assume responsibility for the care of the patient. (1407)

11.   **The answer is (B).**   Potential hazards associated with the administration of antineoplastic agents have prompted the Occupational Safety and Health Administration (OSHA) to set guidelines for compounding, transporting, administering, and disposing of toxic chemotherapy agents. (1421)

12.   **The answer is (D).**   It is important for the patient and/or family to know at what temperature to store the medication since consideration needs to be given to the stability of the drug. Signs and symptoms are important to know since the nurse will not be present at most infusions. Withdrawal of heparin and heparin administration are required following drug administration in order to keep the VAD patent. Infusion therapy agencies with pharmacies will prepare and deliver the antibiotics and the supplies on schedule. (1424)

13.   **The answer is (A).**   The husband is not becoming addicted but might be experiencing some degree of drug tolerance. This is normal, and it is not uncommon for drug doses to increase over time. He also might be having increased bone metastasis or other sites of pain; further assessment is required. Sleep is often the first sign of pain relief since patients may have been unable to rest comfortably with pain. Patients and caregivers often negatively influence the treatment of pain because of their fears about potent narcotics. They may increase the dose interval, withhold doses, or refuse certain medications or certain routes as they attempt to prevent dependence, addiction, somnolence, or sedation. The wife needs education regarding cancer pain and relief methods, as well as a great deal of support. (1426)

56 Hospice

STUDY OUTLINE

I. INTRODUCTION

1. Hospice care was developed to meet a simple objective: to facilitate a comfortable and natural death.

A. DEVELOPMENT OF HOSPICE CONCEPT

1. Developers of the hospice concept recognized that allowing a "natural death" requires **preparation** of the patient and family, changes in medical practice, and redesign or circumvention of some aspects of the existing health care system.
2. When hospices first began to appear as organized programs, they were commonly **volunteer programs** with lay volunteers and a few nurses, organized from a church basement or around someone's dining room table.

B. ROLE OF NURSES IN THE DEVELOPMENT OF HOSPICE

1. In the late nineteenth century hospice was applied to the care of the dying by Sister Mary Aikenhead, a colleague of Florence Nightingale, who opened Our Lady's Hospice, in Dublin, the first facility dedicated to care of the terminally ill.
2. Florence Wald resigned as dean of the Yale School of Nursing to participate in the development of the first American hospice, Connecticut Hospice Inc.
3. In 1984, the **Joint Commission on Accreditation of Hospitals (JCAH)** published its first standards manual for hospice programs.
4. Another factor influencing the development of palliative care was the ground-breaking work in the 1960s of **Elisabeth Kübler-Ross,** who pointed out that health care professionals, due largely to their own ineffectual coping with the subject of death, isolated dying patients.

II. PALLIATIVE CARE APPROACHES

1. Palliative management involves a **shift** in treatment goals from curative toward providing relief from suffering.
2. The emotional, spiritual, and existential co-components of suffering and pain must also be addressed.

A. PRINCIPLES OF PALLIATIVE CARE

1. See **text page 1434,** column 1, which lists the principles of palliative care, including
   a. Optimizing the quality of life.
   b. Death as a natural process.
   c. Minimizing tests and procedures.
   d. Discouraging the use of heroic measures.
   e. Appropriate pain relief.
   f. Symptom management.
   g. Individualized care.

B.   **PALLIATIVE VERSUS ACUTE CARE**

    1.   In a palliative care situation, the etiology generally is either already known or unimportant if the patient has a short time to live.

    2.   In an acute care situation, a patient will have diagnostic studies to determine the etiology of the problem.

C.   **PATIENT CRITERIA FOR HOSPICE CARE**

    1.   Each program determines its own criteria for selecting patients to receive hospice care.

    2.   To qualify for the **Medicare Hospice Benefit,** two physicians must certify that a person is terminally ill and has less than 6 months to live.

    3.   Another criterion under Medicare and most state hospice regulations is that the patients sign a consent form or election statement declaring that hospice and palliative care are their choice of treatments and that they have the right to elect out of hospice at any time.

    4.   Additional criteria required by most hospice programs:

        a.   The patient must have a primary caregiver.

        b.   The patient needs to reside in the hospice program's geographic area.

        c.   The patient must agree to palliative, not curative treatment.

        d.   Some programs require that the patient have a DNR status prior to admission to the hospice program.

III.   **HOSPICE CARE IN THE PRESENT**

    1.   Development of a hospice program is not as simple as it was in the early phases of the hospice movement.

    2.   Hospice programs have been affected by mandated guidelines of **federal** and **state legislation.**

A.   **MODELS OF HOSPICE CARE**

    1.   A recent National Hospice Organization (NHO) study indicated that 40% of all hospices were **independent, community-based programs.**

    2.   Hospice progams may contract with hospitals for inpatient care.

        a.   Beds in the **hospital** for hospice patients may be scattered in the medical or oncology units.

        b.   Care is focused on **symptom management** and limiting invasive or painful procedures, and often patients **return home** after symptoms have been alleviated and they are medically stable.

    3.   According to Medicare's guidelines, at least 80% of an individual hospice's **aggregate patient days of care** under the Hospice Benefit must be provided at home.

    4.   The **annual per-patient reimbursement cap** is applied on an aggregate basis.

    5.   The NHO study found that two of every three hospice programs were **Medicare certified.**

    6.   Medicare guidelines **dictate** that a full-service hospice be a medically directed, nurse-coordinated program that incorporates social services along with pastoral counseling and trained volunteers to complete the nucleus of its core services.

        a.   See **Figure 56-1, text page 1436,** for a diagram of various disciplines and services involved to provide hospice care.

B.   **REIMBURSEMENT AND FUNDING METHODS**

    1.   **Per diem** is a system of reimbursement that pays a flat daily rate for all services provided to a patient, rather than paying for the individual services or items.

    2.   The per diem for the Medicare Hospice Benefit is **reimbursed on four levels** as defined by the Health Care Finance Administration (HCFA).

        a.   A routine rate.

        b.   A continuous rate for home care.

        c.   An inpatient rate for acute care, and an inpatient rate for respite care.

    3.   **Recertification** of the patient's appropriateness for hospice care is required three times under the benefit.

    4.   **Eighty-nine percent of current hospices** are operated **not** for profit.

C.   **PATIENT POPULATION**

1.   Of 206,000 patients and families who received hospice care in 1990, 84% were diagnosed with cancer; 4% had AIDS; 3% had cerebral vascular disease; the remaining 9% had other terminal conditions.
2.   Hospice is **evolving** to include patients of differing age groups who have more complex physical and psychosocial concerns.
      a.   See **Tables 56-1 and 56-2, text pages 1437–1439,** for a case study that demonstrates some of the unique challenges presented by a young patient with AIDS.

IV.   **NURSING AND HOSPICE CARE**

A.   **NURSE'S ROLE**

1.   The nurse works cooperatively and communicates effectively within a **multidisciplinary framework** actively to promote holistic palliative care for hospice patients and their families.
2.   The nurse demonstrates self-direction and **initiative** in the role as practitioner, educator, and consultant.
3.   Good **communication skills,** both verbal and written, enable the nurse to foster cooperation within the team and to fulfill federal and state medical record documentation requirements adequately.
4.   The ability of the nurse to **foster** a relaxed, warm, personal relationship with the patient, family, and other team members helps to promote confidence in achieving the goals of care.

B.   **MANAGEMENT OF CARE ISSUES**

1.   The nurse often provides **basic nursing care,** such as skin care, care of central venous lines, checking compliance with medication regimens, and indwelling catheter management.
2.   **Ongoing assessment of pain** is an activity best accomplished with a formal assessment tool.
3.   The nurse performs a general assessment of body systems with each home visit.
4.   The **goal of hospice** is to provide palliative care in the home; therefore, effective physical assessment skills can make a difference in identifying a potential problem early enough for timely intervention to occur.
      a.   See **Tables 56-3 and 56-4, text pages 1440–1442,** on selected principles and approaches for symptom management in palliative care: pain, dyspnea, seizures, diarrhea, and constipation.
5.   The **consultative** role of the nurse comes into play when a patient is referred to hospice to be assessed for potential admission into the hospice program.
6.   The attending physician is contacted to determine **reason for referral, do-not-resuscitate status, expected prognosis,** and **appropriate medical information.**

V.   **DEATH IN THE HOME**

1.   The hospice care philosophy is uniquely characterized by its approach to facilitating a person's death at home.
2.   It is common, if not universal, for patients and families to respond initially to the idea of death at home with **fear** and **anxiety,** because many adults have never seen anyone die.
3.   Patients' overriding concerns about death at home often revolve around being a **burden** to their family.
4.   Family caregivers are concerned about their **emotional ability to cope** with a home death and the potential effects on other family members, particularly when children are in the home.
5.   For most families, the ability to provide care for a home death will **require teaching** them about the death event itself, immediate signs of death, how to relieve symptoms and suffering, and how to access professional help if needed.

A.   **ADVANTAGES OF HOME DEATH**

1.   The approach of death evokes **feelings of loss** in a dying person.
      a.   **Loss of control** may be the most overwhelming and distressing feeling, which can be further intensified by hospitalization.
      b.   The patient at home maintains the opportunity to interact with neighbors, children, and pets.

    c.   Rather than being protected from the illness and death, children can benefit from being involved in very concrete ways to understand the dying process better and facilitate their own grief.

  2. Another major loss for patients is **diminishment of their role** as a contributing, social being.

    a.   Being cared for at home can afford the opportunity for an alert patient to maintain his or her family role.

  3. A final and obvious advantage of home death is that it is much less likely that unwanted medical intervention will be ordered for a terminally ill person at home than for one in a hospital or nursing home setting.

  4. The **greatest potential risk** for a home patient to receive unwanted medical intervention arises if the Emergency Medical System (EMS) is accessed, since this can result in unplanned and unwanted resuscitation and, ultimately, ventilator care.

B.   DISADVANTAGES OF HOME DEATH

  1. Caregivers, particularly those **lacking social outlets** or family support, may find the physical and emotional task of home care and home death too difficult.

  2. A patient may be **too acutely ill** at the end of life to be comfortably cared for at home.

  3. A **psychosocial assessment** should address the emotional and physical health of the caregiver and explore social and financial resources.

  4. Even an in-depth assessment by experienced staff may not provide a reliable **predictor** for whether a patient will remain home to die.

  5. At each subsequent home visit, the hospice staff must **reevaluate** the patient/family situation and revise plans as necessary.

C.   PREPARATION OF THE PATIENT AND FAMILY

  1. Once home death has been established as a desired goal, an individualized home care plan is developed with the patient and family. They need to know **specifically** what the hospice team can and will provide.

  2. The primary caregiver is continually and carefully assessed as to what he or she **wants** to and is **capable** of doing for direct care.

  3. Support to the primary caregiver and other family members includes **acknowledging** how physically and emotionally exhausting caring for someone ill at home can be.

  4. **Knowledge and preparation for the death event**

    a.   Families need to be prepared for the actual time of the patient's death and the time immediately preceding it.

    b.   There are some **universal signs** that families can anticipate and on which they can receive instruction.

      (1) See **Table 56-5, text page 1444,** for an example of a patient/family instruction sheet that lists many of the common signs seen in patients who are imminently dying.

    c.   **Emotional care** of the patient and family around the time of death occurs as the opportunity arises.

      (1) The family is instructed to **listen** to the patient carefully, even if it appears that the patient is confused.

      (2) Many times patients will speak in symbolic language.

  5. **Funeral arrangements**

    a.   In most situations a home death will go more smoothly if the patient and/or family chooses a funeral home **before** the death occurs.

      (1) Beyond choosing the funeral home, no other arrangements need be made prior to death.

    b.   Important factors that differentiate funeral homes are **religious affiliation, financial considerations,** and **policies about home death.**

D.   AVAILABILITY OF THE HOSPICE TEAM

  1. Of utmost importance in supporting families through a patient's home death is instructing them on **how to access the hospice team** at any time on any day as needed.

  2. The time of instruction regarding accessing the hospice team is also a good time to **remind** families not to call the emergency medical system, and to inform them of the possible consequences of such an action.

E. **FACILITATING GRIEF**

1. As family members prepare for the death of a loved one at home, they are also preparing themselves for the loss that is often referred to as **anticipatory grief.**
2. This can be a time of opportunity to **resolve** certain issues, so that after death there are no regrets on the part of the family.
3. Asking a couple how they met or going through a family photo album with them is a good way to facilitate grieving and therapeutic review of life.
   a. An example of facilitating grief is in a case example on **text page 1445,** columns 1–2.

VI. **BEREAVEMENT CARE**

1. Bereavement support is a **required** component of hospice care under Medicare and most state licensing regulations.
2. Grieving is a **normal reaction to loss,** with a wide variety of **physical** and **emotional manifestations,** which include loss of appetite, sleeplessness, heart palpitations, lack of energy, sadness, and anger.
3. Four tasks necessary for the normal grief process to progress:
   a. **To accept the reality of the loss.**
   b. **To experience the pain of grief.**
   c. **To adjust to the environment in which the deceased is missing.**
   d. **To withdraw emotional energy,** and **replace it in another relationship.**
4. The goal of bereavement care or counseling is to **assist** and **support survivors to move through the loss** and **toward resolution.**
   a. Hospice programs generally follow survivors for **1 year,** although there is no mandated standard time for follow-up.
   b. This is a period in which the most acute grief can occur, **not** for mourning to be completed, for grief resolution is a very individualized process that takes place gradually over time.
5. **Methods** of bereavement follow-up can vary, but generally include a bereavement assessment, contact of survivors at regularly scheduled intervals, and, as necessary, additional referrals for professional counseling for those with complicated or abnormal grief reactions.

A. **ABNORMAL GRIEF**

1. Survivors **unable to progress** through the tasks of mourning will develop some form of abnormal or complicated grief that can manifest itself in one of three ways.
   a. First, the grief reaction may be **prolonged.**
   b. Second, the grief reaction may be **masked** in behavioral or physical symptoms, even such seemingly unrelated symptoms as pain, sexual impotence, and behavioral "acting out."
   c. Third, abnormal grief may manifest itself in **exaggerated** or **excessive expressions** of normal grief reactions, such as excessive anger, sadness, or depression.
2. Because unresolved grief has been associated with multiple physical and emotional illnesses, including increased risk of suicide, facilitation of anticipatory grieving and bereavement can be viewed as **preventive health care** for survivors.

VII. **STRESS AND THE HOSPICE NURSE**

1. Providing compassionate care to the terminally ill and their loved ones can create **unique stressors** for the hospice team.
2. Staff attitudes toward death can be greatly **influenced** by unresolved grief issues in their own personal or professional life. Stress can be increased due to unrealistic expectations of ourselves, our coworkers, or the therapy we use to manage symptoms.
3. Several methods for coping with stress that have been used successfully by hospice staff members are seen in **Table 56-6, text page 1446.**

VIII. **LEGAL AND ETHICAL ISSUES SURROUNDING HOSPICE CARE**

A. **ADVANCE DIRECTIVES**

1. The federal Patient Self-Determination Act enacted in December 1991 **requires** hospices, hospitals, and other health care agencies to provide patients, on admission, with written in-

formation about two key areas describing **their right to accept or refuse treatment under state law** and **ways to execute advance directives such as a living will** and a durable **power of attorney for health care.**

2. The nurse provides whatever information is needed to assist the patient in making an informed decision, especially when it affects the patient's decision not to have CPR, intravenous fluids, or tube feedings.
3. Hospice patients and families may **need reassurance** that their focus on comfort and quality of life is being reinforced by their decision not to have CPR or not to have intravenous fluids or tube feedings.
4. **Fluid depletion has the following benign effects** on quality of life:
   a. Urine output is decreased, so there is **less incontinence.**
   b. Gastric secretions lessen, so **episodes of vomiting decrease.**
   c. Pulmonary secretions lessen, resulting in **less congestion.**
   d. Peripheral edema secondary to tumor subsides, resulting in **decreased pain from nerve compression.**
   e. Although the **sensation of dry mouth** and **thirst may increase,** this can be relieved by good mouth care and small amounts of oral fluids.
5. Life-and-death decisions depend on the availability of **written evidence of the patient's wishes.**
   a. In general, the power of attorney for health care is **more useful** than the living will.
6. Through the **power of attorney** for health care, the patient chooses an agent to act on the patient's behalf if the patient is no longer competent to make decisions.

B. EUTHANASIA AND SUICIDE

1. The moral, ethical, and legal questions surrounding terminal illness and methods used to hasten death have their origins in ancient times.
2. In modern times **euthanasia has come to mean the intentional taking of the life of a terminally ill person for purposes of compassion.**
   a. The modern concept is more accurately described as **active euthanasia,** for it is achieved by **"doing something."**
   b. **Passive euthanasia** can be described as "not doing something" that would preserve life, yet without being significantly burdensome.
3. In many states suicide is not against the law; however, encouraging or aiding suicide is a criminal act.
4. For many, the **fear of pain or suffering** associated with dying or the burden that it places on others can stimulate thoughts of ways to hasten death.
5. Euthanasia is quite different from refusing to receive medical treatment that will not contribute reasonably to improved quality of life and/or that proves to be gravely burdensome.
6. Pain medication or other symptom management measures that are used in **unusual quantity** to improve comfort but could lead to an early death should not be considered euthanasia.
7. Hospice philosophy **does not promote** involvement in either the act of suicide or euthanasia.

IX. FUTURE TRENDS AND CHALLENGES FOR HOSPICE CARE

A. UNDERSERVED POPULATIONS

1. The **African-American** and **Hispanic populations are underrepresented,** or totally lacking among hospice staff and volunteers, even in urban hospice programs.
2. Children represent another nationally underserved population.
3. It is difficult to find a hospice program that will acknowledge denying services to those with an AIDS diagnosis; however, there remains the opinion among some in hospice leadership that AIDS **does not "fit in"** to current hospice practice.
   a. AIDS patients **utilize more resources** than have been the norm for hospice patients.
   b. AIDS **care is more complex** and requires more frequent nursing and social work visits.
   c. AIDS patients require **more attendant or custodial care** due to the lack of primary caregivers and limited finances.
   d. **Medications** and **supplies** used are move varied and expensive.

4. With AIDS, a more **flexible interpretation of symptom management** and a **creative approach to quality-of-life issues** are needed.

5. Others who are **"outliers"** confronting hospice care include the rapidly aging population with either no primary caregivers or immediate support persons too frail to provide care.

B. **RESEARCH ISSUES**

1. Palliative care **research topics** could include volunteerism, spiritual care, suicidal ideation in the terminally ill, emotional factors hindering pain management, and long-term effectiveness of bereavement care.

2. Limited funding and the relative lack of hospice and palliative care programs associated with academic institutions provide additional barriers to research.

C. **INTEGRATION INTO HEALTH CARE PRACTICES**

1. Hospice in the United States began as an anti-medical establishment and anti-physician movement. This antagonistic bias has unfortunately been a major factor preventing hospice and palliative care principles from being applied to terminally ill patients on a wider scale.

PRACTICE QUESTIONS

1. The basic medical and nursing approach toward patients in a hospice program is
   (A) acute care.
   (B) curative care.
   (C) palliative care.
   (D) euthanasia care.

2. When caring for the patient in a hospice setting, who is the "expert" on whether pain and/or symptoms have been adequately relieved?
   (A) the primary caregiver
   (B) the attending physician
   (C) the primary nurse
   (D) the patient

3. The hospice nurse decides in the initial interview that patient criteria for hospice care will not be met because
   (A) the patient's spouse expresses his wish to be involved in his wife's care.
   (B) the patient shares her plans of having entered a clinical trial through the National Cancer Institute.
   (C) the patient's home is 5 minutes from the hospice offices.
   (D) the patient does not wish to be resuscitated if she stops breathing at home.

4. The husband of a woman with end-stage breast cancer is concerned that his wife is sleeping more and is not even waking to eat or drink. The hospice nurse would explain to the husband that
   (A) these are signs of approaching death.
   (B) the pain medication has reached a high blood level and needs to be reduced.
   (C) there is no reason to be concerned.
   (D) her oncologist should be called in order to obtain some direction for her care.

5. Which of the following grief reactions of an elderly woman who has lost her husband of 40 years would prompt the hospice nurse to suggest counseling?
   (A) She takes out 40 years worth of photograph albums and wants to review her marriage and life with her deceased husband with the hospice nurse.
   (B) She refuses to let her sister and brother-in-law into her home anymore, blaming them for buying her husband cigarettes "all those years."
   (C) She plans her husband's funeral by herself, listens to all his favorite classical music pieces and chooses passages from his bible.
   (D) She delegates all the responsibility for disposition of her husband's belongings to the children.

6.   Which of the following "directions" provides patients who are at risk for loss of decision-making ability the **best** chance of having their health care wishes carried out?
(A)   power of attorney for health care
(B)   verbal instructions to the attending physician
(C)   a living will
(D)   a do-not-intubate/ventilate order on admission

ANSWER EXPLANATIONS

1.   **The answer is (C).**   Hospice care pivots around the idea of palliative medical management. Palliative management involves a shift in treatment goals from curative toward providing relief from suffering. Euthanasia means active interventions to hasten a person's death and this is NOT the philosophy of hospice care. (1433–1434)

2.   **The answer is (D).**   The patient is the "expert" on whether pain and symptoms have been adequately relieved. This is a principle of palliative care. (1434)

3.   **The answer is (B).**   Clinical trials are experimental medical trials often developed to see if there is any disease response to a new antineoplastic regimen. Patients and their families often turn to an experimental procedure when there are limited, if any, options remaining that might halt their disease progress. This choice suggests that the patient has not agreed to palliative care and is still pursuing curative treatment. Further assessment is indicated here to make sure this is not the case, because a patient criteria for hospice care is that the patient is agreeable to palliative and not curative care. The remaining three options are actually patient criteria for hospice care: the patient has a primary caregiver; the patient resides in the hospice program's geographic area; and some programs require that the patient has a DNR status prior to admission to the hospice program. (1434)

4.   **The answer is (A).**   The hospice team's goal is to help the family prepare for their loved one's death. Families need to be prepared for the actual time of the patient's death and what universal signs they can anticipate. Increasing sleep, a gradual decrease in need for food and drink, increased confusion or restlessness, decreasing temperature of extremities, and irregular breathing patterns may occur. Calling the oncologist would be indicating the need for intervention, when in fact the goal of care is purely palliative. The pain relief regimen should not be altered if the patient is comfortable, even if the patient is sleeping more and death is approaching. (1443–1444)

5.   **The answer is (B).**   Abnormal grief may manifest itself in exaggerated or excessive expressions of normal grief reactions, such as excessive anger, sadness, or depression. For most hospice programs, therapy for abnormal grief extends beyond the scope of the bereavement care services provided. The hospice program staff should be able to identify and recommend competent referrals for abnormal grief syndromes. It is therapeutic to review a person's life with their loved one. Listening to a family member share stories of their life with the loved one honors the meaning of their relationship and their life together. Funeral planning can be therapeutic and facilitate someone's loss as they do one last thing in a special way for their loved one. Delegating responsibilities that can be overwhelming or too painful might actually be an indicator of the grieving party being aware of their limitations and calling on their resources and support systems. (1444–1446)

6.   **The answer is (A).**   A living will may be applicable only when it pertains to a terminal illness but not for a patient whose health is declining for medical reasons other than those that can be classified as terminal or if the patient is in a vegetative state. In general, the power of attorney for health care is more useful than the living will. The living will does not identify another person who can act as the agent for a disabled patient. Verbal instructions are of little value if a family member or anyone else chooses to argue against what has been reportedly verbally communicated. Written instructions are necessary. An order that instructs not to intubate does not address any other interventions that might be suggested. (1447)

57 Quality of Care

STUDY OUTLINE

I. CONCEPTUAL FOUNDATIONS OF QUALITY CARE

A. HISTORICAL CONTEXT AND ORIGINS

1. During the past 10 years, a science of caring has emerged as a discrete theme in the nursing literature, but only recently has care been accorded the major importance recognized by Nightingale a century ago.
2. The relevance of care to society's health is changing because of advanced treatment techniques and the increasing elderly population. The concept of cure has been replaced by that of **prolonged remission with maximum quality of life.**
3. **Quality of care** is challenged by a system that has decreased hospital length of stay and cost coverage and, at the same time, has given proportionally less coverage to those most vulnerable members of society (nonwhite, poor, less educated) who have the greatest need and the least access to health care.
4. The Oncology Nursing Society (ONS), in 1988, revised and expanded its scope of practice statement to recognize that persons with cancer and their families need to be active participants in their care and treatment as the owner-manager of his or her total health, with the nurse as coordinator and advocate for the patient's needs.
5. **Care and caring**
   a. Nurse practice acts are determined by the state. Most legislate nursing as the diagnosis and treatment of human responses in health and illness, regulated and standardized by education, registration, certification, standards of practice, and quality assurance.
   b. **Diagnostic taxonomies** generally allow for a clear definition of professional purpose and for faster communication among the practitioners of a discipline. They become the basis for a profession's research and development.
   c. The next step is the **integration of standards of practice and nursing diagnoses to foster relevant research, promote therapeutic interventions, and, ultimately, advance the quality of care.**
      (1) See **Table 57-1, text pages 1455–1456,** for a complete list of functional health pattern categories and nursing diagnoses. These categories include **health perception–health management, nutrition-metabolic, elimination, activity-exercise, sleep-rest, cognitive-perceptual, self-perception–self-concept, role-relationship, sexuality-reproductive, coping-stress tolerance,** and **value-belief** patterns.
6. **Quality**
   a. **Quality** is a set of properties, attributes, and capacities that are essential and unique to the focus of evaluation. Beyers defines the correlates of quality as **cost, productivity,** and **risk.**
   b. The "new" approach to quality recognizes four important factors:
      (1) Consumer need and response.
      (2) Integrated service teams.
      (3) Standards of practice, organization, and professional performance.
      (4) Data management systems that document structure, process, and outcome elements.
   c. These factors interact and have the potential for a positive effect. Thus, quality embraces the dimensions of **structure** (patient and environment norms), **process** (strategies of quality management), and **outcome** (documentation of clinical outcomes and patient satisfaction).

B. **QUALITY OF CARE MODEL**

1. **Structure**
    a. A **model of quality of care** incorporates the major goals in cancer care and treatment, as well as standards for oncology nursing practice and for the professional performance of the nurse. See **Figure 57-1, text page 1457,** for a representation of this model.
    b. Major **structural** elements that promote quality of care are **clinical research** and the **development of nursing technology** to test and improve interventions and maximize positive results.
        (1) Clinical research involves keeping up with the literature in the field and taking part in research projects of one's own or of the staff.

2. **Process**
    a. The **process** variables in the quality of health care model are **cancer prevention, detection, treatment,** and **nursing care.**
    b. Most often, nursing care revolves around medical treatment but extends itself beyond the immediate goals of interest to the physician, e.g., the management of side effects and the promotion of functional recovery.
    c. Care augments and enhances cure and in the process humanizes the total outcome.

3. **Outcome**
    a. Cancer treatment today has a cure rate of approximately 50%. Therefore, much of the outcome of cancer care is related to extension of life and improved quality of life.

C. **STANDARDS OF CARE**

1. In 1979, the Oncology Nursing Society and the American Nursing Association (ANA) jointly published the *Outcome Standards for Cancer Nursing Practice,* which was integrated into the *Standards of Oncology Nursing Practice* in 1987.
2. There are 11 Standards of Oncology Nursing Practice, 6 that address professional practice and 5 that concern professional performance. See **Table 57-2, text page 1458,** for a list of these standards and their purpose.
3. **Standards of Oncology Nursing Practice**
    a. These six standards focus on the **process** involved in patient care and include
        (1) A **theoretical framework** derived from the biological, social, behavioral, and physical sciences; the most frequently used nursing theories are **Orem's self-care deficit theory** and the **Johnson behavioral system model.**
        (2) **Data collection** to reflect current and accurate clinical status.
        (3) **Nursing diagnosis** for problems in 11 high-incidence parameters: prevention, information, coping, comfort, nutrition, protective mechanisms, mobility, elimination, sexuality, ventilation, and circulation.
        (4) **Planning** for goals and methods of dealing with the 11 parameters above.
        (5) **Intervention,** in which the oncology nurse implements the nursing care plan to achieve the identified outcomes; the nurse functions autonomously yet in a team framework.
        (6) **Evaluation,** including updates, revisions, documentation, and analyses.
4. **Standards of professional performance**
    a. These include
        (1) **Professional development,** in which nurses are responsible for keeping up with advances in the field.
        (2) **Multidisciplinary collaboration,** including communicating and collaborating with team members.
        (3) **Quality assurance** involving peer review and program evaluation systems.
        (4) **Ethics,** which includes use of the Code for Nurses and the Patient's Bill of Rights.
        (5) **Research,** which involves keeping abreast of literature, and perhaps being a part of a research team.

II. **RESEARCH AND EVALUATION IN QUALITY OF CARE**

A. **BACKGROUND AND CONTEXT**

1. The nursing literature of the 1970s saw a significant expansion in standardized approaches to measuring the quality of nursing care. As early as 1966, Donabedian identified structure,

process, and outcome variables in medicine as the three classic approaches to patient care evaluation.

2. Two important journals that marked the beginning of oncology nursing literature are *Cancer Nursing* and *Oncology Nursing Forum.* Since 1985, coincident with the establishment of oncology nursing standards, an increasing number of authors integrated patients' clinical problems with diagnoses, assessment parameters, interventions, and plans, so that the articles became more useful for the practicing nurse.

B. **APPROACHES TO MEASURING QUALITY OF CARE**

1. The three major approaches to measuring quality of care are
   a. **Quality assurance programs.**
   b. **Clinical research that includes both program evaluation and experimental studies of interventions.**
   c. **Measurement tool or instrument development that involves both quantitative and qualitative measures.**

2. **Quality assurance**
   a. **The Joint Commission on Accreditation of Health Care Organizations** publishes standards used in the accreditation of hospitals and other health care facilities, including hospices and home care organizations. They distinguish between standards of care and standards of practice.
   b. Patterson described standard of care as what the patient outcome should be and what the patient can expect from nursing service; standards of practice relate to what and how the nurse provides care to achieve the patient outcome.
   c. Findings by Oleske revealed that some improvement in nursing performance and outcome followed nursing consultations and continuing education. However, the outcomes were improved only in certain clinical aspects of care.
   d. Stephany tested the reliability and validity of the **Hope Hospice Quality Assurance Tool (HHQAT),** which assesses physical concerns, patient and caregiver education, and emotional and spiritual support. The report concluded that an effective tool had been created for measuring the quality of hospice care.
   e. Dudjak described the **Radiation Therapy Nursing Care Record,** which is used to justify care costs and to further establish standards of practice.
   f. Gullo, in reviewing safe handling practice of antineoplastic agents, estimated that more than 60% of nurses were not using safe handling techniques.
   g. Gray et al. published a clinical database, and generated more than 400 variables on problem areas related to cancer metastasis. Since symptom management is a cornerstone of nursing care, this database facilitates the identification of nursing diagnoses and related nursing practices.
   h. Moore et al. studied three classes enrolled in a graduate oncology program, using an instrument called the **Appraisal of Practice Behavior Instrument.** They found that the nurses' proficiency increased as they went through the educational program.
   i. In an interesting contrast to many studies, McGee et al. found that the attitudes of greatest importance to oncology nurse specialists had to do with ethical practice, respect for humanity, responsibility for behavior, and commitment to continued learning. The identification of nursing diagnoses and commitment to cost-effective practices ranked last.

3. **Clinical research**
   a. In **clinical research,** optimal outcomes are defined in terms of cost-effective patient outcomes and consumer satisfaction. Examples include the following studies.
   b. Oberst polled a large number of nurses, asking them what they felt were their greatest problems in everyday practice and care. Their priorities were **chemotherapy- and radiation-induced nausea and vomiting, pain, discharge needs, grief, stomatitis, venipuncture in long-term therapy, dignity of the dying, analgesia, providing effective pain management,** and **their own attitude toward that pain.**
   c. A similar study from Canada listed as major problems **relaxation and biofeedback to reduce pain, ways to improve patient teaching, improved discharge planning, ways to improve primary care,** and **therapy for relief of treatment- and disease-related symptoms.**

   d. **Table 57-4, text pages 1464–1469,** summarizes a large number of studies of cancer nursing practice from 1984 on. These studies reflect a growing sophistication in research design and measurement, i.e.,
      (1) Scott et al. used **Progressive Muscle Therapy (PMR),** guided imagery, and slow back massage, and compared them to drug antiemetic regimens. The relaxation group had reduced total duration; the drug group had reduced peak vomiting phase.
      (2) Parker used scalp hypothermia to reduce alopecia. Treatment was successful and is in clinical use.
      (3) Winningham and MacVicar used aerobic exercise as antiemetic therapy. Treatment was significantly better than controls. Further studies were suggested.
      (4) Jones, examining catheter care procedures in central venous catheter infection, compared two types of catheters and found no differences in rate of infection. Jones suggested further studies to refine predictive risk factors.
   e. **Table 57-5, text pages 1471–1473,** summarizes 20 studies of cancer care. Of the programs studied, six assisted patients and families to cope with their experience with cancer.
      (1) The programs studied focused on prevention, education, coping, comfort, and nutrition.
      (2) The care programs were studied for effectiveness; the results of these studies are included in **Table 57-5, text pages 1471–1473.**
4. **Measurement tool development: Quantitative**
   a. Some nursing studies have a long list of limitations because they are flawed by faulty design, inadequate sampling techniques, and use of untested measurement tools.
      (1) Sound quantitative measurement includes adequate **reliability** and **validity** of the instrument used.
      (2) Reliability serves to test both the stability (test-retest correlations) and the internal consistency (intercorrelations among items) of an instrument.
      (3) Interrater reliability is defined as consistency among users of the instrument.
   b. **Table 57-6, text pages 1474–1475,** provides a list of cancer nursing measurement tools, what each measures, the kinds of results each looks for, and how the tool is used. For example, the **Quality of Life Index (QLI)** looks at satisfaction in 18 important life areas and establishes norms for these areas.
5. **Measurement tool development: Qualitative**
   a. The most recognized qualitative approaches include **case study, grounded theory, phenomenology,** and **ethnography.**
   b. The results of the qualitative method may include (1) operationalizing a single concept; (2) developing a conceptual framework; (3) establishing guidelines for practice; (4) creating portraits, paradigm cases, or typologies; and (5) forming theory. These processes are no less rigorous than the quantitative approach and may be the best approach to a given problem.
   c. **Indicators** are a set of variables that empirically describe an important clinical manifestation. For example, Saunders and Valentine's article on suicide contains empirical knowledge and general information on the topic, along with a useful *Brief Suicide Assessment Guide* for practitioners.
   d. **Predictors** are variables that have been tested to determine their ability to predict a future event with some degree of accuracy.
   e. **Guidelines for care** include topics such as nursing care, nursing interventions, the nursing role, nursing assessments, nursing management, and nursing plans.
   f. See **Table 57-7, text page 1476,** for indicators, predictors, and guidelines for quality of care.

III.   **QUALITY IN PERFORMANCE: APPLICATIONS IN PRACTICE**

   1. No discussion of care is complete without a look at **process**—the performance of nursing care and its meaning for both patient and nurse. Measuring quality of care by documented patient outcome is only one aspect of the approach demanded.
   2. There are four important patterns to the process of giving and receiving care: **mutuality, contextuality, competence and proficiency,** and **intentionality of caring.**
   3. **Mutuality**
      a. **Mutuality of roles** between the caregiver and the care receiver are complementary in that the relationship works in a nondissident, harmonious way.

b. Jennings and Muhlencamp found that caregivers' perceptions were significantly different from patients' self-reports on anxiety, hostility, and depression. In each case, the patient reported feeling better than the caregivers had thought.

c. Larson interviewed patients and nurses to determine what behaviors were most and least important in making the patients feel cared for. The highest ranked behaviors for the patients were competence, monitoring and follow-through, and accessibility. Actions rated highest by the nurses were comfort factors such as listening and touch. Both groups gave high ratings to accessibility, giving good physical care, listening, and putting the patient first.

d. Mayer basically agreed with Larson. Patients seemed to value the instrumental, technical caring skills, whereas nurses are more attuned to expressive, caring behaviors. Both viewed cheerfulness and appearance as least important.

e. Dyck and Wright found that the needs of family members are emerging as important factors, especially as more and more care is given by them in the home. While the caregivers expected nurses to care solely for the patient, their own needs were also documented.

4. **Contextuality**

a. Communication is important in shaping the illness experience. Patients reported that physicians communicated more about the disease, and that nurses communicated more about treatment and the illness.

b. The more uncertain a patient's condition, the more vulnerable he/she was to the feeling of lack of concern.

5. **Competence and proficiency**

a. Nurses advance with experience from novice to advanced beginner, competent nurse, proficient nurse, and expert.

b. The nurse gathers personal knowledge through a series of steps that involve
   (1) Paradigms of various care issues.
   (2) Changing and refining those paradigms.
   (3) Viewing only those relevant elements and having confidence in intuitive interpretations.
   (4) Having involvement as a confident, effective partner.

6. **Intentionality of caring**

a. This concept links the science and art of nursing knowledge and skill and represents the matrix holding together mutuality, contextuality, and competence and proficiency. Its most overt manifestation in practice is known as **clinical judgment.**

PRACTICE QUESTIONS

1. One factor contributing to a change in the relevance of **care** to society's health is the emergence of advanced treatment techniques. Another is the
   (A) emergence of the concept of cure.
   (B) increasing elderly population.
   (C) recent adoption of a universal definition of care.
   (D) realization that prolonged remission is seldom possible.

2. In 1988, the Oncology Nursing Society (ONS) revised and expanded its scope of practice statement to recognize that
   (A) persons with cancer and their families need to be active participants in their care and treatment.
   (B) cure is the fundamental concept in disease treatment.
   (C) the role of nurse administrator is vital to any program or therapy designed to provide high-quality care.
   (D) delivery of quality care is inseparable from an ongoing pursuit of nursing research.

3. Memory deficits and chronic pain are part of which of Gordon's functional health pattern categories and nursing diagnoses?
   (A) coping-stress tolerance pattern
   (B) cognitive-perceptual pattern
   (C) health perception–health management pattern
   (D) role-relationship pattern

4. Clinical research and the development of nursing technology to test and improve interventions are part of which aspect of the quality of care model?
    (A) process
    (B) outcome
    (C) structure
    (D) practice

5. The *Standards of Oncology Nursing Practice,* co-developed by the Oncology Nursing Society and the American Nursing Association, primarily address the broad issues of
    (A) professional practice and performance.
    (B) quality assurance and research methodology.
    (C) nursing standards and continuing education.
    (D) ethics and legal considerations in nursing.

6. Standards of professional performance, as outlined in the *Standards of Oncology Nursing Practice*, include
    (A) diagnoses and analyses of data.
    (B) evaluations.
    (C) outcome care planning.
    (D) ethics and the use of the *Patient's Bill of Rights.*

7. In clinical research, optimal outcomes are defined in terms of
    (A) fulfillment of institutional goals in keeping with societal priorities.
    (B) the development of new therapies and procedures.
    (C) cost-effective patient outcomes and consumer satisfaction.
    (D) widespread dissemination of research findings.

8. Which of the following is a quantitative measurement tool used in nursing studies?
    (A) indicators
    (B) reliability tests
    (C) case studies
    (D) predictors

9. A major goal of qualitative research in nursing is to
    (A) produce precise and replicable data that predict patient outcomes.
    (B) test the validity and reliability of an instrument used in clinical research.
    (C) assess the ability of a research instrument to measure the construct of interest accurately and objectively.
    (D) shape a representation of the patient's experience from available data.

10. The four important patterns to the process of giving and receiving care are mutuality, contextuality, competence and proficiency, and intentionality of caring. Which of the following pairings involving these four patterns is **incorrect?**
    (A) mutuality: care behavior that is reciprocal and complementary
    (B) contextuality: care behavior that involves a shared meaning of circumstances
    (C) competence and proficiency: care behavior that requires patient involvement
    (D) intentionality of caring: care behavior that requires sound clinical judgment

ANSWER EXPLANATIONS

1. **The answer is (B).** The relevance of care to society's health is changing because of advanced treatment techniques and the increasing elderly population. The concept of cure has been replaced by that of prolonged remission with maximum quality of life. (1454)

2. **The answer is (A).** The ONS revised and expanded its scope of practice statement on the basis of a philosophical recognition that persons with cancer and their families need to be fully informed and to participate actively in their care and treatment and, further, that competent, humane care demands a complementary team of specialized practitioners who communicate with one another and augment one another's efforts. Increasingly, the notion of the patient as the owner-manager of his or her total health, with the nurse as coordinator and advocate for the patient's needs, has been gaining acceptance. (1454)

3. **The answer is (B).**   An important aspect of the nursing profession's research and development activity is the integration of standards of practice and nursing diagnoses to foster relevant research, promote therapeutic interventions, and, ultimately, advance the quality of care. These categories include health perception–health management, nutrition-metabolic, elimination, activity-exercise, sleep-rest, cognitive-perceptual, self-perception–self-concept, role-relationship, sexuality-reproductive, coping-stress tolerance, and value-belief patterns. The cognitive-perceptual pattern incorporates memory deficits and chronic pain. (1455)

4. **The answer is (C).**   A model of quality of care incorporates the major goals in cancer care and treatment, as well as standards for oncology nursing practice and the professional performance of the nurse. Major structural elements that promote quality of care are clinical research and the development of nursing technology to test and improve interventions and maximize positive results. (1457)

5. **The answer is (A).**   Of the 11 Standards of Oncology Nursing Practice, 6 address professional practice and 5 address professional performance. See **Table 57-2, text page 1458,** for a list of these two groups of standards. (1458–1459)

6. **The answer is (D).**   Standards of professional performance include professional development, in which nurses are responsible for keeping up with advances in the field; multidisciplinary collaboration, including communicating and collaborating with team members; quality assurance involving peer review and program evaluation systems; ethics, which includes use of the Code for Nurses and the Patient's Bill of Rights; and research, which involves keeping abreast of literature, and perhaps being a part of a research team. The other choices are aspects of the standards of professional practice. (1459)

7. **The answer is (C).**   Research offers a means of improving and refining practice to ensure optimal outcomes. The desired result of practice is usually defined as a valuable change in the patient for the better. In most institutional settings, this means cost-effective patient outcomes and consumer satisfaction. (1462)

8. **The answer is (B).**   Sound quantitative measurement includes adequate reliability and validity of the instrument used. Reliability serves to test both the stability (test-retest correlations) and the internal consistency (intercorrelations among items) of an instrument. A third type of reliability, interrater reliability, ensures that all persons using a set of evaluation criteria have closely correlated results. Validity testing offers a way to assess the ability of the instrument to measure the construct of interest accurately and objectively. The other choices are all qualitative measurement tools or approaches. (1470)

9. **The answer is (D).**   Qualitative research in nursing begins with carefully stated and clearly articulated research questions to guide data collection and later interpretation. The motive is to understand an aspect of the patient/nursing experience and to shape a representation of it from the data. The results of the qualitative method may include (1) operationalizing a single concept; (2) developing a conceptual framework; (3) establishing guidelines for practice; (4) creating portraits, paradigm cases, or typologies; and (5) forming theory. These processes are no less rigorous than the quantitative approach and may be the best approach to a given problem. (1470, 1473, 1475)

10. **The answer is (C).**   Competence and proficiency involve care behavior that is based on practical knowledge and imbedded in expert nursing. Nurses advance with experience from novice to advanced beginner, competent nurse, proficient nurse, and expert. The nurse gathers personal knowledge through a series of steps that involve paradigms of various care issues, changing and refining those paradigms, viewing only those relevant elements and having confidence in intuitive interpretations, and having involvement as a confident, effective partner. (1478)

58   Cancer Economics

STUDY OUTLINE

I. **INTRODUCTION**

    1.   Nurses today must be prepared to consider **cost requirements** as well as standards of excellence in administering patient care. A cost-effective approach is one that emphasizes **balancing cost requirements and standards of excellence.**

II. **SCOPE OF THE PROBLEM**

    1.   Since the early 1980s, major changes due to **new technology, innovative therapy,** and **economic conditions** have resulted in a much greater emphasis on the cost of cancer care.
        a.   Expenditures for health care grew from **4.5%** of the U.S. gross national product (GNP) in 1960 to **12.3%** in 1992.
        b.   For the federal government health care costs are the fastest growing major budget item, increasing annually at approximately 8%.
        c.   There are pressures from politicians, business leaders, and consumers to cut back on the use of health care resources, and to do more with less.

III. **ECONOMICS THEORY**

    1.   In most areas of business, prices are established by the **law of supply and demand:** pricing is established to balance the supply and demand of goods and services.
        a.   See **Figure 58-1, text page 1486,** for a schematic description of the normal economic environment based on supply and demand economics.
    2.   This law does not apply to health care, however, because the **consumer does not pay for services,** so price does not provide a balance between supply and demand.
    3.   During the 1950s and 1960s, most employed Americans believed that health care was a right, not a privilege, because insurance coverage was a part of their employee benefit package.
        a.   Unemployed persons not covered by insurance were usually covered by Medicare or Medicaid, which are **retrospective and cost-based** in terms of payment for services. The more money a hospital spent, the more the government paid.
        b.   Because neither the consumer nor the health care professional was concerned with the price of services, **demand became unlimited.**
        c.   The method of payment caused overutilization of resources and soaring costs.
    4.   In response to soaring health care costs, Congress passed the **Tax Equity and Fiscal Responsibility Act (TEFRA)** in 1982. This law changed the method of providing inpatient services for Medicaid and Medicare from a retrospective, cost-based payment system to a **prospective payment system.**

IV. **PROSPECTIVE PAYMENT SYSTEM**

   A. **HISTORY**

    1.   The **prospective payment system (PPS)** reimburses hospitals with a fixed payment depending on the complexity of the problem that precipitated the hospitalization.
        a.   The exact amount reimbursed is determined by using one or more of nearly 500 **diagnosis-related groups (DRGs).** DRGs determine the amount that a hospital will be reimbursed for a patient's care, and not the actual cost that the hospital incurred.

    b.   The **Health Care Financing Administration (HCFA)** now assigns the weighting factors, such as laboratory tests, medical and surgical supplies, room, and medications for each DRG.

B. CALCULATION

1. See **Figure 58-4, text page 1489,** for a sample calculation of a prospective payment.

C. EXEMPTIONS

1. DRGs were developed with a primary orientation toward **short-term, acute-care hospitals.** Application to specialty hospitals is limited.
2. Some hospitals, including NCI-designated comprehensive cancer centers, are not reimbursed under the PPS system. See the list of exempt facilities on **text page 1488,** column 2.

D. HOSPITAL COST-PER-CASE COMPARISONS

1. A variety of factors determines the payment a hospital receives per case, including the case mix of **patient population, number of low-income patients served, labor costs, urban versus rural location, teaching intensity,** and **outlier cases** (cases with extremely long length of stay or extremely high costs when compared to others classified in the same DRG).
2. Variations in cost per case that are not accounted for by the adjustment factors described above are due to **differences in hospital efficiency.**

E. MONITORING ACTIVITIES

1. Hospitals are required to contract with a **peer review organization (PRO),** established by the U.S. Department of Health and Human Services, to insure that quality care is provided and that the duration of the hospital stay is appropriate to the required level of care.
2. The **Health Care Financing Administration (HFCA)** periodically reviews hospital records and will deny payment if PPS preregulations are not followed.
3. Another agency established by Congress, the **Prospective Payment Assessment Commission (PROPAC),** makes recommendations annually to Congress for the annual percent increases in Medicare expenditures, and also for the DRG patient classifications and weights. PROPAC also analyzes and develops prospective payment policies for all facilities under Medicare and examines and reports on broader issues regarding the effectiveness and quality of health care delivery in the United States.

F. IMPACT OF PPS

1. The impact of PPS on the health care system has been enormous.
   a. If the cost of a patient's care is less than the DRG amount, the hospital keeps the difference.
   b. Conversely, if the costs exceed the pay scale, the hospital absorbs the difference.
2. **Changes in the hospital industry**
   a. The major objectives of PPS were to **reduce the rates of increase in the Medicare inpatient payments** and to **decrease hospital costs overall.**
   b. As hospital operating margins became tighter, other significant changes in the hospital industry developed.
      (1) Soon after the implementation of PPS, hospital **inpatient admissions declined** and continued to do so until about 1987, when such admissions stabilized.
      (2) Approximately 500 hospitals closed their doors between 1980 and 1991.
   c. By contrast, the **utilization of hospital-based outpatient services has grown steadily.**
   d. The shift to outpatient services has allowed patients with less complex cases to be treated in outpatient facilities.
      (1) Those patients that continue to need inpatient care frequently are severely ill and in need of complex services.
   e. The severity of illness or amount of services provided to patients is measured by the case-mix index (CMI), which is the average DRG weight for all cases paid under PPS.
      (1) The CMI index has been **increasing** each year since the implementation of PPS.

f. Medicare spending continues to rise, despite a decade of intensified attempts to control costs.
   (1) Medicare costs per enrollee increased at a slower rate than the national health care costs per person during the late 1980s.
g. **The hospitals that have done well under Medicare's PPS reduced their length of stay, controlled their labor costs in relation to other hospitals in their market area,** and **offered more services to attract patients.**

3. **Decrease in length of stay**
   a. Historically, the length of stay (LOS) has been associated with several dependent variables, including the **patient's age,** the **presence of other diseases or conditions, complications,** and the **use of surgery.**
   b. Many other factors also affect a person's LOS, such as the **severity of the condition,** the **socioeconomic status of the patient** (disadvantaged patients may need more social services and nursing care), and the uniqueness of the physician's practice.
   c. Current trends are in the direction of **decreasing days spent in the hospital.** Since 1984, Medicare's reimbursed LOS has decreased an average of 2.1% per year.
   d. The job of PROs is to make sure LOS is not shortened inappropriately for those who need longer care, especially the elderly.
   e. Hospitals are examining closely their practices and eliminating inappropriate or ineffective services. Many hospitals have concentrated their resources in a few specialties, increasing profitability and quality of patient care.
   f. **Nursing implications**
      (1) Nurses have an increasing role in educating patients, so that their self-knowledge can facilitate their long-term care.
      (2) Coordinated discharge planning is crucial so that home care agencies or the patient's family can continue needed care.
      (3) A case management model to maximize resources is the **group practice,** a specific group of nurses linked to a specific physician. Together, this group is responsible for developing standards, management tools, and designs for delivery of care. The entire plan functions within the DRG LOS framework, with a goal of **minimizing LOS while maximizing quality of care.**
      (4) One tool for case management and managed care is the **critical pathway (CP),** which is an abbreviated version (usually a one-page outline) of the clinical practices for the physicians and nurses involved in the case management plan of a particular DRG.
         (a) See **Figure 58-6, text page 1493,** for an example of a critical pathway.
         (b) The **development** of a critical pathway starts as a collaborative effort among physicians, nurses, and other supportive services, targeting a specific DRG in the institution that is high-volume, high-cost, and problem-prone.
         (c) Next, a retrospective chart review is done of patients with the targeted DRG, and an outline of current clinical practices is established.
         (d) A collaborative team then considers adding, excluding, or adjusting tasks in the critical path in order to help reach patient goals sooner.

4. **Restraining technologic advances**
   a. **History**
      (1) It is now necessary to **justify the purchase of items using new technology** such as drugs, devices, diagnostic equipment, and any equipment needed for medical and surgical procedures that prevent, diagnose, and treat disease.
      (2) These items account for a large part of the increase in health care costs.
      (3) Historically, these items were included as capital expenditures and treated as a "pass-through." Currently, these items **must be calculated in the hospital's indirect costs and therefore must count against the DRG.**
      (4) Congress continues to mandate percentage reductions in hospital capital payments.
      (5) The federal government influences development and utilization of technology through
         (a) The NIH, which supplies financial support for both basic and applied research related to the development of new medical technologies.
         (b) FDA reviews of the safety and efficacy of the new medical technologies, drugs, and medical devices.
         (c) State government regulating, in many states, the purchase of new equipment through a certificate of need program.
         (d) Medicare and Medicaid influencing indirectly the availability of new technology through decisions regarding reimbursement.

(e) The Office of Technology and Assessment providing congressional committees with objective analysis of the emerging, difficult, and often highly technical issues of our time; also indicating the beneficial and adverse impacts of the applications of technology.

(f) Patent law providing manufacturers a monopoly for a period of several years.

(6) Insurance companies have also developed techniques to control costs. These mechanisms include technological assessment, utilization review, case management, and selective contracting and price discounting.

(7) In 1989 the DHHS created the Agency for Health Care Policy and Research to enhance quality and promote appropriate and effective health care services through research and dissemination of information.

(8) At the request of HCFA, the **Office of Health Technology Assessment (OHTA)** evaluates the safety and effectiveness of new or not-yet-established medical technologies that are being considered for coverage under Medicare.

(9) The **Medical Treatment and Effectiveness Program (MEDTEP)** is involved in four major activities: data development, outcomes of research, clinical guideline development, and dissemination of research findings and practice guidelines.

(a) Integrating these activities provides, for practitioners, consumers, employers, educators, and insurers, scientific information about the most effective medical strategies.

(10) The development and review of clinical practice guidelines are facilitated by the **Office of the Forum of Quality and Effectiveness in Health Care.**

b. **Current trends**

(1) **"High tech" has become synonymous** with everyday medical practice in the United States, and America is the world's acknowledged high-tech leader.

(2) As the economy and median income in our nation rise, Americans tend to spend **more on health care,** demanding more and different kinds of health services.

(3) **Americans expect nothing but the best in health care** and react negatively to any efforts to slow technologic advancement.

(4) The state-of-the-art **cancer therapies increasingly drive the development of and rapid changes in technology.**

(a) The 1990s have witnessed an explosion in highly sophisticated new treatment modalities.

(b) Examples include colony stimulating factors, genetic engineering, monoclonal antibodies, new antiemetic and chemotherapy agents, and revolutionary bone marrow transplants.

c. **Nursing implications**

(1) In today's environment of cost containment, nurses must assume that resources are scarce relative to demand.

(2) More and more, nurses are being called on to justify the resources that are needed for improving patient care.

(3) Some techniques at the nurse's disposal are **feasibility studies** and **cost analysis studies.**

(4) **Feasibility studies** determine whether a new program should be developed and implemented in a health care agency. The basic steps are bulleted on **text page 1186,** column 1.

(5) Nurses may also be involved in cost analysis techniques such as **cost-benefit analysis (CBA)** and **cost-effectiveness analysis (CEA).**

(a) **Cost-benefit analysis** assigns monetary value to all costs and benefits of a potential program or practice, resulting in a cost-benefit ratio.

(b) **Cost-effectiveness analysis** is all the costs, measured in dollars, necessary to achieve a certain benefit, calculated and expressed as cost/unit of effectiveness. This technique is used to compare relative costs of several alternatives.

(6) Nurses may be involved in a **product evaluation committee (PEC)** responsible for controlling which product or service will be used by the agency.

(7) With the creation of the **Clinical Practice Guidelines by the Agency for Health Care Policy and Research (AHCPR),** nurses have an opportunity to inform patients about their development and use.

(8) Nurses involved with the updating of **products** or the purchase of new products should collaborate with many hospital departments: materials management, biomedical engineering, central supply, and research and development.

(9) Besides the internal health care system's serving as a resource for nurses responsible for product changes, an external nonprofit agency, Emergency Care Research Institute (ECRI), can be contacted.

5. **Limiting access to health care**

   a. Before the great depression of 1929, health care was paid out of pocket by the patient. Care was therefore highly inequitable, though proportionally less expensive than now.

   b. During the depression, costs rose sharply and people could not pay most doctors or hospital bills; Blue Cross was promoted by the American Hospital Association to pay for hospital stays.

   c. During World War II, health care coverage grew as an **employee benefit,** because it was not counted as a wage during the wage and price freeze.

   d. Health care costs continued to grow, but no major changes in policy were made until 1965 when **Medicare** and **Medicaid** were started. Federal and state governments now paid 26% of all money spent for health care.

   e. In the 1970s medical care costs rose sharply, faster than the general rate of inflation. The government's share of the total payments rose to **43%.** Health care costs as employee benefits also rose to **one-quarter of corporate after-tax profits.**

   f. In 1982 TEFRA was passed by Congress. PPS was established for the national Medicare program.

   g. In 1992, the Resource-Based Relative Value System (RBSIS) was implemented. This reimbursement system for Medicare recipients establishes national rates for each physician procedure, activity, and patient visit.

      (1) Hospitals treated people who could not pay and then charged higher rates to insured patients to cover the costs of the charity patients.

      (2) Insurance costs rose about 400% in the 1980s, and companies could no longer go on paying these increasing premiums.

      (3) Hospitals were also working to contain costs and could not cover the uninsured any longer.

   h. **Current trends**

      (1) Hospitals are squeezed as more and more Americans are uninsured at the same time that cost of care is still increasing.

      (2) Approximately 90% of uninsured Americans are in the active workforce but are employed by small companies that do not offer health coverage benefits. This category of worker will continue to increase as small service-oriented companies increase and large manufacturing companies decline.

      (3) **Alternative care delivery systems**

         (a) Several options of "managed care" are currently available.

         (b) **Health maintenance organizations (HMOs)** were started in the 1940s to emphasize preventive health maintenance.

            i. Members pay a **fixed price** and must receive care from only those doctors and hospitals designated by the HMO.

            ii. HMOs provide corporations the financial advantage of **fixed rates of reimbursement.**

         (c) **Individual practice associations (IPAs)** are a type of HMO in which the physician may accept HMO patients as well as fee-for-service patients.

            i. The physician is paid for care of the HMO patients according to a set fee schedule.

            ii. If the care costs less than the set fee schedule, the physician keeps the difference; if the care costs more, the physician must pay the difference.

         (d) **Preferred provider organizations (PPOs)** are another popular alternative plan, in which a group of providers joins a network and provides a discounted fee for service.

            i. The physicians and hospitals can charge the discounted fee in return for a guaranteed volume of patients.

            ii. The PPO offers the employer cost-controlling mechanisms.

            iii. The PPO has a prospective review process and will not do any procedures deemed unnecessary.

         (e) The percentages of insured people in alternative plans is growing.

            i. The greatest concern for alternative plans is that there is a strong incentive to reduce overall spending, potentially leading to poor health care.

ii.   However, studies have shown that the level of care for two types of cancers, breast cancer and colorectal cancer, was not statistically different from care provided to fee-for-service patients.

(4)   **National Health Care**

(a)   Many Americans, including some politicians, are proposing some kind of nationalized health insurance system.

(b)   Health care plans from other countries are being carefully studied. In some countries, including Great Britain, costs are low, but people wait long times for elective procedures, and high-technology treatments are often not available.

(c)   Other countries, such as Canada and Germany, have somewhat more services available, but salaries and operating costs are significantly lower than in this country.

(d)   Several detailed proposals have been outlined by politicians and by health-care-policy think tanks.

(e)   Most Americans agree that the time is right for significant health care reform in this area.

(f)   A key issue will be quality of care in relation to cost-effectiveness.

(g)   The American health care system was founded on the principle of universal access, but runaway health care costs have eroded the system's ability to deliver care to all.

(h)   In an effort to respond to the ailing American health care system, approximately **40 different reform proposals** that discuss possible solutions have been developed by individuals or organizations.

i.   The **AMA Plan** proposes to achieve universal access through reform of he existing system of health care. The first point is reform of the Medicaid program, requiring the use of only one national formula for eligibility, in place of the existing method of state discretion in setting the economic level for eligibility. Added coverage for prescription drugs, rehabilitative services, and emergency services will be provided. Medicaid reimbursement levels are increased to the Medicare level. This reform requires employer provision of health insurance for all full-time employees and their families, with tax help to employers. Legislatively created insurance programs would extend coverage to individuals without coverage or health insurance. Long-term care for senior citizens would be expanded.

ii.   The **Nursing Plan** calls for a basic core of essential health care services to be made available to everyone. All U.S. citizens would be provided a standard package of essential services. Employers without private coverage would pay into the public plan for their employees. The Medicare and Medicaid systems would be replaced by a single program administered by the state but based on federal guidelines and eligibility requirements. The plan encourages managed care, private plans through lower deductibles, and copayments.

iii.   The **AHA Plan** discusses a basic benefit that would cover preventive care, inpatient and outpatient care, and long-term care. It sets no fixed limits on the types or quantities of service; rather, coverage is based on medical necessity and reasonableness. Medicare and Medicaid would be replaced by a public plan financed through federal taxes and premium contributions. The plan would be financed half by employers and half by employees. Quality of care would be ensured by establishing medical practice parameters and by providing to the public information on the practices of individual practitioners, costs of services, and quality outcomes.

(5)   In addition to national proposals, several **states have initiated legislation** in response to the struggle related to access of care and allocation of resources.

i.   **Nursing implications**

(1)   Nurses can play an important role in defining the issues in the changes that are coming about in delivery of health care by

(a)   **Investigating strategies to reduce costs without compromising care.** This can be done by finding and recommending removal of those procedures that have a negative or minimal effect on quality of care.

    (b)   **Improving education of the public,** so that consumers can weigh their choices of type of insurance and their health care providers.

    (c)   **Assisting patients as their advocates in the decision-making process.** See **text page 1503,** column 1, for a list of questions for consumers to consider in choosing an HMO or PPO.

    (d)   **Keeping abreast of studies in cancer nursing,** through the American Society of Clinical Oncology and the Oncology Nursing Society. New studies are defining needs and standards for patient care in oncology.

    (e)   Engaging in political activities to influence how tax dollars are spent on health care.

    (f)   **Helping consumers select a care system** that meets their needs.

    (g)   **Helping patients understand,** and cope with, newly evolving **reimbursement restrictions.**

    (h)   Developing ways to **document, in financial terms, the nursing care needed for indigent patients.**

    (i)   **Researching strategies** for cost effectiveness and quality services.

    (j)   Keeping abreast of work by the Joint Committee on Accreditation of Healthcare Organizations for the Study of Change.

V.   RESOURCE-BASED RELATIVE VALUE SYSTEM

A.   HISTORY

1. In 1965 the Medicare program established the physician payment policies, Part B, which was modeled after plans developed by private insurers.
   a. Payments were based on what the law considered to be the usual, customary, and reasonable (UCR) charge.
   b. The amount of the government's payment was based on the lowest of the following:
      (1) The physician's actual charge.
      (2) The physician's customary charge.
      (3) The prevailing charge.
   c. Medicare paid the doctor **80% of the approved charge.**
2. Reasonable charges were established to try to rectify the problem of the aging population in the 1960s, for many of these individuals lacked health insurance.
   a. Within a short period, spending for physician services under Medicare began to **rise,** jumping by more than double-digit rates each year.
   b. In 1972 the laws changed, and the government would pay no more than what 75% of the practitioners in the geographic area were charging for the same services.
3. Over the years, Medicare began delaying recognition of physician fee increases, and payment amounts lagged behind market value.
   a. In 1988 the commission reported to Congress that the current **"reasonable charge"**-based system for the reimbursement of Medicare Part B payment needed to be replaced.
4. In 1989 a law was announced that had three major new elements: establishment of **Medicare Volume Performance Standard (MVPS),** replacement of the "reasonable charge" payment mechanism with a fee schedule for physician services, and replacement of the maximum actual allowable charge (MAAC) with a new limiting charge.
   a. The MAAC is the total amount that nonparticipating Medicare physicians could charge Medicare patients for their services.
5. In November 1991, the HCFA issued its final rules to implement the new Medicare physician fee schedule, **Resource-Based Relative Value Scales,** by January 1992.
   a. The new scale is **based on resources** such as the time, mental effort, judgment, technical skill, and physical effort involved in the patient procedure or treatment.
   b. The intent of this new system is to **raise reimbursement for primary care physicians,** who evaluate and manage patient care, and to offer less reimbursement to procedure-oriented physicians, pathologists, radiologists, ophthalmologists, and thoracic surgeons.

B.   CALCULATION

1. A relative value for each **Current Procedural Terminology (CPT) code** has been established.
   a. CPT provides a list of descriptive terms and numeric identifying codes and modifiers for reporting medical services and procedures performed by physicians.

2. The **total relative value unit (RVU)** is based on three separate units: the amount of physician work, practice expenses, and professional liability insurance or malpractice costs.

3. The relative value for each of the three separate units is multiplied by a conversion factor (CF) and a geographic adjustment factor (GAF).
   a. A sample computation of an estimated payment amount for a specific service in 1992 is presented in **Figure 58-7, text page 1506.**

4. Another important element of the new system is the CPT codes used by physicians for reporting evaluation and management (E/M) services.
   a. Every time a physician visits a patient in a hospital or outpatient setting, a CPT code must be selected that **reflects the care the patient received** from the physician.
   b. **Table 58-2, text page 1505,** presents a tool designed to help physicians determine the appropriate code for the services provided to their patients.

VI.   SPECIFIC ECONOMIC ISSUES IN CANCER CARE

1. Cancer treatment used to be seen as an opportunity to spend unlimited resources, i.e., a sacred cow. All this has changed; all costs must now be justified.

2. Cancer is now seen by some hospitals and administrators as a losing proposition, due to its **hospital intensive, high acuity care needs,** its **chronicity,** its **need for intensive monitoring throughout treatment,** and its **use of abundant psychologic interventions.**

A.   CANCER-SPECIFIC DRGs

1. The information concerning cancer-related DRGs has been compiled by the Association of Community Cancer Centers (ACCC).
   a. Cancer or cancer-related DRGs are listed in **Table 58-3, text pages 1506–1507.** DRGs that deal purely with cancer are indicated in the table with the letter "P."
   b. The cancer or cancer-related DRGs with the highest total gross reimbursement are listed in **Table 58-4, text page 1508.**
      (1) These high grossing DRGs do not necessarily represent money-making situations for the hospital; in fact, lung cancer is the cancer with the highest incidence, but it is a money loser for some hospitals.
      (2) This is because hospital care for these patients is usually more expensive than the allowed DRG reimbursement.

2. There are **regional variations** in the cost of treating cancer-related diseases.
   a. Some DRGs can be a moneymaker in one area of the country but a money loser in another.
   b. Individual hospitals can compare their cost data against other hospitals in the region. They can then ask which of their DRGs are costly in comparison to other hospitals and make changes in the procedures and protocols or length of stay.
   c. The **oncology clinical nursing specialist (OCNS)** can assist in reviewing and analyzing this type of information.

3. Other important factors in the cost analysis of a cancer program are
   a. Making sure that the unit of analysis is **cancer admissions** and not **cancer patients.** One patient may eventually have several admissions.
   b. Looking at several DRGs to get the **total number of admissions from one disease entity.** This combined DRG may represent the true profit or loss figure.

B.   CLINICAL TRIALS

1. **Clinical trials** are very costly for the hospital. One study showed that the loss per patient for those in a clinical trial was **30 times the loss for a patient not in a clinical trial.**
   a. This extra money was spent on **increased laboratory and radiology tests,** the need for a **special unit and/or a more highly educated interdisciplinary team, higher staff/patient ratios, nutritional support,** and **data management.**
   b. Research funding is available through the National Cancer Institute (NCI) for some of these studies, but not for all of them.
   c. Medicare will no longer pay these costs, as they did before PPS.

2. Exemptions are allowed for nine comprehensive cancer centers: MD Anderson Cancer Hospital, Houston, TX; Fox Chase Cancer Center, Philadelphia, PA; City of Hope National Medical

Center, Duarte, CA; Kenneth Norris, Jr., Cancer Center, University of Southern California, Los Angeles, CA; Fred Hutchinson Cancer Center, Seattle, WA; Memorial Sloan-Kettering Cancer Center, New York, NY; Roswell Park Memorial Institute, Buffalo, NY; Dana-Farber Cancer Institute, Boston, MA; and Ohio State University Arthur G. James Cancer Hospital, Columbus, OH.

   a. Other hospitals cannot afford the cost of investigational drugs for patients with advanced cancer.
   b. Some insurance companies are denying claims whenever investigational drugs are part of the therapy.
3. Treating cancer patients with stage III or stage IV disease is viewed by some as a financially ineffective use of health care resources, since the treatment most likely does not cure but only prolongs life and wastes resources, especially for those near death.
4. Pharmaceutical companies may contribute to the funding of clinical trials that test their products.
5. Patients may fund some of their own care if they can afford to do so.
6. The debate over reimbursement for clinical trials will continue and raises political, ethical, and financial issues.

C. UNLABELED USE OF FDA-APPROVED CHEMOTHERAPY DRUGS

1. In the late 1980s, the government and insurance companies began to deny reimbursement for uses of drugs that did not fall within the package insert guidelines.
2. As many as half of all approved drugs are used for unlabeled indications.
   a. It is time consuming and costly for the manufacturers to get FDA approval for all possible use indications. This situation has yet to be resolved.
3. In February 1991, after much public awareness and pressure from lobbyists, the Senate Committee on Labor and Human Resources asked the General Accounting Office (GAO) to **examine off-label drug use in the treatment of cancer.**
   a. The findings were that off-label drug use among oncologists is **widespread;** more than half (56%) of the patients studied had at least one off-label drug as part of their chemotherapy drug regimen **(Figure 58-5, text page 1512).**
4. The reimbursement problems for off-label drug treatments seem to be **increasing** today, and attempts are continually being made to challenge payment denials for chemotherapy off-label drug use.

D. OUTPATIENT ONCOLOGY CARE

1. Due to the fact that patients are being discharged earlier in their treatment, there has been an **accelerated growth of outpatient care facilities.**
2. Management of complicated care and toxic side effects has become possible on an outpatient basis by increasing the education and responsibility of the patients and their families (see **Chapter 54, Ambulatory Care).**
3. One of the most unstable factors in outpatient care is the billing procedures. There have been four different types of coding for physician insurance payments, which can be found on **text page 1512,** column 2.
4. Nurses must keep abreast of the changes.

E. PREVENTIVE CANCER CARE

1. An example of a **wellness program** sponsored by many of the larger companies is one to stop smoking. Industry also sponsors **cancer screening programs.**
2. These kinds of programs help prevent the development of cancer in the first place.
3. Close to half the states require insurance companies to pay for screening mammography.

F. CANCER AND THE SOCIOECONOMICALLY DISADVANTAGED

1. **Overall 5-year cancer survival** among African Americans is 38%, compared to 50% among Caucasians.
   a. The racial differences in cancer statistics are due **primarily to differences in socioeconomic status,** not to racial differences per se.

2. **Poor Americans, regardless of race, have a 10%–15% lower 5-year cancer survival rate,** as well as a higher overall incidence, compared to other Americans.
3. **Basic features of the poor** that affect the problems of early cancer detection, treatment, and survival are unemployment, inadequate education, substandard housing, chronic malnutrition, and diminished access to medical care.
    a. The **expanding number of legal and illegal immigrants** entering the United States is a major factor contributing to the increased number of people living below the poverty level.
4. The ACS and NCI both prioritized activities to eliminate this gap in cancer survival between the economically disadvantaged and other Americans.
5. The United States medical system does little to encourage preventive health care for the poor.
6. See **text page 1514,** column 1, for the five most critical issues related to cancer and the poor outlined in "Cancer and the Poor: Report to the Nation."
7. The ACS responded to the report by identifying 10 specific challenges (**text page 1514,** column 2) that address the problems poor people encounter when seeking cancer education, prevention, detection, and treatment services.
8. The ACS authorized $1.8 million in grants to initiate demonstration projects. A pilot project's goal was to provide a full spectrum of cancer prevention services to persons who are not normally receiving such services.
    a. Initial results show that the **poor are interested in receiving cancer-prevention-related services** and will use them if they are available.
    b. Also, there are **professionals extremely interested in working with the poor** to help them prevent cancer.

VII.   **NURSING'S FUTURE IN THE ECONOMICS OF HEALTH CARE**

1. It is important for nurses to be aware of the cost containment procedures that are now in place and that will continue to exert pressure on types of cancer care that can be provided. Nurses must become more proactive, creative, and open-minded.
2. While nursing costs are not calculated separately in determining DRGs, studies have shown that these costs account for **between 20% and 28% for two-thirds of the DRGs in the study.**
    a. There has been a great deal of interest in charging separately for nursing costs, but this is not yet a reality in most geographic areas.
3. The PPS will change over time to further restrict health care payments. This fact presents cancer nurses with an opportunity to be a significant part of the clinical research needed to determine which nursing interventions are most beneficial from a cost-benefit perspective.

PRACTICE QUESTIONS

1. The law of supply and demand does not apply to health care because
    (A) hospital fixed costs are inelastic.
    (B) demand has risen faster than supply.
    (C) physicians order too many tests due to fear of malpractice.
    (D) the payer is not a direct part of either supply or demand.

2. Which of the following statements about TEFRA is true?
    (A) It covers both private insurers and Medicare.
    (B) It was created before Medicaid.
    (C) It created a prospective payment system (PPS).
    (D) It allowed hospitals to be reimbursed based on actual costs.

3. One of the positive effects that the prospective payment system (PPS) has had on health care in the United States is that
    (A) technologic advancement in health care has been encouraged.
    (B) a greater number of Americans now have access to the health care system.
    (C) hospital bills have decreased as a result of reduced LOS.
    (D) federal funding of clinical trials has been encouraged.

4.   Which of the following types of health facilities is reimbursed under PPS?
     (A)   rural hospitals
     (B)   children's hospitals
     (C)   Veterans Administration hospitals
     (D)   comprehensive cancer centers

5.   PPS takes into account all of the following **except**
     (A)   urban versus rural setting.
     (B)   labor costs.
     (C)   the family's ability to care for the patient at home.
     (D)   the patient's need for ancillary services.

6.   Which of the following is true as a result of PPS?
     (A)   Many insurers have developed formal procedures for evaluating the effectiveness of new technologies.
     (B)   Capital expenditures can be reimbursed according to cost, but patient care costs cannot.
     (C)   States have very little regulatory power over the purchase of new equipment by hospitals.
     (D)   Hospitals may only purchase new equipment for which they have a large number of DRGs.

7.   Nurses may use all of the following to justify needed resources **except**
     (A)   feasibility studies.
     (B)   cost-benefit analyses.
     (C)   standards of quality of care.
     (D)   cost-effectiveness analyses.

8.   Cost shifting is defined as
     (A)   transferring excess funds from Medicare to Medicaid.
     (B)   paying for charity cases by overcharging privately insured patients.
     (C)   providing government-funded insurance for unemployed persons.
     (D)   sending uninsured patients to the nearest municipal hospital.

9.   The demand for charity care is steadily increasing at a time when many hospitals have negative operating margins. A significant reason for the increased need for charity care is the
     (A)   dramatic growth in ambulatory, hospice, and home care.
     (B)   number of people who are employed but not covered by employer health insurance.
     (C)   trend toward reduced Medicare and Medicaid coverage for outpatient services.
     (D)   change in federal and state guidelines regarding reimbursement to physicians for charity cases.

10. Preferred provider organizations (PPOs) control costs by
     (A)   allowing member physicians to overcharge patients with other forms of insurance.
     (B)   not covering the cost of annual physical examinations.
     (C)   requiring subscribers to use their own salaried physicians.
     (D)   offering discounted fees for service in exchange for a guaranteed quantity of patients.

11. Cancer treatment services generally are not regarded as moneymakers by hospitals for all of the following reasons **except**
     (A)   the elderly take up a disproportionate share of hospital costs.
     (B)   chemotherapy drugs are costly.
     (C)   intensive monitoring and high acuity care are needed.
     (D)   only investigational drugs are covered by Medicare.

12. One reason why the future of some clinical trials is in jeopardy is that
     (A)   most individuals are unable to pay their own costs for clinical trials.
     (B)   an increasing percentage of patients have stage III or stage IV disease.
     (C)   National Cancer Institute funding to the nine comprehensive cancer centers has been drastically cut.
     (D)   a lack of travel funds is limiting the presentation of research findings.

ANSWER EXPLANATIONS

1.   **The answer is (D).**   The law of supply and demand does not apply to health care because the consumer does not pay for services, so price does not provide a balance between supply and demand. In normal

supply and demand, a decrease in price would be followed by an increase in demand. With health care, there has been an increase in demand with little concern for price because a third party (the insurer) is paying. (1486–1487)

2.   **The answer is (C).**   TEFRA, the Tax Equity and Fiscal Responsibility Act passed by Congress in 1982, changed the method of providing inpatient services for Medicaid and Medicare from a retrospective, cost-based payment system to a prospective payment system. TEFRA created a PPS for Medicare and Medicaid reimbursement. It pays hospitals a certain amount per patient per admission based on a formula, as opposed to reimbursing actual costs. (1487–1488)

3.   **The answer is (C).**   The prospective payment system (PPS) reimburses hospitals with a fixed payment depending on the complexity of the problem that precipitated the hospitalization. The amount reimbursed is determined by using one or more of nearly 500 diagnosis-related groups (DRGs), which determine the amount that a hospital will be reimbursed for a patient's care and not the actual cost that the hospital incurred. One effect of the PPS has been to reduce patient length of stay (LOS) in hospitals and thereby reduce the overall hospital bill. Since 1984, Medicare's reimbursed LOS has decreased an average of 2.1% per year. (1488)

4.   **The answer is (A).**   All of the other types of facilities represent exceptions to the program of PPS reimbursement under Medicare. DRGs were developed with a primary orientation toward short-term, acute-care hospitals; application to specialty hospitals is limited. Among the other hospitals that are not reimbursed under the PPS system are long-term care hospitals, psychiatric hospitals and units, rehabilitation hospitals and units, and hospitals located in states with state-regulated PPS plans. (1488)

5.   **The answer is (B).**   A variety of factors determine the payment a hospital receives per case, including the patient population, labor costs, location, and teaching intensity. Variations in cost per case that are not accounted for by the adjustment factors described above are due to differences in hospital efficiency. (1489)

6.   **The answer is (A).**   Under PPS, it is necessary to justify the purchase of items using new technology, such as drugs, devices, diagnostic equipment, and any equipment needed for medical and surgical procedures that prevent, diagnose, and treat disease. Historically, these items were reimbursed on the basis of actual costs, a "pass-through." Currently, these items must be calculated in the hospital's indirect costs and therefore count against the DRG. The other choices are incorrect: hospitals cannot pass through either capital or treatment costs; many states regulate the purchase of new equipment through a certificate of need (CON) program; and cost-effectiveness is not correlated with numbers of patients. (1494)

7.   **The answer is (C).**   Increasingly, nurses are being called on to justify the resources that are needed to improve patient care. Feasibility studies and cost analysis studies, including cost-benefit analysis and cost-effectiveness analysis, are some techniques at the nurse's disposal. Feasibility studies determine whether a new program should be developed and implemented in a health care agency. Cost-benefit analysis assigns monetary value to all costs and benefits of a potential program or practice, resulting in a cost-benefit ratio. Cost-effectiveness analysis is all the costs, measured in dollars, necessary to achieve a certain benefit, calculated and expressed as cost/unit of effectiveness. This technique is used to compare relative costs of several alternatives. (1496)

8.   **The answer is (B).**   Historically, those who could not pay hospital costs were covered via cost shifting. Hospitals treated people who could not pay, and then charged higher rates to insured patients to cover the costs of the charity patients. Insurance costs rose about 400% in the 1980s, and companies could no longer go on paying these increasing premiums. Hospitals were also working to contain costs and could not cover the uninsured any longer. (1497–1498)

9.   **The answer is (B).**   Approximately 60% of uninsured Americans are in the active workforce but are employed by small companies that do not offer health coverage benefits. This category of worker will continue to increase as the number of small service-oriented companies increases and that of large manufacturing companies declines. The other factors are real, but less important. (1498)

10.   **The answer is (D).**   Preferred provider organizations (PPOs) are a popular alternative health care plan in which a group of providers joins a network and provides a discounted fee for service. The physicians and hospitals can charge the discounted fee in return for a guaranteed volume of patients. The PPO

offers the employer cost-controlling mechanisms. The PPO has a prospective review process and will not do any procedures deemed unnecessary. (1498–1499)

11. **The answer is (C).** Cancer is now seen by some hospitals and administrators as a losing proposition, due to its hospital-intensive, high-acuity care needs, its chronicity, its need for intensive monitoring throughout treatment, and its use of abundant psychologic interventions. Cancer patients require a great deal of labor-intensive care for a long period of time. The nonreimbursement of investigational drugs makes this situation worse. (1506)

12. **The answer is (A).** Clinical trials are costly both for the hospital and the patient. Patients often must pay for the cost of clinical trials, since they are frequently not reimbursed by third-party payers, including Medicare. (1509–1510)

59   Ethical Issues in Cancer Nursing Practice

STUDY OUTLINE

I.   **INTRODUCTION**

    1.   In addition to the many physical and emotional challenges faced by oncology nurses, many different ethical issues arise in caring for patients with cancer.

II.   **GENERAL ETHICAL ISSUES**

    A.   **AUTONOMY**

        1.   **Autonomy** is a principle that compels us to respect the **self-command** of the individual.
        2.   Autonomy is part of what makes us moral. It is more than simply patients' rights or even the freedom to choose. The core of what it means to be a person is **moral responsibility to oneself and to others.**
        3.   Caregivers have a **duty** to respect the **moral origins of the person, not just to respect the choices the person makes.**
        4.   For centuries, health care practitioners practiced a form of **paternalism, acting in the best interests of others without asking their preferences, or even explicitly acting against their preferences.**
        5.   Caregivers are often reluctant to accept the wishes of individuals with serious illness, especially if they think something still might be done to improve either longevity or quality of life. This can create a conflict between the caregiver's **duty to protect and prolong life and the autonomy and privacy rights of the individual patient.**

    B.   **BENEFICENCE**

        1.   **Beneficence** is the principle of **altruism,** that is, to act in the best interests of others. This leads to the maxim in health care **"the patient comes first."**
        2.   Self-interest is a part of duty to oneself, yet the principle of **beneficence** creates an expectation that health professionals have promised and will take exceptional steps to **place their patients' interests above their own.**
        3.   While beneficence is a good thing, it can become problematic if it takes a **paternalistic** form of doing good without attention to the **wishes of the other person.**
        4.   Beneficence does not rule out trying to persuade patients to overcome their fears and to help them choose what is in their best interests. In the final analysis, however, it is **unethical to act against the wishes of patients** if they continue to refuse the offerings of modern health care.
        5.   It may be difficult to determine what is in the patient's best interest. There may be **conflicting courses of treatment** or only **statistical or epidemiological information** that may or may not apply to the circumstances.

    C.   **NONMALEFICENCE**

        1.   When caregivers find that there is confusion or disagreement about what is in the patient's best interest, they must fall back to a position of **nonmaleficence: "at least do no harm."**
        2.   Nonharm is a minimalist beneficence position. **Respecting the personhood of the patient**

requires an attempt to honor autonomy and to act in **his or her best interests.** At the very least, however, it means **never harming intentionally.**

3. It may be difficult to **define harm.** The definition may span **physical to psychological and even spiritual harm.**

D. JUSTICE

1. The principle of **justice** requires that we give each person **his or her due.**
2. There are competing opinions of **how to measure what is due.**
3. Approaches to measuring what is due include **equity** (attempt to equalize the inequities of life) and **egalitarian** (everyone is entitled to exactly the same treatment) approaches. Libertarians argue that justice requires a **fundamental respect for autonomy** and that one cannot alter the social situation without the consent of those being governed.
4. Different views of justice have little bearing on clinical decisions at this time, although they do influence various proposals for **access to care** and the design of **social programs.**

E. ALTERNATIVE ETHICAL THEORIES

1. The difficulty in clinical ethics is rooted in the tendency of ethics to require **abstract thought,** which often contrasts sharply with the **concrete** individual problems encountered by professionals who must make **quick decisions about very complex issues in order to benefit their patients.**
2. **Ethical analysis** must take careful note of numerous ethical theories, axioms, and other concerns in order to conduct a conceptual and problematic analysis. This process takes time and, by necessity, can become quite abstract. Health care professionals, on the other hand, must do **ethics on the run,** and they may lose interest in abstractions and theories that are not decisively and explicitly linked to their immediate need to provide patient care.
3. Dissatisfaction with **principle-based ethical theories** has led to new proposals for moral analysis, such as **casuistry, hermeneutics, and "ethics as story."** Each of these approaches stresses the **concreteness** of the individual situation and the importance of **interpreting values** of those involved in the case.
4. **Casuistry** is a methodology by which each case is analyzed on its own merits. No overarching principles will lead to a conclusion from one case to another.
5. **Hermeneutics** means interpreting the case in its whole context, including the individuals' **life plans and values, the family's values, and social and cultural factors.**
6. **"Ethics as story"** relies on narrative to discover the interests and values in each instance, especially with relationship to **caregivers themselves.**
7. **Virtue theory** is also an alternative that may complement principle-based ethics. Virtue theory assumes that **no principle could be implemented without the commitment of caregivers or patients to the good as they perceive it.** Even the most rule-bound person must have virtues of interior commitment to the rules.
8. Relying solely on the virtuous caregiver or patient, without a set of objective moral guidelines or principles, can lead to difficulties and, without some limits, could result in abuse.
9. There is a need for a relationship between **objective standards** and the **virtue of the nurse** (his or her own conscience and personal standards).

F. RECONCILIATION EFFORTS

1. Concerns about the increased role of the health provider's values in caring for the dying patient, greater attention to the relation between physician and patient, and questions about what kind of society we want have focused attention on both medical ethics and ethics theory.
2. It has been proposed that the goal of health care ought to be **"beneficence in trust,"** wherein the caregiver holds in trust the **values of the patient** in making **joint decisions with the patient about best interests.**
3. **Libertarianism** is another approach to reconciling medical ethics and ethics theory. Libertarianism is based on an assumption that a **fundamental rationality all humans beings share can enlighten them in their pursuit of consensual agreements in bioethics.**
4. Regardless of the approach taken, it is important that **individual moral commitments** are not separated from **ethical decision making.** Approaches to resolving ethical dilemmas must also

remain sensitive to the concrete situation and to the uniquenesses of both the patient and the nurse.

5. Given the nature of our society, a rationalistic approach to bioethical decision making must also be met with some reservation. Further, this approach ignores the potential for us as human beings to identify with a vulnerable individual through **compassion.**

6. **Casuistry**

   a. **Casuistry** is the theory that each case is unique and from that each case certain norms can be developed that may or may not be applicable to analogous cases.

   b. The goal of casuistry is to establish the **paradigm case,** in which a certain norm predominates. Other cases are then **compared** to the paradigm case and analyzed for the extent to which they match.

   c. One of the problems with casuistry is that it presupposes a **unified theory of human nature** by which one case can logically be compared to another. In addition, casuistry neglects the importance of ethical theory in case analysis and ethical decision making.

7. **Contextualism**

   a. A middle ground between a generalist application of ethical theory and specialized case-by-case analysis is possible with a **contextual grid** for ethical analysis.

   b. **Contextualism** seeks to place a moral problem in context by describing the hierarchy and particular emphasis or weighting given to the values and principles at issue in a particular case. Having established the context and the weighting of the various values and principles, the discussion can proceed toward a means for resolving the case by protecting the interest and values of those affected by it.

   c. Variability in the context of a case describes the unique **weighting of values and principles** as determined by the **medical specialty** involved; the **personal values of patient, family, or social group;** the personal and professional **values of the health professionals** involved; and the **institutional setting** in which the problem arises.

   d. The contextual grid rests on two distinctions: a distinction among **primary, secondary, and tertiary care settings** and a distinction between the individual and the number of persons affected by the problem. When we consider the values of different persons whose interests are affected by the outcome of the case, **we tend to protect the common good.**

G. **ETHICAL WORK-UP**

1. A tool developed to facilitate case analysis is presented on **text page 1525.** The **Ethical Work-up Guide** is designed to try to **examine as many values** as possible within the specific **context** of a case and to reach a resolution that respects as many of these values as possible.

III. **NURSING ETHICAL ISSUES**

1. Beneficence must go well beyond the minimalistic interpretation of avoiding harm. It entails helping others even when that involves inconvenience, sacrifice, and risk to self-interest. Conflicts occur between the obligation to help others and self-interest.

A. **THE VIRTUE OF COMPASSION**

1. Compassionate care was traditionally supported by ensuring that sick persons were surrounded by those who loved them the most and knew their values.

2. In contrast, our community of today seems more concerned about the resources the sick **divert** from other projects, and **rationing care appears to be more valued than providing it.**

3. With rationing of care comes a danger of shrinking from the sacrifice of time, emotions, energies, and money that are required in the care of sick persons.

4. Compassion is more than pity or sympathy. It is the capacity to feel, **to suffer with the sick person, to experience something of the fears, the assault on the whole person, the loss of freedom and dignity, and the vulnerability that the illness experience produces.** It flows over in a willingness to help, to make some sacrifice, and to go out of one's way.

5. Compassion entails a **comprehension of the suffering experienced by another,** and thus compassion enriches understanding of what we ourselves must some day pass through.

6. Compassion is the quality that keeps health professionals from operating solely on the basis of **objectivity and rationality.**

7. Compassion enables health professionals to assist in **healing,** if by healing we can mean the **reconstruction of the person.**

8. True healing and appropriate decision making can take place only when all the **particulars and values of the individual and all the parties involved in the process of caring are taken into account.**

9. Compassionate care means that patients who cannot be cured by medical sciences may still be "healed" if we help them to **express the meaning of their lives** by respecting, insofar as possible, their own **values and commitments.**

B. **CLINICAL ETHICS AND THE RELATION TO THE PATIENT**

1. The connection between clinical judgment and clinical ethics can help reveal structures of good decision making in patient care that are not simple products of contractual models of the provider-patient relationship.

2. Traditional commitments to the value of human life within the patient care relationship are important. As persons, patients are owed **humanity,** not just "humaneness," since the relationship between the healer and the ill person rests on the desire of both to promote the **wholeness of the one who is ailing.**

3. As a society, we are tempted by **technical rather than personal solutions to problems. However, responsible use** of technological intervention requires **rational analysis,** as well as **sensitivities to the particulars of the case** and to the **value commitments of the parties involved.**

4. The responsible **use of power** is a clinical ethics judgment about the best balance of interventions and outcomes, and this provides **counterpressures** to a **straightforward honoring of patient wishes and autonomy.**

5. The **virtue of compassion** requires awareness of the **physical condition of the patient (to assess outcomes)** and the **values of patients or of those speaking for them (to assess the quality of those outcomes measured against patient values).**

C. **THE PATIENT SELF-DETERMINATION ACT**

1. This act, which went into effect in December 1991, requires all health care institutions to notify patients on admission of their rights under state law to execute an advance directive.

2. Other provisions of the law include
    a. Asking patients whether they have issued an advance directive or wish to do so.
    b. Asking for a copy of the advance directive if one exists.
    c. Placing a copy of the advance directive prominently in the patient record.
    d. Notifying the patient of the institution's commitment to honor the patient's wishes.

3. Honoring patient wishes would not only show **respect for persons** but would also help save critical health care funds.

4. **Difficulties can arise when the wishes expressed do not anticipate future events.** For example, if the patient who develops a reversible sepsis has said earlier that she does not want to "be on a respirator," but that treatment is required to treat the sepsis, can her wishes be disregarded in this instance?

5. Nurses are usually **caught in the middle** on issues like this, as they find it difficult to interpret the treatment plan if the physician chooses to ignore advance directives for any reasons. In such cases, an **ethics consult** or patient-care discussion is recommended.

D. **COMPASSIONATE ANALYSIS**

1. Advances have occurred in **emphasizing the rights of patients not only to determine the treatments they desire** and do not desire **during the dying process** but also to **choose treatments at any time during life,** not just while dying.

2. The principle underlying instruments such as the **Living Will** and the **Durable Power of Attorney** is essentially to **increase the role of compassion in decisions about life-prolonging technology.**

3. A **Living Will** gives advance directives for the **final period of terminal illness.** In most states it is interpreted to cover only the last few weeks of a person's life. Consequently, the Living Will is a limited instrument.

4. The **Durable Power of Attorney** is a much more favored document. This instrument gives another person **authority to make health care decisions for an individual who becomes incompetent to do so.** Not only would this person know the **patient's wishes,** but he or she could also **communicate with caregivers to determine the best treatment or nontreatment options during the course of temporary or permanent incompetence.**

5. The Durable Power of Attorney covers **any treatment decisions,** formally anticipated or not, and at **any stage in life, not just a terminal situation.**

6. These documents are important because of the tendency of our **"technofix" society** to prolong suffering in conditions of **"hopeless injury."**

7. **"Hopeless injury"** is a condition in which there is **no potential for growth or repair, no pleasure or happiness from living,** and a total **absence** of one or more of the following **attributes of quality of life:** cognition or recognition, motor activity, memory or awareness of time, consciousness, and language or other intelligent means of communicating thoughts and wishes.

IV. **CANCER ETHICAL ISSUES**

A. **THE DYNAMICS OF CANCER**

1. The **dynamics of cancer** refers to the spiritual struggle of the patient to come to terms with the diagnosis of cancer. The term **spiritual** refers to the **inner realm of fundamental values** each person possesses.

2. The spiritual realm is often neglected in daily life because external matters and concerns so easily obscure it. Serious trauma in the external life is often necessary before people face their spiritual realm directly.

3. For the patient with cancer, the spiritual struggle may be intensified by confusion about **goals of treatment, longevity concerns,** doubts about the most effective therapy, problems of **cost and benefit,** and the relation of these difficulties to the patient's longstanding **system of values.**

4. The dynamics of cancer has its own structure. At first patients may feel **guilty.** Cancer is seen as **self-destructive,** almost as if the body is eating itself. Later, patients come to see that they are not usually responsible for their cancer. Even if they risked cancer through smoking or other bad habits, they might forgive themselves.

5. In the next phase of the dynamic, cancer is made into an **object,** an "it," an invading army of cells. Depending on age, habits of resiliency, and the individual's assessment of his or her own life span, patients may choose to do battle with their cancer.

6. **Guilt reemerges** when individuals decide not to continue against the odds. This guilt is attached to the patient's worries about loved ones.

7. The likelihood of participating in research therapies for cancer treatment may decline in elderly cancer patients because of lowered life span expectations, poorer prognosis due to more advanced stages of the disease, the body's inability to cope with the collateral effects, and (very importantly) a value hierarchy that may place continued economic security for their family over their own continued life.

8. The dynamics just outlined represent a **spiritual struggle,** and an important component at each step of the dynamic is the patient's own ranking of values.

B. **CANCER AND AUTONOMY**

1. **Autonomy is often identified with decision making,** but patients themselves seldom make this identification.

2. Patients are engaged with at least three **struggles:**
   a. With the body, often leading to **physical exhaustion.**
   b. With the **environment,** their family, community, etc.
   c. With their own **values,** including their life plans, expectations, the hierarchy of their values, etc.

3. While the cancer dynamic continues, the patient identifies autonomy with **reshuffling a hierarchy** of values. **These values can easily be missed** in well-intentioned but ineffective efforts to respect the patient.

4. In making quality-of-life decisions, **the patient's value hierarchy is of prime importance.**

5. By **respecting the patient's value hierarchy, we can best prevent paternalistic overtreatment against a patient's wishes** and any biased undertreatment of cancer patients.

6. **Eliciting patients' values is part of the process of respecting them as persons.**

C.   **CANCER AND SUFFERING**

1.   Pain is a major consideration in caring for any cancer patient. It can so preoccupy caregivers that concomitant **suffering is masked.**
2.   The first **source of suffering is the division of the person** into an ego, often isolated and alone, and the body that has betrayed that person by being taken over by the disease.
3.   There is a documented disparity between patients' and physicians' evaluations of the quality of life.
4.   **Involving patients in decisions about the therapeutic plan can help heal** the suffering caused by the division of the self into ego and body.
5.   Concern with both **eliciting patient values** and **using them to design a humane treatment plan** is fundamental to quality care.
6.   The biggest danger a cancer patient faces is that of being **stripped of his or her values** in the face of the vast array of interventions we have available to us. The **emotional roller coaster** of promises and hopes versus outcomes and despairs can disrupt the relationships people have constructed all of their lives.
7.   The **primary task** of caregivers is to ease suffering by **working to promote synthesis of the human entity.** Recommendations for **promoting synthesis** include
     a.   Providing excellent pain control, as well as attempting to meet the suffering person as a person, thus minimizing the suffering caused by withdrawal and fear.
     b.   Making every effort to **understand the patient's value system,** so that it can be respected and employed in the treatment plan.
     c.   Implementing the care plan consistently as a means to minimize suffering.
     d.   Continuing to respect the patient's values, even when the patient can no longer feel pain and is in a comatose state near the end of life.

D.   **TERMINATION OF TREATMENT**

1.   Decisions about the termination of treatment involve the **proportionality of the treatment to the expected and sometimes realized outcomes of the treatment for the individual in his or her specific circumstances.** There is **no** absolute **objective standard by which to measure this proportionality,** and each instance must be judged on its own characteristics.
2.   The physical condition of the body, personal demographic factors such as age, and an individual's life plans, goals, and values can all contribute to individual differences in decision making about the termination of treatment.
3.   **Withholding and withdrawing**
     a.   Caregivers today seem more willing to withhold and withdraw major interventions deemed "heroic," but the **reasoning behind the intent** of withholding and withdrawing major interventions seems to be confused. There are two possible lines of reasoning:
          (1)   The withholding or withdrawing is done with the **goal of bringing about the patient's death.**
          (2)   The withholding or withdrawing is done with the **goal of removing treatments that prolong the patient's suffering, while not intending the patient's death.**
     b.   Although the action of withholding or withdrawing will be the same in either case, the second intent is entirely different from the first. With the first intent, death is seen as good, and actions are taken to bring about that good. The second intent assumes that death is either neutral or an evil and that one cannot will such an evil and still maintain purity of heart.
     c.   In the past, the distinction in intent between aiming at the patient's death and aiming at reducing suffering was used to distinguish between active and passive euthanasia. However, **ethicists argue that if the intent is that bringing about the patient's death would be a good thing, there is no difference between withholding and withdrawing on the one hand and actively bringing about death on the other.**
     d.   If our intent in withdrawing care is to bring about death, then other, more direct forms of euthanasia may seem much more appropriate.
     e.   Currently, Americans are hotly debating whether to legalize active euthanasia, aid in dying, and physician-assisted suicide. Of major concern is allowing physicians to kill patients out of mercy in the context of a society that has so little respect for human life in other areas.

4. **Control of dying and life support**
   a. In addition to concern about active euthanasia, we must also be concerned about meeting the physical and social needs of the dying individual.
   b. One "technofix" solution to patient anguish is to prolong suffering in conditions of hopeless injury. Much technological intervention is not so much **life-supporting as organ-supporting.**
   c. **The effect of employing life-prolonging technology on dying individuals without their involvement in its application is to increase patient and family suffering.** It both prolongs the personal suffering of the dying and promotes social suffering by wasting resources that might benefit those with potentially reversible diseases.
   d. In order to protect human dignity, societies must maintain constant vigilance about protecting persons from both undertreatment and abandonment and inappropriate overtreatment.
   e. Undertreatment occurs when the "bottom line" predominates over benefit to the patient.
   f. Overtreatment occurs through the technological enthusiasms of caregivers, the fear of "letting go," or appeals for unreasonable treatments from patients.
5. **Nutrition and hydration**
   a. Those who oppose the withdrawal of nutrition and hydration do so on the grounds that providing food and water to the dying is a **special obligation and that beneficence should overrule patient autonomy.** They argue that withdrawing or withholding these **leads directly to the death of the patient,** since the patient does not die from the underlying disease process but rather from starvation and dehydration.
   b. There are two problems with this contention:
      (1) Patients have a common law right and probably a constitutional **right to refuse treatment even if they are dying.**
      (2) **Patients may request aid in dying on the grounds that death is a good** and that others have a duty out of compassion to bring about such a good.
   c. Bringing about a death does not necessarily entail active, direct euthanasia or even physician-assisted suicide. However, it does require that all interventions, including fluids and nutrition, be **examined for their impact on the desired goal of treatment.**
   d. It is also important to **consider the expressed wishes of the individual** with regard to food and fluids, so that in the absence of expressed wishes, vulnerable persons are not "put to death" by such actions.
   e. In making decisions about the withholding or withdrawing of fluids and nutrition, consideration must be given both to the **objective criteria (medical indications)** for such an action as well as the **context, life plans, or values of the individual patient.**
6. **The role of the family**
   a. In light of recent court decisions, **it is unclear what the role of the family or guardian is in speaking for patient values** when the patient is incompetent.
   b. It is very important to **obtain advance directives from all patients,** especially seriously ill ones.
   c. Despite the cautions noted by the court about family surrogacy, most persons feel comfortable about naming a family member to make decisions since such a person knows them and their values best.
7. **Access to care**
   a. Some argue that beyond a certain point, expensive medical technology should not be offered to persons over the age of 80; however, this point **should not** be set by **ageist limits** but rather by **the limits of medicine** to provide any meaningful change in the **outcome** for patients during their last years.
   b. It may not be necessary to set such limits on the basis of age, if we first try to respect a patient's value system.
   c. Many older patients are more ready to die than to fight cancer. It is not an instance of wanting to die. They still regard life as precious, but it is a matter of proportion. Older patients are more accustomed to thinking that they will soon die anyway.
   d. Other important **issues regarding access to cancer care** include the rights of all persons to **expensive interventions,** the right to request **experimental therapy,** allocating **scarce resources,** large-scale **distribution of health care among competing health needs,** and the **distribution of funding for other human needs versus health care needs.**
8. **Playing God**
   a. Modern technology **empowers us beyond our normal capacities** and tempts us to exceed the bounds of moderation. This leads to a kind of **paternalism** in which an individual

comes to believe that due to superior technical knowledge, he or she knows best what is good for another person.

   b. This kind of paternalism can result in the overzealous application of interventions or, more rarely, undertreatment or abandonment of patients.

   c. There is **nothing intrinsically wrong with the application of technology** to improve our lives; on the contrary, it is part of the mission of all human beings to use their talents to **bring about the good in their lives and in society.**

   d. It is important for health care that providers understand the risks and benefits of technological interventions they propose.

9. **Euthanasia**

   a. The problem of euthanasia and many difficult questions about human reproduction all involve the question of **dominion over life.**

   b. Our technology makes the temptation to take control over life itself almost overwhelming.

   c. A distinction must be drawn between **objective evaluation of interventions and outcomes on the well-being of the patient** and subjective quality-of-life judgments in which physicians and other caregivers **judge that the life the patient is now living is not worthwhile for that person.**

   d. Given today's economic conditions, there is a danger that it will be easier to eliminate those persons whose care costs too much, or who are now considered to be a burden on society, than to address their suffering.

   e. It is important to maintain compassionate respect for human life in our society.

   f. Some argue that **actions to eliminate burdensome life,** even if requested by the patient himself or herself, are a form of **"privatizing life,"** denying its social and communal dimensions as both a private and public good.

   g. Others argue that euthanasia and/or assisted suicide are **appropriate and important forms of caring** for persons whose lives, by their own assessment, have become too burdensome to continue.

V.   CONCLUSION

1. The duty to protect a patient's life lies primarily in **protecting his or her autonomy and value hierarchy.** Values assessment and constant discussion with the patient and family throughout the course of treatment are methods of achieving this objective.

2. Institutions should require that each patient prepare an **advance directive** prior to or on admission to the facility.

3. Teaching guides should be developed for all health care professionals that would train them in the processes of **implementing patient advance directives.**

4. The current **default mode of health care delivery,** in which it is **assumed that everyone desires technological support of life,** should be changed and the opposite assumption made unless the patient has issued advance directives to the contrary.

5. **Utilize a process** like the Ethical Work-up Guide to **analyze and discuss cases** that arise in one's service. By doing this, one not only gains greater critical awareness of one's own assumptions and values but also becomes more able to discuss the deepest commitments of one's profession.

PRACTICE QUESTIONS

1. As an oncology nurse, you frequently make decisions and act to promote the best interests of others. You are using which of the following ethical approaches?
   (A) nonmaleficence
   (B) justice
   (C) beneficence
   (D) utilitarianism

2. A nurse states that she is always truthful in dealings with patients, since truthfulness is part of respecting the self-command of the individual. She is applying which of the following fundamental ethical principles?
   (A) autonomy
   (B) beneficence
   (C) compassion
   (D) informed consent

3.   Ethical theories recently advanced as **alternatives** to principle-based ethics include
     (A)   nonmaleficence, libertarianism, and virtue theory.
     (B)   contextualism, beneficence-in-trust, and hermeneutics.
     (C)   ethics as story, hermeneutics, and contextualism.
     (D)   casuistry, hermeneutics, and ethics as story.

4.   Which of the following statements about casuistry is true?
     (A)   Casuistry is an ethical theory that provides a means to identify and examine the values, issues, and variables in a case and to describe the values that are most likely to take precedence over others.
     (B)   Casuistry challenges the deductive model of ethical reasoning and describes realistically how good decisions regarding the resolution of ethical dilemmas can be made.
     (C)   Casuistry emphasizes the practical importance of ethical theories in the examination and resolution of ethical dilemmas in clinical practice.
     (D)   One of the strengths of casuistry as a basic model for ethical decision making lies in the assumption of a unified theory of human nature by which one ethical dilemma can be compared with another.

5.   Which of the following statements about compassion is **false?**
     (A)   Compassion is the capacity to feel and suffer with the ill person; it is more than pity or sympathy.
     (B)   Compassion enables caregivers to facilitate healing by reuniting the separated body and ego, respecting patient values and commitments, and helping the patient to express the meaning of his or her life.
     (C)   Compassion is the quality that helps health professionals balance a tendency toward overinvolvement, which can result in a loss of objectivity and rationality.
     (D)   Compassion includes both a comprehension of the patient's suffering, fear, vulnerability, and loss and a willingness to take action to help.

6.   The **primary** goal of the Patient Self-Determination Act is to
     (A)   facilitate a systematic process of eliciting and honoring patient wishes.
     (B)   control health care costs in the last 6 months of life.
     (C)   require health care institutions to notify patients on admission of their rights under the law to execute an advance directive.
     (D)   facilitate a responsible use of technological intervention.

7.   Which of the following statements about Living Wills and Advance Directives is true?
     (A)   A Durable Power of Attorney gives advance directives for the final period of terminal illness.
     (B)   The underlying principle of any advance directive is the prevention of suffering and the enhancement of the role of compassion in decisions about life-prolonging technology.
     (C)   A Living Will identifies a specific person who can express the wishes of the individual should she or he become incompetent or ill.
     (D)   In some states, the Living Will is also called a Durable Power of Attorney.

8.   A mentally competent 71-year-old patient receiving chemotherapy treatment for her newly diagnosed breast cancer expresses her worry that she will receive treatments at the end of her life that prolong her suffering. She is not married and has no children. Although she has nieces and a nephew, they live across the country and are not involved in her care. She considers the woman with whom she has shared a house for the past 25 years her closest "relative." In providing counseling to her regarding her concern, you would
     (A)   discuss the meaning of a DNR order and the Patient Self-Determination Act.
     (B)   encourage her to consider a Living Will.
     (C)   explore her wishes and preferences about end-of-life decisions, and provide information about a Durable Power of Attorney.
     (D)   contact her physician so that he or she can discuss DNR with the patient.

9.   The "cancer dynamic" involves the following four processes:
     (A)   guilt, fighting the cancer, betrayal, and depression.
     (B)   guilt, objectification and struggle against the disease, relapse and betrayal, and reemergence of guilt.
     (C)   guilt, struggle against the disease, anger, and betrayal.
     (D)   denial, depression, struggle against the disease, and guilt.

10. Which of the following statements about the termination of treatment is **false?**
     (A)   In some states, family members may not be able to authoritatively articulate the wishes of a patient

who has become incompetent unless such wishes are documented in writing through an advance directive.
- (B) The termination of treatment and/or limiting options for intervention should be considered most relevant in decision making for patients who are over 80 years old.
- (C) Decisions about the termination of treatment involve the proportionality of the treatment to the expected or realized outcome for the individual in his or her specific circumstances.
- (D) Employing life-prolonging technology on the dying without patient involvement in its application serves to increase patient and family suffering.

11. In our current health care environment, the **greatest** danger regarding euthanasia is that
- (A) it will be used as a simple method of eliminating persons whose care costs are too much or who are considered a burden to society.
- (B) caregivers will be tempted to regard certain individuals' lives as not worthwhile.
- (C) it will discourage caregivers from proposing aggressive treatment for the seriously ill older person.
- (D) it is inconsistent with the position of nonmaleficence.

ANSWER EXPLANATIONS

1. **The answer is (B).**   Beneficence is the principle of altruism, that is, to act in the best interests of others. Nonmaleficence is the principle of never harming the patient. Justice is the principle that requires that we give each person his or her due. Utilitarianism is an ethical principle that states that an action is morally right if it brings about good consequences. (1521–1522)

2. **The answer is (A).**   Autonomy is the principle that compels us to respect the self-command of the individual. Beneficence is the principle of acting in the best interests of others. For centuries, health care practitioners practiced a form of paternalistic beneficence, acting in the best interests of others without asking their preferences, or even explicitly acting against their preferences. Compassion and informed consent are not fundamental ethical principles, but both compassion and the requirement for informed consent support truthfulness with patients. (1521–1522)

3. **The answer is (D).**   Casuistry, hermeneutics, and ethics as story are three new proposals for moral analysis. Contextualism utilizes principle-based ethics as it locates a moral problem and describes the values and principles at issue within the moral problem. It is a middle course between generalist application of ethical theory and specialized case-by-case analysis. Beneficence-in-trust and libertarianism are approaches that attempt to reconcile the emphasis on personal autonomy with the need for beneficence, questions about the kind of society we ought to be, and greater attention to the health provider's values in the interaction. Nonmaleficence is the principle of "at least do no harm." (1522–1524)

4. **The answer is (B).**   Casuistry is the theory that each case is unique and that from that case are developed certain norms that may or may not be applicable in analogous cases. Casuistry is therefore unconcerned with formal ethical theory. One of the difficulties with casuistry is that it presupposes a unified theory of human nature by which one case can be logically compared to another. This unified theory, as it was employed in the past, is now discredited. (1523–1524)

5. **The answer is (C).**   Compassion entails a comprehension of the suffering experienced by another. It is the quality that keeps health care professionals from operating solely on the basis of objectivity and rationality. (1526)

6. **The answer is (C).**   The Patient Self-Determination Act may also serve to control health care costs in the last 6 months of life and to facilitate a responsible use of technological intervention. However, these are not the primary goals of the act. The act does not necessarily facilitate a systematic process of eliciting and honoring patient wishes. (1527).

7. **The answer is (B).**   The principle underlying any advance directive is the prevention of suffering and the enhancement of the role of compassion in decisions about life-prolonging technology. A Durable Power of Attorney, not a Living Will, gives another person authority to make health care decisions for an individual who becomes incompetent to do so. A Living Will is a much more limited document than the Durable Power of Attorney. The Living Will gives advance directives for the final period of terminal illness,

interpreted to mean the last few weeks of a person's life. The Living Will and the Durable Power of Attorney are not the same. (1528)

8. **The answer is (C).**   Although part of the counseling process to address this patient's concerns might include discussing DNR, such a discussion may not be comprehensive enough to address the patient's presenting concern since DNR is concerned essentially with the withholding of cardiopulmonary resucitation. Discussion of the Patient Self-Determination Act is only a launching point for an exploration of the patient's wishes and preferences regarding end-of-life decisions and for discussion of the concept of a Durable Power of Attorney, which names an individual who will speak for the patient when the patient is incompetent to make decisions about health care. A Living Will tends to be a more limited document covering only the terminal phase of an illness. Discussion with the physician about DNR orders may or may not be appropriate, depending on the nurse's discussion with the patient about her wishes.

9. **The answer is (B).**   The cancer dynamic refers to the spiritual struggle of the patient to come to terms with the diagnosis of cancer. (1529).

10. **The answer is (B).**   Although some have proposed that options for intervention should be limited in patients beyond the age of 80 years, this point should not be set by ageist limits but rather by the limits of medicine to provide any meaningful change in the outcome for patients during their last years. It may not be necessary to set such limits if we first try to respect a patient's value system. (1532)

11. **The answer is (A).**   In today's cost-driven health care climate, the biggest danger of euthanasia is that it will be used as a simple method of dispatching persons whose care costs too much or who are now considered to be a burden on society. For many theorists, the principle of nonmaleficence is not consistent with euthanasia. However, others argue that euthanasia is an appropriate and important form of caring for persons whose lives, by their own assessment, have become too burdensome to continue. It is possible, though less likely, that if euthanasia were permitted, over time caregivers would be encouraged to regard certain individuals' lives as not worthwhile or to refrain from proposing certain treatments for certain groups of individuals, such as the elderly. (1533)

60 Questionable Methods of Cancer Therapy

STUDY OUTLINE

I. **INTRODUCTION**

    1. Each year thousands of cancer patients and many others who merely fear they might develop cancer devote countless hours and invest billions of dollars in the use of questionable cancer remedies outside the realm of mainstream medicine.

        a. Whether labeled **"unconventional," "unsound," "unproven," "unorthodox,"** or **"alternative,"** these treatments range from those that are both fraudulent and dangerous to those that are hazardous mainly to the pocketbook.

        b. Often these treatments offer individuals a chance to participate in their own care, reflecting the **naturalistic approaches** so popular with the public today.

    2. **Questionable methods** of cancer management include diagnostic tests or therapeutic methods that have not shown activity in tumor animal models or in scientific clinical trials but are promoted for general use in cancer prevention, diagnosis, or treatment.

        a. Such methods do not protect the consumer because they have not met the requirements of the U.S. Food, Drug and Cosmetic Act.

    3. Each year Americans spend $10 billion on unscientific remedies and $4 billion to $5 billion on fraudulent ones.

        a. Various studies have reported that 9%–50% of cancer patients admitted using an unproven remedy.

II. **HISTORICAL PERSPECTIVES**

    1. For thousands of years, individuals in need have turned to people offering what they hope will be an answer to their medical problems.

A. **LEGISLATION**

    1. Before the Food and Drug Act of 1906, thousands of unproven treatments were promoted to the American public.

    2. In 1906 President Theodore Roosevelt signed into law the **Pure Food and Drug Act,** which forbade misleading or false statements on the labels of remedies.

    3. In 1912 Congress passed the **Sherley Amendment,** which made it a crime to make false or fraudulent claims regarding the therapeutic efficacy of a drug.

        a. This legislation was limited, in that it was still necessary to prove that the promoter intended to defraud the public.

    4. In 1962 Congress clarified some of the language of the previous legislation and further added that drugs must demonstrate efficacy in addition to safety before they could be marketed.

B. **PAST UNPROVEN METHODS**

    1. Examples of unorthodox approaches, arranged according to their years of popularity, are identified in **Table 60-1, text page 1538.**

    2. Many of the popular questionable methods of cancer treatment parallel the most promising developments in scientific clinical trials.

    3. **Koch antitoxin therapy: 1940s–1950s**

    a. The Koch antitoxin treatment consisted of pure **distilled water mixed with one part per trillion of a chemical called glyoxylide,** which is merely glyoxylic acid (a normal body constituent) with water removed.

    b. Over 3000 health practitioners in the United States employed this regimen, paying $25 per ampule and charging patients as much as **$300 for a single injection.**

    c. In 1943 the Canadian Cancer Foundation reported that no patients on a clinical trial using the Koch method benefited from the treatment.

    d. Although Koch antitoxins are illegal in the United States, they can still be obtained through the underground medical community or in Mexico.

4. **Hoxsey method: 1950s**

    a. Hoxsey maintained that cancer was a result of a chemical imbalance in the body that caused healthy cells to mutate and become cancerous and that his therapy restored the chemical environment and killed the cancerous cells.

    b. Hoxsey's Herbal Tonic consisted of several different formulas: the "black medicine" was composed of cascara in an extract of licorice root, alfalfa, burdock root, red clover blossoms, buckthorn bark, barberry root, pokeweed, and prickly ash bark; the "pink medicine" contained potassium iodine and lactated pepsin.

    c. Today, Hoxsey's medicines are available at the Biomedical Center in Tijuana, Mexico, and a special diet and an attitudinal approach have been added.

5. **Krebiozen: 1960s**

    a. Krebiozen allegedly was first produced by a Yugoslavian physician who developed the substance from blood extracted from horses.

    b. In 1961 the National Cancer Institute (NCI) obtained a sample of Krebiozen, and the substance was identified as a creatine monohydrate, an amino acid found in all animal tissue.

    c. The Krebiozen Research Foundation submitted 504 case records to the NCI in an effort to demonstrate therapeutic efficacy in justification of a clinical trial, but a panel of 24 scientists reviewed these records and concluded that Krebiozen was an **ineffective drug.**

    d. The treatment was available until 1977.

6. **Laetrile: 1970s**

    a. Laetrile is a general term for a group of cyanogenic glucosides, derived from several different seeds, e.g., apricot, peach, cherry, and almonds.

    b. Claims have been made that laetrile is a nontoxic form of **"vitamin B$_{17}$"** and that taking this vitamin can prevent cancer, but no reputable scientist accepts the existence of vitamin B$_{17}$.

    c. Evidence suggests that laetrile has **toxic effects.**

        (1) A number of deaths attributed to **cyanide poisoning from oral laetrile** have been reported, and laetrile by **enema is also poisonous.**

    d. Laetrile in the United States is either imported illegally or brought in under court order.

    e. Numerous animal studies and two retrospective studies have shown no therapeutic benefit.

    f. In 1980 the **FDA gave approval to the NCI for the first prospective clinical trial** of laetrile, and once again it was demonstrated that laetrile is ineffective against cancer.

    g. Laetrile was still a billion-dollar-a-year industry in 1983.

    h. Today, many of the proponents of laetrile have changed their strategy of using it as a single agent and are combining it with vitamins, enzymes, or so-called metabolic therapy.

III. **POPULAR QUESTIONABLE METHODS OF TODAY**

1. Questionable methods of cancer treatment during the 1980s and into the 1990s are primarily related to **lifestyle** and as such cannot be regulated by the FDA.

    a. Many of the unproven methods place responsibility for a healthy lifestyle on the patient and have an aura of respectability in relation to conventional scientific medicine that is concerned with diet, environmental carcinogens, lifestyle, and the relation between emotions and physiologic responses.

2. The most commonly used remedies in a study of 669 patients who had utilized questionable treatments were, in order, metabolic therapy, diet therapies, megavitamins, mental imagery, spiritual or faith healing, and "immune" therapy.

3. **Nutritional therapy** represents a major type of questionable cancer treatment.

A. **DIETARY THERAPY/METABOLIC THERAPY**

1. Many questionable cancer therapies emphasize **natural cure through dietary manipulation or "metabolic" approaches.**
   a. There are approximately 20 different types of metabolic regimens for the prevention of cancer and for cancer treatment, including **restricted diets, specific dietary modification, enzyme therapy, cellular therapy, megavitamins, detoxification with colonic irrigations,** and the **development of an appropriate mental attitude.**
   b. The concepts of metabolic therapy are based on the **theory that cancer is a result of impaired metabolism that causes a buildup of toxins in the body.**

2. **Gerson regimen**
   a. Gerson's **"metabolic" therapy** proposes that constipation or inadequate elimination of wastes from the body interferes with metabolism and healing.
   b. Cure can be achieved through **manipulation of diet** and **"detoxification,"** or purging the body of so-called toxins.
   c. Gerson's approach includes avoidance of exposure to carcinogens, positive mental outlook, and the elimination of wastes from the body.
   d. See **text page 1540,** column 2, for the specifics of the regimen.
   e. Promotional brochures cite cures of 90% of patients with early cancer and 50% of patients with advanced cancer; however, these claims are **not** supported by data or statistics.
      (1) What has been reported is that **repeated enemas** and **purgatives** are more likely to lead to **metabolic imbalance,** and coffee enemas have killed people.

3. **Manner metabolic therapy**
   a. The "Manner cocktail" consists of an **intravenous solution of dimethyl sulfoxide (DMSO)** and **massive doses of vitamin C, vitamin A,** and **laetrile.**
      (1) Various protocols may also include coffee enemas, fasting, and a highly restricted diet that advocates raw milk, megavitamins, live-cell therapy, and **enzymes.**
   b. There is no objective evidence that this metabolic therapy has any benefit in the treatment of cancer.

4. **Macrobiotic diets**
   a. The macrobiotic diet probably is the **most popular diet therapy** both for curing cancer and for preventing cancer.
   b. The diets have their origins in Zen mysticism, which proposes **two antagonistic and complementary forces, yin and yang,** that govern all things in the universe.
      (1) Each food is classified as yin or yang, whereas each tumor is classified as being caused by an imbalance of either yin or yang.
      (2) **Balance is also achieved through cooking techniques** and **attitude toward life.**
      (3) See **text page 1541,** column 1, for the details of the diet.
   c. Macrobiotic therapy can result in **malnutrition** and cause a variety of serious health problems.
   d. There are no valid data on the efficacy of **macrobiotic diets in the prevention or treatment of cancer.**

B. **PHARMACOLOGIC AND BIOLOGIC APPROACHES**

1. **Antineoplaston therapy**
   a. Stanislaw Burzynski, M.D., originally isolated the **antineoplastons from blood** and then from the **urine of individuals without cancer.**
   b. He claims that antineoplastons are **natural peptides** and **amino acid derivatives that cause cancer cells to change to normal cells, inhibit the growth of malignant cells,** and are also **useful in diagnosing cancer.**
   c. His product is not a naturally occurring peptide, and he does **not claim to cure cancer but reports complete remissions with minimal side effects.**
   d. Based on an **NCI site-visit team review** of a best-case series of seven patients prepared by Burzynski, the NCI plans to conduct a **phase II study** in patients with brain tumors.

2. **Cancell**
   a. Cancell, also known as Entelev, Jim's Juice, Croinic Acid, and Sheridan's Formula, is a **mixture of synthetic chemicals created for their electrical properties.**

  b. It is claimed that the **formula reacts with the body electrically** and **lowers the voltage of the cell structure and converts cancer cells to waste material.**

  c. Cancell is more effective if **taken internally and externally at the same time** and must be taken for a minimum of 45 days.

    (1) See the specific details of Cancell on **text page 1542,** column 1.

  d. Although the **FDA obtained a permanent injunction prohibiting the distribution of Cancell** in interstate commerce, it is being distributed as "a gift" to anyone who requests it.

3. **Dimethyl sulfoxide (DMSO)**

  a. DMSO is an agent that has been used as an **industrial chemical solvent** and as a **preservative for culture cells.**

    (1) It is rapidly absorbed through the intact skin.

  b. The industrial form has been used **alone** or **in combination with laetrile and other forms of "metabolic" therapy,** with claims that it will restore the cancer cell to being a normal cell.

  c. A review of the literature by the American Cancer Society revealed no evidence that DMSO results in objective benefit in the treatment of cancer patients.

4. **Live-cell therapy**

  a. Live-cell therapy (fresh-cell therapy or cellular therapy) is the **injection of cells from animal embryos or fetuses.**

  b. The **type of cells given supposedly matches the diseased tissue or organ in the patient.**

    (1) Proponents claim that the **live cells contain active agents that stimulate the immune system** and **repair** and **regenerate the host cells.**

    (2) Cellular therapy is promoted for a variety of indications (menstrual disorders, premature aging, sterility, neoplastic conditions).

  c. In a review of the literature, the American Cancer Society found **no scientific evidence that live-cell therapy was effective in the treatment of cancer.**

    (1) More important, **serious side effects** have resulted from the application of live-cell therapy.

5. **Megavitamins**

  a. Whereas certain cancers have been associated with low intake of some vitamins, there is **no** clear-cut evidence that high doses of vitamins prevent cancer.

  b. Excessive vitamin intake is **useless** against cancer and, more important, may be **toxic.**

  c. **Vitamin C**

    (1) Megadose vitamin C probably is the most popular self-administered vitamin supplement.

    (2) A series of three NCI-funded randomized trials of vitamin C documented no consistent benefit from vitamin C in patients with cancer.

    (3) **Megadoses** of vitamin C can cause **severe kidney damage, release cyanide from laetrile,** and **may cause death if administered intravenously.**

  d. **Vitamin A**

    (1) Doses of vitamin A supplements, as low as five times the recommended dietary allowance (RDA), may be **toxic** and have no clear value in the treatment of cancer.

  e. **Pangamic acid ("vitamin B$_{15}$")**

    (1) Pangamic acid or "vitamin B$_{15}$" is not a vitamin, has no standards for use, and is not recognized by the FDA as a drug.

    (2) Even though it is **illegal** to sell it as either a drug or a food supplement in the United States, it is still available in many health food stores.

    (3) There is evidence that the chemicals in products labeled "B$_{15}$" or "pangamate" **may promote the development of cancer.**

6. **Oxymedicine**

  a. Oxygen treatments have gained popularity among the promoters of questionable cancer regimens.

  b. **Hydrogen peroxide** is administered by various routes: **oral, rectal, intravenous,** and **vaginal.**

  c. Promoters claim that it **stimulates immunity, oxidizes toxins,** and **kills bacteria** and **viruses.**

  d. Ozone gas can be administered by rectal infusion, intramuscularly, or in blood transfusions.

  e. Oxidizing agents such as hydrogen peroxide and ozone can be **harmful, causing oxygen emboli** and **death.**

C. **IMMUNOLOGIC APPROACH: IMMUNOAUGMENTATIVE THERAPY (IAT)**

1. IAT is based on the theory that **stimulation of the immune system will enable the body's normal defenses to destroy tumor cells.**
2. Treatment regimens are based on the determination of the individual's daily or twice-daily blood levels of "tumor antibody," "tumor complement," "blocking protein factor," and **"deblocking protein factor."**
3. An **NCI analysis** of the IAT materials revealed that the materials were dilute solutions of blood plasma, with no biologic activity.
4. **Safety concerns** have arisen over the years:
    a. The unopened vials of treatment materials examined by NCI were found to be **unsterile** and **contaminated with various bacteria.**
    b. **Skin abscesses** at the injection site of IAT have been reported.
    c. In 1985, **antibodies to hepatitis B** and **acquired immunodeficiency syndrome (AIDS) were found** in the IAT serum.
5. IAT remains a **hazardous** approach to the treatment of cancer, with no documented clinical activity or scientific rationale.

D. **BEHAVIORAL AND PSYCHOLOGICAL APPROACHES**

1. **Mental imagery**
    a. The **Simonton method,** a program of relaxation and imagery, is a self-help approach that has been popular since the 1970s.
    b. **It is the Simontons' belief that attitude and stress are crucial** in causation and cure of cancer and that relaxation and imagery will enhance the immune system and alter the course of malignancy.
    c. Cancer patients and their partners are taught to use mental imagery and relaxation techniques to visualize cancer cells as weak and sick and to imagine body defenses as a powerful army that attacks and eliminates the cancer cells.
    d. The Simontons **strongly advocate** that participants in their counseling sessions continue to receive conventional medical treatment.
    e. The following **problems** remain concerning the Simonton method:
        (1) There are no carefully controlled clinical studies that show objective benefit.
        (2) The method may be harmful, in that individuals may be made to feel guilty because their particular personality type was responsible for the development of cancer.
        (3) If individuals become overly reliant on the Simonton method, they may be encouraged to abandon standard medical therapy.
    f. Bernie Siegel also places **responsibility on the individual** by emphasizing a positive attitude toward survival.
    g. Both these approaches allow individuals' participation in care; however, they **suggest** that those patients who do not survive may not have been strong enough or had a good attitude.
2. **Spiritual, faith, or mind healing**
    a. Many people find empowerment and comfort through various aspects of spiritual or faith healing.
    b. Many patients resort to **commercialized faith healers** who defraud people of their money by claiming they can cure cancer.
    c. Some methods that require patients to accept the idea that emotions contributed to their cancer may render patients **vulnerable to guilt** and **depression.**

IV. **QUESTIONABLE TREATMENT FACILITIES**

1. Unorthodox clinics are flourishing in Tijuana, Mexico, which has become a haven for promoters who treat cancer patients with unconventional therapies.
2. Patients arriving at these clinics encounter not only dubious cancer treatments but also dubious diagnostic tests.
    a. See **Table 60-2, text page 1545,** for information on the major Tijuana clinics.

V.   **PROMOTERS AND PRACTITIONERS OF QUESTIONABLE METHODS**

    A.   **STRATEGIES USED BY PROMOTERS**

        1.   Promoters of questionable cancer remedies survive, thrive, and grow rich.

        2.   Much effort and money are devoted to **public relations** and **media presentations** that use scientific words or phrases in a misleading and deceptive manner while exploiting their emotional impact.

        3.   Highly motivated and better-educated individuals are more likely to turn to questionable methods because of the promise that "you control your disease."

    B.   **ORGANIZED ADVOCATES OF QUESTIONABLE CANCER THERAPY**

        1.   See **text page 1545,** columns 1 and 2, for a list of the organizations most active in promoting questionable methods of cancer treatment.

VI.   **WHO SEEKS QUESTIONABLE CANCER TREATMENTS, AND WHY**

        1.   Patients who seek questionable therapies are more likely to be Caucasian, to be asymptomatic, to have localized disease, and to be better educated.

        2.   Many patients seek unconventional therapy **after** completing their mainstream treatment regimens, when they have no evidence of disease.

    A.   **MOTIVATIONS AND REASONS FOR USE**

        1.   **Fear**

           a.   Cancer creates many fears. Many individuals with cancer are in **great need of hope** and may seek unproven therapies that are offered as "nontoxic" therapies that will "cure" their disease.

           b.   Resorting to some dietary or enzyme therapy that **promises no side effects** or uses **"the body's natural defenses" may coincide with the person's fantasies about being cured.**

        2.   **Desire for self-control**

           a.   Use of an unproven method may provide an individual with a greater sense of self-control.

           b.   **Better-educated** and **highly motivated patients** are more likely to turn to unproven methods, because the methods **falsely promise** to give the patient control over the disease.

        3.   **Isolation/antiestablishment**

           a.   The promoters of questionable methods frequently suggest that the government and organized medicine are in a **conspiracy** against curing cancer.

           b.   The isolation that is **projected by the purveyors** of questionable treatment methods may be easy for cancer patients to identify with, because they too may feel isolated.

        4.   **Social pressures**

           a.   The **family has many of the same fears** as the patient.

           b.   They may feel that the best course is to try everything, with the hope that something will work.

           c.   It may also help them feel less guilty if the treatment does not work or the patient does not recover.

VII.   **CONTROL OF QUESTIONABLE METHODS**

        1.   Any new method of cancer management in the United States must meet certain **scientific standards.**

        2.   See **text page 1546,** column 2, for the standards of scientific investigation.

        3.   Recently, the National Institutes of Health (NIH) were congressionally mandated to establish the **NIH Office of the Study of Alternative Medicine.**

           a.   The pivotal issue for the NCI in trying to improve cancer therapy is **whether the treatment in question is effective, regardless of the source.**

           b.   The NCI participates in best-case series reviews and the conduct of pilot clinical trials.

        4.   The federal and state governments participate in the regulation of questionable treatment methods.

5. Education plays a major role in the control of questionable cancer treatment.
   a. Private and government organizations provide information to health professionals and the public.
   b. See **Table 60-3, text page 1547,** for sources of information on questionable cancer remedies.

VIII. **ROLE OF NURSES/NURSING INTERVENTIONS**

1. Nurses must deal realistically with the complexities and limitations of modern cancer care as well as the subtlety and seductiveness of the unorthodox cancer treatment industry.

A. **IDENTIFICATION OF QUACKERY (LEGITIMATE VS. FRINGE CARE)**

1. The health professional must be **informed** regarding the most frequently encountered unproven methods and the particular aims of a given individual's therapy.
2. The health professional should be able to **explain the risks of unproven methods.**
   a. For individuals using an unproven method in combination with standard therapy, it is still important to know what **side effects** to look for.
3. The Subcommittee on Unorthodox Therapies of the American Society of Clinical Oncology has listed 10 questions to ask in making a decision as to whether a treatment should be suspected of being questionable (**Table 60-4, text page 1548**).

B. **ASSESSMENT OF COMMUNICATION CHANNELS AND PATIENT MOTIVATIONS**

1. **Communication patterns** between the patient and family must be **evaluated.**
   a. The family may become preoccupied with seeking different therapies as a means of coping with stress.

C. **MAINTENANCE OF POSITIVE COMMUNICATION CHANNELS**

1. It is important for the physician and health care professional to discuss questionable methods of cancer management with patients.
   a. **Table 60-5, text page 1549,** identifies some potential questions to ask in order to assess a patient's risk and possible motivations for seeking questionable methods of cancer therapy.
   b. By initiating such a discussion, the health care professional helps keep the **channels of communication open.**
2. A nonjudgmental attitude facilitates the assessment of the patient's and family's motivations for wanting to try an unproven method.

D. **MAINTENANCE OF PATIENT PARTICIPATION IN THEIR HEALTH CARE**

1. Many patients turn to questionable cancer remedies because they **do not feel like active participants** in their care and have lost hope that their conventional therapy will work.
   a. It is important for patients and family to **participate** in health care.
   b. Patients will be less likely to seek questionable cancer care remedies if such needs are met.
2. **Patient education** can increase patient satisfaction, increase patient knowledge, and enhance self-care.
3. The patient should be urged to continue standard medical care.

PRACTICE QUESTIONS

1. Which of the following does the federal government insist on before a drug can be marketed?
   (A) the safety of the drug only
   (B) the efficacy of the drug only
   (C) the safety and the efficacy of the drug only
   (D) the safety, efficacy, and long-term value of the drug

2. One of the principal appeals of most questionable methods of treatment to the cancer patient is their
   (A) perceived absence of risks and side effects.

(B)   ready availability and modest costs.
(C)   level of acceptability to family and friends.
(D)   high degree of efficacy and safety.

3.   Which of the following reasons is **least** likely to explain a decision by a cancer patient to explore a questionable method of treatment?
(A)   a desire for greater control over the treatment process
(B)   pressure from family and friends
(C)   valid data on the efficacy of the method
(D)   resentment toward an impersonal medical system

4.   One problem that may arise in the Simonton method of cancer treatment, which relies on mental imagery and relaxation techniques, is that
(A)   the Simonton method excludes standard cancer therapies.
(B)   patients may be made to feel that their mental attitude caused their cancer.
(C)   the long duration of the treatment causes patients to lose faith in its therapeutic value.
(D)   other aspects of patient care, notably nutrition, are overlooked.

5.   Which of the following questions would a nurse be **least** advised to ask the cancer patient or family member who desires to use a questionable treatment method?
(A)   "What do you know about this method?"
(B)   "How do you think this method will help you [or your loved one]?"
(C)   "Have you [as a family member] discussed this method with your loved one?"
(D)   "Are you aware of the potential dangers of this treatment?"

ANSWER EXPLANATIONS

1.   **The answer is (C).**   The Food and Drug Act of 1906 called for the truthful labeling of ingredients used in drugs but did not ban false therapeutic claims on drug labels. The Sherley Amendment in 1912 made it a crime to make false or fraudulent claims regarding the therapeutic efficacy of a drug, but proof of intent to defraud the customer was needed. Finally, in 1962, Congress added that drugs must demonstrate efficacy in addition to safety before they can be marketed, and a process was created by which a substance can become approved for prescription use. (1547)

2.   **The answer is (A).**   Individuals use questionable methods for a variety of reasons, such as "I have nothing to lose" or "If it won't hurt me, why not try it?" Often they are confused by conflicting reports of cure rates of standard treatments and frightened by treatment risks and possible side effects. Many unproven methods promise no side effects and draw on the patient's fantasy of cure involving "the body's natural defenses." By using an unconventional therapy, the patient hopes for an unconventional cure. (1546)

3.   **The answer is (C).**   In theory, valid data on the efficacy of a questionable method would be the **best** reason for a patient to choose that method, but then the method would no longer be "questionable." The fact remains that none of the various questionable methods discussed in this chapter has stood up to scientific scrutiny, especially the requirement of proven efficacy in human subjects. The reasons stated in the other choices are among the most likely to motivate the cancer patient to seek an alternative therapy. (1546)

4.   **The answer is (B).**   The Simonton method is based on the idea that a positive mental attitude can improve an individual's physiologic responses, resulting in improved response to standard therapies. Patients are taught to use mental imagery and relaxation techniques to visualize cancer cells as weak and sick and to imagine body defenses as a strong army that attacks and eliminates cancer cells. Patients are encouraged to continue conventional treatment, however. Besides the problem of patient guilt, other problems with this method are that objective benefits have yet to be documented by clinical studies, and individuals may become overly reliant on the method to the exclusion of standard medical therapy. (1543)

5.   **The answer is (D).**   The first job of the nurse is to assess the underlying motivations of a patient or family member who wishes to discuss an unproven method. This can be done by asking questions such as those in choices (A)–(C). The individual is usually aware that such techniques are not likely to be approved by

the professional. Asking questions such as those in choices (A)–(C) may help the professional to discover unmet needs of the patient and family and to assess their understanding of the therapies that have been administered. A nonjudgmental attitude on the part of the professional also may make the patient and family more receptive to the information provided by the caregiver. A question such as that in choice (D), on the other hand, may be regarded by the patient as negative and judgmental, and it may serve to cut off further discussion. (1547–1549)

61 Teaching Strategies: Public Education

STUDY OUTLINE

I. **INTRODUCTION**

    1. Educating the public in the area of health has been a nursing responsibility for many years. Health care professionals in the cancer field view themselves as role models, not only to the patients they serve but also to the public at large.

II. **DEFINITION OF TERMS**

    1. There are many definitions of health education. The broadest definition is **"any combination of learning experiences designed to facilitate voluntary adoption of behavior conducive to health."**

III. **THEORIES AND MODELS**

  A. **HEALTH BELIEF MODEL**

    1. The **health belief model** establishes a framework for explaining why people engage in specific preventive behaviors. It combines variables such as the person's perception of being susceptible to some health problem, the perceived seriousness of that problem, and the availability of specific actions that prevent or treat the problem.

  B. **PRECEDE**

    1. The **PRECEDE (predisposing, reinforcing, and enabling causes in educational diagnosis and evaluation) model** for health education focuses on **interventions.**
    2. It provides an organizing framework and seven phases from which a health education program can be planned and carried out, including
      a. Assessment of social problems of concern.
      b. Identification of specific health-related problems.
      c. Identification of specific health-related behaviors linked to the health problems.
      d. Categorization of factors that have direct impact on these behaviors (predisposing, enabling, or reinforcing factors).
      e. Assessment of relative importance of factors and resources available to influence them.
      f. Development and implementation of programs.
      g. Evaluation.

  C. **TRANSTHEORETICAL MODEL OF BEHAVIOR CHANGE**

    1. This theory states that people who are changing their health behavior move through a series of **stages.**
      a. **Precontemplation** is when people are not thinking seriously about changing.
      b. **Contemplation** is when people are thinking seriously about changing an unhealthy behavior in the next 6 months.
      c. **Action** is a 6-month period in which an overt modification of an unhealthy behavior occurs.

    d. **Maintenance** is from 6 months after an overt behavior change until the problem is finally terminated.

    e. **Termination** is a stable period of zero temptation and maximum confidence in ability to resist relapse.

2. When this model is applied to smokers, the data have shown that approximately twice as many smokers in the contemplation stage took action during the first 6 months of a self-help intervention study as did those in the precontemplation stage.

D. COMMUNICATION THEORY

1. **Communication theory** focuses on elements that are essential to successful communication and incorporates communication skills, attitudes, knowledge level, and social or cultural systems of both the communication source and the receiver.

E. SOCIAL MARKETING THEORY

1. The **social marketing theory** introduces the principles and practices of marketing to social issues, causes, and ideas.

2. The **attitudes and needs** of the target audience are taken into account when programs are planned.

3. Because health behavior is caused and determined by many factors, education must incorporate different methods and channels to effect changes in behavior.

IV. DEVELOPMENT OF PROGRAMS

1. The NCI outlines six stages in developing health communications programs.

A. STAGE 1: PLANNING AND STRATEGY SELECTION

1. Stage 1 is an **assessment and planning phase** to determine whether a health problem can be addressed by communication strategies, and which strategy should be employed.

B. STAGE 2: SELECTING CHANNELS AND MATERIALS

1. In Stage 2, the **method** for reaching the target audience (the **channel**) and the **materials** to be used are determined.

C. STAGE 3: DEVELOPING MATERIALS AND PRETESTING

1. Stage 3 is essential if new materials need to be developed. As these materials are produced, they are **pretested** with members of the target audience to be sure they clearly convey the desired message.

D. STAGE 4: IMPLEMENTING THE PROGRAM

1. During Stage 4, the **program is introduced** to the target audience. Periodic **assessments** are incorporated into planning to determine how effective the program is at reaching the audience and time schedule as well as other goals previously set.

E. STAGE 5: ASSESSING EFFECTIVENESS

1. Stage 5 determines the **outcome** of the program—whether the target audience learned, acted, or made a change.

F. STAGE 6: FEEDBACK

1. Using data gathered during the other stages, Stage 6 prepares to **improve an ongoing program, revise it,** or **plan a new cycle of program development.**

V.   **BARRIERS TO EDUCATING THE PUBLIC**

1. The **National Cancer Institute (NCI)** has identified several barriers to public acceptance to health messages. These include the following:
    a. Health risk is an intangible concept.
    b. The public responds to easy solutions.
    c. People want absolute answers.
    d. The public may react unfavorably to fear.
    e. The public doubts the verity of science.
    f. The public has other priorities.
    g. The public holds contradictory beliefs.
    h. The public lacks a future orientation.

VI.   **OPPORTUNITIES AND CHALLENGES**

1. The NCI established a **Year 2000 goal** to achieve a 50% reduction in the 1985 cancer death rate.
2. Cancer control objectives to meet this goal fall under the categories of **prevention** (with smoking and diet targets), **screening** (of breast and cervical cancer), and **treatment.** These objectives are outlined in **Table 61-1, text page 1557.**
3. The **U.S. Public Health Service** sets out agendas for 10-year periods.
    a. Its Health People 2000 is an expansion of its 1980 objective-setting document.
4. The **American Cancer Society (ACS)** set its priorities for the 1990s along with measures on which it will judge its success in 2000.
    a. The ACS set a narrowed agenda, with **three cancer control core programs** to be accomplished in each of its 3600 local units: **comprehensive school health education, comprehensive year-round tobacco control,** and **breast cancer detection.**
    b. These objectives form a strong basis for program planning and offer widespread opportunities.
5. The Behavior Risk Factor Surveillance Survey (BRFSS) is used in 35 states to collect data through telephone surveys, give comparable data on behavior risk factors such as smoking, dietary habits, and alcohol consumption.

A.   **SEGMENTING TARGET AUDIENCES**

1. A major challenge in public education is to identify the main audience for the program. **Audience segmentation** has become so complex that it encompasses an entire new field of study called psychographics.
2. **Need for targeting**
    a. The NCI reinforces the need for segmenting audiences to increase the likelihood that the targeted learner is reached by the particular educational program.
    b. The NCI outlines **several opportunities** for health education in cancer prevention.
        (1) The lung cancer rate is rising for **women** much faster than for men and has surpassed the death rate for breast cancer.
        (2) Cigarette smoking among **adolescent girls** is now greater than among boys in the same age group.
        (3) **Low-income Americans** have a higher incidence of cancer as well as lower survival rates.
        (4) Since nearly 60% of all cancers occur in **Americans age 65 and over,** a group that represents only 12% of the U.S. population, this age group is a primary target for early-detection tests.
        (5) The proportion of **women who have ever had a mammogram** decreases with age and is lower among Hispanic and African-American women.
3. **Using psychographics**
    a. **Psychographics,** sometimes referred to as attitudinal or lifestyle research, segments the country into neighborhood types, personality types, media users, product and brand buyers, and benefit seekers.
        (1) It identifies **small, targeted clusters** in the population so that programs can be delivered in the appropriate areas.
        (2) Psychographic techniques are used in oncology to identify targeted learners and what message should be delivered to learners.

(3) The NCI outlines several opportunities for health education in cancer prevention based on identification of targeted groups. These include **smoking habits of females, mammography and breast exams for women,** and **early detection tests for people over 50.**

4. **Primary and secondary targets**
   a. A **"primary" target audience** is one that will be affected in some way by the messages given (e.g., women over age 50 who are the target for a mammography education program).
   b. A **"secondary" target audience** is one that has some influence on the primary target audience or that must do something to help cause change in their primary audience (e.g., physicians who serve this population of women and who can be reminded to refer these women for the screening test).

5. **Obtaining information about audiences**
   a. **Demographic information** about audiences (e.g., age, sex, ethnic background, area of residence and work) is available in census data, reports from Chambers of Commerce, health departments, etc.
   b. New data may need to be obtained to pinpoint specific information about a target audience.
      (1) **Focus group interviews** provide insight into the beliefs, perceptions, and feelings about a topic among a particular group of people. They can also be used to clarify the results of survey research, to generate hypotheses, and to give depth to feelings about health-related issues.
      (2) **Personal or telephone interviews** can also be used to gather vital data but are more expensive to conduct.
      (3) **Mailed questionnaires** are relatively inexpensive but minimum information may result because of low response and because the sample may not be representative of the whole population.
   c. Whatever method is chosen, it is useful to identify the people who are most important to reach so that pertinent messages can be developed and communication channels established. This assures that the available resources will be used in the most cost-effective manner.

B. REACHING THE DISADVANTAGED

1. The NCI's National Advisory Board has recommended intensified efforts to provide cancer information, prevention, and early detection programs to certain disadvantaged subgroups whose access to health care is poor. Groups to be included are the **poor, older Americans, blacks, Hispanics, Asian-Americans,** and **native Americans.**
2. Serious cancer problems exist in disadvantaged populations. Both the incidence and mortality of some cancers is higher in these populations, and knowledge about cancer prevention and early detection is poor.
3. **Identifying leaders** in a given target community can give planners of health education programs crucial access to and information about the community.
4. **Social service agencies and health organizations** are an important point of entry into these communities.
5. **Addressing cultural characteristics**
   a. Certain **socioeconomic** and **cultural characteristics** should be considered when designing health education programs for minorities, including the role of the family, the community, the language, folk beliefs and traditions, and the influence of poverty.

C. REACHING THE ELDERLY

1. Older people are at greater risk for developing cancer, though many are not aware they are at risk. In addition, the elderly are more likely to present to the health care system with more advanced disease.
2. Some of the topics that need to be addressed in educating the elderly are
   a. **The increased risk of cancer with advancing age.**
   b. **The seven warning signals of cancer.**
   c. **Normal vs. abnormal changes of aging.**
   d. **Health maintenance practices recommended by the ACS.**
   e. **The benefits of early detection in relation to reduced morbidity and mortality.**

      f.   **The acceptability and management of cancer treatments.**
      g.   **The skills and coping strategies needed to make the elderly more successful as patients in the contemporary health care system.**
      h.   **The community resources available to provide early detection services and assistance in developing better self-care skills.**
   3.   Several strategies that should be used when producing materials for older learners and lower socioeconomic groups are listed in **Table 61-3, text page 1564.**

D. SPECIFIC BARRIERS TO GETTING MAMMOGRAPHY AND PAP TESTS AMONG SPECIAL POPULATIONS

   1.   A study completed for the U.S. Centers for Disease Control and Prevention concluded that the **two major barriers** causing underuse of mammography are **an absence of physician referrals** and a **lack of perception that going without mammography involves risk.**
      a.   **Cost** is also a barrier for some women, though not as much as physician referral and perception of risk.
      b.   **Table 61-4, text page 1565,** summarizes tactics to be used in overcoming barriers to women obtaining mammography.

E. LOW LITERACY AND READABILITY

   1.   There is a wide gap between the readability level of commonly used health teaching materials and patients' reading comprehension.
   2.   **Performing readability tests**
      a.   **Readability testing** measures the approximate level of education needed to understand the written material.
      b.   The **SMOG grading system** for testing materials is used by the NCI because it is easy to use and accurate. See **text page 1567,** column 2, for a description of this system.
   3.   Some **guidelines for producing simpler material** are to
      (1)   **Use short words, short sentences, short paragraphs, and simple language.**
      (2)   **Write to one person, using conversational style and action verbs.**
      (3)   **Repeat the same information in several ways. Use examples.**
      (4)   **Do not abbreviate.**
      (5)   **Summarize major points.**

VII. THE MEDIA AS GATEKEEPER

   1.   **Mass media** transmits information quickly to a broad audience and is probably the public's main source of information.

A. DRAWBACKS OF MASS MEDIA

   1.   Some of the drawbacks of mass media when used for public education about cancer are that
      a.   Its main purpose is to inform and entertain rather than educate.
      b.   It is difficult to use for transmitting complex messages.
      c.   It has major constraints on space and time.
      d.   It carries a high risk of miscommunication, especially with complex messages.
   2.   Well-planned and well-produced **Public Service Announcements (PSAs)** can be an effective way to educate the public about cancer. However, PSAs have diminished since deregulation of the media.
   3.   Other media opportunities include news programs, public affairs programs, interview and talk shows, local television panels, call-in programs, editorials, letters to the editor, and health and political columns.
   4.   **"Media gatekeepers"** determine what gets seen and when. Educators are challenged to produce materials that are appealing to these gatekeepers as well as to target audiences.

B. BELIEFS AMONG GATEKEEPERS

   1.   Stuyck and Chilton examined the role of mass media gatekeepers in disseminating cancer information. Among their findings were that

a. Disease mortality and morbidity in themselves do not guarantee media interest.
b. Health professionals should be aggressive if they wish to achieve results and should be well informed before approaching the media.
c. The media are more likely to pay attention to information from **credible sources.**
d. The information should be perceived as useful to the gatekeeper's audience and should be clearly written and brief.

VIII. **EXAMPLES OF PUBLIC EDUCATION ACTIVITIES**

A. **HELPING PEOPLE TO STOP SMOKING**

1. Despite the large number of smoking cessation programs, over 50 million Americans continue to smoke.
2. A comprehensive review of smoking cessation programs was carried out in the mid-1980s. Some of the conclusions reached by this study were that
   a. Smokers prefer to quit **on their own** with the help of instructions, medicines, and guides.
   b. Many people who quit act on the advice or warning of a **health professional.** Nurses are ideal people to provide counseling support.
   c. **Nicotine chewing gum** can be a useful adjunct.
   d. Success of **media instruction** has been low but may be improved when combined with group or individual instruction.
   e. The **worksite** offers an excellent opportunity for implementing strategies that lead to smoking cessation.
   f. **Maintenance support is critical** for long-term success: leading causes of relapse are anxiety, stress, weight gain, and a lack of inner resources.
   g. The highest median quit rates were scored by **physician intervention programs** for cardiac disease patients.
   h. A significant trend is the increased negative attitude toward cigarette smoking.
3. **Smoking, Tobacco, and Cancer Program (STCP)**
   a. The primary thrust of the STCP is the development of intervention activities to reduce the incidence and/or prevalence of smoking and tobacco use.
   b. The results of the first set of large-scale community initiatives are providing the rationale for the next step in the strategic plan–the American Stop Smoking Intervention Study for Cancer Prevention (ASSIST).
4. **COMMIT trials**
   a. The COMMIT trials were conducted in several areas: **adolescent tobacco use prevention; the use of the mass media; physician, dentist, and self-help/minimal interventions; smokeless tobacco use; and black, Hispanic, and women smokers.**
   b. The data from these and more than 100 controlled intervention trials sponsored by the NCI during the 1980s have been used to formulate a national smoking strategy.
5. **National smoking strategy**
   a. The national strategy recognizes that **no single approach is best for all individuals,** that no one intervention channel is capable of effectively reaching all smokers, and that no single time is best for individual smokers to attempt to quit.
   b. The STCP research has shown that different programs have **an impact on different points in the process of initiation, maintenance,** and **cessation of smoking behavior.**
      (1) See **Table 61-6, text page 1572,** for planning smoking cessation programs for selected target audiences.
   c. The **COMMIT trials** are providing the scientific foundation for the largest, most comprehensive smoking control project ever undertaken–(ASSIST).
6. **The ASSIST/2000 program**
   a. The ASSIST/2000 program supports large-scale demonstrations in states and large metropolitan areas. Activities of the program include **training health care professionals for cessation counseling, workplace tobacco cessation programs,** and **antismoking curricula in schools.**
   b. The ACS and local health departments are leading the effort.
   c. A **collaborative effort** between the NCI and the ACS, working with state and local health departments and other voluntary organizations, ASSIST will develop comprehensive tobacco control programs in 17 states.

    d.   It is estimated that some **91 million Americans,** including **18 million smokers,** will be reached by ASSIST.

    e.   The ASSIST interventions are based on proven smoking prevention and control methods developed within the NCI's intervention trials and other smoking and behavioral research.

        (1)   The primary objective of ASSIST is to **demonstrate and evaluate ways to accelerate the decline in smoking prevalence,** in all ASSIST sites combined, to less than 15% of adults by the year 2000.

        (2)   The secondary objective is to **reduce by 50% the numbers of new smokers among adolescents,** in all award sites, by 2000.

    f.   Groups with high smoking rates and groups that have displayed slower rates of decline will be targeted.

7.   **California's experience**

    a.   In 1988, Californians passed **Proposition 99**—an initiative to increase the excise tax on tobacco by 25 cents per pack, with tax monies earmarked for tobacco-related health, research, education, and environmental activities.

    b.   The program is simultaneously pursuing four strategies: to **raise the priority of smoking as a public health issue; to improve the ability of communities to change smoking behavior; to increase the influence of the existing legal and socioeconomic factors that discourage tobacco use;** and to **strengthen social norms and values that discourage tobacco use.**

    c.   Cigarette consumption in California has gone **down** by 7% and continues to drop since the passage of Proposition 99. The decline is on track for reaching the goal of 75% reduction in smoking prevalence by 1999.

B.   **THE CANCER INFORMATION SERVICE (CIS)**

1.   **CIS as public educator**

    a.   The **Cancer Information Service (CIS)** is a toll-free telephone service sponsored by the NCI that answers questions about cancer prevention, control, diagnosis, treatment, and rehabilitation.

    b.   CIS counselors use the NCI's **computerized database, PDQ (Physician's Data Query),** to provide state-of-the-art information to callers.

    c.   Evaluation of the service shows that it has been overwhelmingly successful at providing clear, easy to understand, and helpful information to callers.

2.   **CIS as change agent**

    a.   The CIS functions as a **change agent** in providing information about varied techniques to quit smoking, including basic strategies for behavior change.

    b.   Counselors also are being trained to provide information about clinical trials.

    c.   A program at the CIS in Los Angeles focuses on the use of CIS to **increase breast screening among female callers.**

IX.   **CHALLENGES FOR THE FUTURE**

1.   The NCI and ACS have led the way in the public education of cancer-related issues.

2.   Some of the challenges facing us as we near the year 2000 are

    a.   **Developing interventions to reduce cancer risk.**

    b.   **Implementing the interventions to reach the greatest number of people at risk.**

    c.   **Using resources to their maximum benefit.**

    d.   **Attending to the needs of minorities and other target populations.**

PRACTICE QUESTIONS

1.   The broadest definition of health education is

    (A)   a form of communication in which a target audience takes in health information and then demonstrates an appropriate understanding of it.

    (B)   a combination of activities leading to a situation where people know how to obtain health.

    (C)   any combination of learning experiences designed to facilitate voluntary adoption of behavior conducive to health.

    (D)   an organizing framework from which teaching can be planned.

2. According to the NCI, health education program planning should proceed, in order, through which of the following stages?
   (A) developing and pretesting materials, selecting channels and materials, implementing the program, evaluating the program
   (B) planning and selecting a program strategy, selecting channels and materials, developing and pretesting materials, implementing the program, assessing program effectiveness, generating feedback to the program
   (C) planning the program, selecting the audience and materials, delivering the message
   (D) segmenting the target audience, determining the psychosocial characteristics of the audience, planning the program, selecting teaching materials, delivering the health education message, evaluating the program

3. The purpose of segmenting target audiences is to
   (A) identify the target audience for a program.
   (B) separate the interests of several different potential target audiences to determine who would be most interested in a given program.
   (C) determine which members of a population would be most likely to participate in a program.
   (D) determine the demographics of a given population.

4. Two special population groups that have been singled out by the NCI's National Advisory Board for intensified programs of cancer education are
   (A) young black men and heavy smokers.
   (B) the elderly and the disadvantaged.
   (C) elementary school children and urban teenagers.
   (D) poor women and individuals at risk from radon.

5. Guidelines for producing more understandable written materials for public education include all of the following **except**
   (A) using short words, short sentences, short paragraphs, and simple language.
   (B) writing to one person, using conversational style and action verbs.
   (C) repeating the same information in several ways.
   (D) using abbreviations where possible in order to simplify language.

6. Mass media has been widely used in programs of public education about cancer. One **disadvantage** of the use of mass media for this purpose is that it
   (A) places so few constraints on time and space.
   (B) is difficult to use for transmitting complex messages.
   (C) tends to transmit information slowly.
   (D) reaches a narrow audience with attitudes and needs that are often inappropriate to the message.

7. The primary function of the Cancer Information Service (CIS) is to
   (A) perform diagnostic screening on large numbers of high-risk individuals.
   (B) investigate suspected carcinogens in the workplace and home.
   (C) set standards on potentially hazardous products.
   (D) answer inquiries from the general public concerning cancer-related issues.

ANSWER EXPLANATIONS

1. **The answer is (C).** The broadest definition includes learning experiences designed to effect behavioral changes in the learner. Inherent in most definitions of education is the notion of behavioral change as an indication that learning has occurred. (1554)

2. **The answer is (B).** The most complete health education program plan would include all of these phases in the order they appear. Of particular importance are the last two—assessing effectiveness and feedback—as they are barometers of the success of the program. (1555)

3. **The answer is (A).** Segmenting is done to identify the target audience for the program. A type of segmenting, psychographics, describes a population in terms of neighborhood types, personality types, product and brand buyers, etc. (1557–1558)

4.   **The answer is (B).**   The NCI's National Advisory Board has recommended intensified efforts to provide cancer information, prevention, and early detection programs to the elderly and to certain disadvantaged subgroups whose access to health care is poor. Older people are at greater risk for developing cancer, though many are not aware they are at risk. In addition, the elderly are more likely to present to the health care system with advanced disease. Serious cancer problems also exist in disadvantaged populations. Both the incidence and mortality of some cancers are higher in these populations, and knowledge about cancer prevention and early detection is poor. (1558, 1562)

5.   **The answer is (D).**   Simpler written materials can be produced by using short words, short sentences, short paragraphs, and simple language; writing to one person and using action verbs and a conversational style; using the same word to describe an item; repeating the same information in several ways; using examples to illustrate important points; breaking up text with subheads and graphics; avoiding abbreviations; and summarizing at the end of major points. (1564–1567)

6.   **The answer is (B).**   Some of the drawbacks of mass media when used for public education about cancer are that its main purpose is to inform and entertain rather than educate, it is difficult to use for transmitting complex messages, it has major constraints on space and time, and it carries a high risk of miscommunication, especially with complex messages. However, it reaches an enormous audience, is fast, and can deliver a powerful message if that message is properly packaged (e.g., a television drama focusing on AIDS). (1568)

7.   **The answer is (D).**   The Cancer Information Service (CIS) is a toll-free telephone service sponsored by the NCI that answers questions about cancer prevention, control, diagnosis, treatment, and rehabilitation. CIS counselors use the NCI's computerized database, PDQ (Physician's Data Query), to provide state-of-the-art information to callers. The CIS also functions as a change agent in providing varied techniques to quit smoking, including basic strategies for behavior change. A new program at the CIS in Los Angeles focuses on its use to increase breast cancer screening among female callers. (1573)

62 Teaching Strategies: Patient Education

STUDY OUTLINE

I. **INTRODUCTION**

    1. Within the broader context of cancer education, patient education has been overshadowed by preventive efforts and education of the public-at-large.

II. **HISTORICAL PERSPECTIVE**

    1. Patient education has always been conducted, but efforts were sporadic and inconsistent.

    2. A prime factor responsible for increased attention to patient education was the **development of prepaid health care plans** and the idea that **informed self-care could reduce the cost of long-range patient care.** Patient education was viewed as a factor that facilitated self-care.

    3. Since 1964, the American Hospital Association has served as the primary advocate for the development of patient education programs. Out of their efforts came *A Patient's Bill of Rights*, approved by the Association's House of Delegates in 1973.

    4. Both the National Cancer Institute's document entitled *Adult Patient Education in Cancer* and the Oncology Nursing Society's *Outcome Standards in Cancer Patient Education* identify a number of tasks for patient education. These include helping patients and family members **adjust to disease, participate in treatment, carry out treatment regimens, manage stress, recognize and control side effects, prevent social isolation and strengthen relationships with significant others, mobilize and manage resources,** and **adapt to a life of uncertainty.**

    5. Other factors responsible for stimulating patient education are

        a. The rise in the number of Americans with chronic disease.

        b. An active consumer rights movement.

        c. Rising health care costs and changing medical reimbursement policies.

        d. The need for greater accountability by health care providers.

  A. **RECENT LITERATURE**

    1. Studies by Dodd, Beck, and others have documented the role of cancer education in improving knowledge, attitudes, behavior, and health status.

    2. Johnson's work demonstrated that patients who were **informed** of sensations involved in medical procedures experienced less stress than their uneducated cohorts.

    3. The trend toward briefer hospital stays and outpatient therapy administration has resulted in greater need for information related to self-care management.

    4. **Self-regulation theory** as developed by Leventhal and Johnson recognizes patients as active problem solvers.

    5. On the basis of their review of the literature on patient education, Rimer and colleagues suggest concise considerations for patient education programming that include

        a. Use of a combination of education methods.

        b. Enhancement of education methods through combination with behavioral modalities such as relaxation, guided imagery, and/or hypnosis.

        c. Use of repetition to improve the generally compromised recall facilities of those with cancer.

        d. Preparation of informed consent forms at a reading level and in a format conducive to their use as education vehicles.

e. Development of programs with the objective of teaching self-care as part of treatment regimens.

f. Development of programs targeted at the special needs of the older patient as well as other high-risk audiences.

6. Specific areas emphasized in the recent literature include **AIDS, patient information needs, self-care,** and **chemotherapy.** The cancer that received the most attention in terms of patient education publications was **breast cancer.**

B. **PROGRAM PRIORITIES**

1. A list of national priorities in patient education programming is given on **text page 1578, column 2.**

2. Since the 1950s the **ACS patient service programs** have provided information to patients and their families.

3. The **I Can Cope program** responded to the growing awareness that, with advances in cancer treatment, cancer was becoming a chronic rather than a fatal disease.

4. To further emphasize the importance of patient education, the ACS has established a **Patient/ Family Education Work Group** under the direction of the Service and Rehabilitation Department.

a. They have been charged with overseeing the review and revision of the existing materials and programs of the ACS.

5. Other current ACS projects include new materials on **sexuality** and information on **insurance concerns** and **employment discrimination.**

6. The Oncology Nursing Society has addressed patient education through their special-interest-group structure.

a. The mission of this group is to promote highly **effective education** for patients and families who are actually and/or potentially afflicted with cancer.

7. The educational needs of two audiences—the **elderly** and **cancer survivors**—take on greater importance as more people, and more people who have cancer, live longer.

a. Specific educational needs of the **elderly** focus on their peculiar beliefs, myths, and misconceptions about cancer, information style preference, and concomitant medications and diseases.

III. **CANCER SURVIVORS**

1. Educational needs of the **cancer survivor** are seen in the context of a continuum ("seasons of survival") that include

a. The **medical or acute stage,** commencing with diagnosis and focusing on containing the disease; education focuses on the medical and psychosocial needs for information and self-care and on fostering a "surviving" attitude.

b. The **"watchful waiting" stage,** during which the governing force is the patient's fear of recurrence; education addresses both the need for continuing medical surveillance and ways to live as normal a life as possible; teaching strategies incorporate health-promotion behavior and a wellness concept.

c. The **"permanent survival"** or cure stage, characterized by concerns about employability, insurability, and long-term effects of treatment; educational concerns include teaching people to be their own advocates and to feel empowered to speak for their rights.

2. The American Cancer Society's *Cancer Survivors' Bill of Rights* calls attention to the specific needs of the cancer survivor in areas that include excellence in acute cancer care, ongoing lifelong medical care, health insurance, job opportunities, and interpersonal happiness.

IV. **DEFINITIONS**

1. Patient education can be defined as a **series of structured or nonstructured experiences designed to help patients**

a. Cope voluntarily with the immediate crisis response to their diagnosis, with long-term adjustments, and with symptoms.

      b.   Gain needed information about sources of prevention, diagnosis, and care.

      c.   Develop needed skills, knowledge, and attitudes to maintain or regain health status.

  2. Patient education is able to accomplish all of this by enabling patients and their families to

      a.   Plan strategies for change.

      b.   Interpret and integrate needed information for achieving the desired attitudes or behaviors.

      c.   Meet patients' specific learning needs, interests, and capabilities.

  3. Patient education through a combination of learning experiences derived from joint planning by patients, significant others, and health care professionals is considered part of total health care.

V.   RATIONALE FOR PATIENT EDUCATION

  1. **Structured patient education,** including courses and classes, enhances the patient's process of adapting to disease by

      a.   Ensuring that important medical and psychosocial information is made available to the patient in a consistent manner.

      b.   Providing the patient with options, choices, and ways to engage self-care and to develop a proactive stance in their treatment decisions.

      c.   Broadening the opportunity for patient and provider to interact and to form a partnership in health care.

VI.   DEVELOPING PATIENT EDUCATION MATERIALS AND PROGRAMS

  1. Integral to the success of any patient education material is the **extent to which the needs of the intended audience are met.** This means assessing audience needs at particular points in the development and implementation process.

  2. The development process is illustrated by **Figure 62-1, text page 1581.** Key to this process is **pretesting,** a qualitative research method that systematically gathers target audience reactions to draft concepts and materials before final production and implementation.

      a.   Pretesting helps identify strengths and weaknesses during the early stages of development.

      b.   It also provides diagnostic information that can lead to improvements in materials and programs before they are made widely available.

A.   PRETESTING TECHNIQUES

  1. The **method of pretesting** chosen depends on the target audience, the concepts being tested, the objectives of the pretest, the best mode of access to the target audience, and the time and resources available.

  2. The techniques most conducive to pretesting of patient education materials and programs include

      a.   **Readability testing,** which is used to predict the level of reading comprehension necessary to understand a particular written piece.

      b.   **Focus group interviews,** which are guided group discussions with a group of 8 to 10 individuals who share specific target audience characteristics. This technique is especially valuable during the concept-development stage and provides insights into audience beliefs and perceptions.

      c.   **Individual in-depth interviews,** which use a prepared questionnaire to address sensitive subjects or subjects that require in-depth probing.

      d.   **Self-administered questionnaires,** which are used to gather reactions to draft materials. Various techniques are used to encourage a high rate of return of completed questionnaires.

      e.   **Gatekeeper reviews,** which solicit comments and suggestions from the health professionals who will be using the materials or adopting the program.

B.   THE DEVELOPMENT PROCESS

  1. During the **planning and strategy selection stage** of the development process, a concise definition of what the material or program will address is formulated and its objectives and target audience are identified. This process includes

a. A **needs assessment,** often involving a needs assessment survey.
b. Perusal of literature in the field and identification of other analogous materials and programs.
c. A more formal assessment to determine education needs and strategies that have the greatest potential for meeting needs.
d. The application of such pretesting techniques as in-depth interviews, focus group interviews, and small-scale surveys.

2. During the **concept-development stage,** draft educational resources are developed on the basis of concepts that appear to have the greatest potential for educating the target audience.

3. During the **message-execution stage,** draft educational resources are pretested before final production. Both gatekeeper review and self-administered questionnaires are typically employed during this stage.

4. During the **implementation stage,** the material or program is used with the target audience, with initial reaction monitored closely.

5. During the **assessment of in-market effectiveness stage,** the effectiveness of materials and programs in terms of stated objectives is assessed. Often this process utilizes self-administered questionnaires completed before and after exposure to the material or program.

6. During the **feedback stage,** the information gathered during pretesting, process, and outcome evaluations is critically assessed for the purpose of replanning. Problems, strengths, and other feedback related to the material or program are examined in terms of changes necessitated by actual implementation.

VII. CLIMATE FOR LEARNING

1. Studies of the clinical practice of health care show that more emphasis needs to be placed on the "how" of patient teaching.

2. Factors that must be considered if a climate for learning is to be created can be summarized by the following "HOPE" mnemonic:

> **H**uman
> Interpersonal relations
> Individual needs and wants
> **O**rganization
> Policy
> Structure
> **P**hysical
> Environmental factors
> **E**ducational options
> Methods
> Materials

3. The **human factor (H)** involves offering learners ways to participate throughout the educational process. To maximize readiness to learn, teachers must ascertain the concerns people have at that particular moment. Consideration also must be given to
a. A **person's age,** which directly affects his or her ability to understand and master information and skills.
   (1) Intellectual development in **children** moves from the concrete to the abstract as they mature, and they move toward a clearer distinction between what is internal and what is external to themselves.
   (2) **Adult learners** are motivated to learn when they recognize a gap between what they know and what they want to know. The learning process in adults capitalizes on their past experiences.
   (3) In **older people,** the speed of learning, and not the ability to learn, declines. Frustration and anxiety may occur if they are asked to learn too much too quickly. Reinforcing learning and building confidence in learning abilities are vital to the teaching process. Consideration is also given to such issues as print size, the volume and speed of visual presentations, and the amount of information given at one time.

      b. **Differences in culture, language, level of literacy, and physical impairment,** which means accounting for

         (1) The importance of the person's **family and immediate community** as a support system.

         (2) Culture-specific **medical and religious beliefs and practices** and attempting to incorporate these into educational opportunities.

         (3) Subtleties of **language and dialect** that may change the patient's expression of symptoms and his or her level of comprehension. Using a variety of teaching methods (e.g., visual aids) can help convey information in an understandable way, as can translating material into the patient's primary language.

         (4) The **literacy level** of the patient, which may mean simplifying written and spoken language for the benefit of patients with poor reading skills.

4. Factors related to **organizational or institutional support (O)** must also be considered when establishing a climate for learning.

      a. Quality patient education is nurtured by a supportive administrative and medical staff.

      b. Often, however, patient education is given only lip service by an institution. Strategies for gaining support and recognition in such cases include

         (1) Knowing the state-of-the-art literature.

         (2) Supporting claims of effectiveness with research data.

         (3) Presenting a cost-effective plan for implementing a program that addresses quality patient care.

      c. Patient education addresses issues of concern to the institution, including accreditation standards, requirements for informed consent, self-care interests of consumers, and trends of earlier discharge with home care collaboration.

5. Factors related to the **physical environment (P)** for learning are focused on mutual respect, acceptance of differences, and freedom of expression and include the availability of

      a. **Adequate time, space, privacy, quiet, lack of interference,** etc., for individuals to learn.

      b. A **learning resource center** to facilitate self-initiated learning.

      c. **Visual aids,** such as anatomic charts or a human torso, to heighten peoples' interest in their own body parts.

      d. Adequate **equipment,** including chairs, tables, microphones, lighting, and audiovisual equipment.

6. Factors related to the **choice of educational methods and materials (E)** focus on the ways to best present the content to be taught. People tend to learn better when

      a. More than one of their senses is involved in the learning process.

      b. They are active participants in this process.

      c. Learning materials are chosen that enhance teacher-student interaction.

7. The computer revolution has increased interest in the use of computers in patient education.

8. Computer-based education and interactive videodiscs can benefit patient education in the following ways: reduces learning time by one-third, offers privacy for user learning, provides personal control of the instructional pace, accommodates a variety of learning styles, reduces teaching time required of care providers, and offers options for teaching patients of low literacy.

PRACTICE QUESTIONS

1. A major factor in the trend toward an increased emphasis on patient education was

    (A) the development of prepaid health care plans.

    (B) passage of the Long-Term Health Care Act of 1981.

    (C) the formation of a national consortium of patient educators in 1963.

    (D) the decision by many private insurers to reimburse patient education costs.

2. On the basis of their review of recent literature, Rimer and colleagues suggested a number of considerations for patient education programming. These included all of the following **except**

    (A) use of repetition to improve the generally compromised recall facilities of those with cancer.

(B)   simplification of the teaching-learning process through the adoption of a single educational method.

(C)   development of programs with the objective of teaching self-care as part of treatment regimens.

(D)   development of programs targeted at the special needs of the older patient as well as other high-risk audiences.

3.   For which of the following groups is patient education considered to be a national priority?
(A)   children and cancer survivors
(B)   recently diagnosed cancer patients and the elderly
(C)   children and recently diagnosed cancer patients
(D)   the elderly and cancer survivors

4.   The primary goals of patient education include all of the following **except**
(A)   helping patients cope voluntarily with the immediate crisis response to their diagnosis.
(B)   helping patients gain needed information about sources of prevention, diagnosis, and care.
(C)   helping patients to communicate more effectively with the family and with health care providers.
(D)   helping patients develop needed skills, knowledge, and attitudes to maintain or regain health status.

5.   Pretesting is used during the development of patient education materials and resources in order to
(A)   help identify strengths and weaknesses of the materials and resources during the early stages of development.
(B)   produce findings that are reportable in terms of their statistical significance.
(C)   predict the potential success or failure of the materials and resources in terms of variables pretested.
(D)   provide a quantitative basis for necessary revisions of the materials and resources.

6.   The pretesting technique that would **most** likely be used in the development process when the subjects addressed are sensitive or require in-depth probing is the
(A)   individual interview.
(B)   self-administered questionnaire.
(C)   gatekeeper review.
(D)   focus group interview.

7.   Which of the following activities takes place during the message-execution stage in the development of patient education materials or programs?
(A)   The material or program is used with the target audience, with initial reaction monitored closely.
(B)   The effectiveness of materials and programs in terms of stated objectives is assessed.
(C)   Draft educational resources are pretested before final production.
(D)   The information gathered during pretesting, process, and outcome evaluations is critically assessed for the purpose of replanning.

8.   Providing the appropriate climate for patient education involves consideration of all of the following factors **except**
(A)   human factors, including the concerns people have at the moment.
(B)   environmental factors, including time, space, privacy, quiet, etc., for individuals to learn.
(C)   organizational factors, including the patient's age, culture, level of literacy, and any physical impairments.
(D)   factors related to the choice of educational methods and materials, including ways to best present the content to be taught.

9.   An example of a human factor that must be considered in providing an optimal climate for patient learning is the
(A)   type of learning method used.
(B)   patient's age.
(C)   content of the learning materials used.
(D)   organization's patient education policy.

ANSWER EXPLANATIONS

1. **The answer is (A).** Patient education has always been conducted, but efforts were sporadic and inconsistent. Associated with the development of prepaid health care plans was the idea that informed self-care could reduce the cost of long-range patient care. Patient education was viewed as a factor that facilitated self-care. Other factors contributing to a greater emphasis on patient education included the activities and publications of the American Hospital Association, National Cancer Institute, and Oncology Nursing Society; the rise in the number of Americans with chronic disease; the consumer rights movement; rising health care costs and changing medical reimbursement policies; and the need for greater accountability by health care providers. (1577)

2. **The answer is (B).** Rimer et al. suggested that a combination of education methods, and not one single method, be used in patient education. Other suggestions were enhancement of educational methods through combination with behavioral modalities such as relaxation, guided imagery, and/or hypnosis and preparation of informed consent forms at a reading level and in a format conducive to their use as education vehicles. (1578)

3. **The answer is (D).** As more people live longer, and as more of those who have cancer experience long-term control or cure, the educational needs of two audiences—the elderly and cancer survivors—take on greater importance. Specific educational needs of the elderly focus on their peculiar beliefs, myths, and misconceptions about cancer, information style preference, and concomitant medications and diseases. Educational needs of the cancer survivor are best seen in the context of a continuum ("seasons of survival") that include the acute stage following diagnosis, a period of "watchful waiting" during remission or completion of the treatment course, and the stage of "permanent survival" or cure. (1579)

4. **The answer is (C).** Communication, while important in patient education, is more accurately seen as a means to an end and not an end in itself. (1580)

5. **The answer is (A).** Integral to the success of any patient education material is the extent to which the needs of the intended audience are met. This means assessing audience needs at particular points in the development and implementation process. Key to this process is pretesting, a qualitative research method that systematically gathers target audience reactions to draft concepts and materials before final production and implementation. Pretesting helps identify strengths and weaknesses during the early stages of development, and it provides diagnostic information that can lead to improvements in materials and programs before they are made widely available. It is a qualitative method, however, and does not yield findings that are reportable in terms of their statistical significance. (1581)

6. **The answer is (A).** The method of pretesting chosen depends on the target audience, the concepts being tested, the objectives of the pretest, the best mode of access to the target audience, and the time and resources available. Individual in-depth interviews or one-on-one discussions are carried out by an interviewer who uses a prepared questionnaire that consists of both open-ended and closed-ended items. The technique is appropriate when the subjects addressed are sensitive or require in-depth probing. Self-administered questionnaires are used to gather reactions to draft materials. Gatekeeper reviews solicit comments and suggestions from the health professionals who will be using the materials or adopting the program. Focus group interviews are guided group discussions with a group of 8 to 10 individuals who share specific target audience characteristics. This technique is valuable during the concept-development stage and provides insights into audience beliefs and perceptions. (1581–1582)

7. **The answer is (C).** Choice (A) refers to implementation; choice (B) refers to assessment of in-market effectiveness; choice (D) refers to feedback. During the message-execution stage, both gatekeeper review and self-administered questionnaires are typically employed. (1583)

8. **The answer is (C).** Differences in culture, language, level of literacy, and physical impairment are all important considerations in providing the appropriate educational climate for each patient, but they are human factors and not organizational factors. Organizational (or institutional) factors refer to the need for support from the organization or institution in order to provide quality patient education. (1583–1584)

9.   **The answer is (B).**   A person's age directly affects his or her ability to understand and master information and skills. Ability to learn depends on maturation, e.g., as children mature, their intellectual development moves from concrete to abstract. Changes brought on by aging are particularly important to acknowledge in patient education. Frustration and anxiety may occur if older patients are asked to learn too much too quickly. Reinforcing learning and building confidence in their learning abilities are vital to the teaching process. (1584–1585)

63　Cancer Nursing Education

5. **Association of Pediatric Oncology Nurses**
   a. Among its objectives are to **promote excellence in the care of children with cancer,** provide communication for nurses, disseminate information about care of patients, encourage publication in professional lay literature, and support research in pediatric oncology.

B. **SCHOLARSHIPS**

1. By 1992, 256 **ACS scholarships** had been awarded at the master's level, while 22 students had received doctoral scholarships.
2. Since the **ONS scholarship programs,** which offer bachelor's and master's degrees, have been in existence, many recipients have benefited from the opportunity to attend school.
3. The **NCI offers fellowships** at the predoctoral, doctoral, and postdoctoral levels.
4. In addition, both the ACS and the NCI have offered 6–10 week courses for baccalaureate level nursing students to encourage them to enter the field of cancer nursing.

C. **CERTIFICATION**

1. Certification **acknowledges** nurses' additional education or experience.
   a. The level of knowledge of certified nurses is **above** the level required for licensure, thus protecting the public by demanding a certain level of excellence in those who are certified.
2. The **Oncology Nursing Certification Corporation (ONCC),** in conjunction with the Educational Testing Service (ETS), offers a certification examination open to nurses who have a current license, have two and a half years of experience as a registered nurse over the 5-year period prior to application, and have at least 1000 hours of oncology nursing practice within two and a half years prior to application.

III. **CANCER NURSING EDUCATION TODAY**

A. **CONCEPTUAL FRAMEWORK**

1. A conceptual framework has been developed by the Education Committee of the ONS consisting of four concepts: **individual and family, health-illness, health care system,** and **community-environment.**

B. **STANDARDS OF ONCOLOGY NURSING EDUCATION**

1. The ONS has developed
   a. *Outcome Standards for Cancer Nursing Education at the Fundamental Level*
   b. *Scope of Advanced Oncology Practice*
   c. *Standards for Oncology Nursing Education: Advanced Level*
2. The ultimate goals of the standards are to **enhance the quality** of oncology nursing education and to improve health care for the public.
3. Guidelines for all levels of educational preparation are published in the *Standards of Oncology Nursing Education: Generalist and Advanced Practice Levels.*
4. The purpose is to provide guidelines to
   a. Plan and evaluate generalist education encompassing diploma, associate, and baccalaureate programs.
   b. Plan and evaluate advanced education at the master's, doctoral, and postdoctoral levels.
   c. Plan and evaluate continuing education programs at all levels.
   d. Assess individual knowledge of oncology nursing care.
5. **Generalist level**
   a. The generalist level of cancer nursing, originally referred to as the fundamental level, provides a **core of knowledge, skill,** and **attitudes for beginning practice. Although it encompasses diploma, associate,** and **baccalaureate educational programs, the literature deals only with baccalaureate education.**
   b. In a 1983 study Brown, Johnson, and Groenwald found that an average of **14.5 classroom hours** were devoted to cancer nursing, with numerous content areas inadequately covered.
   c. Pope found similar results in a study conducted in Switzerland. On surveying the wishes and needs of oncology students, it was found that students could not agree as to **what areas** in oncology were most important in preparing them for care of patients with cancer.

d. Another European study came to the conclusion that education follows the **medical model, the faculty is without oncology experience, there is paucity of teaching materials,** and **there is little connection between theory and practice.**

e. Findings by Pope and Fanslow suggest that a lack of oncology content **leads to negative attitudes** on the part of students.

f. Many creative ways to improve curricula in cancer nursing and promote positive attitudes about cancer at the baccalaureate level have been attempted and are discussed on **text page 1591.**

    (1) Programs are scarce, and only limited numbers of students are able to benefit. In many other programs, glaring **deficiencies** still exist.

6. **Advanced level**

a. Graduate education is concerned with the development of a **broader scope of practice, coordination, continuity,** and **evaluation of care.**

b. The **Master's Degree with a Specialty in Oncology Nursing** provides a role definition and curriculum guide for educators in planning educational offerings as well as a program selection guide for students.

c. At the end of 1991, there were 45 graduate oncology programs listed by the Education Committee of the ONS, each with its own qualities.

    (1) See **text page 1592,** column 1, for a list of questions potential students should ask when assessing a program.

d. Piemme identified the most **significant problems** of graduate oncology programs to include recruitment of students, lack of financial support, pressures on faculty time, and a need for faculty prepared in oncology nursing.

e. In a survey of 185 clinical nurse specialists (CNSs) who were ONS members employed in oncology, Yasko found that **69%** of the specialists reported they did not have theoretical content or planned experiences in oncology nursing in their graduate programs.

C. CONTINUING EDUCATION

1. Many continuing education (CE) programs are sponsored by the ONS and ACS at both the national and the local levels.

2. In order to ensure successful CE program planning, the ONS conducted a needs assessment of its membership to determine learning needs.

a. The top five topics about which the members said they definitely would attend a seminar were the clinical practice issues of oncologic emergencies, pain, critical care, legal issues, and advanced practice roles.

3. Bushy and Kost confronted the issue of **inaccessibility** of CE programs in rural North Dakota and came up with a successful model for delivering CE programs by utilizing Knowles' model of adult learning.

IV. CRITICAL ISSUES AND CHALLENGES

A. INVITATIONAL CONFERENCE ON THE CLINICAL NURSE SPECIALIST ROLE

1. A **study on burnout** among oncology CNSs was an outgrowth of the first invitational conference on the role of the oncology CNS.

2. Among the recommendations for oncology education at the undergraduate level were the following:

a. Cancer nursing content needs to be emphasized in the classroom and clinical settings using the Standards of Oncology Nursing Practice and Education.

b. Faculty need updates.

c. Hospitals need to use the Standards of Nursing Practice.

3. Recommendations also were made for oncology nursing education at the **graduate level** with stong emphasis on

a. Physical assessment.

b. Clinical decision making.

c. Prevention, screening, and early detection.

d. Care of high-risk and underserved clients, such as the elderly and socioeconomically disadvantaged.

e. Public health policy.

f. Basic sciences, especially immunology.

B. **CONTINUING EDUCATION**

1. Continuing education (CE) must provide some of the content that cannot be covered within the confines of a baccalaureate or master's curriculum.
2. Separate standards may need to be developed for informal and formal educational programs.

C. **RECRUITMENT OF STUDENTS**

1. Because admissions to nursing programs at both the undergraduate and graduate levels have decreased over the past few years, effort must be made to try to attract the traditional as well as the older, nontraditional student.
2. A critical mass of minority nurses who can work with minority populations to encourage prevention and early detection practices is needed to make an impact on cancer care in this group of patients and reduce high mortality rates.

D. **PREVENTION AND EARLY DETECTION**

1. More emphasis must be placed on prevention, risk reduction, and early-detection activities.
2. Nurses can have a powerful impact on prevention and early detection.

E. **PRACTITIONER OR SPECIALIST**

1. A combined clinical nurse specialist with nurse practitioner skills is essential to meet future challenges.
2. These combined skills will require changes in graduate programs that focus on clinical nurse specialists.

F. **STANDARDS AND THE CURRICULUM**

1. Faculty should be familiar with the recommended curriculum and follow the guidelines set forth in the *Standards*.
   a. Perhaps more definitive guidelines at the undergraduate level need to be written, similar to the master's degree guidelines.
2. The nursing curricula should include content on **publishing,** to teach nurses to share their knowledge, skills, and expertise with others.
3. Students also need **public-speaking skills** and **media awareness training** and should be well versed in the **legislative process** and **public policy issues.**
4. It is imperative that graduates of nursing programs be **computer literate** and knowledgeable about using information by way of **electronic networks.**
5. Students should be encouraged to participate in local and national ACS and ONS activities or, if in pediatrics, APON activities.

G. **TEACHING APPROACHES**

1. Adult learning concepts—including **problem-centered approaches to teaching, immediate application of knowledge, recognition of individual experience, flexible scheduling,** and **self-directed learning**—must be incorporated into educational offerings.

H. **FACULTY COMPETENCE**

1. Faculty at all levels need to be prepared in oncology nursing, be knowledgeable in the latest trends in oncology as well as clinically competent.
2. New forms of **collaboration** between faculty and clinical staff could be developed to provide faculty entrance and exposure to the clinical arena.

I. **PROGRAM EVALUATION**

1. Evaluation of oncology programs should be an ongoing process.

J.   **PRECEPTORS AND CLINICAL FACILITIES**

    1.   Nursing educators must continue to nurture clinical preceptors to act as role models for students in clinical agencies.

K.   **DOCTORAL EDUCATION**

    1.   Doctorally prepared oncology nurses are needed to ensure high-quality education, research, and practice in the future.

L.   **COMPLEX CARE**

    1.   Advances in technology and early-discharge practices have changed both inpatient and outpatient care, calling for **changing roles and responsibilities of nurses** in ambulatory and home settings. More emphasis on these roles must be given in curricula.

M.   **CERTIFICATION AND RECERTIFICATION**

    1.   The question of **recertification** may need to be explored further to determine if reexamination is the best alternative for keeping knowledge and practice current.

N.   **MEETING NEW HEALTH CARE CHALLENGES**

    1.   It is expected that by the twenty-first century over 65% of persons diagnosed with cancer will survive longer than 5 years.
        a.   This will have enormous impact on delivery of **services, rehabilitation,** and **quality-of-life issues.**
    2.   Nurses must be prepared to meet the challenges of a **diverse** spectrum of patients and problems.

PRACTICE QUESTIONS

1.   Which group has been the **most** active over the years in establishing standards of cancer nursing practice as well as guidelines for cancer education?
    (A)   the Oncology Nursing Society (ONS)
    (B)   the American Cancer Society (ACS)
    (C)   the National Cancer Institute (NCI)
    (D)   the American Nurses' Association (ANA)

2.   Within the conceptual framework for cancer nursing education developed in accordance with the Outcome Standards for Cancer Nursing Practice, which of the following concepts is central to oncology nursing practice?
    (A)   community-environment
    (B)   health care system
    (C)   individual and family
    (D)   health-illness

3.   Which of the following generally applies only to the advanced level of nursing education and not to the generalist level?
    (A)   a baccalaureate degree
    (B)   a discrete area of practice
    (C)   clinical experience
    (D)   conceptual knowledge and skills

4.   The **best** teaching approach to enable the cancer nurse to keep up with the changing health care environment, treatment modalities, and the nurse's numerous roles and responsibilities is
    (A)   didactic lecture.

    (B)   hospital training with minimal lecture.
    (C)   self-directed learning.
    (D)   structured, inflexible coursework.

5.   Faculty consultation in clinical sites, faculty-clinical staff research projects, and faculty-clinical staff manuscript preparation are all examples of efforts to:
    (A)   identify new research topics.
    (B)   maintain faculty clinical competence.
    (C)   increase academic and hospital revenue.
    (D)   recruit students.

6.   The political implications of cancer care are **most** likely to be covered at what level and under what concept within the conceptual framework of cancer nursing education referred to in practice question 2?
    (A)   generalist level, health care system
    (B)   generalist level, health-illness continuum
    (C)   specialist level, individual-family
    (D)   specialist level, community-environment

7.   Which of the following is **not** required for use of the designation Oncology Certified Nurse (OCN)?
    (A)   3 years' experience as an RN within the last 5 years
    (B)   a baccalaureate degree with credits toward a master's degree
    (C)   a minimum of 1000 hours of cancer nursing practice within the last 3 years
    (D)   a passing score on the ONCC certification examination

ANSWER EXPLANATIONS

1.   **The answer is (A).**   The ONS has been promoting excellence in oncology nursing by setting standards, studying ways to improve oncology nursing, encouraging nurses to specialize in oncology nursing, and fostering the professional development of oncology nurses. In addition, the Education Committee of the ONS has been active over the years in developing standards of education that have had significant impact on cancer nursing education. (1588–1589)

2.   **The answer is (C).**   Central to cancer nursing practice is the individual-family concept. The health-illness concept is the adaptation of the individual and family along a continuum. The practice of cancer nursing occurs in the health care system. The community-environment concept provides the resources and support necessary for individuals with cancer. (1590)

3.   **The answer is (B).**   Cancer nursing is practiced by both nursing generalists and nursing specialists. Nursing generalists have conceptual knowledge and skills acquired through basic nursing education, clinical experience, and professional development and updated through continuing education. They meet the concerns of individuals with cancer and provide care in a variety of health care settings. Nursing specialists have substantial theoretical knowledge gained through preparation for the master's degree. They meet diversified concerns of cancer patients and their families and function in a discrete area of practice. (1591–1592)

4.   **The answer is (C).**   Adult learning concepts, including problem-centered approaches to teaching, immediate application of knowledge, recognition of individual experience, flexible scheduling, and self-directed learning, must be incorporated into educational offerings. (1595)

5.   **The answer is (B).**   Faculty need to be prepared in oncology nursing and need to be both knowledgeable in the latest trends and clinically competent. In addition to joint appointments, new and different ways to ensure competence must be explored. (1595)

6.   **The answer is (D).**   The political implications of cancer care constitute an area that should be addressed in graduate education within the framework of the community-environment concept; in the future the politics of cancer care will play an increasing role in cancer nursing. Other content areas associated with the community-environment concept are cancer-related resources, including home care and bereavement services; economic and legal implications of cancer nursing practice; issues of employability and insur-

ability; the identification of environmental carcinogens; knowledge of safety measures related to hazards of cancer treatment; and the fostering of empathy in those who will care for individuals with cancer and their families. (1590, 1595)

7. **The answer is (B).**   The Oncology Nursing Certification Corporation (ONCC) administers a certification program for cancer nurses. A certification examination is offered twice yearly. Nurses with an RN license, 3 years' experience as a registered nurse within the last 5 years, and a minimum of 1000 hours of cancer nursing practice within the last 3 years are eligible to take this examination. Certification is valid for 4 years. Renewal of certification involves a process similar to the initial certification process. Candidates must meet the same criteria as before, and an examination will constitute the requirements for re-certification. (1590)

64 Cancer Nursing Research

STUDY OUTLINE

I. **INTRODUCTION**

1. An examination of the role of the cancer nurse in the implementation of medical research and in the development, implementation, dissemination, and application of cancer nursing research provides a basis for understanding the rapid development of nursing research in the provision of care for today's cancer patient.

II. **RESEARCH DEFINED**

1. **Research is a structured approach to answering questions or discovering new knowledge.** Among its fundamental aspects are that
    a. It can be considered valid only when it is replicated.
    b. It involves an orderly and standardized series of steps, similar to those in the nursing process.
    c. It focuses on groups of patients and includes the obligation to disseminate the results for critique by others.
2. See **Table 64-1, text page 1600,** for a comparison of clinical nursing and research processes.
3. In the development of cancer treatment, **medical research** is used to describe the natural history of the diseases, to test new treatment approaches, and to evaluate the value of singular and multimodal approaches to cancer treatment.
4. It is through **research endeavors** that surgical, chemotherapeutic, radiation, biologic, genetic, and supportive care approaches to cancer treatment have been developed.

III. **CLINICAL TRIALS**

A. **THE CLINICAL TRIALS APPROACH**

1. The medical research approach to clinical investigation of cancer treatment methods has resulted in a specialized approach called the **clinical trials approach.**
2. This approach involves **several phases of study on human subjects,** each designed to answer specific clinical questions.
    a. **Phase 1 clinical trials determine the maximum tolerated dose (MTD) and drug toxicities.** They are initiated only after testing of treatment approaches with appropriate animal or cell models.
        (1) **Pharmacokinetic data on the medication being tested may be conducted as well.** Thus the collection of time specimens is common and requires precision by the nursing staff implementing the research protocol.
        (2) **Test subjects are those for whom standard therapy has failed.** Frequently the only benefit to these patients is the satisfaction of having contributed to scientific knowledge for treatment of other cancer patients, although patients often view participation in a phase 1 study from a hopeful perspective.
        (3) **Phase 1 trials are implemented only at NCI-designated cancer centers,** so as to assure the full spectrum of clinical support needed in studies in which toxicities are unpredictable and close monitoring of patients is critical.
    b. **Phase 2 trials focus on the specific tumor types for which the treatment appears promising.**
        (1) Patients are eligible if they are not able to participate in standard therapy or have failed to respond to standard therapy.

        (2) **Specific tumors are selected that have shown some positive responses in preclinical or phase 1 trials,** e.g., the use of LAK cells and IL-2 for patients with colorectal cancer and renal cell carcinoma.

        (3) Depending on the nature of the treatment being tested, **toxicities are frequently profound, and close monitoring of patients is necessary** to provide data for evaluation of patient response and early detection of toxicities.

    c. **Phase 3 trials determine**

        (1) **The effects of treatment relative to the natural history of the disease.**

        (2) **Whether a new treatment is more effective than a standard therapy.**

        (3) **Whether a new treatment is as effective as a standard therapy but is associated with less morbidity.**

    d. Phase 3 trials require the greatest number of subjects and are conducted in large medical centers, university hospitals, and community centers.

  3. Participation of cancer patients in all three kinds of clinical trials has been the critical element in the rapid development of current cancer treatment options, e.g., new treatments for breast cancer and Hodgkin's disease.

B. SETTINGS FOR MEDICAL RESEARCH

  1. Four types of cancer centers are defined by the NCI.

    a. **Basic science centers** conduct laboratory research.

    b. **Clinical cancer centers** conduct a combination of basic and clinical research.

    c. **Comprehensive cancer centers** include the same research as clinical cancer centers, plus cancer-control research.

        (1) Cancer-control research focuses on the reduction in incidence of cancer by primary and secondary disease-prevention activities.

    d. **Consortium centers** involve clinical and cancer control research, plus cancer-control activities.

  2. Medical research related to cancer treatment may be conducted at any of these settings.

  3. **Oncology nurses have been involved in all aspects of cancer research,** ranging from extravasation studies that use animal models, to clinical trials of experimental therapies, to research and activities on cancer prevention and early detection.

  4. Although phase 1 studies are restricted to NCI-designated centers, phase 2 and 3 studies may be conducted at institutions with cooperative arrangements with NCI-designated centers.

    a. This is done to increase the number of test subjects, as well as to provide patients with options that are not available through their private physicians.

C. THE CANCER RESEARCH TEAM

  1. The multidisciplinary research team includes a **principal investigator, co-investigators,** a **research** or **protocol nurse,** a **data manager,** an **investigational pharmacist,** a **statistician,** and a **clinical nursing staff.**

  2. The **principal investigator** is responsible for the scientific integrity of the study, as well as the development of the protocol, presentation of the study to the institutional review board, and implementation of the study.

  3. The **co-investigators** may include other physicians whose patients may be eligible for the study and other scientists (e.g., molecular biologists, psychologists) interested in other aspects of cancer patients' responses.

  4. **The research nurse is responsible for patient accrual, implementing the physician's orders as described in the protocol, and observing patient responses and toxicities.** In implementing this role, the nurse is involved in informed consent issues, astute clinical care, and education of supporting nursing staff.

    a. Involvement in **informed consent** means ensuring that patients understand

        (1) What has been defined as the treatment.

        (2) What the risks and benefits are.

        (3) What alternative treatment approaches are available.

        (4) What the probability is that the patient will benefit from the treatment.

        (5) This is especially important in phase 1 or 2 clinical trials, when benefits may be nonexistent. The research nurse notifies the principal investigator if any patient does not understand any of the above information.

    b. **Astute clinical care** includes monitoring the patient's symptoms and reporting toxicities that are a threat to the patient's life or comfort.

    c. **Education of the patient's caregiver** includes educating the clinical nursing staff, the patient, and/or family or significant other.

       (1) When the research or protocol nurse is not present, responsibilities must be delegated to someone else. The patient and the caregiver need to know when to notify the physician or the research nurse of side effects.

5. The role of the **data manager** is to collect the information on toxicities from the chart and to enter these data into the computer for statistical analysis. Laboratory responses, pathology reports, and physician's progress notes are frequent sources of data.

6. The **investigational pharmacist** is a part of the team when the focus of the clinical trial is chemotherapy. Many phase I and II trials involve investigational drugs, which are not available for public use and for which specific records need to be kept. The investigational pharmacist is responsible for dispensing these medications and for making sure that the records on the drugs are in order.

7. The **statistician** is responsible for a variety of activities in relation to a clinical trial. These include determination of initial sample size, study design and protocol review, data evaluation and analysis, interpretation of findings and preparation of manuscripts.

8. The **clinical nursing staff** has a major contribution to make in terms of patients' response to the research therapy.

    a. While many of the patients in medical research protocols are hospitalized, other settings may be used as well. Thus, staff includes nurses in hospital units, ambulatory care settings, physicians' offices, and home care agencies.

D. THE CHEMOTHERAPY RESEARCH NURSE

1. **The chemotherapy research nurse assumed one of the first specialty roles in the development of cancer nursing practice.**

2. Nurses were responsible for the administration and monitoring of chemotherapy, and they accrued patients for medical protocols, administered medications, counseled patients on management of side effects, collected data, and kept the physician informed of the patient's condition.

3. Out of this role grew an increasing familiarity with the research process as used in clinical chemotherapy research. **These nurses were among the first nurses to participate as collaborators in cancer research,** and many of them sought further education and developed into primary researchers interested in either medical or nursing aspects of cancer care.

4. The first survey of research skills of ONS members revealed that a large proportion of oncology nurses had participated in a variety of steps in the research process.

5. Research grants, publications, abstract sessions, and the success of the Advanced Research Special Interest Group and the research Mentorship Program of the ONS Research Committee all provide **evidence of the rapid development** of the **independent research role** for the oncology nurse.

IV. NURSING RESEARCH

1. **Nursing research is defined as the systematic investigation of the responses of patients to actual or potential health problems.**

2. The focus of nursing research differs from that of medical research. **Nursing research focuses on the patient rather than on the disease and may encompass biologic, psychological, and social aspects.**

3. The **profound effect of cancer and cancer treatment** on the patient provides a **rich source of questions** and problems for cancer nursing research investigators.

4. The inclusion of a large proportion of data-based articles in cancer nursing journals attests to the flourishing amount of nursing research relevant to cancer care.

A. THE ROLE OF THE NURSE IN CLINICAL RESEARCH

1. Currently the nurse has several roles in the implementation of research for cancer patients.

    a. The **protocol nurse** serves as a member of the medical research team, as discussed above.

    b. Other nurses **initiate studies that are conducted along with a medical protocol.** This arrangement has been useful in the testing of a variety of nursing approaches.

    c.   Still others act as **principal investigators,** initiating studies, writing protocols, selecting the subjects, and evaluating the results. Results can expand the knowledge basic to the development of nursing science.

  2. Several **recent developments** have made the **expansion of cancer nursing research** possible.

    a. **Priorities** have developed that reflect clinical needs.

    b. **Resources** for nursing research have increased and include financial as well as knowledge dissemination opportunities.

B. PRIORITIES FOR CANCER NURSING RESEARCH

  1. One method that has proved useful in the development of the scientific foundation for nursing practice has been a **systematic targeting of researchers and resources to areas of needed knowledge.**

  2. The National Center for Nursing Research has been involved in **identification of clinical nursing research priorities** through the development of a **national nursing agenda.**

  3. **Cancer nursing research priorities** have been identified and revised over the years.

  4. In one of the first published reports of oncology nursing research priorities, the following **five top-priority areas** were identified:

    a. **Relieving nausea/vomiting induced by chemotherapy/radiation.**

    b. **Pain management.**

    c. **Discharge planning and follow-up.**

    d. **Grief and death.**

    e. **Stomatitis.**

  5. **Table 64-3, text page 1606,** compares the top 10 cancer nursing research priorities from 1981–1991. Changes that have occurred include the rise of **quality of life,** the persistence of **symptom management, pain control and management, prevention and early detection, cancer rehabilitation, and economic influence on oncology.** Newcomers to the priority list include

    a. **Quality of life.**

    b. **Outcome measures for interventions.**

    c. **Cancer survivorship.**

    d. **Cost containment.**

    e. **Research utilization.**

C. MAJOR AREAS OF CURRENT CANCER NURSING RESEARCH ACTIVITY

  1. **Most of the oncology nursing research studies between the years 1989 and 1992 focused on pain, quality of life, patient education, coping, stress, home care, and self-care.**

  2. **Quality-of-life research**

    a. The 1980s and early 1990s witnessed a growing nursing interest in quality-of-life research.

    b. Oncology nursing investigators have provided **conceptual definitions of quality of life,** examined the **domains of the concept of the quality of life,** and led the effort to develop **reliable and valid instruments to measure quality of life.**

    c. Oncology nursing studies have focused on several significant clinical objectives related to quality of life. One important objective concerns the description of **patient psychosocial and physical responses to specific diseases such as melanoma, cancer pain, and non-small-cell lung cancer.**

    d. Cancer nursing has played a prominent role in encouraging **clinical interest in quality-of-life research.** For example, nursing played an important role in the introduction of quality-of-life measures in cancer clinical trials in the Southwest Oncology Group.

    e. The Oncology Nursing Society leads the way in support of research and offers an annual Quality of Life Award and an annual Quality of Life Lecture at its Fall Institute.

    f. Oncology nursing maintains a vital interest in quality-of-life issues, as reflected in numerous articles in scientific journals. The scope of cancer nursing's commitment to promoting quality-of-life research includes **studies to describe quality of life, develop measures, and test interventions to promote it in different cancer populations; conferences to disseminate information; pre- and postdoctoral training programs to foster research interest; and awards for excellence in research.**

3. **Cancer nursing research on pain**
   a. Advances in pain management have been influenced by knowledge derived from nursing research. Oncology nurses have made important contributions in the areas of pain assessment, interventions, and eradication of factors that impede pain relief.
   b. **Table 64-4, text pages 1608–1609,** outlines examples of the vast contributions nurses have made to the research on the topic of cancer pain in the areas of:
      (1) Pain as a component of oncology nursing.
      (2) Pain assessment.
      (3) Nursing knowledge and attitudes regarding pain.
      (4) Pharmacologic interventions.
      (5) Nursing models of pain interventions and other contributions.
   c. The first important contribution to pain research by nurse investigators was the identification of **pain as a component of oncology nursing.**
   d. The identification of **comfort as a basic goal of cancer nursing firmly established pain as a dimension of oncology nursing.** The ONS Standards of Practice identify 11 high-incidence problem areas for oncology, of which comfort is one.
   e. The commitment to pain management by the profession was reinforced by the publication of the comprehensive **ONS Position Paper on Pain.**
   f. A major contribution by oncology nursing researchers has been made in the area of **pain assessment,** including the assessment of pain in populations with special needs such as children and the elderly.
   g. Research in pain assessment has also been extended to include more complex issues such as the **role of biobehavioral and environmental factors and affective states associated with pain.**
   h. Continued evaluation of the **validity and reliability of assessment tools** has been an important component in the progress of pain research.
   i. Research in the area of **nursing knowledge and attitudes regarding pain** and the resulting effect on pain relief is an area where oncology nurses have made key contributions.
   j. Nurses have been involved in investigating **pharmacologic interventions** to manage pain, including patient education, appropriate dosing, conversion between drugs, route of administration, and evaluating the impact of various drug interventions on the patient in pain.
   k. An important yet understudied area of pain research has been the evaluation of **nursing models of pain intervention.**
   l. Several other contributions include the role of the patient's family in pain management, evaluation of patient education related to pain, and **ethical issues.**

D. **RESOURCES FOR ONCOLOGY NURSING RESEARCH**

1. **Financial support** for oncology nursing research has **expanded** and is a **major resource for cancer nursing research activities.**
2. One source of support is **internal support at one's own institution.** This is an especially valuable resource for the investigator with limited or no grant-writing experience.
3. **Biomedical support grants from the federal government** are available for both educational and clinical institutions that have already achieved a specific level of research support from the government.
4. **External funds** are available for individual investigators from the **government** and from **private foundations.**
5. Two major sources for federal funds are the National Center for Nursing Research and the National Cancer Institute.
6. A valuable resource for cancer nurses seeking federal funds is the **NIH Guide for Grants and Contracts, published by the National Institutes of Health.**
7. **Private funds** for cancer nursing research have expanded and include the Oncology Nursing Foundation, Sigma Theta Tau, American Cancer Society, and Robert Wood Johnson Foundation.
8. The education and experience of oncology nurses reflect increased academic preparation for research and increased involvement in a variety of research activities.

E. **FUTURE DIRECTIONS FOR CANCER NURSING RESEARCH**

1. Review of cancer nursing research reveals areas where **clusters of studies** have begun, such as quality of life and pain, and **areas where much work is still needed,** such as prevention and early detection, management of symptoms such as fatigue and anxiety, and approaches to nursing care for special populations such as ethnic minorities, the young, and the elderly.

2. Development of **programs of research** where studies build on one another provides for **sequential scientific knowledge.**

3. **Research utilization** cannot be emphasized enough as the critical step to applying findings of studies to the daily care of patients.

PRACTICE QUESTIONS

1. Which of the following is **not** true of research?
    (A) It can be considered valid only when it is replicated.
    (B) It involves an orderly and standardized series of steps.
    (C) It includes the obligation to disseminate the results for critique by others.
    (D) It focuses on individual patients rather than on groups of patients.

2. Which of the following pairings of trial phases and their functions in the clinical trials approach to clinical research is **incorrect?**
    (A) phase 1: determine drug toxicities
    (B) phase 2: determine the activity of a new agent in specific types of cancers
    (C) phase 2: determine maximum tolerated dose
    (D) phase 3: determine whether a new therapy is more effective than a standard therapy

3. Phase 2 and phase 3 studies are often conducted at institutions with cooperative arrangements with NCI-designated cancer centers. **One** reason for this is to
    (A) provide the full spectrum of support services needed in studies in which toxicities are not predictable.
    (B) increase the number of test subjects, thus speeding up the process of developing new therapies.
    (C) provide closer monitoring of patients.
    (D) increase the participation and involvement of the patient in the selection of medical treatment.

4. With which of the following issues or activities is the research nurse in the medical research team **least** likely to become involved?
    (A) acute clinical care, including monitoring the patient's symptoms
    (B) education of the patient's caregivers, including the clinical nursing staff
    (C) managing data, including collecting information on toxicities from the chart
    (D) informed consent issues, including ensuring that patients understand the risks and benefits of the treatment

5. The focus of nursing research **differs** from that of medical research in that it
    (A) involves a greater amount of detail and accuracy of measurement.
    (B) focuses on groups of patients rather than on individual patients.
    (C) involves a greater degree of collaboration among various members of the research team.
    (D) focuses on the patient rather than the disease.

6. Assume you are interested in conducting a research study in cancer nursing, and you want to find out if federal funding is available for the study you have in mind. Probably your **best** approach is to
    (A) write or phone the National Cancer Institute for a copy of their *National Nursing Agenda* publication.
    (B) prepare a request for federal seed money through your school or college of nursing.
    (C) contact the Oncology Nursing Foundation or Robert Wood Johnson Foundation for information concerning available grants.
    (D) get a copy of the publication entitled *NIH Guide for Grants and Contracts.*

7. Probably the most significant step in the evolution of cancer nurses into primary research was the
   (A) collaboration of the chemotherapy nurse in clinical research.
   (B) formation of the Clinical Nursing Research Alliance (CNRA) in 1974.
   (C) adoption of the clinical trials approach by the Oncology Nursing Society.
   (D) rise of surgery as the primary approach to the treatment of cancer.

8. Which of the following is **not** evidence that more cancer nurses than ever are participating in cancer research?
   (A) the higher percentage of cancer nurses with baccalaureate and advanced degrees
   (B) a shift in the focus of cancer research from the educational to the clinical setting
   (C) an increase in the number and variety of research roles held by cancer nurses
   (D) an increase in support for cancer research from nursing administration

ANSWER EXPLANATIONS

1. **The answer is (D).** Research involves a structured approach to answering questions or discovering new knowledge, and is conducted for the broad purpose of increasing scientific knowledge. Among its characteristics are that it can be considered valid only when it is replicated; it involves an orderly and standardized series of steps, similar to those in the nursing process but involving greater detail and accuracy of measurement; and it focuses on groups of patients (rather than on individuals) and includes the obligation to disseminate the results for critique by others. (1600)

2. **The answer is (C).** Phase 2 trials focus on the specific tumor types for which the treatment appears promising. Maximum tolerated dose (MTD) and drug toxicities are established in preclinical and phase 1 trials. Phase 3 trials determine the effects of treatment relative to the natural history of the disease, whether a new treatment is more effective than a standard therapy, and whether a new treatment is as effective as a standard therapy but is associated with less morbidity. (1601)

3. **The answer is (B).** Phase 2 and 3 studies may be conducted at institutions with cooperative arrangements with NCI-designated centers both to provide for a larger number of patients available for research accrual, thus speeding up the development of new therapies, and to provide patients with options that are not available through their private physicians. Choices (A) and (C) are both advantages of conducting trials at the NCI-designated centers themselves. (1601)

4. **The answer is (C).** Managing data is the usual responsibility of the data manager in the medical research team. The data manager, who may or may not be a nurse, collects information on toxicities from the chart and enters these data into the computer for statistical analysis. The research or protocol nurse is responsible for patient accrual, implementing the physician's orders as described in the protocol, and observing patient responses and toxicities. In implementing these roles, the nurse is involved in informed consent issues, astute clinical care, and education of supporting nursing staff. (1603–1604)

5. **The answer is (D).** Nursing research, defined as the systematic investigation of the responses of patients to actual or potential health problems, focuses on the **patient** rather than on the **disease** and often encompasses biologic, psychologic, and social aspects of patient care. Nurses have several roles in the implementation of research for cancer patients, including that of protocol nurse, clinical staff nurse, initiator of a study conducted along with a medical protocol, and principal investigator. (1604–1605)

6. **The answer is (D).** One of the most valuable resources for cancer nurses looking for federal funds is the publication entitled *NIH Guide for Grants and Contracts*, which lists grant programs and deadline dates for grants and contracts administered by the National Institute of Health (NIH). Two other major sources for federal funds are the National Center for Nursing Research and the National Cancer Institute. Private funding may be available through various organizations, including the Oncology Nursing Foundation, Sigma Theta Tau, the American Cancer Society, and the Robert Wood Johnson Foundation. Funds may also be available at one's own institution. (1610–1611)

7. **The answer is (A).** The development of chemotherapy for cancers (e.g., leukemia) that were not amenable or responsive to either surgery or radiation gave the nurse a primary role in implementation of medical research. The chemotherapeutic agents were administered intravenously over a course of therapy given on a regular basis. Thus, the chemotherapy nurse assumed one of the first specialty roles in the development

of cancer nursing practice. Out of this role grew an increasing familiarity with the research process as used in clinical chemotherapy research, and many chemotherapy nurses sought further education and developed into primary researchers interested in either medical or nursing aspects of cancer care. (1604)

8. **The answer is (B).** More cancer nurses than ever are participating in cancer research as a result of enhanced educational preparation, as evidenced by the growing percentage of cancer nurses with baccalaureate and master's degrees; an increase in the number and variety of research roles, including those of proposal development, individual investigation, and statistical analysis, as well as data collection; and support from nursing administration in both educational and clinical settings. Dissertation research involving cancer patients has increased with the increasing number of doctoral programs. In clinical settings, a recent trend is toward the establishment of a specific position or department for nursing research. (1611)

65 Thriving as an Oncology Nurse

STUDY OUTLINE

I. STRESS

1. Stress is a pervasive human problem associated with all of life's major institutions.
2. The cost of not effectively coping with stress effectively can be high and may include compromised patient care, job burnout, and even physical and psychological deterioration.
3. The nurse must recognize potential sources of stress and implement coping strategies that permit continued job and life effectiveness.
4. Stress has been variously defined as a response, as a stimulus, and as a transaction.
5. Selye defined stress as a response to events in the environment, a response that is physiological and therefore unrelated to the nature of the stressor, the individual's thoughts and beliefs, or the situational context.
6. Stress has also been characterized as the potential residing within the stimulus or as something that results because of the event itself, unmediated by personal factors or variations in the setting.
7. People respond differently to external events, both interpersonally (between people) and intrapersonally (within individuals at different times). Stress does not reside solely in the event or in the response of the person. It reflects some transaction between the two that is modified by a third factor or set of factors.
8. The transactional model of stress views stress as the tension that results when the **perceived** demands of a situation (whether imposed from within the person or by the environment) are out of balance with the perceived resources available to the individual.

II. INDIVIDUAL APPRAISAL

1. The central focus of the transaction model of stress is the nature of the transactions between the person and the environment. **Figure 65-1, text page 1615,** presents a pictorial representation of the transactional model of stress.
2. Stress arises from a transaction between the individual and the environment when the individual judges the stimuli as damaging, threatening, or challenging in relation to whether the demands tax or exceed appraised available resources.
3. Stress is the perceived imbalance between demands and abilities or resources.
4. Cognitive appraisal refers to evaluations and judgments of events and one's reactions to those events.
5. Primary appraisal refers to a person's judgment about the significance of a stressor. It determines "what is at stake" in the situation and whether the person is in trouble or deriving benefit.
6. Primary appraisals of the transaction take three forms: irrelevant, positive (benign), or stressful.
   a. The encounter is irrelevant if it carries no implications for a person's well-being.
   b. The encounter is positive if it preserves or enhances well-being.
   c. Encounters appraised as stressful involve judgments of harm or loss, challenge, and threat.
7. In secondary appraisal, judgments are made about resources and options available for coping, constraints on using these resources, and consequences.
8. If the individual believes he or she can handle most stressful situations (secondary appraisal), then most transactions will be judged as nonthreatening (primary appraisal).

9. The relationship between an individual and the environment is ever-changing, and as a consequence, appraisals change. This process of changing judgments or appraisals is called reappraisal.

III. PERSON-ENVIRONMENT FIT

1. Within the transaction model of stress, adaptation is conceptualized as a function of the **"goodness of fit"** between the person and the environment.
2. Fit is determined by the extent to which environmental supplies are able to meet individual needs (demands) as well as the ability (supplies) of the person to manage the demands imposed by the environment.
3. If demands exceed supplies, or vice versa, adjustment is required to create a good fit.
4. A job is stressful to the extent that it does not provide supplies to meet the individual's motives and to the extent that the ability of the individual falls below the demands of the job, which are prerequisite to receiving supplies.

IV. DEMANDS—SOURCES OF STRESS

1. In general, stress in nursing generates from mismatches between efforts and results, mismatches between nurse and environment leading to role ambiguity and conflict, and mismatches between people leading to interpersonal conflict.
2. The stress experienced by cancer nurses involves an interplay between intrapersonal (self-concept, motivations, and personal needs), interpersonal (relationships with recipients of care and coworkers and the nature of cancer care), and environmental factors.

A. INTRAPERSONAL FACTORS

1. Individuals bring into relationships and situations personal characteristics that influence their perceptions of other people and events as well as their reactions.
2. Self-concept, personal needs, and motivations have the potential both of providing interpersonal demands and supplies and of playing a significant role in the mediation of a stress response.
3. **Self-concept**
   a. How we see ourselves plays an important role in our relationships with other people and our appraisal of events.
   b. Self-concept is developed through self-appraisal as well as through appraisal by others.
   c. Negative self-talk ("People don't like me," "I am incompetent," "I can't do that procedure," etc.) can inadvertently encourage a person to meet the expectation of the negative statement.
4. **Personal needs**
   a. Most people want approval, praise for accomplishments, love, and respect. These are basic human needs.
   b. The strength of an individual's motivation to fulfill these needs and where the individual looks to have them fulfilled have implications in helping relationships and work environments.
   c. Individuals with intense needs for **approval and affection** may work exceedingly hard to be pleasing and to satisfy the demands of recipients of care and coworkers.
   d. People vary in the expectations about the extent to which they have **control and autonomy** over their lives.
   e. An **internal locus of control** is the tendency to perceive that actions and outcomes are correlated and that one is in control of one's life.
   f. Individuals with an **external locus of control** tend to expect little control over events.
5. **Personal motivations**
   a. An individual's behavior is influenced by the expectation that behavior will bring about need fulfillment.
   b. Failure to fulfill the motivation that prompted the decision to enter a helping profession can generate a great deal of stress.
   c. Motivation or drive for need fulfillment influences how an individual appraises situations (whether or not needs will be fulfilled). As a result, motivations influence stress reactions (behavior).

    d. Motivations are modified by the expectations of self and others. These expectations influence appraisal.

    e. Expectations modify motivations and influence appraisal; if expectations are unrealistic, feelings of anger and hostility (external expressions of unmet needs) can result, as can depression, a sense of failure, and low self-esteem (internal expressions of unmet needs).

B. **INTERPERSONAL FACTORS**

  1. **Helping relationships**
    a. The very structure of the helping relationship can promote a negative view of people or a shift from a positive to a negative view.
    b. This shift from a positive to a negative view of people can frustrate the helper, dampen the helper's sensitivity, diminish the helper's sense of accomplishment, and cause general emotional and physical exhaustion.
    c. **Four aspects** of the helping relationship are **pivotal** in this **positive-to-negative shift:**
      (1) **Focus on the problem.**
      (2) **Lack of positive feedback.**
      (3) **Level of emotional stress.**
      (4) **Perceived possibility of change or improvement.**
    d. By definition, **the recipient of care** in a helping relationship **has a problem** (weakness, deficiencies, illness) that is the **focus** of the relationship. What is normal or healthy is often ignored.
    e. In most helping relationships, when the problem is resolved, the recipient goes away; the relationship is over. **It is easy to see how helpers can shift to a negative view of people in such settings.**
    f. **Most helpers want both feedback about the quality of their efforts and appreciation.** If complaints or criticism from recipients or coworkers are the norm, a negative view of helping can result.
    g. **Lack of positive feedback** is a source of stress, and helping relationships that offer no positive feedback over time are viewed negatively.
    h. The diagnosis of cancer generates a great deal of **emotional distress.** Helpers may attempt to decrease the emotional distress of care recipients by encouraging disclosure of feelings. However, there are consequences to the helper of being on the receiving end of emotional disclosure or catharsis.
    i. When the nature of contact with patients is upsetting, depressing, or difficult, the helper may develop a negative, even dehumanized perception of the care recipient.
    j. Another way to handle the feelings is by distancing oneself emotionally and/or physically, creating a shelter by adding a layer of callus.
    k. The recipient's responsiveness to the helper influences the helper's view of the recipient. Helpers can react not only to a lack of personal responsiveness, but also to a **lack of change or improvement** in the recipient's condition. In the absence of change or improvement in the patient's condition, the helper may have feelings of personal failure and ineffectiveness.

  2. **Cancer trajectory**
    a. Each cancer diagnosis has a unique trajectory. Some patients will be cured, others will live with a chronic illness with periods of remission and recurrence, still others will die quickly.
    b. Trajectory variability creates demands on care providers as variability creates uncertainty.
    c. The unpredictability of cancer leaves the cancer nurse with the dilemma of what messages to convey to patients and family members.

  3. **Prolonged involvement**
    a. Cancer nurses are often involved with patients and their families for extended periods of time. This is a double-edged sword, because prolonged involvement provides both rewards for and demands on cancer nurses.
    b. During sustained relationships, patients and families may manifest a kaleidoscope of emotions, including anger, frustration, grief, and fear. The demands expand exponentially as the nurse cares for multiple patients and families experiencing different emotions.
    c. Being faced with human suffering and distress of the spirit places the listener in a vulnerable position.
    d. One way to lessen the intensity of the relationship is to withdraw physical and emotional support. Withdrawal may include emotional distancing, avoidance, and task orientation, which tend to increase rather than reduce stress for the care provider.

4. **Treatment sequelae**
   a. Feeling as though one, as a nurse, is contributing to the suffering of patients is distressing, because it is not in keeping with an idealized image of the nurse as professional provider of comfort and help.
   b. If therapy causes significant morbidity, ambivalence or cynicism may develop.
   c. The nurse administering investigational therapies may feel incompetent in predicting and managing side effects.
   d. The stress to the care provider associated with disfiguring surgeries stems from the disfigurement itself and, as with other therapies, questioning whether or not the surgery will have a positive impact on the quantity and/or quality of the individual's life.
   e. Lack of consensus among health care providers and patients regarding treatment goals is a source of stress for cancer nurses. Patients may request continuation of aggressive treatment, creating a dilemma for the nurse who believes palliation is the reasonable choice. When palliation is the goal, caregivers may feel helpless and guilty if they are unable to provide relief from symptoms.

5. **Death**
   a. Cancer nurses will encounter physical death and, in a broader context, loss of social worth, value control, energy, relationships, role, life's work, or hopes for the future.
   b. Confrontation or repeated exposure to death causes us to face our own fears about death and contemplate our own mortality.
   c. Continual consciousness of the fear of death impairs functioning; in defence, the fear is repressed. However, continual psychological efforts to repress fear of death demand energy.
   d. When we don't share each experience of death with significant others, the feelings or distress associated with each death accumulate.

6. **Nurses' realities—women's realities**
   a. Caring and feeling cared for are basic human needs that promote personal and societal health.
   b. Caring is devalued in our society in part because it is associated with "women's work" and subservience.
   c. If the essence of nursing is caring, a major source of stress in nursing lies in the devaluation of caring and the lack of recognition and rewards given to the caregiver.
   d. Another societal devaluation of caring stems from the proliferation of codependency theory that calls into question the motive for caregiving. Caring may be perceived as an illness when popularized by definitions such as "any suffering and/or dysfunction that is associated with or results from focusing on the needs and behaviors of others." Such views can cause self-blame for the stress experienced in caring work, doubting caring motivations, and cutting off social support.

C. **ENVIRONMENTAL FACTORS**

1. **Role stressors**
   a. **Role ambiguity** is the extent to which role expectations are not clearly communicated. An individual must understand the expectations that others have of a particular role, as well as the duties, rights, responsibilities, and activities of the role, in order to adequately perform the role.
   b. Role ambiguity experienced by nurses stems from a lack of clear definition of professional nursing as well as the diversity of roles currently enacted by nurses.
   c. In general, the greater the perceived role ambiguity, the greater the perceived stress.
   d. **Role conflict** is the extent to which the expectations of various others are in conflict or incompatible.
   e. The evolving role of the nurse may cause conflicts, particularly with physicians and social workers who feel that nurses are infringing on their traditional roles. The evolving roles of other professionals can create conflict by infringing on the traditional roles of nursing such as patient teaching or symptom management.
   f. **Role overload** is the extent to which a person is incapable of meeting multiple expectations, and may result in physical and emotional exhaustion, negative feelings about patients, coworkers, and the organization, as well as a diminished sense of accomplishment.
   g. **Qualitative** overload implies that the job skills and knowledge exceed those of the individual. **Quantitative** overload implies that there is more work than can be done in a given period of time.

h. The experience of overload can be aggravated by the imposition of tasks that have a high priority for the organization but a low priority for the worker (e.g., completing paperwork versus providing emotional support to a patient). Rather than compromise quality of care, nurses may end up working overtime, often without compensation, and perpetuating the perceived stress.

2. **Control issues: autonomy and authority**
   a. **Job control** is associated with **autonomy and authority,** that is, with the sense that one has control of one's time and activities.
   b. Organizational characteristics such as circumscribed authority, downward channels of commands, specialization, and formal accountability and hierarchy contribute to a sense of lack of autonomy and control.
   c. A lack of autonomy engenders feelings of frustration, victimization, and helplessness.
   d. Nurses can develop feelings of powerlessness as they discover that what happens is independent of their input, expressed concern, or verbal complaint. As a consequence, estrangement from the work environment can occur.
   e. The need for autonomy can also be so great that nurses will blame themselves for problems, errors, and the like just to maintain a sense of control.

3. **Work environment**
   a. Research has demonstrated that the physical quality of the work environment has an effect on performance.
   b. Overcrowded units, noise, poor lighting, poor ventilation, and malfunctioning equipment are physical stressors identified by health care professionals.

4. **Intragroup and intergroup conflict**
   a. Conflict seems inevitable in the dealings of any two autonomous persons whose interests or relationships are interdependent.
   b. Factors that influence intragroup and intergroup conflicts include the scarcity of, or competition for, resources (time, money, people, skills), divergent goals, and group interdependence for work sequencing.
   c. In teamwork, the greater the interrelatedness and dependence on one another, the greater the potential for conflict.
   d. Group cohesiveness, compatibility, and group attitude about conflict influences whether and the means by which conflicts are addressed.
   e. Among the basic commitments for nurses who practice in accordance with generally accepted standards is that they participate as members of the health care team.
   f. Physician-nurse conflict is rooted in historical antecedent, power and status inequity, mutual lack of knowledge of and respect for unique contributions of each role, personality conflicts, and lack of communication regarding treatment goals.
   g. Unresolved intragroup conflicts (nurse to nurse) seem to represent losing sight of the basic idea of nursing as a caring profession that includes caring for both patients as well as fellow nurses.
   h. Intragroup conflicts disrupt team stability, isolate team members, and lessen the likelihood that nursing staff will share feelings related to work experiences.

5. **Organizational climate**
   a. Size, structure, goals, and organizational climate are organizational factors that can serve as sources of stress.
   b. Hospitals have characteristics that foster stress:
      (1) Multiple levels of authority.
      (2) Heterogeneity of personnel.
      (3) Work interdependence.
      (4) Specialization.
   c. Ambiguity of organizational structure, procedures and policies, and conversely overregulation can both be perceived as stressful. Precise organizational charts, a chain of command, and detailed job descriptions and procedures can create stress due to perceived inflexibility and lack of individual control.
   d. Organization goals may be in conflict with the goals of the individual. The organizational goal may be to provide care at minimal cost, whereas the goal of the caregiver may be to do everything possible. Goals of the organization are both explicit and implicit.
   e. Organizational climate can support or diminish nurse-patient relationships. Nursing is a people-oriented profession, and thus nurses who work in an organization that places a higher value on technology would be expected to experience job stress due to the devaluation of their patient-centered orientation.

6. **Management strategies—rewards**
   a. Reward, recognition, praise, encouragement, expressions of appreciation, and clear feedback are extremely powerful incentives. Research has shown that employees are better equipped to handle work stress when these kinds of rewards are available, and that they experience increased stress when there is a noticeable lack of these rewards.
   b. Health care professionals gauge their relative worth in the organization by making inferences about the extent to which they are compensated for their contributions. Lack of differentiation of rewards (everyone receives a merit increase regardless of efforts) encourages only average performance as the high contributor concludes that there is no need to work harder. And the low contributor, seeing that the high contributor gets equal reward, concludes that hard work does not pay off.
   c. Recognition and appreciation often are more important than dollars. People who receive recognition, appreciation, satisfaction, and a sense of significance from their work are more likely to be content with their income.
   d. Lack of feedback, as well as a mismatch of work performance expectations between nurses and managers, can create conflict.

V.   SUPPLIES—STRESS MANAGEMENT STRATEGIES

1. Stress results from a mismatch or discrepancy between environmental demands and individual supplies or between environmental opportunities and individual needs and goals.
2. Efforts to reduce stress must alter either environment or self or both, by either reducing demands or increasing supplies or altering one's interpretation of demands and supplies.
3. Coping embraces actions to reduce the mismatch between self and environment. There are two general types of coping: problem-focused and emotion-focused.
   a. **Problem-focused coping** targets the environment of self for direct action by changing one's behavior or environmental conditions.
   b. **Emotion-focused coping** attempts to palliate or eliminate distressing emotions elicited by the stressor. Emotion-focused coping does not change the self or environment, only the way one feels.
   c. When a situation is assessed as having the potential for change, a person typically will use problem-focused coping, whereas emotion-focused coping is employed if the harmful or threatening situation holds little potential for change.
   d. The challenge is to learn to manage effectively those things that can be controlled, to accept the things that cannot be controlled, and to recognize the difference.
4. The **characteristics of effective coping** include
   a. **An active exploration of reality issues and a search for information.**
   b. **A free expression of positive and negative feelings. Feelings are mastered where possible; and where mastery is not possible, the inevitable is accepted.**
   c. **An active effort to engage the help of others.**
   d. **Problems are broken down into manageable bits and worked through one at a time.**
   e. **A fundamental trust in oneself and others and a sense of optimism that something can be done to bring about a positive outcome.**
5. Because stress is a personal experience, stress prevention and management strategies begin with the individual.
6. Self-regulation enables nurses to reappraise self and environment, evaluate the supplies and demands of the work environment, and develop problem- or emotion-focused coping strategies. Self-regulation involves knowing one's self and one's personal values, priorities, and beliefs.
7. Concrete **strategies for coping** with stress include
   a. Reappraisal of goals.
   b. Time management.
   c. Acknowledging vulnerabilities.
   d. Compartmentalizing life and work.
   e. Self-reinforcement.
   f. Change in attitudes.
   g. Creating balance.
   h. Accentuating the positive.
   i. Adopting a wellness philosophy.
   j. Relaxation.
   k. Establishing a sense of control over one's practice.

A.   **INTRAPERSONAL COPING STRATEGIES**

1.   **Recognizing stress responses**
   a.   It is essential that an individual begin to recognize the triggers and signs of physical, emotional, and mental stress. These manifestations of stress are listed in **Figure 65-2, text page 1623.**
   b.   Self-understanding begins with self-observation. It is suggested that individuals keep a daily stress and tension log, as shown in **Figure 65-3, text page 1624** (Maslach). Recording this type of information can provide insight into emotional and cognitive coping responses, the precipitator of responses, and styles of coping.

2.   **Setting realistic goals**
   a.   Unrealistic self-expectations are a formula for defeat, and can cause self-doubt, self-blame, and lowered self-esteem.
   b.   It is imperative to examine self-expectations and goals.
   c.   Reappraisal of goals involves knowing what you want from your life and work, evaluating whether or not the goals are realistic, and redefining the goals as necessary.
   d.   Goals need to be specific, realistic, and measurable. Setting realistic goals improves the probability of success.

3.   **Time management**
   a.   Time management is vital to self-management and essentially involves structuring time in order to meet goals.
   b.   Time waste is caused by self, by others, and by the organization.
   c.   Self-generated time wasters include lack of self-discipline, worry, always saying "yes," procrastination, disorganization, and an unwillingness to delegate.
   d.   Time problems generated by others might include interruptions, phone calls, inter-dependency of work, and meetings that do not start or stop on time or where people arrive late or come unprepared.
   e.   Time wasters generated by the organization and the nature of nurses' work include ambiguity of roles, lack of clarity regarding goals, redundancy of effort, frequent changes, failure to plan, engaging nurses in non-nursing tasks.

4.   **Tuning into inner dialogue**
   a.   One's perception or interpretation of the stressor is a critical variable in what is experienced as stressful. **These perceptions are given voice in an ongoing dialogue we have with ourselves.**
   b.   **Self-talk** can be rational or irrational. Self-talk based on rational thoughts promotes self-respect and goal attainment. Self-talk based on irrational thoughts tends to sabotage self-esteem, results in negative emotions, and inhibits the realization of goals.
   c.   The A-B-C model can be used to examine the relationship between thoughts, feelings, and behaviors. Event A is the activating event. Event C represents our emotional responses and behaviors as a result of the activating event. Something happens between Event A and Event C, Event B, our self-talk, that influences our feelings and behaviors in response to Event A.
   d.   The technique called **cognitive restructuring** involves learning to listen to self-talk and changing unwanted or irrational thoughts in order to change emotional response.

5.   **Accentuating the positive**
   a.   Helping relationships often have a negative bias, for the recipients of care have problems for which they seek help from the caregiver.
   b.   The negative in helping relationships can be countered by actively emphasizing what is good, pleasant, or satisfying about the helping relationship. For examples of emphasizing the positive aspects of the helping relationship, see **Figure 65-4, text page 1626.**

6.   **Compartmentalizing work and life**
   a.   Another strategy for controlling stress is to create a clear distinction between work and home, including finding a balance between the energy expended at work and home activities.
   b.   One form of compartmentalization is not discussing work-related issues at home, and vice versa.
   c.   Another strategy to create a sense of separation between work and home is to allow for decompression time. A decompression routine is a ritual that signals that one part of daily life is ending and another is beginning, that is, the passage from work to personal life. Examples of decompression activities include making a to-do list for the next day's activi-

ties before leaving work, listening to music on the way home, exercising, meditating, or changing from work into at-home clothes.

7. **Creating balance**
   a. Every helper needs to find a way to be involved emotionally as a caregiver without burning out.
   b. Empathy is a double-edged sword; it is simultaneously the nurse's greatest asset and point of real vulnerability. Creating a balance between overinvolvement and depersonalization involves finding a blend of compassion and objectivity or detached concern.
   c. Most nursing educational programs stress the importance of empathy, but few balance that recommendation with the importance of maintaining emotional and physical distance. Experienced practitioners typically learn detached concern through experience, most likely only after experiencing both ends of the involvement spectrum.
   d. Sharing experiences and seeking the feedback of peers regarding involvements with patients and families can help caregivers to learn about detached concern.
   e. Intellectualization can also help with achieving detached concern. Intellectualization involves dealing with emotionally stressful situations in the abstract or as technical realities. It serves as a defense mechanism in creating psychological or emotional distance from distressing situations.
   f. Exclusive use of intellectualization creates imbalance as one becomes increasingly underinvolved. This underinvolvement creates stress, since most nurses are dissatisfied with underinvolvement. Additionally, suppression of one's emotional experiences requires energy and at some point will require attention.

8. **Creating control of one's practice**
   a. Creating control of one's practice involves developing and maintaining competence, setting limits, and organizing one's work to minimize stress and enhance satisfaction.
   b. Reasonable limits of personal giving must be established if sustained, effective functioning is to be ensured. Limit setting helps to create a mastery over one's work. This involves knowing and respecting one's limits, deciding what one can and cannot do, and deciding what one will and will not do.
   c. Organizing work assignments so the work is varied can counterbalance emotionally draining work with task-oriented work. Strategies to restructure work assignments include job sharing, changing the context of the contact with patients (e.g., cross training staff to work in inpatient and outpatient settings), sharing responsibility for difficult patient care assignments, and creating a balanced mix of the types of patients.
   d. Developing specialized roles can give a sense of control and pleasure from one's work. Specialized roles might include developing an expertise in a particular aspect of care (e.g., mouth care) and taking on special assignments (e.g., developing a patient education tool, serving on a committee).

9. **Relaxation**
   a. Chronic stress often produces tense muscles, increased blood pressure, and fatigue. Relaxation brings mental and physical restoration.
   b. Relaxation is based on the mind-body connection and the premise that a relaxed body is the antithesis of a stressed mind. There are many forms of relaxation techniques: progressive deep-muscle relaxation, biofeedback, guided imagery, meditation, yoga, and autogenic training. The key to the effectiveness of any technique is practice.
   c. Relaxation treats the symptoms, not the cause of stress, but provides renewal to face the next challenge.

10. **Adopting a wellness philosophy**
    a. A wellness philosophy promotes health behaviorally. Healthy choices include eating a balanced diet, limiting alcohol and caffeine intake, ceasing smoking, practicing preventive health care, exercise, rest, recreation, socialization, and development of intimate relationships.
    b. The principal benefit of actively adopting a wellness philosophy is conditioning the body to withstand the deleterious effects of stress.

B. **ENVIRONMENTAL STRATEGIES**

1. Six principles that lead to a more satisfying work environment:
   a. Involvement with establishing work objectives and methods.
   b. Clarity of organization and structure.

    c.   Feedback and information.

    d.   Orientation and training.

    e.   Rewards.

    f.   Supportive culture.

2. An organization-based stress management strategy requires assessment of the nurse's perceptions of

    a.   Discrepancies between accountability and authority.

    b.   Extent to which the job provides variety and challenge.

    c.   Extent to which the nurse's role is clearly defined.

    d.   Extent to which the nurse's role conflicts with purported roles of others of different status and position.

    e.   Opportunities for continued training and development.

    f.   Adequacy of supplies/equipment/space.

    g.   Amount of actual freedom and independence.

    h.   Extent to which the nurse is receiving feedback concerning performance.

3. **Nurse-patient ratios**

    a.   Nurses have a right to work in an environment that minimizes physical and emotional stress. Employers have a legal responsibility to provide sufficient staff to meet the care needs of patients.

    b.   The quality of nurse-patient interactions is influenced by the number as well as the acuity of the people for which the nurse is responsible. As the number increases, so does role overload for the nurse.

    c.   Staff-patient ratios that support the provision of quality patient care and equalization of demands with supplies decrease work load stress.

    d.   One organizational strategy to address nurse-patient ratios is to review the cost of staff turnover and staff burnout.

4. **Organizational flexibility**

    a.   Organizational flexibility implies concern for the individual, the provision of individual freedom, permission to exert some control over his or her practice, and providing variability in routines.

    b.   Distrust and failure to recognize the needs and abilities of the individual employee create an inflexible system.

    c.   A decentralized management system is a means of providing flexibility and control.

    d.   Other areas in which organizations can provide flexibility include self-scheduling, job sharing, involvement with equipment selection, development of ongoing job descriptions that change with the individual's expertise and interests, and clinical ladders.

5. **Creating opportunities for withdrawal**

    a.   The concept of "time out" is important to any work that involves emotional, physical, or mental stress.

    b.   Time-out activities include providing not only for meal breaks but also for breaks from stressful work, for example, through a change in routine or through having staff share the direct care responsibilities for a particularly tedious or arduous patient care situation.

6. **Social support**

    a.   The presence of absence of social support plays a major role in stress.

    b.   Social support is defined as enduring interpersonal ties to a group of people who can be relied on to provide emotional sustenance, assistance, and resources, who provide feedback, and who share standards and values.

    c.   Social support can serve a number of functions, such as providing a listening presence, technical appreciation and affirmation of competence, and emotional support and challenge.

    d.   Some nurses may find that receiving support is difficult, because nurses view themselves as caregivers, not as care receivers. Fear often keeps nurses from seeking support or expressing emotions.

    e.   The fallacy of uniqueness is a phenomenon in which individuals falsely assume they are the only one feeling, thinking, or behaving in a particular way. By expressing feelings and experiences, nurses can learn that others share similar experiences, thus decreasing alienation and isolation.

    f.   It is important to build work-based sources of support, because these seem to be more potent than individual efforts at reducing occupational stress. Work-based supports not only provide for individual support, but also provide a mechanism for institutional change through group problem solving.

7. **Work team development**
    a. An important organizational coping mechanism is the sense of belonging to a team that knows what it is doing, knows how to get members to work towards defined professional and personal goals, and knows how to support one another through professional and personal stressors.
    b. Characteristics of an effective team include
        (1) Clarity of objectives, goals, and priorities that are agreed on by team members.
        (2) Role expectations that are realistic and clearly defined.
        (3) Problem-solving and decision-making skills.
        (4) Group rules that support the objectives.
        (5) Goals and priorities.
        (6) Concern for group members.
        (7) The ability to maximize group resources for the good of the group and the individual.
    c. These characteristics can be used as criteria for the periodic assessment of overall team functioning and effectiveness.
    d. The organizational conditions of scarcity of or competition for resources, ambiguity (in procedures, policies, roles), overregulation, and exceptions to the rules provide rich fuel for conflict.
    e. When people in conflict are able to approach the conflict in an atmosphere of trust and mutual support, the energy that normally would be diverted to defensiveness is freed up for us in resolving the conflict.

PRACTICE QUESTIONS

1. The transactional model of stress views stress as
    (A) a physiological response to events in the environment.
    (B) a transaction between a person and a stressful stimulus.
    (C) the tension that results when the perceived demands of a situation are out of balance with the perceived resources available to the individual.
    (D) the potential residing in certain stimuli to create an adverse physiological response.

2. Primary appraisal differs from secondary appraisal in that
    (A) primary appraisal is focused on what is at stake in the situation and whether the person is in trouble or deriving benefit.
    (B) secondary appraisal may take three forms: irrelevant, positive, or stressful.
    (C) Secondary appraisal is concerned with judgments of harm or loss, challenge, or threat.
    (D) in primary appraisal, judgments are made about resources and options available for coping.

3. In the transactional model of stress, the stress experienced by cancer nurses involves an interplay between
    (A) primary and secondary appraisals.
    (B) intrapersonal, interpersonal, and environmental factors.
    (C) personal motivations, self-concept, and the cancer trajectory.
    (D) primary appraisal, secondary appraisal, and the work environment in which the appraisals are made.

4. Aspects of the helping relationship that can cause a positive-to-negative shift include
    (A) distancing oneself emotionally from the patient's experience of distress.
    (B) prolonged patient involvement.
    (C) role overload.
    (D) lack of patient responsiveness or evidence of change or improvement.

5. Societal devaluation of caring stems primarily from the association of caring with women's work and
    (A) the proliferation of co-dependency theory, which calls into question the motivation for caregiving.
    (B) the somewhat mundane and invisible qualities of true caring.
    (C) the general devaluation of mothering in a society that values the pursuit of a career.
    (D) the fact that the caring professions are in general poorly compensated.

6. Which of the following pairings of role stressors with definitions is **correct?**
   (A) role ambiguity; the extent to which the role of the nurse overlaps with the role of other disciplines/ team members
   (B) role conflict; the extent to which the nurse has tasks imposed upon him or her that have a low priority for the worker but a high priority for the worker's supervisor
   (C) role overload; the extent to which a person is incapable of meeting multiple expectations

7. Health care professionals gauge their relative worth in the organization by making inferences about
   (A) the amount of praise, recognition, and appreciation they receive.
   (B) the extent to which they are compensated for their contributions.
   (C) the amount of power and respect they are given by colleagues and managers.
   (D) the opportunities they are given for continued training, development, and promotion.

8. An example of a problem-focused coping strategy is
   (A) realistic goal setting.
   (B) relaxation.
   (C) social support.
   (D) expressing frustrations and disappointments to a friend.

9. Cognitive restructuring is
   (A) a method of fostering control over one's work.
   (B) designed to provide a clear organizational framework for patient care.
   (C) a method of creating psychological distance between patients and professional caregivers, without compromising patient care.
   (D) a technique that involves learning to listen to self-talk and changing unwanted or irrational thoughts in order to change emotional responses.

10. Job sharing, specialized roles, and limit setting are all examples of which of the following work stress management approaches?
    (A) creating control of one's practice
    (B) compartmentalizing life and work
    (C) organizational flexibility
    (D) creating opportunities for withdrawal

11. Which of the following is **not** a characteristic of effective coping?
    (A) There is an active effort to engage the help of others.
    (B) Problems are broken down into manageable bits and worked through one at a time.
    (C) Feelings are compartmentalized whenever possible so as to achieve detached concern and create a psychological distance from distressing situations.
    (D) There is a fundamental trust in oneself and others and a sense of optimism that something can be done to bring about a positive outcome.

12. Which of the following is an example of an intrapersonal strategy for coping with the stress of oncology nursing?
    (A) setting realistic goals
    (B) creating opportunities for withdrawal
    (C) social support
    (D) organizational flexibility

13. In terms of job-related stress, the **most** compelling reason to examine and optimize nurse-patient ratios is
    (A) the impact on quality patient care.
    (B) the legal responsibility to provide sufficient staff to meet the care needs of patients.
    (C) the cost of staff turnover and staff burnout.
    (D) to promote effective time management.

14. The characteristics of an effective work team include concern for group members and group rules that support
    (A) objectives, goals, and priorities that respond to the changing needs of individual group members.

(B)   centralized problem-solving and decision-making skills.
(C)   the ability to maximize resources for the good of certain individuals.
(D)   clear and realistic role expectations.

ANSWER EXPLANATIONS

1.   **The answer is (C).**   Choices (A) and (D) are incorrect because stress does not reside solely within the event or in the response of the person. Choice (B) is not correct because the transaction model of stress postulates that stress results from a transaction between the person and the stressful stimulus, modified by a third factor or set of factors. (1615)

2.   **The answer is (A).**   **Primary** appraisal may take three forms: irrelevant, positive, or stressful. **Stressful** appraisals involve judgments of harm or loss, challenge, or threat. In **secondary** appraisal, judgments are made about resources and options available for coping. (1615)

3.   **The answer is (C).**   Primary and secondary appraisal simply determine whether the work will be **perceived** as stressful. Personal motivations, self-concept, and the cancer trajectory are just a few of the interpersonal and intrapersonal factors that can influence perceptions of stress. However, the stress experienced by cancer nurses involves an interplay between intrapersonal (self-concept, motivations, and personal needs), interpersonal (relationships with recipients of care and coworkers and the nature of cancer care), and environmental factors. These factors provide the demands and supplies that are appraised as satisfying or discrepant. (1616)

4.   **The answer is (D).**   The very structure of the helping relationship can promote a negative view of people or a shift from a positive to a negative view. This shift tends to frustrate the helper, dampen the helper's sensitivity, diminish the helper's sense of accomplishment, and generate emotional and physical exhaustion. Four aspects of the helping relationship are pivotal in this positive-to-negative shift: (1) focus on the problem, (2) lack of positive feedback, (3) level of emotional stress, and (4) perceived possibility of change or improvement. Prolonged patient involvement, role overload, or emotionally distancing oneself will not necessarily contribute to a positive-to-negative shift, although they may increase the perceived stressfulness of the situation. (1618)

5.   **The answer is (A).**   Co-dependency theory contributes to caring being perceived as a symptom of an illness when it popularizes such definitions as "any suffering and/or dysfunction that is associated with or results from focusing on the needs and behaviors of others." The damage of such labeling may include viewing caring as a symptom of a disease, self-blame for the stress experienced in caring work, and cutting off social support. The devaluation of mother in our society may also result from the general devaluation of women's work. The somewhat invisible qualities of caring may make it difficult to observe and measure caring. The fact that the caring professions are poorly compensated probably results from the association with women's work and/or with the devaluing of bonding, comforting, and generativity in our society, which values individualism, independence, logic, and rational thought. (1620)

6.   **The answer is (C).**   Role ambiguity is the extent to which role expectations are not clearly communicated. An individual must understand the expectations that others have of a particular role, as well as the duties, rights, responsibilities, and activities of the role, in order to adequately perform the role. Role conflict is the extent to which the expectations of various others are in conflict or incompatible. (1620–1621)

7.   **The answer is (B).**   While rewards, recognition, praise, encouragement, expressions of appreciation, and clear feedback are extremely powerful incentives, health care professionals gauge their relative worth in the organization by making inferences about the extent to which they are compensated for their contributions. Lack of differentiation of rewards (everyone receives a merit increase regardless of efforts) encourages only average performance, as the high contributor concludes that there is no need to work harder. And the low contributor, seeing that the high contributor gets equal reward, concludes that hard work does not pay off. (1622)

8.   **The answer is (A).**   Problem-focused coping targets the environment or self for direct action by changing one's behavior or environmental conditions. Emotion-focused coping attempts to palliate or eliminate distressing emotions elicited by the stressor. Emotion-focused coping does not change the self or environment, only the way one feels. (1623)

9. **The answer is (D).** The first step in cognitive restructuring is to look at the event or persons as objectively as possible in order to gain a clearer perspective on the event and any irrational thinking and to consider different responses. Although it is unrealistic to expect to make a positive response to all stressful situations, a sense of mastery and control comes from knowing that one has a choice in how situations are perceived, in addition to choosing the response. (1625)

10. **The answer is (A).** The coping strategy of creating control of one's practice involves developing and maintaining competence, setting limits, and organizing one's work to minimize stress and enhance satisfaction. (1626–1627)

11. **The answer is (C).** With effective coping there is a free expression of positive and negative feelings. Feelings are mastered where possible, and where mastery is not possible, the inevitable is accepted. Distancing oneself from distressing situations may be helpful in coping in the short term, but it requires energy for sustained use and may ultimately serve to increase stress. (1623, 1626)

12. **The answer is (A).** Setting realistic goals, time management, tuning into one's inner dialogue, recognizing stress responses, accentuating the positive, compartmentalizing work and life, and creating balance are all examples of intrapersonal strategies for coping with stress. All of the other answers are examples of interpersonal or environmental strategies for mediating the stress of oncology nursing. (1623–1629)

13. **The answer is (C).** While appropriate staff-patient ratios certainly promote quality patient care, it is the cost of staff turnover and staff burnout that provides the most compelling organizational rationale for examining and optimizing nurse-patient ratios. Replacing an experienced nurse includes not only orientation training costs but also the ongoing cost incurred until the novice nurse becomes expert. (1627)

14. **The answer is (D).** In an effective team, the ability to maximize resources occurs for the good of the group and the individual, and problem-solving and decision-making are not generally centralized. In an effective team, objectives, goals, and priorities are clearly articulated and agreed on by team members; they would not respond to the changing needs of individual group members. (1628)